BAREFOOT RUNNING
STEP BY STEP

Dedicated to the tens of thousands of visitors and contributors to The Running Barefoot website and forum, all of whom helped write this book.

Text © 2011 Roy M. Wallack and Ken Bob Saxton
Photography and Design © 2011 Fair Winds Press

First published in the USA in 2011 by
Fair Winds Press, a member of
Quayside Publishing Group
100 Cummings Center
Suite 406-L
Beverly, MA 01915-6101
www.fairwindspress.com

15 14 13 12 11   1 2 3 4 5

ISBN-13: 978-1-59233-465-0
ISBN-10: 1-59233-465-2

Digital edition published in 2011

Library of Congress Cataloging-in-Publication Data available

Illustrations by Michael Wanke
Photography by Matthew Modoono, except for the following:
Adreah Saxton: page 126; Barefoot Ken Bob Saxton: pages 44, 122, 139, 153, and 210;
Bruce Barnhart: page 170; Cathy Lee-Saxton: pages 10 and 72; Damon Hendricks: page 220;
David M. Wright III: page 167; Eric Vouga: page 222; Getty Images: page 192;
Joseph Drugmand: page 179; Joseph Wallack: page 140; Lindsay Foltz: page 177;
Suzanne Mapes Photography: page 168; and Yvonne Welz, *The Horse's Hoof*: page 49

Printed and bound in the United States of America

The information in this book is for educational purposes only. It is not intended to replace the advice of a physician or medical practitioner. Please see your health care provider before beginning any new health program.

BAREFOOT RUNNING
STEP BY STEP

BAREFOOT KEN BOB, THE GURU OF SHOELESS RUNNING, SHARES HIS PERSONAL TECHNIQUE
FOR RUNNING WITH MORE SPEED, LESS IMPACT, FEWER LEG INJURIES, AND MORE FUN

BAREFOOT KEN BOB SAXTON
THE LEADING INSTRUCTOR OF BAREFOOT RUNNING FEATURED IN *RUNNER'S WORLD*,
THE NEW YORK TIMES, AND THE BESTSELLER *BORN TO RUN*

ROY M. WALLACK
LOS ANGELES TIMES FITNESS COLUMNIST AND AUTHOR OF *RUN FOR LIFE*
AND *BE A BETTER RUNNER*

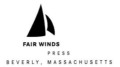

FAIR WINDS
PRESS
BEVERLY, MASSACHUSETTS

CONTENTS

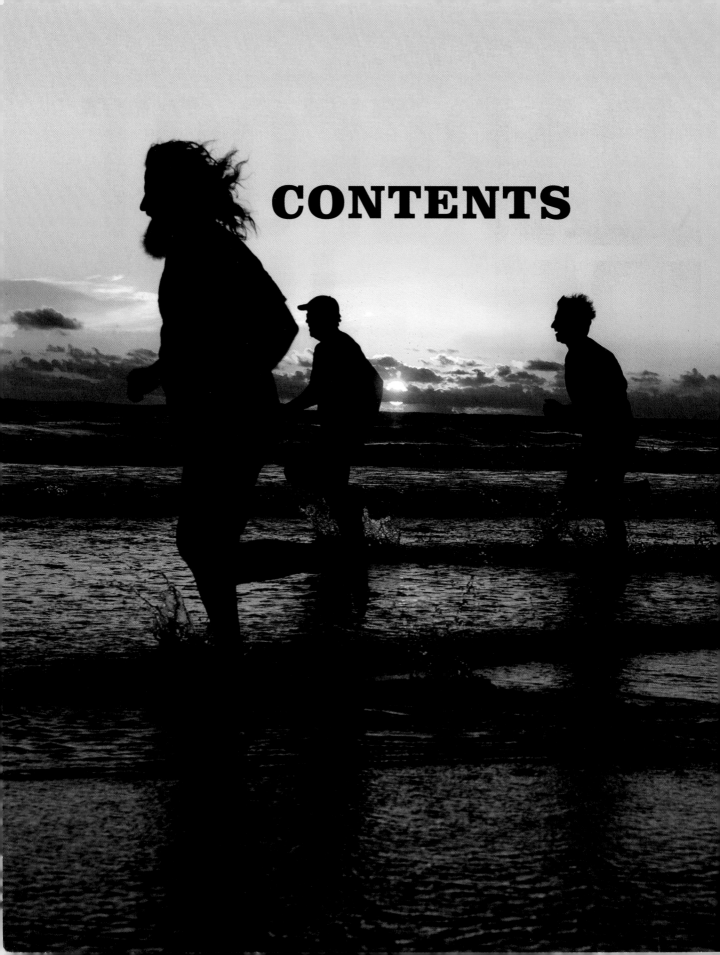

PREFACE
THE JOURNEY

In February 2004, while writing a *Runner's World* story about the Pose method, an impact-reducing running technique then popular among triathletes but relatively unknown to the running community, I googled the words that it reminded me of: barefoot running. The next day, I was on the bike path at Bolsa Chica beach, running barefoot for three miles (4.8 km) alongside the first reference that had come up on my computer screen: Ken Saxton, one of the most unique, friendly, funny, and influential characters I have run across in two decades of writing about sports and fitness.

What happened to me that day isn't unique. Mention "barefoot running" to anyone familiar with it, and chances are that one of their first—and often the first—exposures to it comes through the man I learned later was known as Barefoot Ken Bob. (It's a long story, but christened Kenneth Robert, he was called Bobby by his family and Ken at school. When he was 17, someone who heard both fused the two. "Barefoot" was added in the early 2000s, the practice of all the early barefooters).

Forget six degrees of separation. For many, as you'll see in the stories told throughout this book, it's one degree: search "barefoot running," get Ken Bob's website, and start running barefoot. All barefoot running roads, at least until Christopher McDougall's *Born To Run* tsunami hit in mid-2009, seem to lead directly through Ken Bob.

McDougall's barefooting is, in fact, a second degree of separation, as he learned about it from one of the far-out characters who people his book, Barefoot Ted McDonald, who discovered barefoot running on Ken's website in 2003. From page 156 of *Born to Run*: "Ted stumbled across an international community of barefoot runners, complete with their own ancient wisdom and tribal nicknames and led by their great bearded sage, Barefoot Ken Bob Saxton."

Ken is known far and wide as the "guru," but I like to think of him as the "go-to" guy—the bottomless-pit resource that I always go to first for information about running barefoot. I wrote about Ken and running barefoot in 2005 in *Men's Journal* and later in stories in the *L.A. Times* and my 2009 book, *Run for Life*, discovering along the way that barefoot drills, warm-ups, and cool-downs had been used for decades by Olympic coaches such as Brooks Johnson and Joe Vigil to strengthen, protect, and speed up all kinds of top-level runners, from sprinters to middle distance runners to marathoners. (Incidentally, given that fact, we devoted significant real estate here to the performance-enhancing effect of running barefoot, something we think may come as a revelation to most runners, who only are aware of its well-known injury-stopping and happiness-inducing benefits.)

Of course, I was far from the first to write about Ken. First as a novelty act and then as a trendsetter, he appeared in dozens of magazine and newspaper articles through the decade, including a number in *Runner's World*. Seeing first-hand Ken's deep knowledge and curiosity, his messianic commitment to spreading the word, and his patient, pleasant, and funny ability to explain it, it was natural that I go to him again when I was offered a chance to write a barefoot book in the spring of 2010.

The timing was perfect in several ways. Not only had barefooting gone crazy in the year since *Born to Run* hit the shelves, but Ken was about to embark on a grand tour two-month around the country, with numerous workshops and planned visits with barefoot luminaries such as McDougall, Dr. Irene Davis, and Dr. Daniel Lieberman. It was a unique opportunity to get real-time feedback about the state of barefooting in the county, much in the same way that running barefoot gives you real-time feedback from the ground.

Therefore, our strategy: Talk every day. No matter we each were in June and July (at times, I was in Oregon and Iceland; he was everywhere from New Orleans to Dallas to New York to Michigan to Nebraska to Colorado), I called or emailed Ken to ask how his workshops went, what he learned, and about any unusual people he met or stories he'd heard. I felt like his mother, and soon, his psychoanalyst. The trip was a metamorphosis of sorts for Ken; with far more people interested in running barefoot than he'd ever seen before, he had to raise his game, think about how to explain things better, faster, more thoroughly.

In addition, staying with local hosts who were barefoot enthusiasts, there was a great opportunity to get other points of view. Often, I would call Ken up and he'd be tired or have little to say—and would hand the phone over to someone with interesting revelations to share and/or a great story to tell.

Yes, Ken is the guru. But even he hasn't thought of everything about running barefoot. We got a lot of great of ideas and angles from dozens of other barefooters you'll read about in these pages—most of them, of course, who were first exposed to barefooting through him.

By the time Barefoot Ken Bob's 2010 Summer Tour ended in mid-July, I had notes filling a couple dozen yellow legal pads piled a foot high. Then I metaphorically went back to college, interviewing many academic researchers and digging through the rapidly growing body of published university studies that detail the biomechanics of running, the reduced impact forces of the barefoot landing, and the intricately complex function of things like the mechanoreceptors on the sole of the foot. For this old Political Science–Economics major, it was like cramming for a test in Physiology, Kinesiology, and Evolutionary Biology.

All this is why I think that this book will stand out among the growing number of barefoot running resources. It combines the wisdom of the best barefoot mind out there—Barefoot Ken Bob's—with the ideas of other dedicated barefooters and some of the world's most cutting-edge researchers. In addition, we tapped the power of Ken's website, a vast library of news stories and catalogued emails, and put out the word to his readers that we wanted interesting, insightful stories for the book. We were inundated.

Although you could pretty much sum up the "rules" of running barefoot in a magazine article or page or two (which we do early in chapter 3), really driving the points home required capturing the vast experiences of Ken and dozens more barefooters, each of whom has their

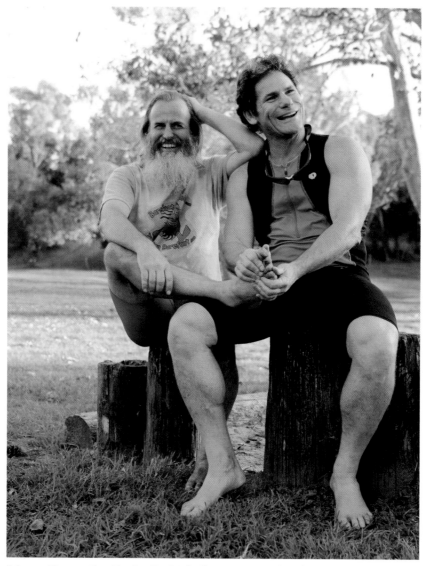

Sole searching: coauthors Barefoot Ken Bob (left) and Roy Wallack (right), getting to the bottom of the guru's barefoot running secrets.

own unique take on it. By the end of the book, if all goes as planned, you will have gotten your barefoot lessons in so many interesting, creative, and funny ways that you simply won't be able to forget them.

You certainly won't forget Ken's story. As with anyone who achieves guru status, there's a "born to do this" fatalism to his life, starting with extraordinary physical sensitivities, that inexorably led him down the barefoot path. I felt surprised, amused, and privileged as I picked through his brain. He was amused, too, by some of the buried treasure we uncovered up there, some of it never discussed before, but all of it abundantly relevant to telling his story and spreading the barefoot word accurately and realistically.

For me, it's been a fun, eye-opening journey that has affected my running and lifestyle in surprising ways. It's a rainy late December as I write this, and about 11 p.m. last night I found myself run-walking my dogs Bruce and Toby, while barefoot. I'd been running barefoot sporadically since I met Ken six years ago, but until a couple months ago never thought about walking the dogs unshod—especially when it's 50°F (10°C) and the sidewalks are soaked and full of downed twigs, leaves, and mud. The neighbors out walking their dogs were amazed— first, that you could actually go barefoot in the cold, and next, that anyone would want to. It felt pretty cool to tell them about the barefoot trend and how I was actually strengthening my feet, fixing my biomechanics, and even straightening my posture just by doing it.

More importantly, perhaps, it also feels pretty cool to fully "get" barefoot running, to understand what Ken means when he says that there's a lot more to it than just taking off your shoes. Through increasing barefoot mileage over the summer and fall, I had good reason to practice everything he'd taught me: the exaggerated knee bend; the straight back; the curved-up toes; the "1-2-3 landing" that brings ball, then toes and heel, down to the ground; the vertical foot levitation (rather than a push-off); the initiation of the levitation before you actually land; and the other stuff you'll see in these pages. I know these rules work; I was extra-sensitive due to a partially-torn ACL in my right knee during the writing of the book, and I could only run pain-free if I observed all of them—and only while barefoot, not in Vibram FiveFingers. (On the long descents in my neighborhood, the lack of true barefoot feel in VFFs seemed to throw me off just enough to hurt my bad knee.)

I also had another lab rat to test them on: My 15-year-old son Joey, who wants to try out for his high school track team. On our first run together, a 4-miler (6 km), I was barefoot and he was in a pair of shoes, but halfway through his knee started hurting and he wanted to stop. "Just take 'em off," I said. Like all first-time barefooters, he was stunned by the automatically gentle ball-of-the-foot landing—and amazed how it minimized his knee pain.

For the last two miles (3 km) I gave him a detailed tutorial on running barefoot. With each instruction, Joey, whose best subject is science, reported the positive effect to me as if it was a real-time physiology-class experiment. The last mile, he had no pain at all and vowed to run barefoot from then on, which he has. "I like running barefoot because it feels so good," he told me. "And because it's like a science."

He's right. Running barefoot is great the minute you take your shoes off. And when you learn the science of it, as taught by Barefoot Ken Bob and friends, it gets better.

—Roy M. Wallack

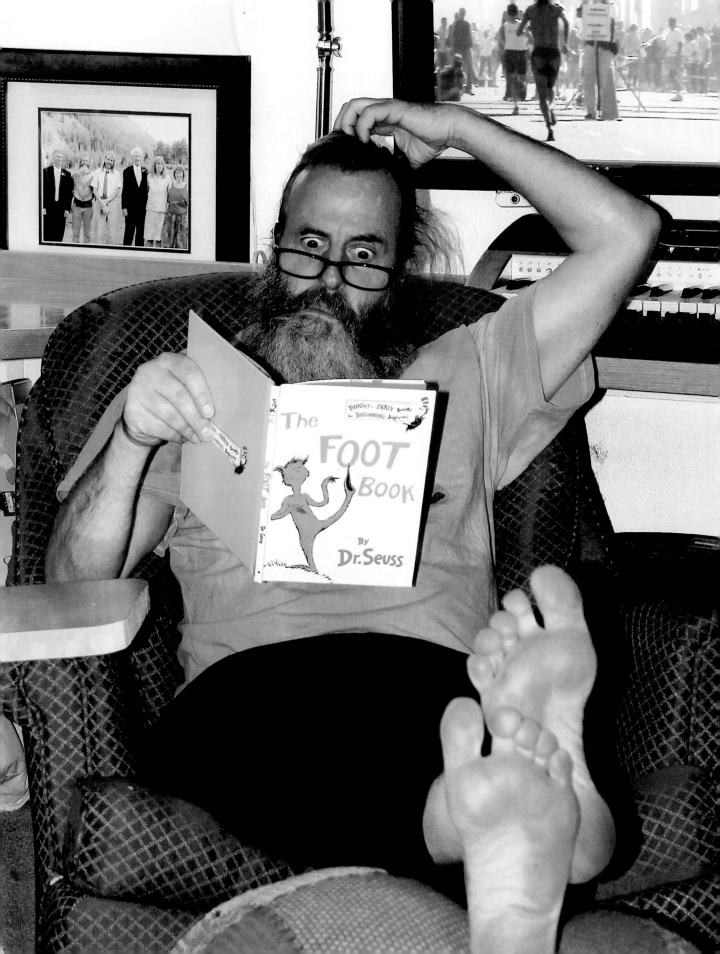

INTRODUCTION
WHY YOU NEED TO LEARN HOW TO RUN BAREFOOT

" **IN THE BEGINNING, WE WERE BAREFOOT. THEN WE SCREWED UP AND INVENTED RUNNING SHOES.** "

—BAREFOOT KEN BOB-ISM #1

Ah, barefoot running, the great panacea that puts an end to running injuries, restores joy to exercise, fixes your posture, keeps you running forever, and even saves you money! And it's so easy to do—just take off your shoes and run. Right?

Wrong!

Do you actually think someone would have paid me the big bucks to write a book about how to run barefoot if all it required was taking off your shoes? Anyone could tell you that. Yes, that's indeed what I did two decades ago when I got sick of the blisters caused by my running shoes, and I haven't looked back. But while starting the first running barefoot website, racking up seventy-six barefoot marathons (as of late 2010), leading dozens of Running Barefoot Workshops, and getting used to being described as "The Guru" of running barefoot, I've come to a realization: Running barefoot is a great thing for all runners, but it has problems. Some people don't get as much benefit from it as they should. Some even give up and go back to shoes. The problem? Lack of knowledge. It's a fact: You need to *learn* how to run barefoot.

That may come as a shock to many. Why would you have to "learn" to run barefoot when we were born that way? The truth is that the only people who don't have to learn how to run barefoot are those who've been doing it their entire lives. Once we start running around in shoes all the time, like most of us do by kindergarten or earlier, our biomechanics change. Add cushiony 1½-inch (4 cm) heels, and it changes even more. By the time we decide to run barefoot, either out of desperation to avoid recurrent injuries or out of mere intellectual curiosity, we simply can't revert to a natural barefoot gait unless we "unlearn" and "retrain" the bad habits, lazy muscles, and screwed-up biomechanics we've picked up in decades of working, playing, and running in shoes.

So that's why I've written this book—to help you get right to the benefits of running barefoot without the frustrating drawbacks and learning curve. Although every body and running form are subtly different, there is a *right way* to run barefoot, with a bunch of important rules. It took me two long, fun decades of trial and error to learn them—a wonderful journey, to be sure, but it would have been better, faster, and easier if I'd known more sooner and had someone (like myself) to learn from.

People have been asking me to write a book for years, but I'm a procrastinator (meaning that I wait until I have a better way of doing things before getting around to them). What finally got the project into gear were three things: a call from my cowriter Roy M. Wallack, who'd been approached about writing a barefoot book; the tremendous amount of knowledge I gained while conducting clinics and meeting with top researchers all over the country during my 11,000-mile (176,000 km) Barefoot Ken Bob's Running Barefoot 2010 Summer Tour (see chapter 3); and finally, a profound sense of urgency.

With the publication of Christopher McDougall's blockbuster *Born to Run* in mid-2009, the interest in running barefoot skyrocketed. Quirky little barefoot running went mainstream, with thousands of runners trying it out for the first time. Suddenly, the litany of problems caused by the cushioned running shoe and the heel strike it encourages—leading to patellofemoral pain, sore hips, aching lower back, black toenails, blisters, iliotibial band (IB) syndrome, plantar fasciitis, Achilles tendonitis, shin splints, general all-body fatigue, and years lost to rehab—seemed solvable. But almost just as suddenly, we started hearing reports of new problems from barefoot runners and even more from minimalist shoe–wearers.

So that's the urgency behind this book: If the thousands of new barefoot runners don't learn how to do it correctly *right now*, they could simply give it up and go back to their injury-riddled shoe-wearing habit. And barefooting, which does indeed have the potential to make life better for nearly all runners, will recede back to a minority of runners.

Certainly, running barefoot is too big now to ever go away or shrink back to a tiny fringe. Too many people know of its power to rejuvenate and exhilarate runners. Barefoot running is out of the bag as a tool for strengthening and injury reduction. But it would be a shame if the great masses of runners dismiss it as an orthotic, or even a fad. It isn't. It's life changing, if you do it correctly.

After spending two decades immersed in the subject and thirty years before that running barefoot occasionally, I'm ready to tell you how. I knew it in the summer of 2010 when McDougall introduced me to a crowd by saying, "This is the guy we've been stealing information from all these years."

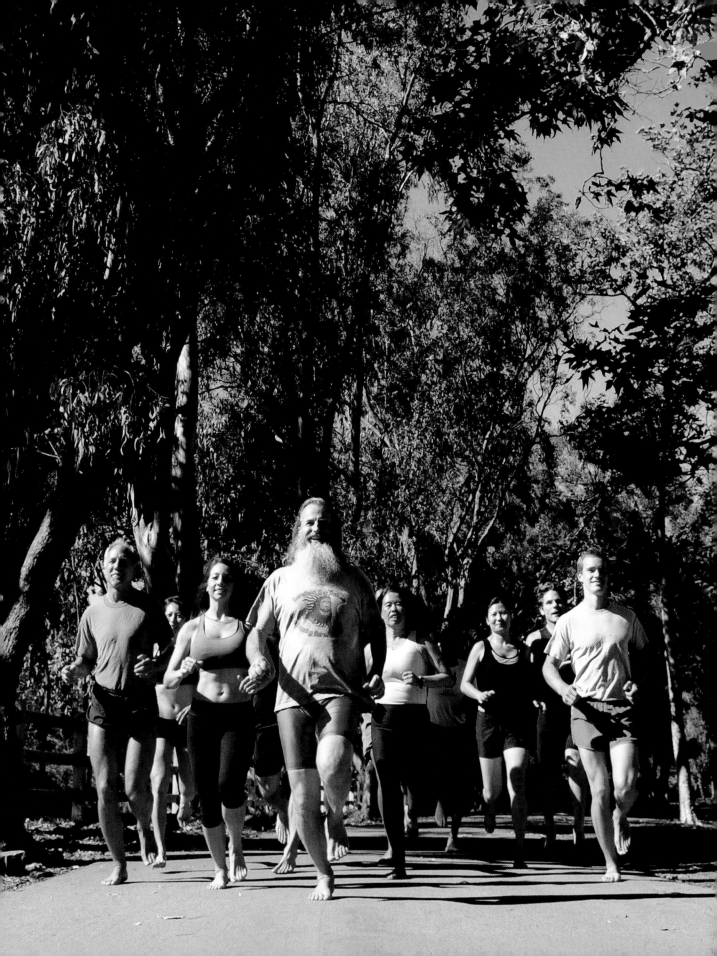

BARE SOLES, OPEN MINDS

I won't spend time here in the introduction telling you the "secrets" to running barefoot properly. The rest of the book is for that. I will tell you that, in some ways, it *is* rocket science, and as with rocket science, the key takeaway is that you need to take it slow, learn the basics, and build gradually. Although barefooting is definitely the antidote to our unhealthy addiction to shoes, going unshod after a lifetime in them is like a heroin addict going cold turkey. It's a shock to our (corrupted) system. Our feet are not only weak and tender, but they are also dumb, blind, and brainwashed. Locked in a shoe prison of covering and cushioning and protection from age four or five or earlier, they are so far removed from their natural movement and function that they need to unlearn decades of bad habits *and* relearn how to act like their natural selves again. It might take weeks. It might take months. For a few, it might never take at all. But everybody will learn something—if not to open (and escape) your shoes, then perhaps to open your mind to other new ideas.

In the pages to come, you'll find profiles of barefoot runners old and young, Olympian and amateur, male and female, slow and fast. You'll find practice sessions and scientific studies. You'll find some pats on the back for Vibrams—and real warnings you ought to heed before putting them on your feet. You'll find proof that running barefoot is a great tool that can make anyone faster—*even in shoes*.

A revelation in this book is that you need not run exclusively barefoot to get the benefits (although you'll probably enjoy it so much you may want to); for some, running barefoot just 10 or 20 percent of the time will bring real speed and the end of injuries. In these pages, you'll find endless stories of neurologically rewired leg muscles, of unbound, exhilarating proprioception, and of lives transformed.

To make this book happen, I dug through the decade-old catacombs of my website, TheRunningBarefoot.com, built a library of barefoot-related books from respected barefoot authorities ranging from Abebe Bikila's coach to Dr. Seuss, and spent hundreds of hours on the phone and in person with my cowriter Roy Wallack. Roy has spent two decades writing about running, cycling, and training for the *Los Angeles Times* and many other publications; has made a career out of covering innovative training techniques; and has served as my student, biographer, and public relations guy in his writings about me over the years in various magazines and newspaper articles. He even wrote an entire chapter about me and running barefoot in his own book about running to age one hundred, *Run for Life*.

Having incubated running barefoot as a lone wolf for many years, then nurtured the trend as it exploded last year, I am thrilled and privileged to be in a position to help expose a vast new audience to an activity that has the potential to turn running into a lifelong, injury-free sport that can vastly add quality, health, achievement, and fun to life.

I use the word *fun* a lot. Ultimately, it's all about fun. Distinguished Road Runners Club of America Hall of Fame member Tom Osler once said (in Roy's first running book, actually), "I love running—it's the most fun I can think of. I'll do whatever it takes to keep doing it." For millions of people, that will be running barefoot.

Have fun,
Barefoot Ken Bob

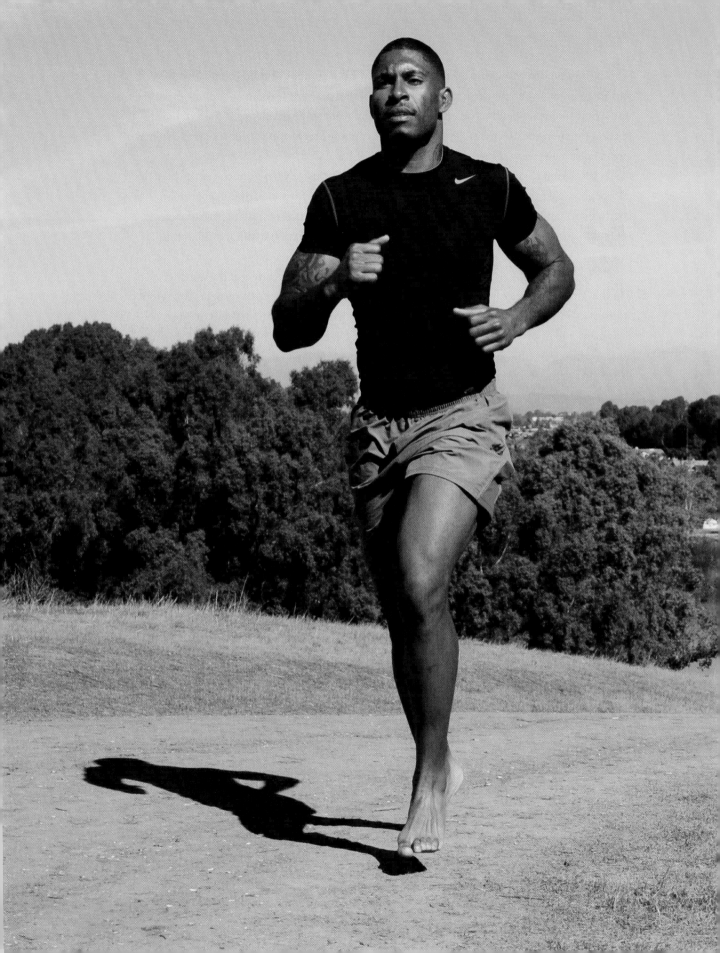

SECTION I:

TAKING FEET AND BODY BACK TO NATURE

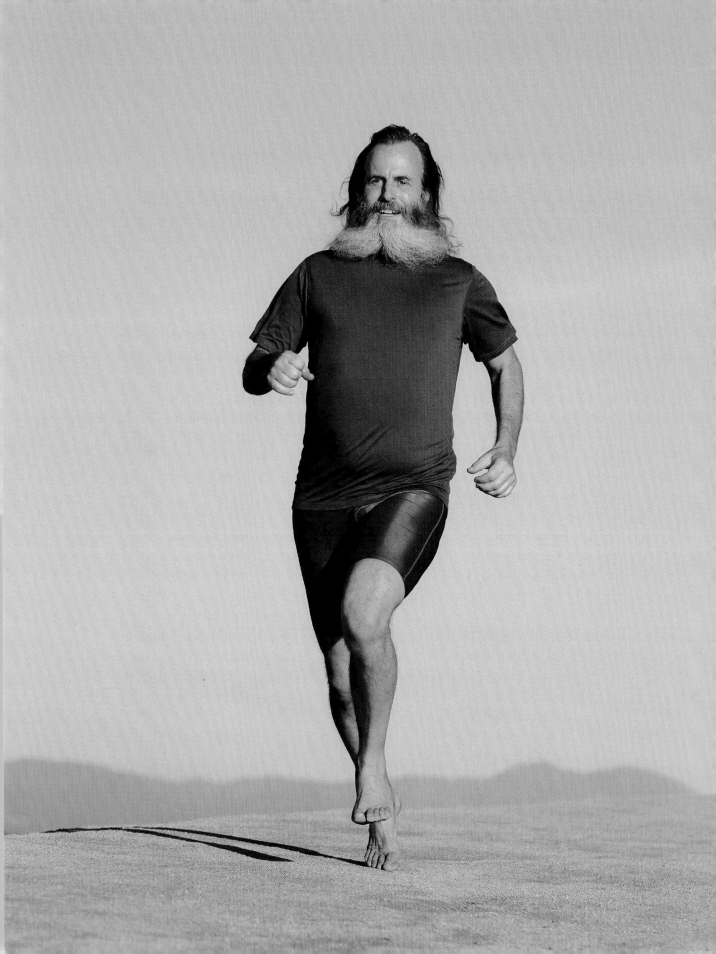

CHAPTER 1

BORN TO RUN BAREFOOT
THE LIFE AND TIMES OF BAREFOOT KEN BOB

How an unusually sensitive boy who couldn't stand tobacco smoke, coffee, polyester disco shirts, or shoes listened to his body and discovered running barefoot rule #1: *Bend your knees!*

> **WE HAVE SENSES TO MAKE THE EVERYDAY THINGS WE DO LESS DANGEROUS AND LESS PAINFUL. TO IGNORE THESE SENSES IS TO LIVE—AND RUN—SENSELESSLY!**
>
> —KEN BOB-ISM #5

Some say that genetics is destiny. For me, looking back on how running barefoot became such an essential part of who I am, and why I think it can make life better for millions of people, it's more like "*sensitivity* is destiny."

When my neighborhood friends in rural northwest lower Michigan were smoking and drinking in their teens, I didn't. When my parents fired up a pot of coffee every morning, I left the kitchen. This was not due to any conservative morality or health obsession. I was just extremely sensitive, and I tried to avoid discomfort and pain.

Cigarette smoke gave me headaches. One whiff of cigar smoke and I felt like puking. Beer just didn't taste good. The scent of coffee made me nauseous; a coffee-flavored milk drink once made me vomit and have diarrhea. Perfume and cologne gave me headaches. The *Lost in Space*–inspired synthetic pullover sweaters of the 1960s made me itch like crazy. My disco-fever polyester shirts of the '70s made my skin feel like it was crawling with bugs.

For a long time, I thought something was wrong with me. I couldn't roller skate for long in my cool skate clothes because they made me uncomfortable. I squirmed in class adjusting my clothing. I'd stay home from school not because I was sick, but because I *felt like* I was going to be; it must have worked because I almost never got truly sick. My shoes blistered and chafed, so I took them off every chance I got.

Running barefoot around the local fields, forests, and swamps, I noticed that my first footfalls seemed to rattle my brain, so I somehow began landing more gently (although I didn't realize how I did this—by bending my knees deeply—until years later). It was a classic feedback loop: if it's uncomfortable or painful, don't ignore it or tough it out; either drop it or figure out a more comfortable way to do it. My body complained about a lot of minor, run-of-the-mill stuff that didn't seem to bother anyone else. But fortunately, I listened to my body—something I advise everyone to do. It forced me to figure out easier ways to get things done, not by cheating or shortcutting but by being more efficient.

Although my hypersensitivity was a hassle as a kid, making it hard to fit in and learn how to socialize, I later began to see it as a gift, an early warning system, a canary in the coal mine. A similar sensitivity motivated my oldest brother to convince our parents to stop smoking.

I would be the only teen not drinking at a party, and I became shy, almost a loner. But as I began to accept myself for who I was, I began to like not fitting in with the crowd; as it turns out, the crowd didn't have any special wisdom. I liked the fact that I was repelled by things that probably aren't great for anybody—such as nicotine, toxic synthetics (the polyester disco shirts, and possibly disco music, too), overly processed foods (I often suffered severe constipation-induced cramps until I figured that one out), and running with stiff legs, which pounds feet into the ground without much shock absorption. It was all about my body giving me a gift of true wisdom. All I needed to do was listen and respond appropriately!

Two decades ago, my odd supersensitivity finally led me to ditch my shoes for good and dedicate my spare time to telling people about the benefits of running, walking, and being barefoot. As I will try to show you, if there is one overriding philosophy that captures the essence of barefooting, it is listening to your body. This can virtually eliminate most common running injuries, improve performance, restore and lengthen your running career, and just feel great. Your body always tells you the truth—if you can develop enough sensitivity over the years to understand it.

No book will substitute for listening to your body and soles. We can give you a head start with basic techniques. Fine-tuning these basics for your own body is up to you.

BAREFOOT FROM THE BEGINNING

Looking back, I've always been a barefooter. I'd go barefoot around the house more than my friends. I would drive barefoot, liking the precise feel of my foot on the clutch, brake, or gas pedal. I was barefoot all summer. Growing up, I wore shoes as an anomaly. My mom, a thrifty farmer's daughter raised during the Depression, was a big influence. When other mothers yelled "put your shoes on" as their kids went out to play, Mom would say, "Don't get your shoes dirty." Going barefoot kept my shoes safe and clean in the closet. We weren't well-to-do; we never had a new car or TV, just sets repaired by my dad, a telephone company technician.

In high school, when we began running long distances in P.E. class, I liked it. "Maybe I'm a runner," I thought. Running only a mile or two (1.6 to 3.2 km)—at a 7:00 or an occasional sub-6:00 pace—was fun. But although I might have had some talent, I didn't join the cross-country team for a couple of reasons: I was a short, late bloomer who didn't feel like an athlete next to the big jocks, and after-school practices would have made me miss the 15-mile (24 km), hour-long bus ride home. I did run a couple of times a week on my own just for fun, and occasionally even ran naked in the dark through the tiny maple grove behind the barn (hey, it was rural). So by the time the running boom started when Frank Shorter won the 1972 Olympic marathon, I was already a runner in my mind, enjoying running a few times a week. Few people ran on their own back then.

I kept running, although not obsessively, while working odd jobs for the next four years before starting college at Northwestern Michigan in 1977 as a twenty-two-year-old freshman. I'd run 5 to 7 miles (8 to 11 km) a week, probably never more than 3 miles (5 km) at a time. I also enjoyed walking, as much as 10 miles (16 km) a day. We had miles and miles of trails through local forests, around lakes and ponds, and past swamps. Sometimes I would run to keep the mosquitoes from swarming around me!

A MOMENT TO REMEMBER

One cold February day in 1978, I was hanging with a friend, talking about running. Like many people, my friend wasn't interested in running himself, but his eighteen-year-old roommate, Gene, seemed interested, so Gene and I decided to go outside and run a couple of miles on the icy roads. He thought I was an experienced runner, and seemed to be looking for advice. So I watched him run, and to get a feel for what he was experiencing, I tried imitating the way he was running. Gene pushed his feet hard into the pavement, his knees barely bending, if at all. He looked and sounded painfully awkward. His heels thudded into the road, cushioned only by thin rubber soles that couldn't possibly absorb the impact.

I winced when I tried imitating his technique. I really could feel his pain. The feeling wasn't as pronounced as stepping on sharp stones barefoot, but with my weird hypersensitivity I could feel my feet pounding. My knee, which I had sprained badly nearly ten years before while being pulled by a horse on skis (how the horse got on skis, I never did figure out!), ached horribly. My bones were jolting all the way from my soles to the top of my head. My brain seemed to be rattling inside my skull.

THE MOST IMPORTANT LESSON IN THIS BOOK

Bending your knees—a little more than you might think necessary—is easily my number-one principle for fun, injury-free, lifelong running, barefoot or not.

This book is full of barefooting dos and don'ts, but it all starts with bending the knees, or at least "unlocking" them as you stand, walk, or run. Doing that effectively turns your whole leg into a spring instead of a rigid stick (as I'll elaborate more on in chapter 3), and changes practically everything.

Bend your knees a little more than you might think necessary. Note the bent knee and slightly squatted position here. More bend means more spring, with no additional effort to push forward.

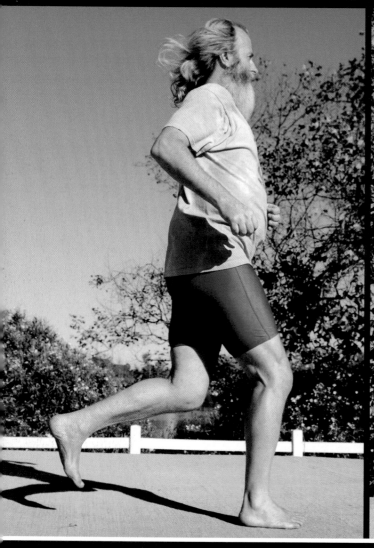
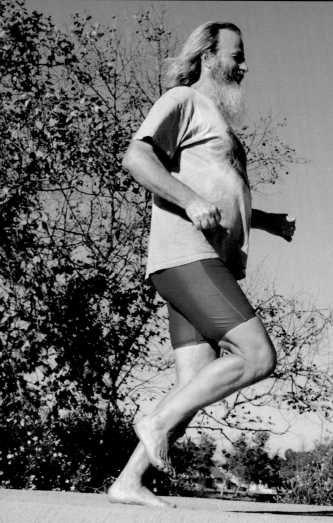

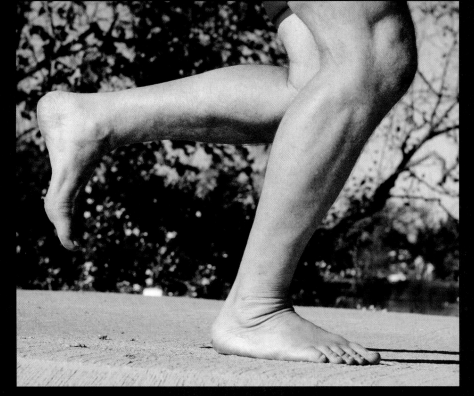

The key movements from the bent knee to the foot. Relax your calves so that after initially landing ball-of-foot-first, the entire sole settles into the ground, distributing your weight evenly across a larger surface.

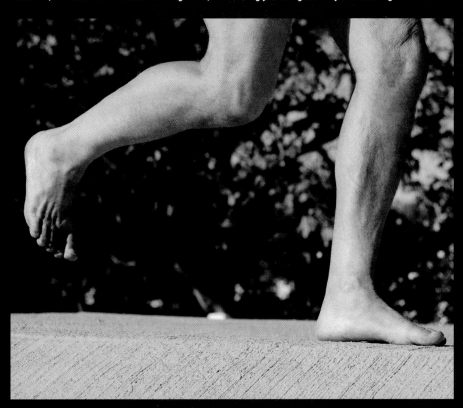

Note the lightness of the feet and the distance from the ground, as the bent knee enables a runner to have softer, lighter landings. And note that the feet are not heel striking!

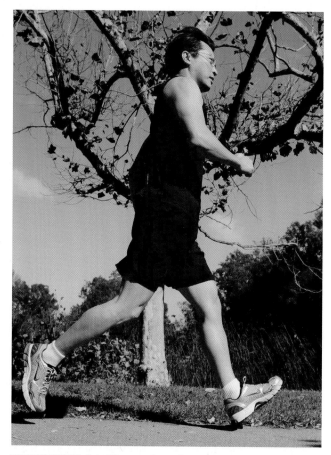

WHAT NOT TO DO: Note this runner's nearly straight legs and unbent knees. The resulting impact would be too uncomfortable without footwear, which is the main reason barefooters run more gently.

Other than slipping and sliding a bit with each step, Gene didn't seem bothered a bit by the pounding!

I started experimenting with the way I ran and the way Gene ran, and compared what we were doing differently. Among other things, I noticed one major change that seemed to have the most effect.

"Gene, try *bending your knees*!" I said.

Because I was respected by many of our friends (who usually only ran if they were being chased by a girlfriend's father) as a "real" runner, he thanked me and started bending his knees. Instantly, Gene's lurch-and-crash stride was transformed into a smooth, springy flow. I basked in the satisfaction of having helped.

Then a lightbulb flicked on in my head: no wonder so few people enjoy running—especially if they're running like Gene was! But then, who was I to tell anyone how to run? I was no expert. Was I? I never had been a coach. I had never even been coached.

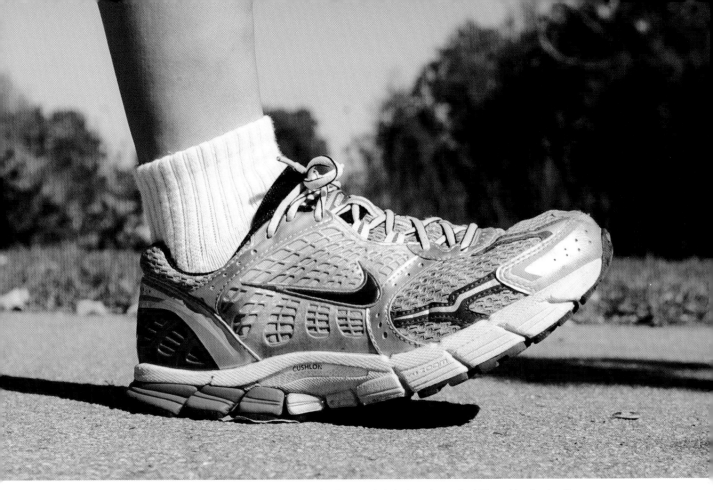

WHAT NOT TO DO: The heel lands hard on the ground in this all-too-typical shod running method. The sudden deceleration (hammering, collision, impact, jolt, jog) is transmitted through the entire body. I can't help but think of a former running partner, about 10 to 15 years younger than myself, who just posted an update on his post–knee surgery recovery. Such reports from shod running buddies are far too common. There can be little doubt that excessive impact (masked by footwear) is responsible for damaging the knees, hips, and backs of countless runners.

But so what? However it was that I came by my knowledge of the importance of bending the knees while running, it worked. Gene improved instantly. I began to realize that my from-the-gut sensitivity—in fact, anyone's sensitivity—was as legitimate as any double-blind Harvard research study. Feeling discomfort and pain is a feedback system; it's how we naturally protect ourselves from injury, toxins, and danger. Our sensitivity tries to teach us how to run, even how to live, without injuring or killing ourselves.

Over the next few days, I paid closer attention to my own running technique. Yes, I did bend my knees and ran somewhat squatted, a bit like Groucho Marx's trademark walk. I must have unconsciously taught myself to bend my knees more, back when my bare soles touched the ground as a child, through the fields and trails behind my house. In my mind, I saw my younger self letting my legs "go limp" when running over sharp rocks and crossing rough tar and gravel roads. I may have incorporated what I learned about bending my knees on the rough surfaces to every surface, even while running with shoes on, during the wintertime.

It was a good feeling to think that I'd actually stumbled upon some basic tenet of proper running technique. My P.E. coaches back in high school told us to run faster or longer, but not *how* to run better, more efficiently, or gently. I'd never heard anyone talk about deliberately running while squatted with bent knees, but as with many things that are not common knowledge, it didn't mean it wasn't true.

Ironically, when I watch small children running barefoot, I often marvel at how perfect their technique is, as bent knees and flexibility transform their legs into shock-absorbing springs. I say "ironically" because I must have been like that, too. I may have occasionally lost the springiness, especially in the first steps of a run, but fortunately, my bare soles reminded me to bend my knees. It was that wonderfully sensitive, almost magical, feedback loop preventing me from injuring myself.

LEAVING SHOES BEHIND FOR GOOD

One day in 1987, one of the most influential days of my life, I got tired of wearing out shoes, and shoes wearing out my feet. So I stopped wearing them. Here's the story:

Throughout my life, shoes had almost always left my feet uncomfortable, chafed, blistered, and in pain. Besides, I like going barefoot. So, after I moved across the country with my associates of arts degree in electronics technology to Southern California in January 1980, I stopped wearing shoes whenever practical. That included while running, which I did on the beach and park trails. But running barefoot for long distances on pavement did not occur to me for another ten years.

As a teenager, I'd set a goal of running a marathon during my lifetime. Being a procrastinator, I eventually got around to it at age thirty-two, when I finished the Long Beach Marathon in 5:05. Unfortunately, it wasn't the joyously pleasant experience I'd planned on. I'd done the training—a few 22-mile (35 km) runs, 14 or 15 miles (22.5 or 24 km) shod and the rest along the beach barefoot—and had the speed from shorter runs and a few 10K and 20K races to do the 26.2 miles (42 km) in about four hours. But by the 18-mile (29 km) mark, my feet were so blistered in their shoes that I had to walk most of the last 8 miles (13 km).

It hadn't occurred to me to take my shoes off during the race, or to run barefoot on the asphalt; I'd never heard of anyone doing that. So I walked slowly and tenderly to the finish line, delicately setting each foot down as gingerly as possible to avoid any further rubbing of the inside of my shoes against the skin on my feet. I walked across the finish line exhausted and in pain, happy to check the marathon off my list of lifetime goals.

"I'm glad I won't need to do this again," I thought as I sat down and painfully peeled off my shoes. Every bit of my skin on the upper portion of both feet had blistered; over the miles, the blisters had worn away, revealing bare dermis (the second layer of skin immediately beneath the epidermis, or outer layer of skin). All of my toenails were solid black (and would fall off within a week). As I later found out, these conditions are considered "normal" for many marathon runners—at least those running in shoes. At least my knees didn't hurt, like several others were complaining about.

As I carefully inspected my feet, I somehow found the energy to be amazed that the soles of both my feet were perfectly intact, as if designed to go the distance, despite being subjected to the same friction against the inside of my shoes that had removed the epidermis on the remaining surface of both feet.

I would not run an official race for another ten years, and would never race in shoes again. But I still loved running barefoot. That was one of the reasons (along with surfing and the Beach Boys) that I'd moved to the land of year-round sunshine, Southern California, in 1980.

Although my suburban paradise might not include the open fields, lush forest, and trails I had back in Michigan, I could run barefoot all year long. For the next few years I didn't run much, but when I did, it was usually barefoot, mostly on the beach, a gravelly dirt trail along the Santa Ana River, or trails in local parks. But that was okay; I wasn't training for or even planning on ever running another marathon. I knew that my life—my running life, anyway— had forever changed. I was just another of many, many unknown recreational runners, except *I was running barefoot.*

I had no more goals of finishing marathons, or even racing any distance again. I wouldn't have guessed that someday I'd be running hundreds of races, including seventy-six more marathons, with fourteen marathons in one year alone, including a 33-mile (53 km) ultramarathon over mountain trails to 9,000 feet (2,743 m), all barefoot. Who knew that I would become known as "the Godfather" or "the Guru" or "the Voice" of running barefoot? From then on, I simply knew that most of my running would be enjoyable, because I wouldn't run if it wasn't—and running in shoes, at least for longer runs, was nearly always uncomfortable, and often painful and injurious.

SOLE SUPPORT: THE NATURAL COMMUTE

In 1990, I started commuting home from work by foot—barefoot!

The normal commute between home and California State University, Long Beach (CSULB)—where I'd been working since 1985 as an electronics technician while simultaneously studying for my BA degree in radio, television, and film—was 10 mostly flat miles (16 km). In the morning, I'd ride my bike or take the bus, and then do the long run home on a slightly more involved 11-miler (17.6 km) after work.

It was on my runs home that I happily discovered my feet would carry me any distance my body was capable of running (I had gained a bit of weight and gotten out of shape over the previous three years) with no problem—and no shoes—over a variety of surfaces. About half of my running route was concrete sidewalks or asphalt. On the rest of the commute, I chose between modern surfaces or dirt along the San Gabriel River bike path, a dirt and gravel shoulder of Pacific Coast Highway from Seal Beach to Surfside, a grassy greenbelt through Sunset Beach, and dirt trails through the Bolsa Chica Wetlands. Carrying shoes in my backpack (just in case), I even ran an extra mile so I could run 1 mile (1.6 km) on the sand at Seal Beach. Every "run" home was an adventure of running, walking, and even stopping occasionally for a dip in the ocean before finishing. If I was tired, I might even catch the bus.

Sometimes I ran the entire distance on pavement or sidewalks, finding it to be the most efficient. These hard surfaces, besides being more consistent, thus making it less challenging, also returned more energy from my natural springs—my bent knees. This practice would also eventually pay off when I started running road races barefoot.

Through those years, there were always lessons to be learned on my barefoot commute. Running home in the dark one winter evening, as I started the short descent under one of the bridges that crossed the river trail, I slammed my heel into a sharp rock. *Ouch!* I managed to run the remaining 8 miles (12.8 km) home, but kept my calf tensed the whole way to prevent my heel from touching the ground. After a few similar incidents, I couldn't keep running with my calves tensed because it was just too much work, and *I hate work!*

So again, I experimented, playing with my technique. At first, I would look for some gravel, so that if I was doing anything wrong, I'd know it immediately from my sensitive soles. I figured out pretty quickly—actually, I had known it all along—that I needed to follow the same old advice I gave to Gene nearly twenty years before: Ken Bob, *bend your knees more.*

Bending my knees changed the angle of my foot, so that my heel couldn't land first, and I didn't even need to tense my calves. In fact, I could now relax my calves, giving them and my Achilles tendons a rest. If I felt my heels pounding or pressing into the sharp gravel, rather than trying to push the balls of my feet into the gravel (which was as painful as pushing the heels into it), all I needed to do was bend my knees more. This automatically changed the way my foot landed, and gave me more spring, so my foot landed more gently.

After several residential moves, I had literally met "the girl next door"—Cathy—and in 1990 married her, barefoot on the beach, naturally. I worked full-time, but soon switched to a ten-month-a-year schedule with additional vacation time. In 2000, we moved to a tiny condo with a tiny mortgage on Pacific Coast Highway. So now I'm with the girl of my dreams, living in Southern California, at the beach. I was truly in paradise!

Starting in 1996, a couple of things occurred that shook up my blissful paradise—in a good way.

BAREFOOT AT WORK

I'd long been kicking off my shoes or sandals in my tech shop, where I worked alone, and putting them on to work on the computers, repair test equipment, and shoot videos in faculty offices and labs. One morning, the dean of engineering called me up to install a new component in his computer. I started to grab my shoes, then thought, "Why?" At worst, he'll just tell me to go put them on. I put them back and went upstairs.

As I entered the dean's suite through the outer office, his administrative assistant, Vickie, gave me a thumbs-up. As I went to his computer and started working, I casually watched as the dean did a double take.

AMUSING REACTIONS

It was interesting to see how different people reacted over the years. When the dean resigned in 1999, his replacement told me that he'd gone five years without shoes in college. A temporary typist expressed her shock ("That guy's barefoot!") to Vickie, the administrative assistant, who laughed when she relayed the story to me. One day, the associate vice president expressed his shock that I had shoes on (I had been working outside in the compound, putting scrap metal, computers, and other components onto pallets for recycling). One custodian, who had bugged me about being barefoot, eventually ceased giving me the old "staples and tacks on the floor" warning each time she saw me. Some students would seem truly surprised that the bottoms of my feet weren't full of holes and sores, especially after they found out I also ran barefoot—in marathons. It became clear that most people overestimate the risks and underestimate the pleasure of going barefoot.

But he never said a word about it, and I've worked barefoot ever since. Working barefoot was even part of the conditions I set before accepting an offer to transfer from the electrical engineering department to the computer engineering and computer science department at CSULB a couple of years later.

In the decade since I'd started running almost exclusively barefoot in 1987, I'd adopted a near-100-percent barefoot lifestyle. I'd become a barefoot worker, barefoot racer, and barefoot webmaster.

NOW A "HARD-CORE" BAREFOOT RUNNER

The next big change in my life was becoming what others might call a "hard-core" runner. In reality, I never was hard-core. I only ran when I felt like it. Whenever running was painful or too much work, I'd take a break. On the other hand, I often ran farther and faster throughout the year than true hard-core runners, because I wasn't getting injured. So, despite not being a naturally gifted athlete, despite that I rarely ran more than 50 miles (80 km) in a week (and when I did, I might not run at all the following week if I didn't feel like it), I was able to do something that many gifted or elite athletes couldn't: run all year without injury.

My serious running started one day in 1996. While biking to work, I stopped on the San Gabriel River and talked with George, a guy who occasionally passed me running in the other direction on my way to or from work. George ran in shoes, but he was curious and wanted to know if I could run barefoot on trails. He invited me to run in the hills on Sunday mornings with Buffalo Bill's Wild West Trail Runners, a group led by "Buffalo" Bill McDermott, who I soon discovered was a Southern California legend who ultimately won the Catalina Island off-road marathon thirteen times and finished it thirty-one years in a row. Staged on an island 26 miles (41.8 km) off the coast, and with free-range buffalos roaming it, the hilly Catalina Marathon is renowned as one of the most difficult races in the country. Bill, known variously as "The Downhill Devil" or "The Human Shock Absorber" for his prowess on the hills, stayed in shape by running thousands of miles a year on the steep dirt, gravel, and asphalt trails around his home in nearby La Habra Heights, where the terrain was very similar to that of the Catalina Marathon. Running these hills took me to a new level.

The first day on the trail, I showed up a little late but still managed to catch up with the "slow" group, which did 13 miles (21 km). The next week, it was 16 miles (25.7 km). Within a couple of Sundays, I was running with the "fast" group. Soon I was totaling 50, 60, and, at least a couple of times, more than 80 miles (80.5, 96.5, and 128.7 km) in a week—13 to 20 miles (21 to 32 km) Sunday on mostly trails, and the rest commuting to or from work mostly on asphalt. There would be weeks that I wouldn't run at all. Still, my average mileage doubled within a few months.

I hadn't planned this. I was running barefoot, over some of the roughest possible terrain, and doing it faster and nearly as far as when I trained for my first shod marathon—and it was all just for fun. I mean, I hadn't set a goal to run this much, I was only running when I felt like it, and like Forrest Gump, quite often, "I just felt like running"—except that I was running barefoot. Perhaps it's true that "you can tell a lot about a person by the shoes they wear."

SPURRED ON BY RUNNING CLUBS

I hungered for more, but the Sunday runs were a long drive from my home and only once a week. So I joined another running club, the local A Snail's Pace Running Club in Fountain Valley. I had run occasionally with this group some ten to fourteen years before, but had never officially joined the club.

Let me warn you right now: If you don't want to ever run in races, do *not* join a running club. Within a year of joining, not only was I racing again, but with a lot of prodding and pushing from other members, so was my wife, Cathy.

I started running with other members down the bike path at the beach, back on the Santa Ana River trail where I had trained for my first marathon in 1987, and in Peter's Canyon on some of the steepest hills I would ever run on.

At Peter's Canyon, I had the opportunity to fully test my "bent-knee" shock absorbers. So one day, running with a group of about ten other runners, there I was on top of one of the steepest hills in the canyon. Large sharp rocks had been uncovered by horses, mountain bikes, and shod runners pounding down that hill. Most of the loose sand ended up at the bottom.

This was the *perfect* place to test my gentle running technique. If I could manage to run down this, letting gravity pull me down the near cliff at full speed, then the soft sand at the bottom would be there to break my fall.

So I set out, letting my knees collapse under me, being extremely careful to plant my feet gently between the sharp rocks, and avoiding pushing my feet into the hard ground as I nearly flew down the hill. It was only about 165 feet (50 m) down, but I was running faster than I had ever run in my life. When the trail suddenly turned up at the bottom, and when I hit the soft sand, my knees collapsed fully, my heels practically touching my butt. But I did not fall on my face! It felt so wonderful that I burst out laughing.

I looked back as the other runners came pounding down the hill, using their stiffened legs, like a pole-vault jumper might, to launch themselves up with each step. Why were they launching themselves up? Didn't they realize that the hill was going down? As they tried to slow their descent in this impractical way, they actually hit harder and harder with each step!

MY FIRST BAREFOOT RACE

On June 14, 1997, I headed to nearby Chino Hills, California, for The Road Less Traveled 10-mile (16 km) trail race. The title was adapted from the poem "The Road Not Taken" by Robert Frost:

> "Two roads diverged in a wood, and I—
> I took the one less traveled by,
> And that has made all the difference."

Hmm . . . sounds a bit like my life . . .

Because this was my first real race in ten years and first "real" barefoot race, I started at the back of the pack and ran a slow first mile on the hilly out-and-back course.

As the only barefooter of several hundred racers, I naturally heard "I could never do that," from some slower runners as I passed by. I started with a Nigerian who'd grown up running barefoot but had lived in the U.S. for twenty years. He was pudgy, like many Americans. He was also wearing shoes and running slow. I left him in the dust on the first climbs.

At the first creek crossing, about a half-mile (0.8 km) from the start, I took advantage of my "water-proofing." As others detoured to a narrow point to jump across the water or step on rocks, I went right through the creek.

After steadily passing people early, the crowd thinned at about mile 4. From that point, I only passed on the downhills, where my deeply-bending knees gave me an advantage. Most seemed afraid of running fast downhill, and unable to make use of gravity's acceleration. I'd pace a runner up the hill, and on the descents, letting my knees collapse under my falling mass, gravity pulled me past him. At least I didn't have to worry about tripping over my shoelaces.

At one point I yelled ahead to warn people that I was "coming through, no brakes!" I heard one woman reply, "No brakes, no knees!" She just didn't get it. As I flew past her, I watched her land stiff-legged, launching herself up into the air away from the hill, only to come down harder with each step as she pounded down it. I wanted to warn her: "Brakes destroy the knees!" But I was already far ahead of her.

Much of the way back, I was alone. I had passed most of the pack, and the leaders were several minutes ahead. I may have gotten some of the spectators wet as I ran through the creek without slowing down. After finishing, I soaked my feet in the cool water and watched many finishers, even after running this far, still worry about getting their shoes wet.

I did pretty well, finishing in 41st place overall and 8th place for my age group (40–45) in 1:11:06 (about 7:07 per mile).

The crowd's reactions after the race were hilarious. I felt like a celebrity, with dozens of people approaching me. Some brave souls inspected my bare soles, surprised that they didn't look like hamburger and were nice and soft, with no hard, dry, calluses. Many "interviewed" me. "Why do you run barefoot?" they asked. "Doesn't it hurt to run barefoot?" Eventually, I decided that my best tack would be to balance the discussion by putting the shoe on the other foot, so to speak. So I'd answer their questions with another question: "Doesn't it hurt to run with *those* on your feet?"

BIRTH OF A WEBSITE

There were so many questions after my first barefoot race (see "My First Barefoot Race" at left) that I decided to start The Running Barefoot website. I'd already gotten my feet wet on the Internet in 1996 by joining the Dirty Sole Society (DSS), later to be renamed the Society for Barefoot Living. In February 1997, convinced that barefooting was a healthy option that others should be made aware of (a fact that the multimillion-dollar advertising campaigns for running shoes were skipping), I organized and hosted a DSS "barefoot gathering" at the Secret Spot, a restaurant next to my apartment complex. About a dozen participants showed up for barefoot walks in the nearby nature preserve and a beachfront 5-miler (8 km) to the Huntington Beach Pier. Over time, however, I realized that the DSS website simply did not have adequate resources for runners. Not only were the same old discussion topics being recycled ("Is it illegal to go barefoot into a restaurant?"), but also the things that I posted on barefoot running never got much response.

The Internet was exploding but still in its infancy in 1997. I'd set up my personal Web page the year before, then got together with Cathy's second cousin, Jonathan, a CSULB student, to set up a server in my office. I was friends with all the network techs, and they assigned our server an address and a name so we could make it accessible to the public. Mine was undoubtedly the world's first running barefoot website.

Later, when I transferred to the computer engineering and computer science department, we renamed the server "barefoot" — still on a sub-domain of the CSULB system. I figured that would soon become inappropriate as more traffic visited The Running Barefoot website, and because I was interested in setting up affiliate advertisements to help pay for running the site. I signed up with a hosting company, and purchased a domain name. The current domain name is TheRunningBarefoot.com. Some of the old addresses, including http://barefoot.cecs.csulb.edu/runbarefoot and RunningBarefoot.org, should still forward to the new address.

When I set up The Running Barefoot website in 1997, of course there was no other information about running barefoot on the Internet to link to. I went to the library and looked up tales of barefoot runners. I titled one of the pages of The Running Barefoot website "WHO: We are not alone," and wrote about anyone I could find who had or was running barefoot. That included Abebe Bikila, who won Olympic gold running barefoot in the marathon at the 1960 games; Zola Budd, the South Africa teenage sensation who ran barefoot in the 1984 and 1992 Olympics; and Ron Daws, an American marathoner who finished 22nd in the 1968 Mexico City Olympics. I found out about Ron Daws, a National Road Runners Hall of Fame member, in his book *The Self-Made Olympian*, which included a photo of him running barefoot over the caption "Running barefoot in the cross-country in Minnesota."

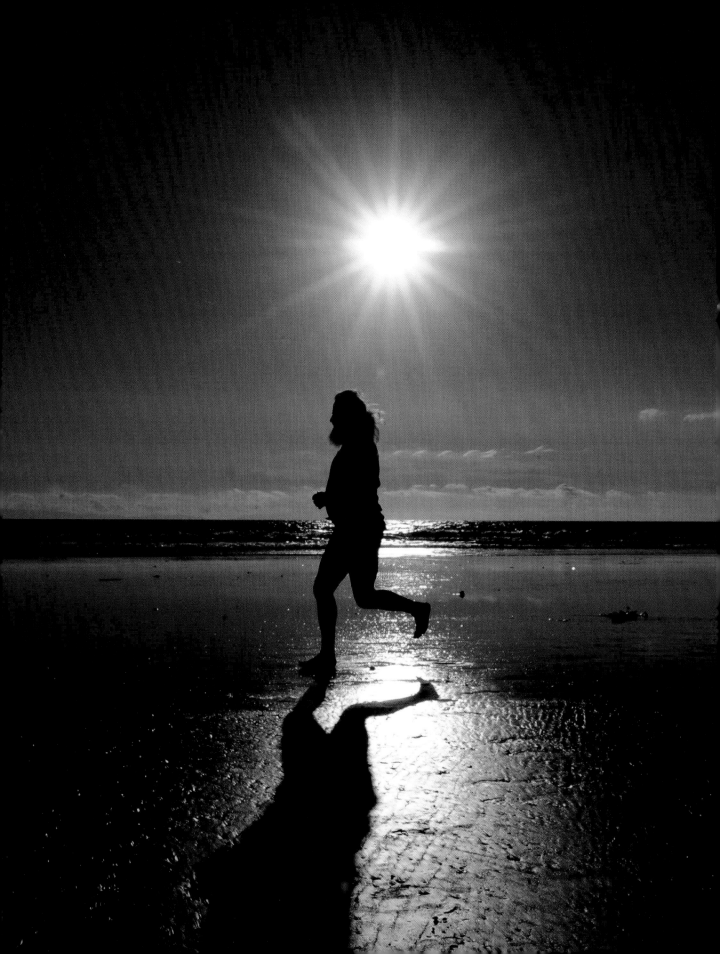

I posted a few pictures of me running barefoot. When my wife saw someone running barefoot in a race and had the camera handy, she would get a photo for my website. Still, there weren't many other barefoot runners locally. I spent most of my lunch hours at the university library looking for books and articles that mentioned anyone running barefoot. I spent several hours each week researching and writing about running barefoot on the website.

Eventually, more people discovered how useful the Internet was for posting and gathering information for their running clubs. Through Web searches, I was able to discover other barefoot runners around the world, and I started posting stories and pictures of anyone and everyone I could find who was running barefoot, such as Ingrid Kupke, the European ultra-running champion.

When curious folks started asking too many questions and wanted more information at races than I could give them, I'd tell them to do a Web search for "running barefoot." The Running Barefoot website would come up first. Other than my own articles posted on the DSS website, for quite a while The Running Barefoot website would yield the only results for such searches. For years, it literally was the only site about running barefoot.

MY FIRST BAREFOOT MARATHON

On April 4, 1998, eleven blister-free years after limping to a blister-riddled finish at my first marathon in shoes, and a year and a half after I began running with Buffalo Bill's group, I raced my second marathon—this time in bare feet. Because I lived in Southern California, I picked a marathon in northern California so I wouldn't embarrass myself in front of anyone I knew. I picked a trail marathon, because I figured—incorrectly, as it turns out—that being more natural, it would be easier on bare feet.

This is what I read on EnviroSports.com: "The Napa Valley Trail Marathon is beautiful, traversing the rock-strewn babbling streams, dirt trails, and majestic hills of redwood, oak, and madrone coursing through Bothe-Napa Valley State Park." On a cold (46°F [7.8°C]), drizzly, northern California day, about one hundred runners competing in the marathon, half marathon, and 10K races forded ice-cold mountain streams, climbed over logs, climbed the side of a mountain, negotiated narrow goat trails on the edge of a cliff, danced around sharp rocks that jutted up from the trail like stalagmites, and slipped on muddy riverbanks. My feet were numb after the first 10K loop.

By the fifth and final loop, cold, tired, and alone, I sat down on a log and tried to peel an orange with numb fingers that refused to function anymore. Then I began the final downhill, used some of the extreme knee-bending skills I'd picked up running in the hills with Buffalo Bill, and began reeling in a few of the thirty-four runners in the marathon, finishing in 4:34.

It was a new marathon personal record (PR)—more than half an hour faster than what I did almost eleven years earlier on a flat, fast course in perfect weather. The difference? Besides the fact that I was now quite well conditioned, with more consistent running and longer distances, it was obviously the lack of shoes. Barefooting motivated me to run more by making running more enjoyable.

I placed 13th out of thirty-five finishers in the marathon. Somewhere along the course I managed to cut my right foot, but because my feet were numb, I didn't notice it. Then, while sitting down at a picnic table afterward to have a banana and chat with Dave, the race director, someone came up and asked to look at my feet. My soles were just fine, but there was a small slice on the side of the foot near the big toe, with a line on the ball of the foot that led directly to the cut. Apparently I stepped on a sharp rock, possibly in one of the stream crossings. My foot probably slipped on the sharp edge, but the rock was only able to leave a line on my toughened sole until it slid over to thinner skin. I still have a ⅝-inch (1.5 cm) scar there.

GOING TOE TO TOE

KEN BOB'S FIRST SHOD MARATHON VS. FIRST BAREFOOT MARATHON

EVENT	LONG BEACH MARATHON	NAPA VALLEY TRAIL MARATHON
DATE	May 3, 1987	April 4, 1998
FOOTWEAR	Saucony	none (barefoot)
AGE	32	42
DISTANCE	26.2 miles (42 km)	26.2 (42 km)
TIME	5:05	4:34
HILLS	practically flat	up, over, and down a mountain—twice!
DESCRIPTION	smooth asphalt	dirt, gravel, logs, mud, pebbles, rock, sticks, streams, twigs
WEATHER	cool (61°F [16°C]), cloudy, perfect for running	cold (46°F [7.8°C]), fog, rain
15 MILES (24 KM)	tired	tired
20 MILES (32 KM)	OWWW!	WOW!
25 MILES (40 KM)	Let this be over	Can I do this again?
POST RACE	couldn't wear shoes comfortably for two weeks	ran 20 miles (32 km), barefoot, comfortably, two days later
CITY	Long Beach	Calistoga
STATE	California	California

The cut was no big deal. Many runners had abrasions from slipping in the mud and the rain. My cut was so minor that I was able to run 20 miles (32 km) two days later.

Dave and I pondered why people run these kinds of crazy events. Then he congratulated me for running such a rough course on bare feet. I told him that I would never have attempted it, let alone completed it, if I had to run it in shoes.

BARE FEET MADE ME A MARATHON MAN

In one day, thanks to a decade-old decision to chuck my shoes, I went from hating the marathon to enjoying the marathon. In shoes, the marathon was drudgery, pain, and injury. Barefoot, it was all fun, excitement, and speed. I wanted more, and I did more because barefooting had changed my running from drudgery to fun.

I ran a 50K trail race in June. The next January, I ran my first barefoot road marathon, the Pacific Shoreline in my adopted hometown of Huntington Beach, in a torrential downpour, in a new PR of 4:10. I finished two more marathons in 1999, including the mostly downhill St. George (Utah) Marathon in 3:20. It was my first Boston Marathon qualifier and a new PR for a few months, until I set my all-time best of 3:18 at my next Pacific Shoreline a few months later.

Old habits don't change easily, though. The big pavement miles started to wear on my soles, but I fixed that by "running lighter"—bending my knees more, picking up my feet faster, and using numerous other technique adjustments that I will detail in chapters 3 and 4.

The 2004 Boston Marathon was one of a dozen marathons—one per month—that I did that year. After taking it easy in 2005, I pushed it hard in 2006, doing sixteen marathons, including four in three weeks. As I write this in late 2010 at age fifty-five, I'm up to seventy-six career marathons, and there's no end in sight. Although I don't race as much now due to time commitments and skyrocketing race fees, I am quite certain of one thing: Running is a lifelong sport—if you run barefoot.

And that's not just because you don't get blisters, which is the only benefit I noticed at first. It is because of something that I frankly didn't think about until I built my website, but is the all-important, number-one reason to run barefoot: Debilitating injuries almost always disappear.

THE INJURY-PREVENTION REVELATION

I did not know that runners frequently got injured. After all, I rarely did (at least not from running barefoot; I might stub a toe around the house, or sprain my finger, and one time I dropped a vacuum cleaner canister on my toe), not counting an occasional thorn or tiny splinter of glass, which I'd just pull out and keep on going. Until the late 1990s, I mostly ran alone and was not networked in with other runners, so I had no clue that shoes might be responsible for running-related injuries beyond the blackened toenails, blisters, and occasional ankle sprains I remembered from my shod days. I didn't know that going barefoot could help cure them, even though it turns out that researchers had been coming to that conclusion for decades. That's why I was so surprised by an email I got on April 5, 1998, the day after I ran the Napa Valley Trail Marathon, about how running barefoot cured the incurable back pain of Luke Finlay, a Tennessee college student and cross-country runner:

The [Running] Barefoot page is worthy of praise . . . I'm glad to see somebody calling attention to what just seems to me to be a natural extension of exercise.

I've heard all kinds of stuff the past couple of years while running cross-country for Austin Peay State University (APSU) in Clarksville, Tennessee. I had been "benched" with a debilitating back problem as a junior, and had given up running altogether.

Before my junior year, I spent the summer on the West Coast, and I started running again on beaches and on grass; of course, this time, it was minus my running shoes. My form improved, my back pain decreased, and I have gone on to have my two best seasons of cross-country ever, while running every race barefoot.

I can't explain it medically; all I know is that I went from being incapable of running to becoming more successful than I had ever been previously. I chalked it up to the barefoot thing, and my teammates believe it. What else could explain my comeback? So they have been really supportive of the whole thing.

I have heard all kinds of wisecracks from spectators, including one who screamed out that the coach at his university had a sufficient budget to buy them shoes . . . Oh, well. I just save Coach the money on a pair of spikes.

The only injuries I have sustained weren't truly injuries, they were just brief moments of inexplicable pain. One was caused by my own stupidity . . . I kicked an immovable cone at the NCAA regionals when it was in the low 40s . . . ouch. But very rarely do I hurt my feet. I haven't mastered running on the road yet, but I am trying it a little bit more. Track running is possible on some tracks, but I haven't got that one completely figured out yet, either.

Anyway, I enjoyed the information on your page. Thanks.

Luke
APSU

I was stunned. What an eye-opener! Running barefoot might actually cure injuries, like it cured Luke. I had posted excerpts and links on my website of studies showing evidence of reduced impact while running barefoot, but until now I hadn't made a connection to anyone I knew, much less thought that removing shoes could reverse impact-related injuries. Until that moment, I thought barefooting only prevented blackened toenails and blisters on the tops of the feet.

Q: WHY DO ELITE AFRICAN RUNNERS DO WELL IN SHOES?
A: THEY ALREADY KNOW HOW TO RUN BAREFOOT

Don't let the use of shoes by elite runners fool you. Yes, the Kenyans, Ethiopians, and other runners from areas where people grow up running barefoot do quite well in shoes. But that's because they learned how to run gently at an early age! They take their amazing running technique for granted because they don't remember learning it. They run in shoes in races because that's how they make a living. Haile Gebrselassie, for example, has spent hundreds of thousands of dollars to help fix up his hometown and build an amazing sports arena, thanks to running shoe endorsement contracts.

Don't get me wrong: I think it's great that he has the opportunity to help his countrymen. I'm just pointing out the reality of why he, and many others, won't be seen racing barefoot any time soon. But Gebrselassie does run barefoot, some of the time, to keep his feet in shape, and, whether he knows it or not, to fine-tune his running technique.

Ultimately, elite athletes do not run fast because of their shoe sponsorships; they get shoe sponsorships because they run fast.

" When I had no shoes I was comfortable—I used to run barefoot. When I wore shoes it was difficult. To run in shoes was okay, but at the beginning of my career it was hard. In our countryside, you see those kids, they are very comfortable with no shoes. It's better to have no shoes than not the right ones. **"**

—Haile Gebrselassie, http://edition.cnn.com/2007/TECH/09/26/revealed.HaileG.qanda

So this was big. I didn't know then, as we do now, that every year half of all runners suffer injuries severe enough to stop them from running—although I *was* getting tired of hearing runners tell me that they couldn't join me for a long run due to an injury. (Maybe they wanted to avoid my witty conversation, and were tired of hearing about the wonders of running barefoot.) I did not know that the numbers of runners practically fall off the table after age fifty, due to accumulated injuries. And I didn't know that barefooting—even just a little barefooting, as you'll see later in this book—might prevent injuries (or at least let them heal), because I'd always run at least some of the time barefoot since I'd been a kid. I did have an inkling that the heel strike encouraged by padded shoes had the effect of adding—not subtracting—shock, and that this shock probably led to injuries. After all, I could certainly hear the pounding shoes of people I was running with.

SCIENTIFIC STUDIES TO BOOT

But Luke's email was confirmation of something more important, which led me to review some studies posted on the barefooters.org site of the Society of Barefoot Living. Sure enough, there was a definite shoes-injuries correlation:

In 1987, a survey of Africans in the article "Running-Related Injury Prevention through Barefoot Adaptations" in the journal *Medicine and Science in Sports and Exercise* by Robbins and Hanna found an extremely low running-related injury rate among runners in barefoot populations.

This was not the first time shoes had been implicated in foot problems.

In 1949, Samuel B. Shulman's "Survey in China and India of Feet That Have Never Worn Shoes," published in *The Journal of the National Association of Chiropodists*, concluded that "restrictive footwear, particularly ill-fitting footgear, cause most of the ailments of the human foot." (Having worked in a shoe store, I knew that many customers, especially women, actually tried to buy shoes that were "ill-fitting." I would attempt, usually futilely, to convince them to do otherwise.) Shulman not only found that there was a lower incidence of foot fungus in barefooters than in shoe-wearers, but also that barefoot feet were "perfect," stronger and tougher, with a bigger space between the first and second toes to handle more weight-bearing loads, or possibly to compensate for variations in metatarsal length.

You could even go back to 1874, when *The Journal of Hygiene and Herald of Health*, volume 45, published an article by Dr. J. William Lloyd recommending that his patients go barefoot to cure their foot problems.

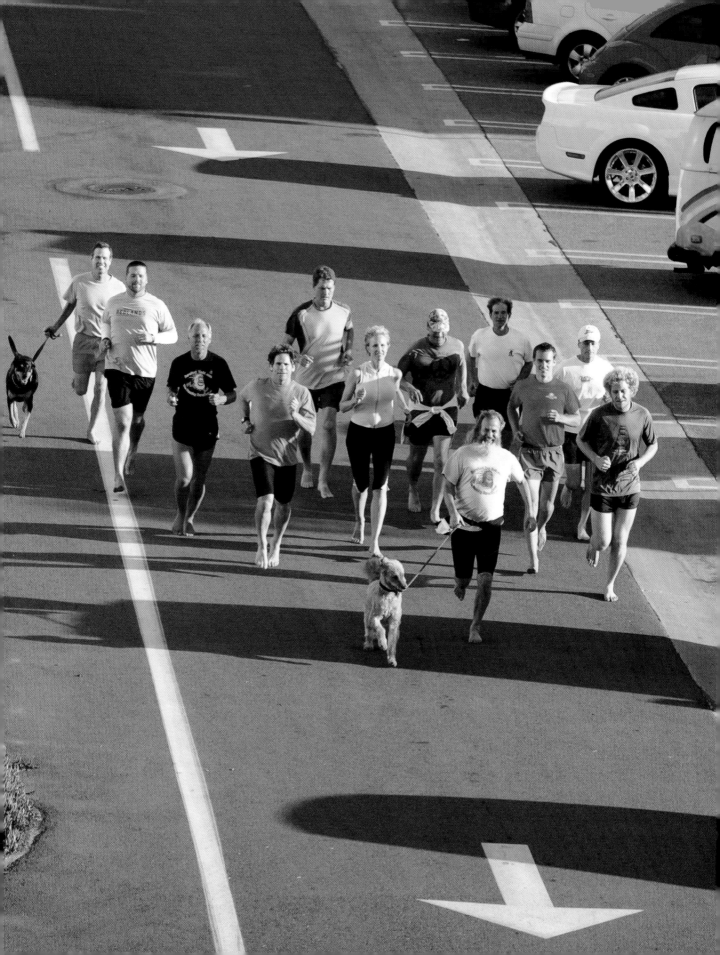

Plenty of new studies basically say the same thing. One of the most recent, a 2010 study of healthy young runners published in *PM&R: The Journal of Injury, Function and Rehabilitation*, found that running in shoes can put more stress on the knee, hip, and ankle joints than running barefoot does. It was even harder on the knees than walking in high heels, they noted.

As The Running Barefoot site ramped up, and publicity started coming in from the numerous articles being written about me in *The Los Angeles Times*, *The Boston Globe*, *Runner's World*, *Competitor*, *Orange County Register*, and *The Wall Street Journal*, as well as stories on National Public Radio and ABC World News, the trickle of messages about shoe-caused injures and barefoot rehab became more like a flood.

I got into this barefoot thing to make running a more pleasurable experience for myself, and I started my website to share my experiences with others because they were curious. But finding out that barefooting curtailed injuries took it to a new level. My website was no longer just a resource for granola-eating vegetarian runners who wanted to peacefully coexist with Mother Earth—to literally walk lightly on the earth without getting blisters. Now the site could be a critical quality-of-life resource for thousands of mainstream runners.

As the new millennium arrived and my running got better and better, I found myself increasingly infused with a messianic zeal, researching articles and devoting hours a day to answering emails, posts, and comments on my website.

Skeptics might choose to focus on the cut I got on my foot in Napa Valley (which didn't slow me down a bit and cost me zero training time) as proof of the dangers of running unprotected by shoes. But I haven't been cut like that since, and the dangers of being "protected" by shoes are far worse than the occasional twig or rock.

I will go into more detail about why shoes cause problems in chapter 2, but the fact is they can wreck your knees, ankles, hips, and back, as well as slow you down. Running on top of pillowy cushions throws off your balance, blocks and eventually deadens the proprioceptors on your feet, encourages joint-jarring heel striking, and—due to the extra weight—eats up more of your oxygen.

But your body already knows that. If you listen to it and dump your shoes (at least some of the time), you'll get a nice reward: nearly injury-free running the rest of your life.

Ultimately, I don't get too hung up on academic studies to justify barefooting. If I'd waited for academic studies, I would probably not be running at all, except for a few times a week at the beach. If I waited for academic studies, I might not be *eating*! Where is the research that demonstrates that we need to breathe? We don't need that research because, when we try not breathing, our body tells us to breathe!

Your best researcher is your own body. Mine told me a long time ago to put more bend in my knees, and it worked. As I've experimented more with various details of my running techniques, some suggested by other runners through my website, and listened more closely to my body in recent years, it's given me more details about how exactly to move my legs, hips, shoulders, arms, and head, so my bare soles will land comfortably, precisely as they should, to give the rest of my body the smoothest ride possible over any terrain—all explained in detail in chapter 3.

The bottom line? Be sensitive to your body. Listen to it. It's always talking to you. If you're like every other mammal on Earth, it'll tell you that barefooting is right.

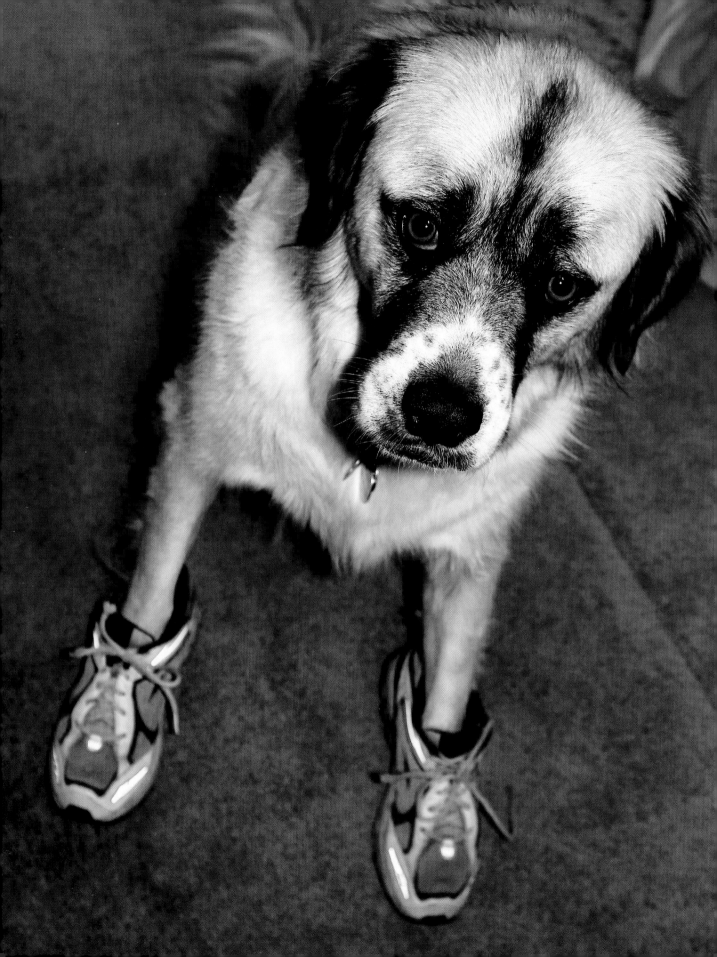

CHAPTER 2

THE "FEETBACK" LOOP
LOSE YOUR SHOES TO GAIN NATURAL SENSORY FEEDBACK

The equation is simple: *Feet + Feedback = Feetback*. Shoes lead to injuries because they deaden sensations, throw you off balance, and encourage a high-impact heel strike. Here's why running barefoot fixes up humans—and other creatures, too.

> **Q: HEY, KEN BOB, DO YOU RECOMMEND WALKING YOUR DOG BAREFOOT?**
>
> **A: OF COURSE. BUT HOW LONG HAS YOUR DOG BEEN WEARING SHOES?**
>
> —KEN BOB-ISM #12

Almost everyone I meet finds out quickly that I like corny puns and twisted-logic comebacks. It's always fun to stop people in their tracks for a second or two. And because I'm a dog person and often bring Herman, my 90-pound (41 kg) Great Pyrenees/Golden Retriever, to my workshops, the above question—and my tried-and-true response—comes up a lot.

Keeping in mind that the great comedians often say that the best humor usually has some truth to it, the "dog-wearing-shoes" line got me thinking of a new approach to explaining the shoes-versus-barefoot issue. Instead of approaching it from the typical Physiology 101 explanation—that running shoes lead to rampant injuries by blocking our natural sensitivity, throwing off our balance, and making us prone to unnatural, high-impact heel striking—I simply looked at Herman and wondered: Why don't we put dogs in shoes? In shoes, would they get faster? In shoes, would their joints get less arthritic, their agility increase, their quality of life improve? Surely, someone has done studies of this!

A quick Internet search was not helpful. Although there are several dog footwear products—such as NeoPaws neoprene shoes for ice and harsh winter weather ($30), and Ruff Wear Grip Trex Bark'n boots for rough gravel and Idaho cheatgrass ($59.95 set of four; choice of obsidian black or currant red)—I found no studies or articles that compared the performance, injury rate, and quality of life of shod verses unshod dogs.

Then it struck me that I was looking at the wrong quadruped. There actually is one animal that wears shoes even more than humans do: horses!

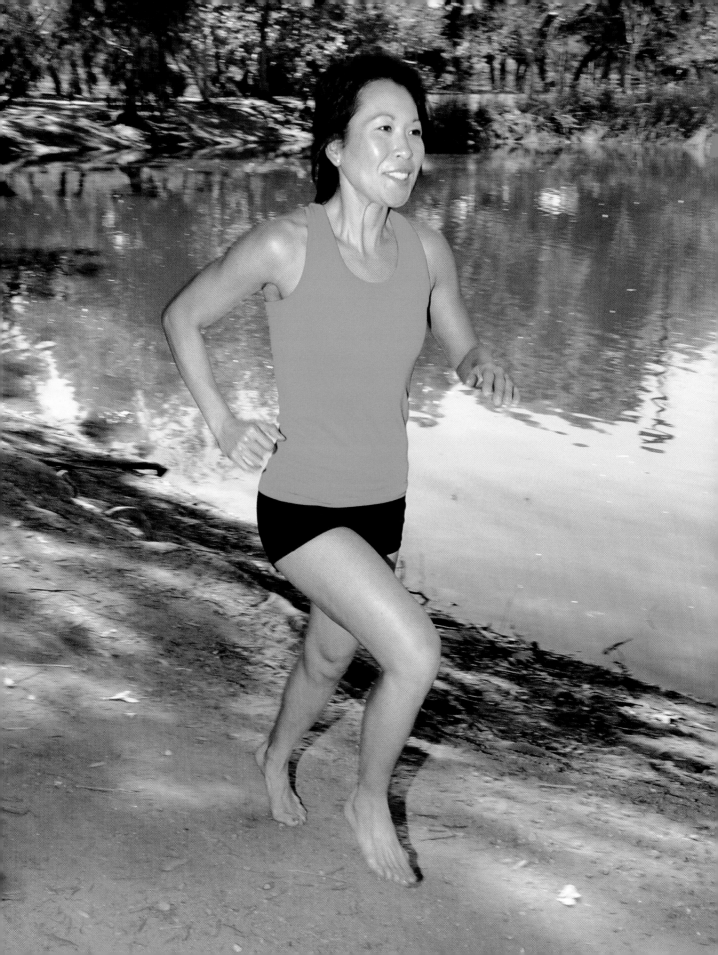

We started putting horseshoes on horses back in the Middle Ages to keep their feet from rotting in dank castle stalls for months at a time, and the practice stuck. But do they actually still need horseshoes in cleaner conditions? It turns out that they often don't. According to Dr. Hiltrud Strasser, author of *A Lifetime of Soundness*, shoes damage a horse's feet, legs, and circulatory system in many ways, the worst being the loss of blood nutrients in the hoof and loss of shock absorption. A movement to remove shoes and restore the natural non-flat hoof shape found in the wild—on so-called "barefoot horses"—is growing. (For more detail on barefoot horses, see pages 48–49.)

The experience of the Mounted Patrol Unit of the Houston Police Department, which converted all of its thirty-six horses to barefooting in recent years, may be instructive. "The hoof is an amazing piece of equipment, and the horse's well-being—and sometimes life—depend on it," said the program leader, Officer Greg Sokoloski, in a 2005 article in *The Horse's Hoof* magazine. "I was stunned and fascinated by the importance of hoof mechanism and how some of the injuries and behavioral problems could be due to the constraints of metal shoes. Since we converted them to barefoot, our horses are so much healthier and happier. People have noticed not only better dispositions, but glossier coats, along with much less downtime."

Now, replace "hoof" with "foot," "glossy coat" with "healthy glow," "downtime" with "running injuries," and "horse" with "human." Then ask yourself: Haven't I heard this before?

WHY THIS CHAPTER IS CALLED "FEETBACK"

This chapter will touch on a lot of ideas: why running in running shoes disrupts the natural function of feet, ankles, knees, hips, and lower back; deadens our sensations; compromises our proprioception (our knowledge of where our body parts are in space); upsets balance; encourages a dangerous change in biomechanics; and increases impact on and destruction of joints. It will reference some studies that show cushioned shoes create more shock than the bare feet and minimalist shoes they replace. And ultimately, it will show that we are a lot like dogs and horses and probably other animals: We function best when our feet are free.

A simple way to remember the main thrust of this chapter is to remember its title, Feetback, which my coauthor Roy and I came up with in a "eureka!" phone moment after days of spirited brainstorming in the summer of 2010. (Or maybe it was just a bad connection.)

Beyond being a remarkably clever pun (at least we think so), this lovechild of "feet" and "feedback" is helpful because it accurately describes the two key benefits of barefoot running: balance and impact reduction. First, it restores *feedback* to your *feet*, which strengthens them; restores body balance; and, as a bonus, simply feels great. Also, running barefoot literally positions your feet *back* under your body, which eliminates heel striking and overstriding, and can reduce impact by 50 percent or more. Feetback gets you back to a natural position that minimizes stress and maximizes efficiency. Consider the following:

← **WHAT TO DO: an example of correct feetback and posture. Note the position of the hips, knees, and ankles.**

HOW HOUSTON'S MANE ATTRACTIONS GOT THEIR HOOVES BACK

THE POLICE HORSES' BAREFOOT BENEFITS—BETTER BIOMECHANICS AND SHOCK ABSORPTION—ARE REMARKABLY HUMAN.

As humans are discovering the benefits of going shoeless, so are horses. The trend of removing horseshoes for the horse's well-being and performance, which started in the late 1990s and reached the Houston Police Department several years ago, illustrates a remarkable symmetry with the challenges and issues humans face in converting to running barefoot.

The thirty-six horses of the Houston Mounted Unit, which patrols the Central Business District, all wore borium-tipped metal shoes until 2004, when officers attended a barefoot demonstration that explained how a correct, unshod hoof results in fewer injuries, fewer diseases, and better behavior.

A natural hoof is a dynamic cone that flexes wider when it contacts the ground and narrows into a "closed" shape as it lifts off the ground. According to barefoothorse.com, this spread-and-squeeze acts like a pump, pulling blood into the foot with each step. But when a horseshoe is nailed onto the hoof, the pump no longer works, circulation suffers, nutrients are choked off, and the horse's feet become painful and slow to heal. It gets worse in two ways that are eerily similar to those of shod runners: The horse's biomechanics suffer because the hoof changes shape and curls the heel inward, and the animal's joints get thrashed because of a radical increase in concussive impact. The naturally flexing hoofs are designed to absorb shock; in shoes, they lose 75 percent of this ability.

A few days before the start of Super Bowl week in early 2004, the first HPD horse to lose his shoes was Shadow, a four-year-old Dutch Warmblood ridden by Officer Greg Sokoloski. The horse had worked two fourteen-hour days before the game with no ill effect other than some soreness, which was addressed by hoof boots, a sort of Vibram FiveFingers for horses. Shadow's good behavior convinced the department to de-shoe other horses with physical problems. After Sokoloski pulled the shoes off of Barney, the chronically lame and abscessed horse was perfectly healthy within a week. Nine other horses with issues like split and contracted hooves were de-shoed and similarly rejuvenated. Boots were used in each case for transitioning into barefooting, long assignments, and protection in large disturbances. The program worked so well that it was soon applied to healthy shod horses.

By 2010, every Houston police horse was barefoot. "The HPD realized huge savings," says Yvonne Wells, editor-publisher of *The Horse's Hoof* magazine. "Common diseases like Laminitis, where the hoof tears away from the bone, disappeared." Houston even replaced its old bacteria-riddled stalls, where horses for centuries have stood and lived in their own feces, with a new free-range facility that lets them socialize, eat, and exercise naturally.

Sokoloski admitted to being shocked at the damage the shoes cause. "As we pulled shoes and began trimming some of the horses, we found very deformed and unbalanced hooves," he wrote in *The Horse's Hoof*. "The horses had compensated for these imbalances for years. The transformation for some begins with relief, and the ability to move without restriction."

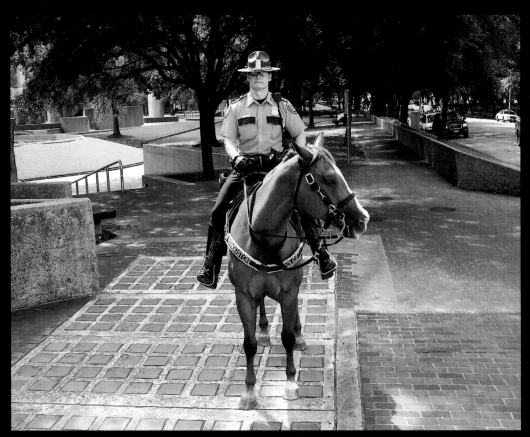
Officer Randy Wallace of the Houston Police Department on barefoot horse Chance

Officers saw the benefits quickly in the form of the barefooters' much improved footing and traction. The enhanced feeling in their hooves gives the horses the ability to adjust quicker to changes of direction and—barefoot runners will relate to this—to walk softer.

"We have a few horses we call 'ground pounders,' who constantly slam their feet into the ground," wrote Sokoloski. "Going barefoot has made these horses walk softer, slower, and much more comfortably in all their gaits. We have also found that horses thought to have 'training' issues could have been that way due to pain and the constant pounding on hard surfaces with steel shoes."

Fitting that description was Cadence, a frequently lame horse with a long list of foot damages and compromised biomechanics. He adjusted well after de-shoeing, but after a month of active duty was bruised, sore, and sent off for some R & R. As with humans, not every horse enjoys a perfect barefoot transition. But the remarkably similar lessons to be learned and the benefits to be gained make it a worthwhile option for quadrupeds and bipeds alike.

1

FEETBACK MEANS THAT BAREFOOTING RESTORES THE *FEEDBACK FROM YOUR FEET,* WHICH RESTORES BALANCE AND COORDINATION.

Like gloves on your hands, shoes attempt to protect your feet. Unfortunately, they also dull the vast array of critical sensors on your soles and feet muscles that guide your balance, weight distribution, muscle-joint coordination, and even warn you when you are getting over-trained. The bigger the cushioning, the more you land out of balance. This imbalance is often imperceptible to runners, but not always. "It's all a matter of angles. Big [cushioned] shoes have too much wobble to them," said Ron Hill, a British running star of the 1960s and '70s who frequently trained barefoot (see his profile in chapter 8), in a *Runner's World* interview with Amby Burfoot. "That increases the strain on your ankles, knees, and hips."

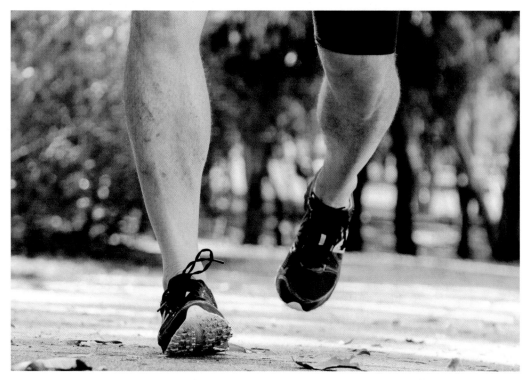

WHAT NOT TO DO: Don't allow shoes to deceive you into developing bad habits, such as excessive loading on one edge of the foot, which adversely affects your balance, weight distribution, and coordination.

Many podiatrists agree. "Turns out that the weight and cushioning of footwear change the way we run—none for the better," says Dr. Paul Langer, author of *Great Feet for Life*, and an avid marathon runner and triathlete. "It disturbs our ability to sense the surface and know how hard or soft we're landing. So in shoes, our gait changes and we actually hit the ground with greater force—unevenly! Increased torque/twisting forces go into the knee, ankle, and hips. That's why, despite the fact that cushioning feels good, you are more prone to injury in shoes."

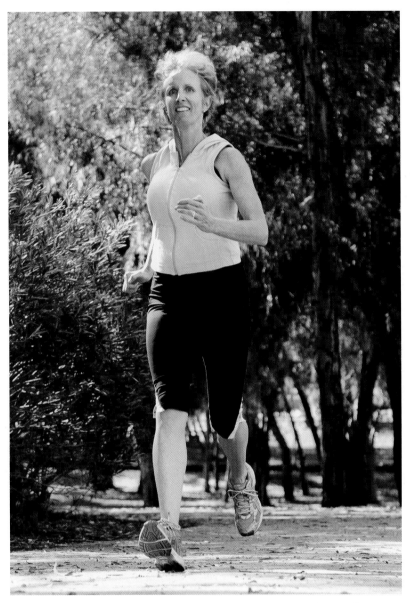

WHAT NOT TO DO: Avoid the stiff-legged landing and heel strike, which cause increased torque at the knee, ankle, and hips. Excess torque, along with excess impact, probably leads to knee injuries.

For some runners, going barefoot stops their aches and pains the very first run. No surprise there; finally getting proper feedback and off of the wobbly cushioning, their body stays calm, balanced, and responsive to the ground, as it was meant to.

Bottom line: "If you numb people's feet, they have poor balance," says Langer, who started weaning himself off cushioned shoes in the mid-'90s and runs in bare feet and minimalist shoes now. "The body can absorb running impact very efficiently if given the appropriate feedback." Or *feetback*.

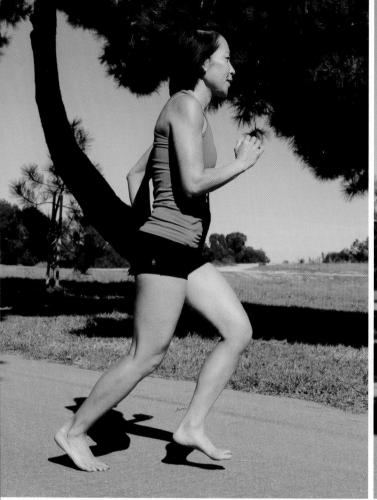

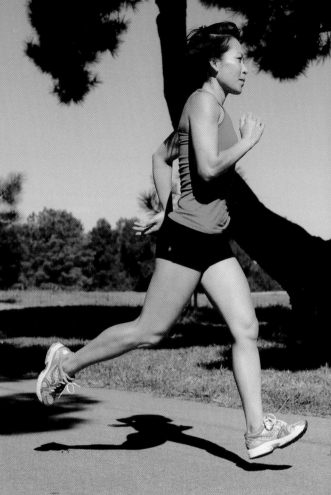

WHAT TO DO: Land with your foot underneath your center of balance, and let your body move in front of your foot, with your legs bent and your strides short and quick. This causes a slight forward imbalance, a falling sensation, which along with your bent knees springs you forward with little effort.

WHAT NOT TO DO: Note the runner over-striding, with long, unbent legs and a heel strike. This is typical of the over-confidence resulting from a lack of feeling/feedback from bare soles letting you know how much damage you are doing to yourself!

2 *FEETBACK* ALSO MEANS THAT BAREFOOTING POSITIONS YOUR *FEET BACK*, WHICH LESSENS IMPACT AND INJURY.

"We were designed to walk on our heels, not run on them," says Irene Davis, director of Harvard Medical School's Spaulding National Running Center. That's because the natural barefoot form immediately and instinctively trains you to let your body lead the way and keep your *feet back* — that is, be positioned under and behind you with a bent leg, moving in quick, short strides, and touching down with a low-impact forefoot landing. In this position, there can be no heel strike, which is the cause of the pounding that leads to endless connective tissue and joint injuries.

The soft, bent-knee, feet-back position of a barefooter contrasts with the harsh, straight-leg, feet-forward position of a shod runner. Barefoot, very few people heel strike. A study of Kenyan adolescent barefoot runners by Dr. Daniel Lieberman found that only 19 percent landed on their heels (and that's on grass and dirt; the percentage surely would be less on concrete). In shoes, the numbers are reversed, as about 80 percent of people tend to overstride (i.e., extend their feet out ahead of the body).

Overstriding is a prescription for injuries because the huge crash of a heel strike sends a massive ripple of shock of up to five times your body weight up the leg. Your leg is meant to be a *shock absorber*, but the heel strike turns it into a *shock producer*.

Of course, encouraging poor positioning isn't the only problem with shoes: Any barrier between you and the ground blunts the function of your foot and sole—which like a horse's hoof is an extremely complex apparatus designed to read the terrain, lead your coordination, and even help pump blood throughout the foot and back to the body. Deprived of information, weakened through immobilization, and undernourished through restricted blood supply, it doesn't work perfectly, initiating a chain of dysfunction that cascades up the body, straining joints and connective tissue like they were never supposed to be strained. Add the extra shock that occurs when the shod foot heel strikes—which the cushioning ironically encourages—and your joints end up pulverized.

Now, we humans are tough enough to handle a little pulverization and imbalance; occasional deviations from ideal natural form might not be a problem once in a while. A few people even run in shoes for decades without injuries. But whether you believe in the popular theory of Dr. Lieberman and others that humans actually evolved as long-distance runners who chased, wore down, and killed their animal prey on 10K and marathon-distance aerobic hunting expeditions (I do), it's logical to assume that too much pulverization and imbalance will usually lead to problems. In a repetitive-motion activity such as running, small discomforts can easily mutate into big injuries. Is a 5-mile (8 km) run in shoes five times a week year after year too much? Hard to say, as every body is different. But we do know that running injuries are rampant, and that the culprits are shoes, overtraining, or a combination of both.

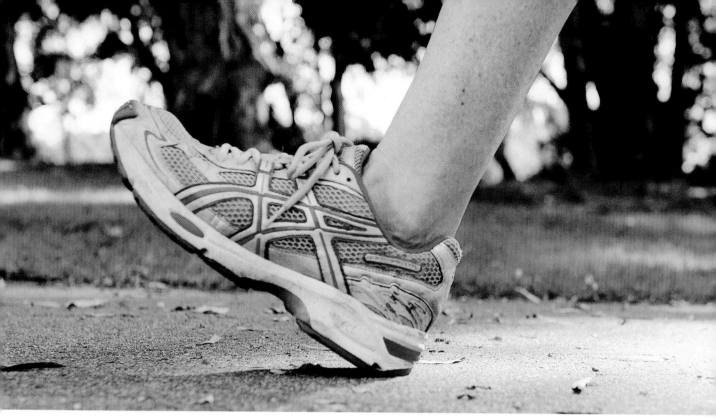

The heel strike is like putting your foot on the brakes—and, not surprisingly, that's exactly what it looks like. This wastes energy, wears out your brakes, and slows your forward momentum.

STUDIES SAY: SHOES = INJURIES; BARE FEET = 50 PERCENT LESS SHOCK—OR MORE

"Rampant" is not too harsh a word to describe the incidence of running injuries. The London-based *Sports Injury Bulletin* reports that 60 to 65 percent of all runners are injured each year, an estimate that is routinely accepted in the running community. As a couple of important studies show, however, it doesn't have to be that way.

A 2003 study led by esteemed South African running researcher Dr. Timothy Noakes, author of *Lore of Running*, a 930-page tome regarded by some as the bible of running, shocked many when it claimed that the heel strike of shod runners transmitted up to 50 percent more shock to the knee than a forefoot landing in or out of shoes. And a study in the December 2009 issue of *PM&R* reported that running in shoes can put more stress on the knee, hip, and ankle joints than running barefoot, and was even harder on the knees than walking in high heels.

First, let's discuss the landmark *PM&R* study. In the article titled "The Effect of Running Shoes on Lower Extremity Joint Torques," a group of authors led by Dr. D. Casey Kerrigan, of JKM Technologies in Charlottesville, Virginia, used detailed motion analysis to observe the form of sixty-eight healthy young adult runners (thirty-one male, thirty-seven female, all averaging over 15 miles [24 km] per week) while they ran alternately barefoot and in shoes. After the runners had warmed up and were feeling comfortable, the camera started recording data points.

The findings were eye-opening, revealing "substantial biomechanical changes," according to Kerrigan. That included "disproportionately large increases" in joint torques at the hip, knee, and ankle with running in shoes compared with running barefoot. When shod, the runners showed an average 54 percent increase in the hip internal rotation torque, a 36 percent increase in knee flexion torque, and a 38 percent increase in knee varus torque when compared with running barefoot.

The researchers concluded that the typical construction of modern-day running shoes provides good support and protection of the foot itself, but also leads to increased stress on each of the three lower extremity joints. These increases are likely caused in large part by an elevated heel and increased material under the medial arch, common characteristics of modern running shoes. They did not test minimalist shoes, which lack these elements, but recommended that shoemakers head more in that direction. "Reducing joint torques with footwear completely to that of barefoot running, while providing meaningful footwear functions, especially compliance, should be the goal of new footwear designs," says Kerrigan.

This study measured "torque"—unnatural lateral pulling on the joint—which may contribute to the eventual destruction of cartilage. Six years earlier, a study led by Dr. Noakes and his University of Cape Town colleague Dr. Regan Arendse rocked the barefoot running world when it measured the other great destroyer of cartilage—impact—and found that running barefoot could save your knees.

In the study, called "Reduced Eccentric Loading of the Knee with the Pose Running Method" and published in the February 2004 issue of *Medicine and Science in Sports and Exercise*, twenty "natural" heel-to-toe recreational runners, male and female, alternately ran in shoes on a treadmill with electrodes attached to their knees. They ran three different ways: first, with their regular heel-to-toe landing pattern; second with a mid-foot landing; and finally with a new style they'd been trained in for five days called the Pose Method, a technique invented by Russian sports scientist Nicholas Romanov that employs a ball-of-the-foot and bent-knee landing like that of barefoot running. In fact, as Noakes told my cowriter Roy in an interview that ran in a lengthy story about Pose that he wrote for the October 2004 issue of *Runner's World*, he viewed the Pose Method to be effectively identical with running barefoot, except that the technique was *more automatic in the latter*. When the subjects were evaluated in barefoot runs, which they hadn't practiced, Noakes found no conventional heel-toe landings, saying, "Runners protect the heel during barefoot running."

After clinical gait analysis was performed for each running style, the team concluded that Pose (barefoot) running "is characterized by a shorter stride length, lower vertical impact forces, a greater knee flexion in preparation for and at initial contact, less eccentric work at the knee, and more eccentric work at the ankle compared with mid-foot and heel-toe running."

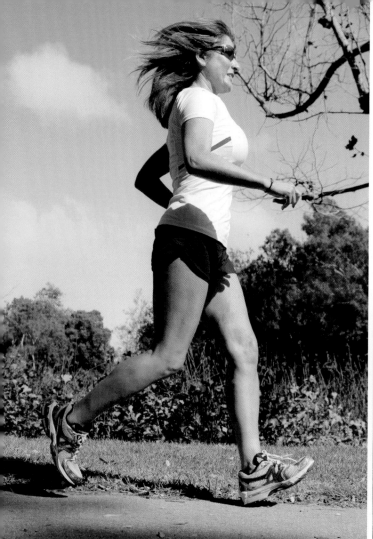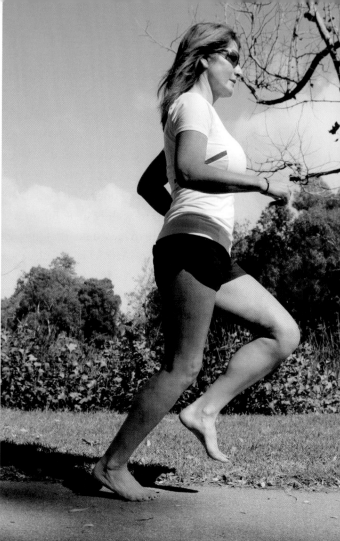

There is excessive up and down bouncing with a heel strike (left), while running correctly with a better foot landing springs you forward (right).

"I was quite surprised at the magnitude of the change to impact," Noakes told Roy. "The average reduction in forces was more than 30 percent, some as high as 50 percent. We have seen nothing else that does this—not shoes, no matter how padded."

Impact reduction as high as 50 percent! That's in italics, to make sure you don't miss it. Fifty percent is huge.

Now, for the first time, we had hard numbers to show that the heel strike, made possible by shoe cushioning and painfully impossible for any normal person to do while running barefoot, was not merely a "normal" landing that was benignly performed by 80 percent of all runners. It was not benign; it was a high-impact hammer that pounds the knee joint and eventually wrecks it.

"My opinion: Romanov really does have something," Noakes said. "I think the Pose and barefoot running are advantageous in preventing injuries, which is important since we know that 60 percent of runners get injured every year. It is highly probable that the Pose and barefoot running would translate to less injuries."

NO IMPACT AT ALL FOR LONG-TIME BAREFOOTERS?

Noakes's findings and conclusion were validated and taken a big step further in research by Dr. Lieberman that was published in the magazine *Nature* in January 2010. Conducted between 2005 and 2009 with barefooters such as my friend Preston Curtis (see more on him in Chapter 10), it was the first to scientifically explain the physics of barefooting by looking at the way that "habitual" (long-term) barefoot runners actually ran, rather than testing shod runners who briefly took their shoes off for testing. Using a high-speed 500-frames-per-second video camera to record subjects running on a sophisticated 25-meter trackway with a built-in force platform that yielded precise measurements of impact and loading, Lieberman discovered something that initially surprised him and finally explained why barefoot running is comfortable and quite safe for joints even on hard modern surfaces such as asphalt.

Importantly, his numbers basically agreed with Noakes's, indicating that the forefoot landing of a barefoot runner delivers less than half the loading of a shod runner's heel strike. Surprisingly, however, he also found that barefooting not only generates far lower collision forces (technically, a rapid and high rate of loading) than a heel strike, but actually had no measurable collision forces at all.

This lack of collision—the sudden, jolting "impact transient" that can make a barefoot heel strike so painful—provides a strong validation of how barefoot running works. A good way to understand it is through an analogy to a plane coming in for a landing. "Think about it: If the pilot brings the airplane in at the proper gradual angle, there literally is no discernable shock to the passengers at touch-down," Lieberman says. "But if she comes in at too steep an angle, the passengers get bumped/jostled at the moment of impact and the airline customer service center gets flooded with complaints. I am sure we can all agree that any collision is worth avoiding." If you need another example, look at the difference between being handed, say, a 10-pound (4.5 kg) weight and having the same 10-pound (4.5 kg) weight dropped on your head. The first is no problem; the second puts you in the hospital.

That difference between a smooth landing and a jarring one is due to the angle and the abruptness. An iron bar that is dropped straight onto the ground with a dead stop has a much bigger impact than that same bar hitting the earth at a 45-degree angle. That's because the percentage of the bar that comes to a dead stop at the moment of collision (the "effective mass" of the object) is much less at a low angle; actually, just the part of the angled bar initially touching the ground stops at that instant because most of the bar is still falling down. The same principle applies to a bare foot landing at a shallow angle on its forefoot. "With a stiff, vertical descent, like in a heel strike, it feels like you're being hit by a sledgehammer every time you land," says Lieberman.

"Technically, a steep-angle landing with a stiff ankle causes an instant and huge exchange of momentum. That hurts," he says. "But a shallow-angle landing, like barefooters tend to do while touching-down on their forefoot or sometimes their midfoot, greatly lessens that exchange." Experienced barefooters are so airplane-smooth that they have virtually no "instant" exchange of momentum. The inherent "compliance" (shock-absorbing characteristic) of the knee bend provides insurance and, as discussed in chapters 1 and 3, sets the foot in proper landing position.

Sports scientists have known since the 1970s that forefoot strikes and some midfoot strikes don't generate impact transients. But the runners in those studies wore shoes. "It's just that no one connected the dot between forefoot (and some midfoot) striking and barefoot running," he says.

Now, the bare truth is out. "If you land on the ball of your foot," says Lieberman, "you don't need any cushioning—because there is nothing (no hard landing) to cushion."

In the final analysis, that makes the cushioning in running shoes at best superfluous (when used with a forefoot landing), and at worst inefficient and potentially dangerous (when used with a heel strike). Cushioning doesn't cushion much more than bare feet do, certainly adds some instability, and doesn't remind you how important a gentle landing is with each and every step.

While it seems logical to assume that this gentle forefoot landing would be safer for joints and would lessen stress on all the structures of the leg, no scientific study has yet proved that heel strikes cause joint injury, says Lieberman. It's all anecdotal and speculative. He did warn, however, that there is a cost to the forefoot landing's lower exchange of momentum: "You need to have strong foot and calf muscles to control the foot and ankle as the heel comes down."

Noakes agrees, issuing a warning about calf pain that was incurred by some of his test Pose/barefooters. Romanov was not surprised, saying that the calf generally takes from two weeks to six months to adapt to the new biomechanics. A lifetime of wearing shoes condition the muscles, tendons, and skeleton to support an injury-causing gait, but changing it is still a shock to the system that requires a gradual readjustment period (see chapter 5 about B.R.E.S., the Barefoot Running Exuberance Syndrome).

"There will be unusual muscles that need to be strengthened [when you make the switch]," says Alex Romero, a Ph.D. candidate in evolutionary biology at Cal Tech who won the 2008 Duke City Marathon in Albuquerque, New Mexico, barefoot in 2:40 (see his profile in chapter 7). "Our calves are actually underused; it's like if you'd been in a wheelchair all your life and started walking. Of course you'd feel muscles you hadn't felt before.

"A nice thing is that those formerly underused muscles—including the muscles of your feet—naturally give you feedback," adds Romero. "The foot tells you when to speed up, when to run softer, when to cool it." And that's because the foot—when not locked into a shoe, that is—is one of the smartest organs in the body.

THE BARE FOOT IS A SUPERSENSORY ORGAN

Yes, the bare foot is an organ—of touch, movement, balance, and survival. In early childhood, toddlers use it as a sensory device to develop proprioception—the relative sense of where, how fast, and with how much effort the body is moving, and where its various parts are located in relation to each other. They learn how hard or soft to step down, push off, or twist. They learn not to land on the heel when running; the pain from one impact is a strong inducement not to do it again.

The foot is quite complex. The foot-ankle assembly has thirty-three joints, twenty-six bones (a pair of feet account for a quarter of the bones in the human body), and more than a hundred muscles, tendons, and ligaments. Those structures and the skin of the sole come loaded with nerve endings and a variety of touch receptors that allow us to feel and respond to pain, itch, tickle, cold, hot, smooth, rough, pressure, vibration, and proprioception as we run, walk, and jump. University of British Columbia researchers P. M. Kennedy and J. T. Inglis found that the sole has 104 mechanoreceptors, a type of receptor that responds to pressure or indentation ("Distribution and behavior of glabrous cutaneous receptors in the human foot sole," *Journal of Physiology*, 2002). The authors discovered that this includes a uniquely high percentage of fast-responding mechanoreceptors that "behave differently" than those on other parts of the body and "probably reflect the important role they play in standing balance and movement control." In fact, besides the inner ear, nothing is more important for balance than the sole; its mechanoreceptors are even more sensitive than those found on muscles and in the ankle joint.

When the feet are functioning perfectly, their mechanoreceptors and other sensors provide seamless feedback to your vision, brain, muscles, bones, and tendons. Without much thought, you instantly adjust your strength, speed, and flexibility to provide protection from the varied forces of running. Sensing a hard landing, for example, you'll reduce overall impact by bending your knees and hips. Afraid of stepping on a sharp twig? The foot, designed to feel pain long before it gets damaged, will minimize the acute discomfort by instantly spreading the load to less-sensitive or untouched areas on the plantar surface. The foot is designed to handle safe, fast movement on naturally-formed animal trails peppered with weathered stones; its sole constantly deforms to flow over these rocks, which may momentarily cause pain, but rarely pierce it and draw blood. The sole's skin, like a thick coat of smart paint, is specially designed to take abuse as it gathers information; with half the mechanoreceptor density of the palm and one-fourth that of the fingertips, the sole isn't as sensitive to touch or temperature, but its high concentration of "rapidly-activating" mechanoreceptors make it more responsive to pressure—which is logical, as it must bear the entire weight of the body and instantly convey instructions about shifting that weight to maintain balance.

Because the feet are so key to safe movement, problems arise upstream when biofeedback is limited and/or the feet get weak though lack of use or age. The big toe, in particular, plays a major role in directional control ability during forward/backward weight shifting. The three arches in each foot (the inner and outer longitudinal arches between the heel and the ball of the foot, plus the traverse arch between the balls of the foot) serve as the foundation of the entire body; that's a big problem for a population where most have lost some or all of their arch support, stressing the knees, hips, pelvis, and spine. Getting old magnifies all problems. Aging adults have significant plantar-surface insensitivity compared to young adults, and it gets worse with time; 70-year-old soles have half the sensitivity of 60-year-olds, according to a study by Stephen D. Perry at Canada's Wilfrid Laurier University (*Neuroscience Letters*, 2006). Weak, desensitized feet increase the risk of falling, putting the brain at risk and your survival on the line. That's why there is evidence that maintaining stability takes priority over foot protection if both are challenged simultaneously, according to Dr. Steven Robbins of McGill University in Montreal, long at the forefront of running shoe research.

In a sense, putting cushy running shoes between you and the earth instantly gives you an inkling of what it's like to have the balance (or imbalance) of an older person. That raises a couple of questions: Do shoes hasten the natural decline in the sensitivity of your mechanoreceptors? And conversely, can barefooting slow the decline down by "re-sensitizing" them—essentially keeping them young through activity? That hasn't been studied, although I believe it. "Use it or lose it" applies to most things about the body; why not your mechanoreceptors? Anecdotally, it seems like many who run barefoot rave about the new sensitivity they develop—and how strong their feet and toes get. That'll come in handy as you age, as studies do show that old folks with the best toe strength are the most stable and have the smallest number of falls.

THE ILLUSION OF SHOES

When you run in socks, shoes, inserts, midsoles, and outsoles, your body's proprioceptive system loses a lot of input. Yes, all that foam padding plus posts, bridges, and dual-density midsoles offer protection from the elements, but they may protect you too much. "They're deceiving the body," says Michael Warburton, a well-respected Australian physical therapist and 2:42 marathoner who writes a lot on barefooting (a link to his excellent paper, simply titled, "Barefoot Running," can be found at BarefootRunningStepbyStep.com). "This has been called 'the perceptual illusion' of running shoes," Warburton says. "We want protection from harmful objects, but scientific studies have not shown that cushioning and/or motion control stop injuries."

In fact, the opposite may be true. In a 1987 study, Robbins and Hanna found that chronic, running-related bone and connective-tissue injuries are rare in developing counties, like Haiti, with large barefooted populations, and that those injury rates were substantially higher in their shod populations. Back in the 1980s, Robbins was one of the first to suggest that the rash of overuse injuries was linked to running shoes—a theory supported by the 2009 study by Kerrigan, et al., cited previously.

What's the problem with footwear? "With shoes, your body switches off to a degree, and your reaction time decreases," says Warburton. Although the foot is a tough cookie built to handle abuse, somehow biomechanists and shoe marketers view it as an inherently fragile object needing protection. So, enclosed in its fabric, leather, and rubber straitjacket, the foot can't help but switch off.

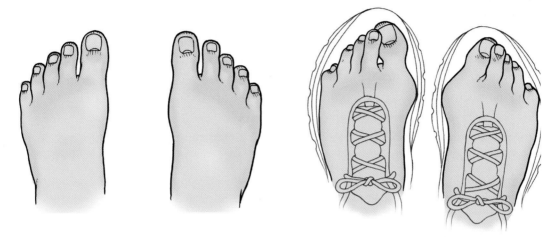

Free bare feet tend to have straighter toes that point forward (the direction we generally want to run). Shoes imprison feet, putting continuous pressure on the toes, deforming them, in some cases, like above, to extreme degrees, resulting in bunions—calcium deposits filling in the space in the gaps of the out-of-line joints.

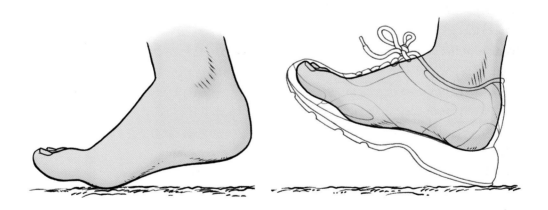

A bare foot in motion. The bent knee, encouraged by the desire for a gentler landing, changes the angle of the foot, resulting in a ball-of-foot first landing. Shoes provide a deceptively comfortable heel-first landing, while sending damaging shockwaves up the leg into the knees, hips, and back.

DUTCH TREAT

"IT JUST FEELS SO GOOD," SAYS HOLLAND'S FIRST BAREFOOTER
BY GEORGE "OERLOPER (PRIMEVAL RUNNER)" KERKHOVEN

In 2002, I didn't know Ken Bob. I didn't know anybody who ran barefoot, not in the Netherlands, not anywhere in the West. One day, without ever hearing anything about it, I just started running barefoot on my own.

I had an injury, Achilles tendonitis, so all I could do was sit on an exercise bike, just to do something for my health in place of running. Pedaling one afternoon, I suddenly heard a voice, like a thought in my head. It simply said, "Run barefoot."

So I made a pronouncement to everybody in that fitness room: I will start to run barefoot from now on, just to heal my tendonitis. And everybody declared me crazy. But I ignored that and started to run barefoot, little by little, step by step. Because I was still injured, I couldn't run much with that pain. But within a month, the injury was gone!

Yet there is far more to running barefoot than that.

I love it, especially the feeling in the feet. Being in touch with the various terrains gave me an almost voluptuous joy. And after eight years, that's what I still enjoy the most, the textures of all kind of ground forms. Most of all, I love to run in the woods, in nature. Only last year I started to run street races. That is okay, but I only did it to show people that it is possible to run without shoes. In the woods, hardly anyone sees me.

After a while back in 2002 I discovered the Yahoo! barefoot group and Ken Bob; I learned a lot from all of the forum members. And I also shared my own experiences.

After being the only barefoot runner here in the Netherlands for a few years, somehow people got inspired by my stories (without me knowing it!) and now we may have thirty barefoot runners here. And we even meet each other now and then during races or organized meetings. It's a lot of fun to share all the remarks one gets from shod people/runners and to share all the different experiences about barefoot running.

So while I am not sure whether barefoot running is better for you (like Dr. Lieberman says), I do know that, for me, it brings so much more pleasure to have better contact with nature. After all these years, I am still astonished almost every day that it is such a joy—which I couldn't say while running in shoes.

George Kerkhoven's website is www.oerlopen.nl ("primeval runner" in Dutch). Reach him at kerkhoven@yahoo.com.

What actually happens inside the shod prison? Instead of being the widest part of the foot, the toes are smushed together and can't splay out like they do barefooted. The heel can't roll normally because the foot is tipped forward and overstabilized by a tall, squared-off heel pad. The big toe, fixed in height with the other toes, can't dig into loose ground when it wants to, inhibiting its balance function. The little toe becomes a useless stub, losing its leading function when changing from supinating to pronating (rolling from outside to inside). The sole gets wimpy; calluses that should protect it from pointed little stones don't develop. Neither does lots of fatty tissue under the skin of the sole for extra cushioning. Less blood is circulated with each foot strike. Instead of dynamic arches that act as springs, they get flaccid and weak from lack of use, being draped over insole arch supports.

What exactly is going on here? Very simply, shoes make feet deaf and dumb, so they can't read the terrain and respond to it. Shoes with soft sole materials, like athletic shoes (including "minimalist" shoes), insulate the receptors on the sole from tactile information about surface position and orientation. For a stable equilibrium, that function now has to be provided by other, less-precise receptors of the foot and ankle muscles.

CUSHIONING THROWS YOU OFF-BALANCE

Next, the highly resilient rubber in shoe soles bounces too much, both up and down and side to side. This amplified impact often overwhelms the imprecise foot and ankle receptors, resulting in a destabilized runner who has lost his foot-position awareness.

Stability is also compromised because the shoe-wearing sole can no longer "flow"—that is, deform as it passes over a pebble in order to spread the load. The cushioning does the deforming, not the foot.

Ironically, more impact may result from more cushioning because, to regain balance, the pillowish pile encourages the foot to plow into the ground like a bull in a china shop. A study Robbins published in 1997 found that runners tend to land harder on soft surfaces to improve stability. He concluded that sports shoes are too soft and thick and recommended they be redesigned to protect the wearer. Most shoes, therefore, are the worst of both worlds: too bouncy, cushioned, and unresponsive. The result is a transformation from a precisely damped and responsive bare foot to an imprecisely underdamped, overcushioned, bouncy, and unresponsive shod foot that ratchets up instability and the risk of falling.

Bottom line: Shielded from the elements, the sensor-rich foot ends up weak and starving for stimuli (which, by the way, is usually feeble anyhow, given that the uniform man-made surfaces of today offer far less stimuli than nature). So is it any wonder that our foot position is often off and we end up with problems like plantar fasciitis (inflammation of the thick connective tissue and contiguous small muscles that help form and support the large arch between the heel and ball of the foot) that simply do not exist in less affluent societies? If our bare feet were once muscular, finely-tuned thoroughbreds, encased in shoes they are now sleepy, flabby cows.

THE "ANGRY PODIATRIST" PROVIDES
A PRO-SHOES COUNTERPOINT

Podiatrists have never been accused of being the glamour boys of the medical world. So when *Born to Run* author Christopher McDougall called Dr. Kevin Kirby the "angry podiatrist who pops up whenever natural-style running is discussed" on his blog in February 2010, the Sacramento foot doc and associate professor couldn't have been happier. "I think I like the new moniker," he crowed on the forum of www.podiatry-arena.com, to applause. "Maybe McDougall just doesn't like someone challenging all the myths he tries to promote in his book."

Kirby, a shod runner for forty years, had already been part of a two-page barefoot running discussion with me that month in the pages of *Runner's World*, and he was clearly establishing himself as the go-to guy for the anti-barefoot point of view.

"Barefooting has some good points," Kirby allowed. "I know more shoe weight makes you less metabolically efficient. I ran a 5:10 repeat on a grassy field in shoes and a 5:05 barefooted. So a little barefooting in moderation is fine; some drills are possibly beneficial. I agree that the tactile experience is nice.

"But the trouble is that in today's population centers, we have a lot more asphalt, concrete, glass, and nails than grassy fields. So I worry that barefoot running is going to produce injuries—puncture wounds, infections, and even lacerations of vital structures at the bottom of the foot.

"Also, consider that not everybody is 150 pounds (68 kg) anymore. As society gets heavier—average males are heading for 200 pounds (91 kg) now—putting more load on your feet is risky. A heavier person needs something to decrease the impact forces—cushioning, beefier, shock-absorbing soles. Either the shoes absorb the shock or the legs absorb it.

"It didn't take the caveman long to find out that the leather skin of an animal helped him walk more. Shoes have been part of civilization forever. I think we humans are smart enough to design an implement to let us do something natural like run. Barefooters and minimalist-shoe runners are getting injured. Metatarsal strains are going up. The bones bend more when you land on the forefoot. Google 'Vibram stress fractures' and you'll see eight or nine guys on different sites.

"Ultimately, what causes injuries is the same force over and over again. That's why you need to run on different surfaces in different shoes. Starting back in college, I'd rotate between three, Brooks, Asics, and Nike, and never use any two days in a row. I'm fifty-three, am a heel striker, run 20 miles (32 km) a week, have a marathon PR of 2:28 in 1980, and have no knee issues.

"One good effect of the barefoot trend will be more variety of shoes. Shoes were all thin-soled when I started running. Then the pendulum swung to thick soles. Now it's swinging back, and there'll be a wider selection at stores, so people can self-select.

"For a few people, barefooting works, but I think that there's more talk about barefooting than people actually doing it. It almost seems like there's a religion to the barefoot running thing, with a limited number of people trying to take the limited evidence and make more of it than it is. They don't mention that Zola Budd said she gets injured running barefoot, so now she runs in shoes."

Of course, Dr. Davis at the University of Delaware puts the blame squarely on shoes: "Our feet react like any other part of our body when you support them: They get weak," she says. "If you hurt your neck, you don't wear a neck brace for the rest of your life—but podiatrists put people in orthotics forever. I seldom recommend orthotics for runners anymore. When muscles don't have to work, they get weaker and more susceptible to injury. And as they make shoes beefier and beefier, injury rates are not declining.

"We have an epidemic of plantar fasciitis because we've taught the feet to be lazy," Dr. Davis continues. "To fix it, go barefoot—a Robbins study in 1986 showed that barefooting raised and strengthened the arch. It's like weight lifting for your feet. You need strong muscles in your feet."

When I visited Dr. Davis at her University of Delaware lab in the summer of 2010 and mentioned how I don't ever wear the most minimalist shoes, even Vibrams, she nodded and noted that anything you put between yourself and the ground changes things for the worse.

GET YOUR FEET BACK

There is a third pun we have derived from "Feetback" that we were saving for the end, and it comes in the form of a command: if you want to improve your running, chuck the shoes (at least occasionally) and *get your feet back*.

Get your feet back from Nike, Asics, New Balance, Etonic, Saucony, Brooks, and K-Swiss. Yes, take 'em back from the shoe companies. All your body parts are important for your body's proper function. Ceding your feet to these cushioned prisons and even to minimalist footwear like Vibrams not only makes them softer and dumber, but also has a ripple effect up the kinetic chain. We land harder and less precisely in shoes, resulting in lesser proprioception, degraded coordination, higher impact, and increased risk to connective tissue and joints.

Barrie Robbins-Pianka, the daughter of the late, great Charlie Robbins (see his profile in chapter 8), describes barefoot running as "feeling more in touch with the road, like a sports car versus a mushy sedan."

You definitely don't want to be a mushy sedan. So get your feet back!

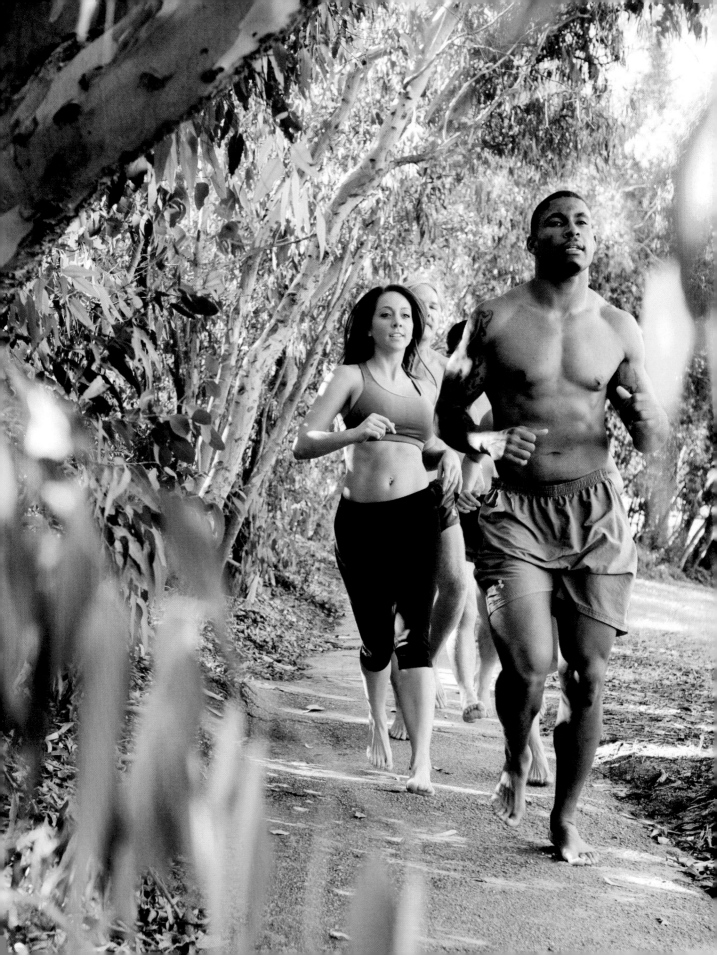

SECTION II:

BAREFOOT TECHNIQUE AND DRILLS

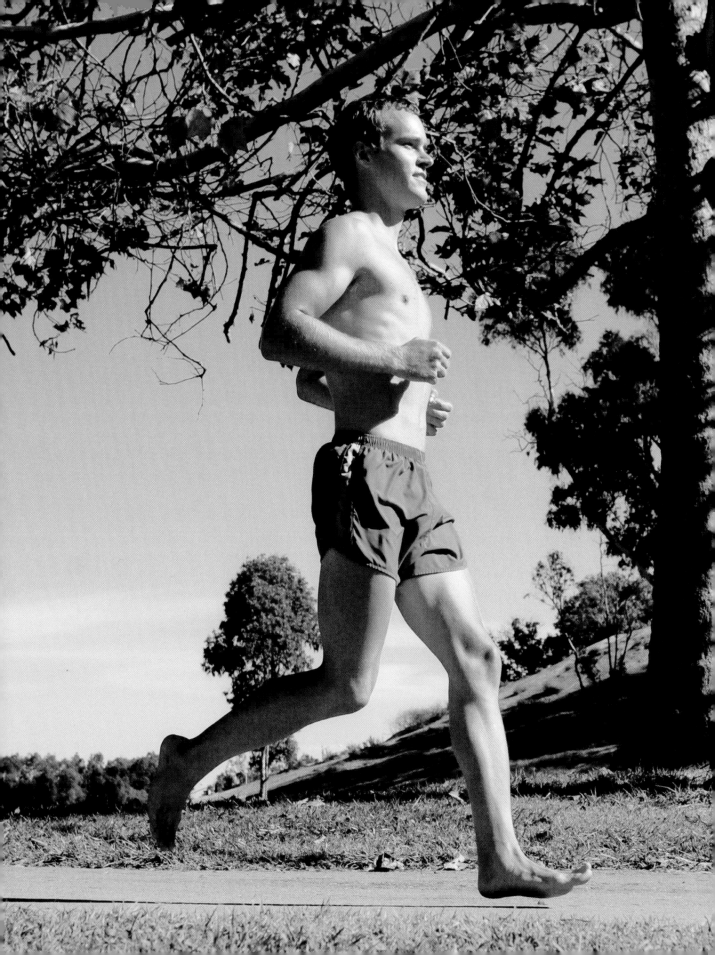

CHAPTER 3

THE BAREFOOT TECHNIQUE
FROM HEAD TO TOE

There's a lot more to running barefoot than the all-important knee bend and forefoot landing. For the safest, most efficient technique, you must start at the top and work down.

> **" I DON'T LIKE TO GENERALIZE BY SAYING THAT 'EVERYONE SHOULD RUN BAREFOOT.' SO I'LL JUST SAY THAT 'EVERYONE *WITH FEET*' WHO WANTS TO LEARN TO RUN THE WAY WE ARE DESIGNED TO RUN SHOULD RUN BAREFOOT. "**
>
> —KEN BOB-ISM #7

Over the years, my discussions and running experiences around the country have led me to look very closely at barefoot technique. Now, if that seems a little odd or oxymoronic—that there would actually be a "technique" to running barefoot when part of the attraction of it is that it is totally natural and therefore "technique-less"—keep in mind two things: Most of us spend our lives in shoes acquiring bad habits and weak feet (see chapter 2), and the caveman probably did not run regularly for fitness like we do, and certainly did not run on a hard, uniform surface such as concrete. There are major differences in the way people learn to run in shoes and those who learn running while barefoot. So we actually have to learn our natural gait, and then tweak it for the conditions of the modern world (i.e., learning to run even "softer" than our ancestors did).

My years of playing with my running and fixing various problems tell me this: For optimal safety and efficiency, for turning your body into a giant shock-absorbing spring that moves forward with little pounding and great exhilaration, there are some universal tenets of running barefoot technique.

Keep in mind that these are from the point of view of the runner (me) and are not those of an observer analyzing a video of someone else. Perception is inaccurate; we think we're copying others, but we often do something completely different. Also, most videos—especially those on the Internet—are so low quality that they show only a couple of frames of each step, which can't accurately capture a runner's movements in great detail. There's no way to see precisely what is happening; for example, most videos might miss the entire landing of the foot, let alone show which parts of the foot are landing in what order, a sequence of milliseconds. My first digital camera shot only 15 frames per second. I have one video from it in which my feet appear to never touch the ground.

By far, the biggest misconception I've seen is that people think running barefoot starts and ends with the bare foot—that proper barefoot technique merely involves taking off your shoes and landing on your forefoot. Some even claim we run "barefoot" in shoes! Even my friend Dr. Irene Davis, director of Harvard Medical School's Spaulding National Running Center, was surprised at how much I bent my knees while running on the treadmill in her lab.

I wasn't surprised. It's easy to oversimplify barefoot running form. But over years and years of races and clinics, it has become clear to me that safe, fun, fast barefoot running actually requires adopting a surprisingly complex technique that, although completely natural, is no longer intuitive to people who've spent a lifetime in shoes. (Those who never wore shoes throughout childhood, especially when taking their first steps, often take running technique for granted, because they perfected their technique without consciously thinking about it, simply by listening to their soles and avoiding techniques that cause pain and eventually injury.) Done right, running (and walking) barefoot involves everything from head to toe. After I finally understood this myself, it took me a few more years to figure out how to articulate it clearly and accurately (which is why I was not ready to publish a book ten years ago, as I alluded to in the introduction).

In fact, it took a grand, coast-to-coast, west-to-east, north-to-south and back loop around the United States in the summer of 2010 for it to all come together for me. What I learned is that the technique of running barefoot, while very dependent on being able to feel the bare soles' precise interaction with the ground, is best learned from the top of the head to the bottom of the toes, in that order. Ultimately, when everything above our feet is moving correctly, the feet should be very pleased. If the feet are unhappy, if we feel excessive pounding or abrasion on our soles, it is an indication that we're doing something wrong somewhere above them.

BAREFOOT KEN BOB'S 2010 GRAND TOUR

On September 7, 2010, I received a CD-ROM from Dr. Daniel Lieberman, the esteemed Harvard researcher known as "The Barefoot Professor," whom I'd spent an entertaining afternoon with earlier that summer, during the grand tour. It contained a video of me running on his treadmill shot at 500 frames per second, slowed down to show the smallest detail of my foot landing.

> *Dear Ken Bob,*
> *Here is the synchronized video of you running on the treadmill in the lab along with the force traces (the graph). As you can see, you have a very elegant, perfect forefoot strike—your foot almost looks like a plane coming in for a landing—and of course, no discernable impact transient. But, you already knew that!*
> *You are welcome to use the video as you wish (e.g., put it on your website, whatever).*
>
> *All the very best,*
> *Dan*
>
> *p.s. You'll be happy to know that we now have a large number of Harvard students barefootin' along the Charles.*
>
> *p.p.s. Say hi to Cathy and Herman for me.*

Cool! I'd never heard that one before—my foot is like *a plane coming in for a landing*. It's so visually accurate—at least up to the point where the wheels start rolling on the runway. I'm going to use it in my clinics from now on! A smooth, almost seamless airplanelike landing is not only a great description of what I hope to convey in this key "technique" chapter, but it also reminds me of the joy I get from traveling. I "met" Dr. Lieberman via email and phone years ago, but had never hung out with him in person until my grand cross-country road trip in the summer of 2010.

I love the excitement of the road. It's very stressful at times, but no matter where I've traveled in the running world over the past dozen years—from the starting line of the Boston Marathon to giving a running barefoot presentation at the Lincoln (Nebraska) Marathon or to Connecticut to present the first-ever Running Barefoot Hall of Fame award to the family of Charlie Robbins for his sixty-eight years of mostly barefoot running and racing (see a profile of him in chapter 8)—it's always great fun to race, swap ideas with locals, and get a sense of what other people (shod and unshod) think about running barefoot. The summer of 2010, which I'll

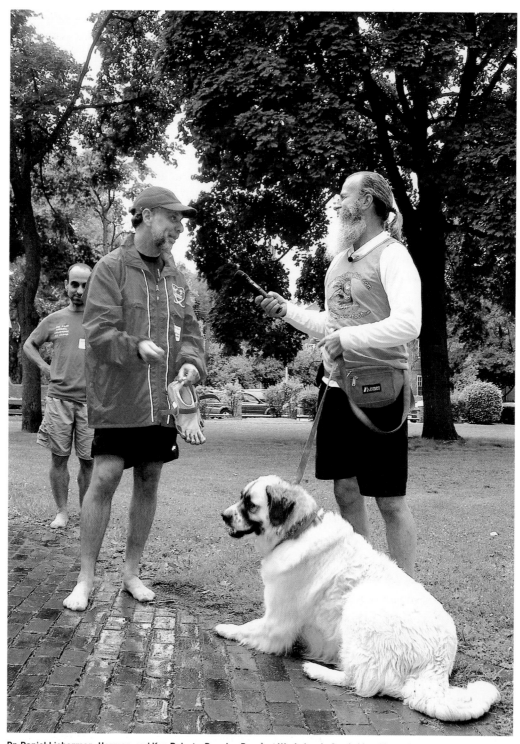

Dr. Daniel Lieberman, Herman, and Ken Bob at a Running Barefoot Workshop in Cambridge, Massachusetts

describe in more detail shortly, was a blockbuster in this regard—a wild 11,000-mile (176,000 km) adventure of barefooting, travel, and learning that included the good Dr. Lieberman and dozens of other thought-provoking people and activities.

We called our great adventure "Barefoot Ken Bob's Running Barefoot 2010 Summer Tour"—me, my wife Cathy, and our dog Herman (the most beautiful, though occasionally psychotic, 90-pound Great Pyrenees/Golden Retriever mix in the world) on the road for two solid months. Along an immense figure eight that started in a workshop in Phoenix, Arizona, on May 17 and ended in a clinic in St. George, Utah, two months later, we drove south to New Orleans, east to New York City, Boston, and Maine, and circumnavigated Lake Michigan as far north as the shores of Lake Superior in Michigan's upper peninsula (the "U.P." to Michiganders). Often staying in the homes of gracious barefoot-runner hosts and accepting donated meals and gas money, we scheduled and held thirty-four workshops in thirty-four cities and twenty-two states. We met in parks and parking lots, rain or shine, in all kinds of structures (once packing a dozen people inside a cottage in Louisiana), and hopefully leaving lots of people with some good advice.

I've been doing presentations, get-togethers, and informal clinics at home and on the road for years, using long weekends and parts of my two summer months off work to spread the word about barefoot running. But my 2010 Summer Tour was my most ambitious trip yet. Although it was rather stressful, often requiring long daily drives to reach consecutively scheduled clinics, I'm very glad we did this. I got to meet prominent author and motivator Lisa Ann McCall, inventor of the McCall Method, who told me she was convinced that barefooting was the way to go after her brother Owen told her about my website years ago; I went for a hike and held a Running Barefoot Workshop with Chris McDougall, now a bona fide international celebrity due to the success of *Born to Run*; ran on a treadmill with infrared sensors attached to various body parts for Irene Davis at her University of Delaware lab; spent some time on a treadmill with accelerometers attached to my head at Harvard with Dr. Lieberman; and even got to visit family and friends in Michigan and Colorado.

In a sign of the times, I got to witness something during the clinics that had rarely happened before: for the first time in two decades of running barefoot in hundreds of races, and talking and writing profusely about running barefoot, people were actually listening to me, almost spellbound, as if they believed I knew what I was talking about!

That may be because running barefoot is red-hot. While growing exponentially for years (from one website—mine—in 1997 to dozens today, and from a few hits a day on my site to a high of 9,280 on August 19, 2010), it exploded like a supernova with the publication of *Born to Run* in May 2009. For hundreds of thousands of people, running barefoot was suddenly real— not a quirky footnote for a hardy (or foolhardy) few, but a legitimate alternative that could bring fun, fast, injury-free running to everyone, even those for whom running had become a chore riddled with chronic pain.

RAPT WITH ATTENTION

The barefoot cat was out of the bag. People finally realized that running barefoot could save and revive their running careers, and even improve healthy ones. That's why hardly anyone at my workshops—from the fifty-plus attendees in New York City's Central Park, to the forty-eight or forty-nine standing patiently in the rain in Cambridge, Massachusetts, to the four in a couple of small towns such as Camden, Maine, and my hometown near Traverse City, Michigan (which included my parents, sister, and brother-in-law)—talked much. In fact, they were absolutely silent when I explained and demonstrated these techniques at my workshops.

That may be because they were no longer just curious about my ability to run barefoot; they wanted some real instruction about how to run barefoot themselves. Many had tried running barefoot, or "barefoot" in minimalist shoes, hoping that changing their foot strike alone (the focus of many recent articles about running barefoot) would be enough to overcome their running injuries, only to suffer new injuries. So they were listening intently to my every word.

That even applied to my friend Jason Robillard, author of the *Barefoot Running Book* and founder of the Barefoot Running University, who hosted a workshop I did in Grand Rapids, Michigan. Unlike a previous workshop host—a coach using similar techniques who kept interrupting me to show some of his drills, reexplain my technique in his words, and, of course, let people know about his own running clinics at his store—Jason didn't say a word. When I asked why, he answered simply, "Because I was interested in what you were saying."

My workshops are free for a reason: I'd never paid a dime to learn how to run barefoot; my sensitive soles have been my teacher for nearly fifty-five years. I can understand the logic of professional coaches charging hundreds of dollars to teach people how to run as if they were barefoot; once you start charging money, then you have to charge a LOT of money, because your disciples are now customers, and as such they expect a professional and polished curriculum, syllabus, insurance coverage, professional support team, and personal instruction, not to mention the added expense of permits to conduct business in a park, or rental of private locations, and so on.

MINISTRY OF SAFETY

But this is my "ministry," not a career—my giving back to the people. Many of my friends volunteer at aid stations in races. I try to help people learn how to run more safely.

I don't use the word *safety* lightly. The main reason I think free workshops are important is because of the epidemic of injuries I'm seeing from people starting out with bad technique, especially if they're trying to run "barefoot" in minimalist footwear. Coaching shouldn't be limited to people who can afford it. My goal is to send you home with your own two coaches, your bare soles, who will accompany you on every barefoot run and let you know, emphatically with every step, when you aren't running correctly.

And finally, because my workshops are free, I don't need to stress out about people complaining they didn't get their money's worth.

Well, apparently they did get their money's worth. Those who could afford it, and felt the workshops were worthwhile, donated enough to cover nearly all of our travel expenses.

Challenged to raise my game by the big turnouts, I refined my approach to explaining proper running and walking barefoot technique so that, most important, it made great sense to me. That seemed to resonate with the attendees.

Instead of starting with the bent knees (which nonetheless is my number-one running barefoot rule), or starting with the more-complex-than-you-think foot landing (which most people focus on), I played around with the order of the various elements of the technique. That's how I discovered that it's best to start from the top and work our way down—the same order I'd been toying with for years on my "How to Run" page at The Running Barefoot website.

Here's why: Every change made above the feet affects how the feet land. Here's an example of the problem: When people focus on how the foot should land, they try to impose a forefoot landing without changing their overall running technique. But to land correctly, you actually first have to move up the body and relax your calves, which will then alter the way the foot lands. Often, correcting one thing is impossible until we move up the rest of the body. Each change above the previous lower body part affects the foot landing. Thus, starting at the top with the head, then working our way down step by step, getting the upper body, arms, hips, legs, and so forth to do what they should be doing, means the feet will naturally land correctly and comfortably.

Ultimately, it comes down to this: rather than trying to force a certain foot landing, we should let our feet land and try to feel whether they are landing comfortably without strain or tension. Instead of trying to change only our foot landing (usually by incorrectly tensing up our feet and calves, resulting in foot and calf pain), we should adjust how the rest of our body is moving. Finally, when everything else is working correctly, our feet will naturally be landing gently and gracefully.

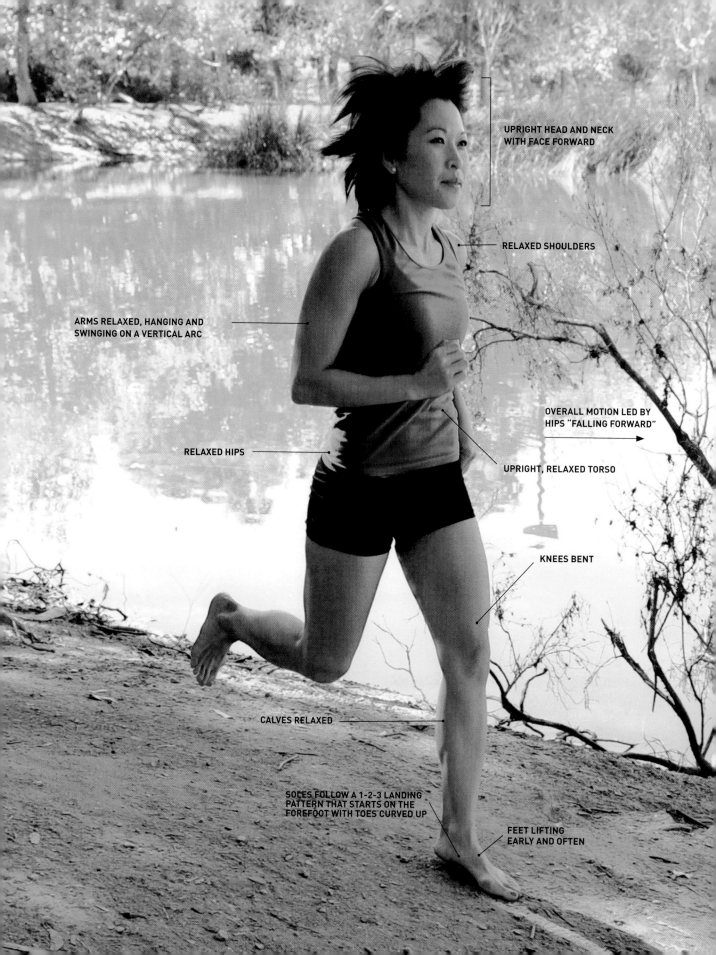

UPRIGHT HEAD AND NECK
WITH FACE FORWARD

RELAXED SHOULDERS

ARMS RELAXED, HANGING AND
SWINGING ON A VERTICAL ARC

OVERALL MOTION LED BY
HIPS "FALLING FORWARD"

RELAXED HIPS

UPRIGHT, RELAXED TORSO

KNEES BENT

CALVES RELAXED

SOLES FOLLOW A 1-2-3 LANDING
PATTERN THAT STARTS ON THE
FOREFOOT WITH TOES CURVED UP

FEET LIFTING
EARLY AND OFTEN

Of course, the key to all this is starting out barefoot, preferably on a surface that will provide adequate feedback. So rather than pussyfooting around on grass or soft sand, or in any kind of footwear (which makes bad technique deceptively comfortable), we would start on the roughest gravel I could find—just standing at first, then lifting our bare feet one at a time, adjusting our body position or movements, while listening to our soles, and figuring out how to best distribute our weight evenly across as much of the surface of our soles as possible. (For gravel-running drills, see chapter 4.)

You'll see below that my ten-step "Head-to-Toe" Guide to Basic Running Barefoot Technique involves the whole body in supporting the key points that you may already know about—the bent knee and the forefoot landing. Naturally, each individual should continue to tweak this form to suit his or her own physiological quirks and capabilities (which will be constantly changing based on how we adapt, grow, age, run on different terrain, and feel that day), but most of it should make sense if you think about it. Changes in running technique will likely feel awkward at first, but they should not be painful.

Steps 1 through 9 can be practiced while standing in place. We'll save moving forward until after we have practiced the first nine steps.

THE HEAD-TO-TOE GUIDE IN BRIEF

I address each step in greater detail below; this is a summary of the technique.

1 **HEAD, NECK, AND FACE:**
Keep them upright, with face forward (not down), to maintain efficient body balance, breathing, and direction.

2 **TORSO:**
Keep it upright and relaxed for the same reasons.

3 **SHOULDERS:**
Keep them relaxed so they can rotate on a vertical axis, counterbalancing opposing hip rotation.

4 **ARMS:**
Relax your arms and let them swing quickly and vertically to serve two functions: encouraging fast leg cadence and reducing excessive torso sway.

5 HIPS:
Relax them and allow natural rotation on a vertical axis to keep the feet under the body's center of balance, so they land along a straight line in the direction you're running.

6 KNEES:
Bend the knee before landing, to lift the foot and turn the legs into shock-absorbing springs that reduce impact and aid propulsion.

7 CALVES:
Relax them to unleash their power. If you keep them tense and loaded all the time, they'll hurt and can't store and release their springlike energy, and eventually they may cause injury.

8 FEET:
Lift them early and often, without pushing the feet into the ground, and curve the toes up (so that they don't land first). Aim for a bicycling-inspired cadence of 180+ steps per minute in order to lessen impact and muscle stress and improve performance.

9 SOLES:
Think "1-2-3" and curve the toes. When the rest of the body is doing all of the above, the foot will correctly land gently by touching down first on the ball, immediately followed by the toes and heel. Don't run on your toes or land flat-footed. To the untrained eye (i.e., someone not shooting high-speed video like Dr. Lieberman) it may look as if the entire foot is landing flat at the same time, but it's not.

10 OVERALL BODY MOVEMENT:
Let the hips and torso lead the way. This should feel a bit like falling forward; you'll need to move the feet quickly under your hips to catch yourself, with each foot landing below—and not ahead of—your vertical body. (A foot-forward landing effectively puts on the brakes with each step, encourages a heel strike, and ratchets up shock and eventual damage to the knees and hips.)

The Head-to-Toe Technique is a lot to think about, but it is simpler to coordinate than it may appear (my fun drills in the next chapter will make it easier to remember). It'll get your muscles to cushion your landing, spare your joints from jarring and rattling, and set up a flowing, economical forward movement that utilizes your body's efficient, built-in "spring" propulsion system and forward momentum rather than the harsh inefficiency of a typical shod runner's long-striding, leaping/braking, push-off/toe-off/heel-strike technique. The ten steps, described in great detail below, can benefit you with or without shoes, although the technique *is* optimized precisely to your own body when coupled with the natural benefits of running barefoot.

THE HEAD-TO-TOE GUIDE IN DETAIL

1 **HEAD, NECK, AND FACE: KEEP THEM UPRIGHT, RELAXED, AND FACING FORWARD**
It's simple: you tend to go the direction you face. So face forward, not down. Besides, if we obsess with looking down at rocks and pebbles, we tense up and often react badly by trying to push up, away from the stones, which never works because it means pushing our sole down *into* the pointy surface. Not holding your head up or not facing forward will wreck your technique, throw off your balance, inhibit your breathing by restricting/compressing your windpipe and lungs, and make more work for your neck muscles.

Relax the throat; this makes for more efficient and quieter airflow—two reasons that I could occasionally overtake better runners than myself: they wouldn't hear me coming, and they were working far harder to breathe than necessary.

" FACE THE DIRECTION YOU WISH TO TRAVEL, OR YOU'RE LIKELY TO END UP SOMEPLACE ELSE. "
—BAREFOOT KEN BOB-ISM #55

Facing down detracts from your running and diverts your attention away from enjoying the beautiful scenery (one of the more important reasons to run). Of course, it's good to scan the ground ahead to avoid large obstacles, but try to do it by moving your eyes, not your head. Scan far enough ahead so that you aren't focused only on the ground just a few inches in front of your toes.

Keeping the head upright is also very important for keeping an upright posture and maintaining balance while running up and down hills. With our head down, our torsos tends to follow and slump over. Keeping the head vertical, therefore, makes it much simpler to follow the next tenet.

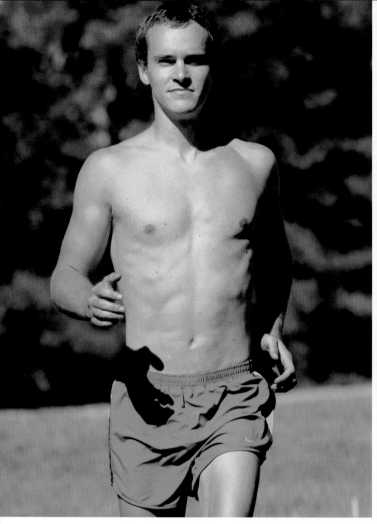

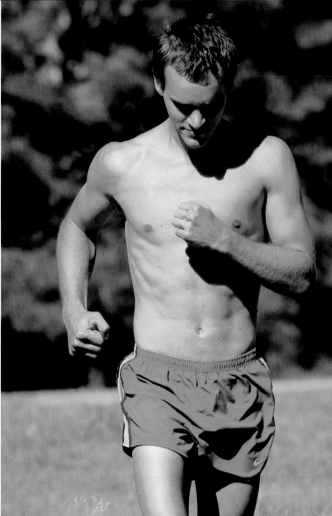

WHAT TO DO: Keep your head and neck upright, face forward, keep your torso upright and your shoulders relaxed, and relax your arms so they can swing freely. Keeping these things upright requires less work than running with your neck kinked or hunching over at the waist, allowing you to relax and enjoy your running even more.

WHAT NOT TO DO: Don't hunch your shoulders or torso, and don't face down—or you might end up there. Don't tense your arms and shoulders.

2 TORSO: KEEP IT UPRIGHT TO MAINTAIN BALANCE

Don't lean your full body forward or bend forward at the waist. The reason? Just as with an upright head, you maintain balance and easier breathing when your body is straight. Also, for the same reason that it takes an intricate series of cables to keep the Leaning Tower of Pisa from falling and none to hold up the Empire State Building, it requires very little effort to maintain an upright posture. When you're straight up, gravity does the work.

This is a point of difference between barefoot running and the Pose and ChiRunning methods, which both advocate a full-body lean (and are discussed in chapter 6). As you'll see when you reach step 10, I believe that you can get the impetus to "fall forward," as those two methods both call it, with a mere forward lean of the legs, while keeping the torso and hips vertical. Only lean your torso forward in two instances: when you want to accelerate, and when running into a headwind. Otherwise, keep the torso upright and balanced. In this position, all

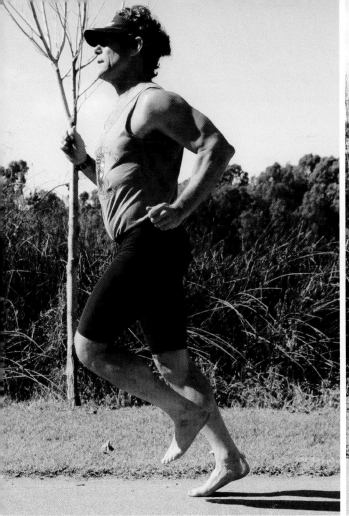 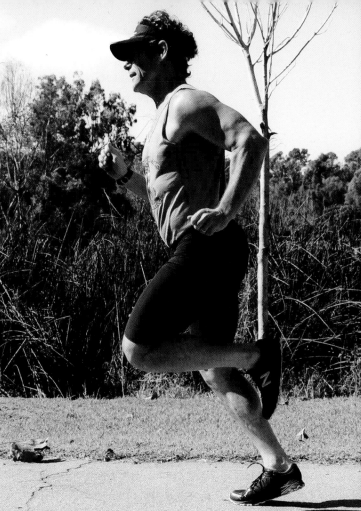

WHAT TO DO: Keep your torso upright and balanced. At a steady running pace (not acceleration, which involves a lean), it requires little effort to maintain an upright position. Imagine balancing a broomstick straight up in your palm.

WHAT NOT TO DO: Don't lean forward with your full body. This is like trying to run with a broomstick held at an angle, like the leaning tower of Pisa. Running at a steady pace with the body tilted forward requires extra work to keep from falling on your face.

forces pull equally in all directions so that there is no need to use muscular force to maintain an upright torso.

Incidentally, because there are other forces besides the Earth's gravity that affect balance, including acceleration and wind, I tend to use the more-inclusive term "center of balance," rather than "center of gravity." Gravity, of course, pulls straight down toward the center of the Earth; so if gravity were the only force at play, as it would be while standing still on a windless day, our torsos would be perfectly perpendicular to the ground. But any body—particularly a lovely one—can have a force that attracts us, and easily throw off our balance. Although a wind-buffeted torso may not be perfectly perpendicular to the ground, it should *feel* like it is vertical from a runner's point of view. Starting with a vertical torso and head as your base, and then factoring in all the other forces at play, you should be doing no extra work in the front, back, right, or left to maintain a balanced body.

3 SHOULDERS: STAY RELAXED, LOOSE, AND UNHUNCHED

In the first few miles of the 1999 San Diego Rock 'n' Roll Marathon, I saw the words "Relax Shoulders" printed on the back of a runner's T-shirt. Sure enough, mine weren't, so I relaxed them. Then five or ten minutes later, I saw "Relax Shoulders" on another runner's shirt. It was interesting how these folks kept appearing just when I needed a reminder to relax my shoulders.

Ten years later, after I held one of my Running Barefoot Workshops in San Diego with Coach Austin "Ozzie" Gontang, I told him the story at lunch. "That was our group," he said.

Tensing the shoulders is common while running, yet it doesn't do you a bit of good, said Ozzie. In fact, it creates excess tension and wrecks your form. That's why his group figured "Relax Shoulders" was the most concise and important message they could convey to runners during the marathon.

Shoulders seem to rise in reaction to stress. As soon as I get folks to stand, walk, or run on sharp gravel, shoulders suddenly rise up involuntarily, as if that would lighten them somehow. It actually does the opposite, effectively pushing our feet down into the sharp stones even harder. The lesson here? If you relax the shoulders, it's much easier to relax the feet so they can mold around sharp objects, instead of pushing into them.

Equally important, the shoulders need to be relaxed so they can rotate and counterbalance hip rotation. (We'll get to that in step 5.) And of course, tensing the shoulder wastes energy.

4 ARMS: RELAXED AND HANGING VERTICALLY

Because there is a direct relationship between arm and leg swing, some people say that we should pump our arms really hard to go fast to force the legs to go faster. But I see that as a lot of unnecessary work.

Pumping the arms in a short sprint may help, but most of our running should be easy and relaxed. I think the kind of work required for pumping the arms is just going to wear us out in the long run.

However, since the arms do counterbalance the legs, slow, rigid, or tense arms *can* slow your legs down. The arms can also be used to maintain balance on varied terrain, such as sharp switchbacks. Watch the tail of a cheetah as it chases its potential dinner. It's amazing how the tail seems to move erratically, but in reality it is helping maintain balance during sudden changes of direction.

Although I have personally not paid much attention to the mechanics of arm swing (besides relaxing them), my cowriter Roy has written quite a bit about the benefits of a vertical pendulum motion in which the hands do not laterally cross the chest, and presented it at one of my running clinics. One attendee, Mike Rose, fifty-seven, a retired naval officer and experienced barefoot runner from San Diego, reported an immediate gain in speed on his first long run after he learned to lift his toes on the landing (see step 9) and maintain a vertical arm swing, believing that it reduced his body sway and tracked his feet in a straighter line. So it may be worth experimenting with. I've found that on flat, consistent terrain, relaxed arms will be swinging vertically.

Whatever you do, don't force your arms into some sort of rigid, robotic path of motion, as that is contrary to listening and responding to varying conditions; keep them loose and relaxed. Whether you are carrying a camera, a phone, or a water bottle, or holding the dog's leash, or find yourself suddenly being chased by a lion or hauling down a switchback, keep your arms and shoulders loose and relaxed, with the arms swinging freely to react and counter-balance changes in direction.

5 HIPS: NATURAL ROTATION ALLOWS FEET TO TRACK IN A STRAIGHT LINE

The ultimate goal of running or walking is to move your body forward in a straight line, not side to side or up and down. So efficiency dictates that our feet touch down fluidly and naturally along a straight line under our center of balance, where one foot is momentarily supporting the weight of the entire body.

In order for us to stay upright when our feet do not follow a straight line, the body will move from side to side (to stay balanced over each foot in turn) or the feet need to push inward to counteract the downward pull of gravity on the tilted body. Neither of those options is all that conducive to forward motion. To help us run forward, we want our feet to land along a single line (visible or invisible) directly below our center of balance.

To allow the feet to land on, rather than straddle, this centerline, the hips must rotate. Keeping our hips relaxed and loose, not stiff, so they can twist on the vertical axis of the body like a swimmer in the water, is therefore essential. The hips will twist naturally if you relax and allow them to rotate, rather than forcing it. So heed one of my key mantras again: relax, relax, relax.

What happens if our hips are held rigid, or we try to track our feet along separate parallel lines? You do the antithesis of an efficient straight line: the John Wayne swagger—swaying from side to side while trying to maintain balance with each alternating step, along two separate lines.

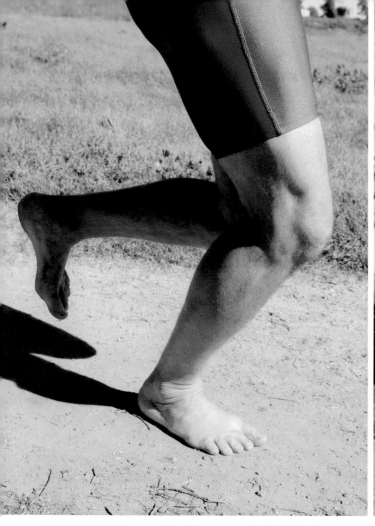 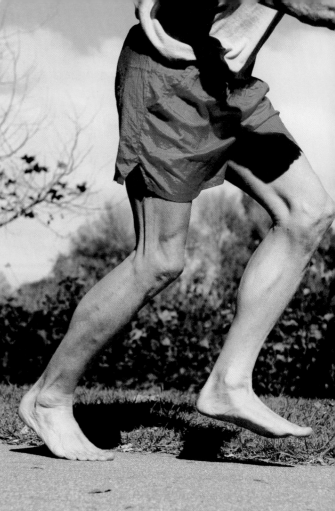

WHAT TO DO: The hips are under the torso on a vertical axis with the knees bent, the legs squatted, and the calves relaxed. This provides a natural spring under your body, which is fully utilized when gravity is pulling all of your torso down on the spring, loading it to help you spring forward on the next step.

WHAT NOT TO DO: Don't lean your torso forward, in front of your hips. When the shoulders are in front of the hips, your springs (in your legs) don't get fully loaded under your torso, making for a mushy spring and less returned energy to move you forward.

Note: Don't overdo the hip twist, which can result in our feet crossing the centerline and an even more ridiculous swaying (to the left over the right foot, and to the right over the left foot). That detracts from the ultimate goal of simply moving forward, and moving forward simply. However, while running in place, some side-to-side stepping may be unavoidable because one foot will be landing exactly where the other foot is/was. Just try to minimize it.

Keep in mind that hip sway and hip rotation are two different things. A good check on excessive movement is linear arm motion that keeps them from crossing the centerline of your body (see step 4).

6 KNEES: KEEPING THEM BENT TURNS LEGS INTO SPRINGS AND PROPERLY POSITIONS THE FOOT

I was a bit nervous about asking Chris McDougall and Irene Davis if they had learned anything new about running barefoot after attending my Running Barefoot Workshops in Pennsylvania and Delaware. After all, Davis is a clinical researcher at the University of Delaware, studying the injury-reducing benefits of running barefoot, and Chris McDougall is the author of what some have referred to as the "Bible" of running barefoot. What could my demonstration possibly teach them?

One important thing, as it turns out: They both noticed that I bend my knees a lot more than they expected.

Of course, that'll be no surprise to anyone who read chapter 1 of this book, where the knee bend is a major theme. The truth is, it's actually very uncomfortable to run barefoot without bent knees. The bent knee is an instinctive response to the pain of excess impact (at least in barefoot children) and makes good things happen. It reduces impact all over—and especially to the knee itself, as well as the heel—by pulling up the heel and preventing a heel-first strike. It aids propulsion, by turning the leg and the foot into "springs" that release and launch us forward as our body moves in front of our foot. Done right, bending our knees allows us to relax our calves and fully utilize the natural spring in our step.

Trouble is, it isn't always done right. Because it requires less effort to stand straight, we often need to remind ourselves that when we aren't simply standing, we should bend more. I've seen many runners, barefooters included, run with legs too straight. However, I've never seen people run with their knees bent too much!

Not bending enough can limit your ability to adapt on rougher and varied terrains. That applies to two of my close friends, Long Beach's Barefoot Todd, known as the Barefoot Coach, and Missouri's Barefoot Rick. Todd has completed more marathons barefoot than I have—at least one marathon each month since 2004—but he has difficulty dealing with rocky trails. (Read about our adventure at the 2007 Park City Marathon in chapter 9.) The problem: After running more than 200 marathons in shoes, like Todd has, it's really difficult to make big changes in the way you run.

Rick had also completed several marathons with shoes by the time he started barefooting. But unlike Todd, Rick was already feeling some knee pain. When he took off his shoes and began running barefoot in 2004, that pain diminished. But both men only made minimal changes in their running form—just enough to run barefoot mostly on fairly smooth roads and sidewalks.

I think that people who run on rough trails seem to have fewer knee problems than those who run similar mileage exclusively on roads. It's not because roads are harder, as I've run barefoot on plenty of trails covered in rocks or made of solid granite. The reason is the varied terrain; besides strengthening your feet and legs at various angles, it's very difficult to straighten your legs out ahead and overstride on uneven terrain.

The bent knee is the absolute key to changing a collision to a gentle landing and probably in preventing running injuries. The huge size and length of the thigh and calf muscles, combined with the knee hinge of the leg, make it our biggest spring, not just absorbing, but storing energy. As the body moves in front of the foot, the energy is released automatically (the spring unloads). A smaller but essential spring is the foot and arch. Both are activated by bending the knee, and are largely nullified when the leg is straightened like a pogo stick.

How huge is the leg spring? Bending at the knee from an erect standing position to a full crouch, is about 24 inches (61 cm). Of course, I rarely use all or even most of that. It turns out that we only compress that spring about 3 inches (7.5 cm)—but that 3 inches (7.5 cm) is a lot more cushioning than the typical running shoe heel's 1½ inches (3.8 cm), which is typically compressed only a fraction of that. (Imagine how much force it would take to compress the rubber in the soles of your shoes to even half of their thickness! With that sort of force, you still only get a spring of ¾ inch (1.9 cm), and the rubber sole won't matter; your leg would probably already be broken!) On the other hand, as I mentioned in chapter 1, while running down a very steep hill I once used the entire 24 inches (61 cm) of my shock absorbers. And it felt so wonderful that I laughed out loud.

As I mentioned earlier, that knee bend also has a critical effect on setting up a soft, shock-absorbing, well-balanced, ball-of-the-foot landing because it lifts and positions the heel off the ground. Speed is a nice side effect, too, because the more you bend your knee, which pulls up your heel, relaxes your calves, and aims you for the ball of your foot, the more spring you get out of the foot arch.

As a test, try to land on your heel with a bent knee. You'll find that it's almost impossible, even in shoes. If you can land heel first, then you're probably not bending your knees enough!

Bottom line: If you run with bent knees, you turn your legs into springs that absorb impact, limit your ability to heel strike, help you make the best use of the spring in your arches, and best of all, avoid pain. Most barefoot runners will instinctively land on the forefoot to avoid the pain of a heel strike. And if you're a coward like me, you try to avoid unnecessary pain.

BENT-KNEE DON'TS

DON'T RUN TALL, DON'T AVOID THE GRAVEL, AND DON'T LIFT THE KNEES

If you're feeling any pain, it may be that you're a bit light on the knee bending and running too "tall," like Barefoot Rick and Barefoot Todd, who perhaps didn't start out barefoot on harsh enough surfaces.

Beginner barefoot runners delay long-term learning when they start on "barefoot-friendly" surfaces. Nothing teaches us the importance of bending knees, relaxing calves, and not pushing off with the feet like a few minutes of standing on some sharp-edged gravel. Once we've mastered pokey gravel, everything else is dessert; having felt the importance of sinking into our springs, we get free insurance when we're on smoother terrain by continuing with that "extra" knee bend. It really comes back to listening to your body. Don't be so mentally tough that you shut out your body's cries for help.

Finally, don't confuse *bending* the knees with *lifting* the knees. You will lift the feet, not the knees. Why expend extra energy raising any body parts up higher than necessary? You really want to run low. So bend the knees, lift the *feet* enough to step over obstacles (it might feel like you're lifting your foot high, but that's only because your body is falling down toward your foot at the same time you are lifting), and imagine pushing your hips forward and *down*. That old myth of running "tall" usually is mistakenly translated to straight, rigid legs. They make for lousy shock absorption!

7 CALVES: RELAX THEM AND LET THE HEEL TOUCH THE GROUND

Stressed-out calves and Achilles tendons are legion among beginner barefoot runners, Pose and Chi runners, and especially minimalist-footwear runners. A big part of that is the return to natural biomechanics, which is less quad-centric and more calf-centric than shod-running biomechanics. But a bigger part of it, possibly, is that many people are doing it wrong. They're either ignoring the resulting pain or hoping the pain will pass when they eventually "toughen up."

Calf pain is not a rite of passage; it is mostly a wrong of technique. If you bend the knees more and learn to allow a heel touch after the ball-of-the-foot landing, you should not suffer much, if any, calf pain. Those who say, "Barefooters must suffer while strengthening their calves"—either through pain on the road or hitting the weight room—are wrong; I say just baby them. Not only will everything strengthen while you're learning how to run barefoot, but also learning to correctly run gently somewhat lessens the need for strength. Good form translates to running barefoot further and faster sooner.

Why is a nonstressed calf so important? I call it the "Spring Theory." We humans are supposed to bounce along in a forward motion like a spring. But the spring only works if you let your calves relax, then load them. If you keep them loaded/tense all the time, they can't unleash their energy.

But that isn't the worst of it. The main reason that I started holding my Running Barefoot Workshops, and why I'm writing this book, is because I'm sick and tired of hearing from all these folks jumping on the barefoot bandwagon and complaining—quite often to me—that they bought the "barefoot" shoes, and they tried running "barefoot" up on the balls of their feet like they thought was correct. And once they "worked through the resulting calf pain," their foot, or both feet, started hurting, really, really badly!

My response: of course your foot hurts. If it isn't "merely" severe tendonitis (enough to stop a runner for a few weeks), then it's probably a stress fracture (enough to stop a runner for a few months). Despite frequent claims by skeptics, these injuries are not limited to barefoot or minimalist footwear running. At least one similar case was reported to me by Dr. Lieberman: One of his research assistants ran through this type of foot pain while training in traditional running shoes for the New York Marathon. He managed to complete the marathon in 3:10 despite breaking a metatarsal bone at mile 13 of the marathon.

Runners do crazy things to get through injuries caused by running badly in shoes. One extreme case happened to a friend. To get through the Boston Marathon, she took new pain-killers (since taken off the market) for her knee injuries. Unfortunately, she spent race day in the hospital with internal bleeding—caused by the painkillers! If it hurts, it isn't because you need painkillers, or artificial cushioning. It's probably because you aren't using the springs you already have.

The coolest thing is, if you bend your knees enough, it's nearly impossible to tense your calves. If you tense your calves, it's nearly impossible to bend your knees. So, if your calves are tense, bend your knees more. And bending the knee is really the same as lifting the foot.

8 FEET: LIFT THEM *BEFORE* YOU LAND.

It's simple: lift the foot, and bend the knee. As you saw in step 6, this is not to be confused with *lift the knee*, a common mistake that is too much work for the hip flexor, not effective in positioning the foot for a forefoot landing, and simply too much work.

One thing I particularly like about lifting the feet early is that it helps stop bare feet from wearing out. I found that out when I started running more road miles in 1997. As I mentioned in chapter 1, that year I quickly upped my mileage from 20 to 30 miles (32 to 48 km) per week to 40 to 80 miles (64 to 128 km) per week within a few months while running with Buffalo Bill McDermott's group. My fitness went through the roof. I started doing marathons, not because I set a goal to complete another marathon, but because I was simply ready to.

❝ LIFTING OUR FEET WHILE RUNNING IS LIKE VOTING IN CHICAGO; DO IT EARLY AND OFTEN. ❞
—BAREFOOT KEN BOB-ISM #66

But there was a problem a couple of years later, when I began training for my first barefoot road marathon. A hard, smooth, man-made surface is no big deal to run on because bent knees make better springs than shoes or soft trails. But my soles were wearing out, getting thinner and more sensitive. Not from impact, but from the friction of the uniform surface of asphalt and concrete. Friction was not an issue on trails, whose varied surface makes every step different. There's no standard landing pattern or muscular pathway used on trails; your foot gets an all-round workout. Also, if your foot skids, scuffs, scrapes, twists, grinds, or spins on a trail (especially a rocky trail), you immediately feel friction. But you feel less feedback on a smooth or comfortable surface. So it's easy to get sloppy.

Fortunately, my hypersensitivity kicked in after a while. When the thinning skin under the balls of my feet made me even more sensitive than usual, I realized that I had to run even more gently. But how? I already knew that tensing up wouldn't help.

Answer: Lift my feet *before* I landed—*before* I touched the ground.

People look at me like I'm crazy when I say that, but the most efficient way to ensure a safe, soft landing when you run barefoot is to lift the foot before touchdown. And that's how I stopped wearing out my soles.

Stay with me for a bit—this is where running technique actually is rocket science, and a bit of relativity, too: Lifting the foot does not mean that it is literally heading in an upward direction relative to the ground; the body is still falling, so when we begin pulling a foot up toward our body (which is falling), we not only manage to reduce the foot's descent toward the ground, but we also reverse the foot's forward motion (unless we make the mistake of lifting our knees), so that the foot lands not only with less impact but also with no friction, skidding, or sliding. Remember that "airplane coming in for a landing" analogy Dr. Lieberman used to describe my touchdown? Well, if my foot had wheels, that description would be perfect.

Although the ground is stationary under us, it is actually moving backward and up relative to our body. Simply by beginning to "lift" our foot before it lands, we are getting the foot to match the speed and direction of the ground as the two initially touch, which is when there is the most potential for wear, besides liftoff (where many people mistakenly "push" instead of lifting or pulling the feet up). That means less pounding of joints and less damage to skin.

I like to use the analogy of the NASA shuttle (i.e., your foot) docking with the space station (the ground). As the space shuttle approaches the space station, it fires its retro-rockets *before* it crashes into the station as it "falls" toward the mother ship.

Lifting the foot, likewise, slows our foot's "docking" maneuver with Mother Earth. Academics such as Dr. Lieberman like to describe this as "reducing our effective mass." Being a romantic, I like to think of it as turning a potential thud into a delicate kiss.

If you need another analogy to picture the mechanics of a soft landing, think of some of the high-bar gymnastics events at the Olympics. Careening toward the mat after a full-twisting triple-flip dismount, the gymnasts lessen their impact and maintain enough control to "stick" the landing by *bending their knees* (which is the same thing as lifting their feet) before touchdown. Relieved to have made a safe landing, they then stand up straight and raise their arms to the roar of the crowd.

Pedal Power to 180+ Steps Per Minute

Lifting the foot early also results in a faster cadence (number of steps per minute).

Roy and I both strongly feel that all runners should bicycle; he's actually edited several magazines and authored a couple of books on the subject. Cycling is great cross-training, prevents us from running too much (something I often warn against) while maintaining aerobic fitness, speeds recovery from hard running workouts, is super fun, and is a great way to get around close to home. Despite some erroneous reports that I run to and from work every day, I actually commute by bicycle more often than by running. And maybe best of all for runners, bicycling can actually teach us to run better—barefoot or not. By that, I'm referring to the classic 180 steps-per-minute minimum cadence, which has benefits I didn't fully understand until I played with its cycling equivalent, 90 revolutions per minute (rpm).

I understood the important concept of gravity and acceleration, and how breaking our footfalls into shorter times could decrease impact. So fast cadence—*not to be confused with fast running*—made sense to me from the beginning.

Fast cadence isn't something to work up to gradually from a slow cadence. We can and should use a fast cadence from the very start, even while running in place. If anything, it would probably be better to start with a fast cadence and work down toward the minimum cadence as we get stronger. Hopefully, you will understand why in a moment.

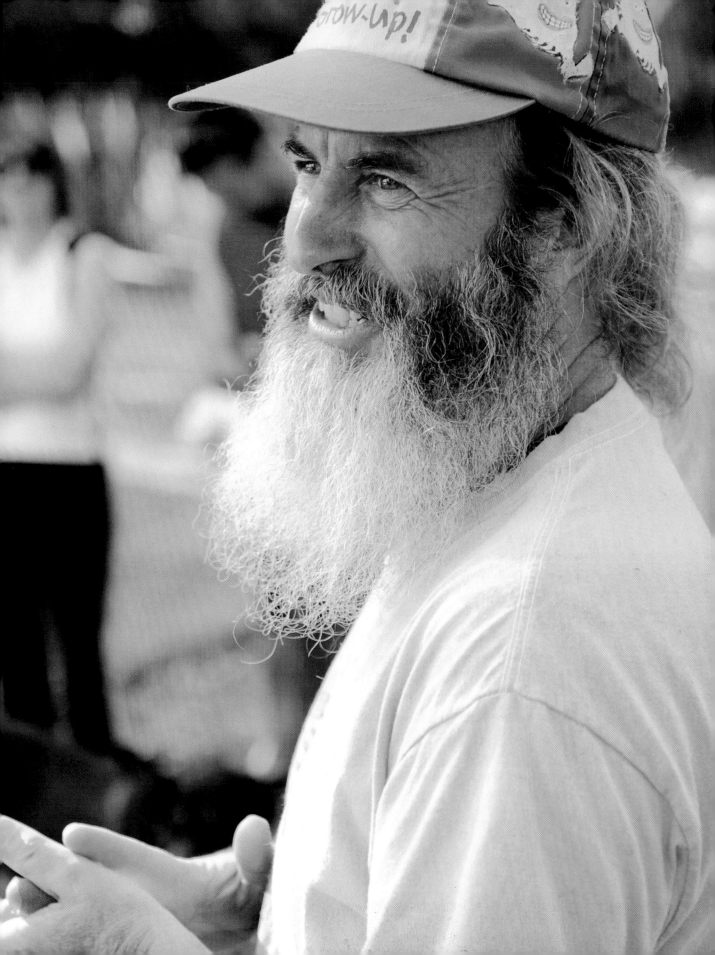

One of my many quirks led me to some experimentation that many may not relate to running. (No, it wasn't drugs!)

Some people like to follow the beeping of a metronome to keep their cadence, and there's nothing wrong with that (unless you're me). But it is important to remember that there is a tendency to emphasize the action on each beat, so use the beeper or flashing light as a cue to *lift* your foot, not push it down. Otherwise, you may end up "playing the drum" and pounding your foot into the ground on each beat.

Now, to my quirk: personally, I don't like being told what to do; maybe that's a big part of the reason, regarding shoes, I do *not* "just do it!" However, I love knowing what I am doing, which is why I prefer a cadence meter like on my bicycle. Rather than imposing a cadence on me, the meter merely reports my cadence. A cadence meter telling me my cadence is so much better than a beeping noise telling me to get in step with it. The meter gives me real information that doesn't impede my freedom to experiment with other cadences. If I want, I can run, literally, "to the beat of a different drummer."

Technically, a fast cadence reduces impact because it limits the time that gravity has to pull us back to earth, which, due to the physics of falling, is accelerating our body toward the earth (we've already slowed the foot's descent some, by lifting the foot early). Now we're going to work from the other end by spending less time falling!

Earth's gravity accelerates any body (us, balls, rocks, etc.) by 9.8 meters per second squared, which means each second we spend falling, we are accelerating *another* 9.8 meters per second. Spend twice as much time falling, and we are falling twice as fast, and therefore, landing with double the impact. If we could reduce the effect of gravity, we could land more gently, *obviously* decreasing the risk of injuries.

Actually, it's not obvious to a few "experts" who offhandedly dismiss the connection of impact with running injuries. They say that there hasn't been enough research proving a cause-and-effect relationship between slamming our foot with a stiff leg into the ground and damage to the joints above the foot! Millions of broken-down ex-runners might argue otherwise. But even if the impact-injury connection is never proven conclusively, it's clear that reducing impact will at least make running more comfortable. So why not do it? I can't think of a good reason not to. It was only because running barefoot was so comfortable for me that I started running marathons again. So let's do as King Arthur suggested in *Monty Python and the Holy Grail*: "run away" from the naysayers.

And a good way to do that is to decrease the time we take with each step.

More Steps Equal Less Work

Another great bonus of "spinning" at a faster cadence (while bicycling or running)—in addition to impact reduction and more comfort—is that it is less work. And since I hate work, I like spinning!

When we lift the foot, we still need to fight gravity, a resistance force that is trying to pull our foot down. Gravity is making us *work* to accelerate our foot upward. By breaking the lift into smaller chunks, it's less work—it's easier to lift the foot a short bit, quickly. My experiments monitoring the cadence meter on my bicycle confirmed my theory.

If we spin at anything less than 90 rpm, it becomes a strength/power workout. But if we downshift and spin at 100 rpm, we could easily go as fast; it's more aerobic, so we strain muscles less and can ride longer (and eventually faster, as Lance Armstrong, a famous high-revolution spinner, proved).

Running works the same way. A cadence above 180 steps per minute cuts the load and stress on each foot landing and, on the other side, the work required to lift your foot. With or without shoes, high cadence lessens impact.

To test my theory, on my next run, I started "pedaling my feet" as I was running. I began "lifting" them even before I hit the ground (that way, they don't "hit" the ground; they gently kiss it), then I sped it up. My feet were landing and lifting, matching the speed of the ground beneath my feet. Then I'd lift my trailing foot, carefully avoiding any push-off. It worked. (Though over the years, I've continued to find even more refinements, such as curving the toes up, which I'll detail in the 1-2-3 foot landing in step 9.)

My soles were happy and repaired themselves faster than I could wear them down. I ultimately completed my first barefoot road marathon in a torrential downpour, with no detectable wear to my soles.

Another way to look at it is that a cadence of 180 breaks up big work into smaller, digestible pieces. Think of trying to lift a 500-pound (227 kg) rock. Few can do that maybe once, and (if not seriously injured) they're still wasted for the rest of the day. But if you break that 500-pound (227 kg) weight into 1-pound (500 g) chunks, then most anyone can lift 1-pound (500 g) weights all day long, maybe a thousand times or more.

I've found that if I focus on a foot lift, not a foot push, it is easy to keep my cadence higher. Here's why: when you try to push your foot into the ground, you are actually launching or pushing your body up into the air, fighting against gravity's accelerating force (which is trying to pull you back down). The harder you push, the higher you launch your body, and the longer it takes for gravity to slow your ascent and to accelerate you back to the earth. You can't take quick steps while you're waiting for your body to crash back into the earth!

BE A "LANDER," NOT A "STRIKER": PRECISE LANGUAGE AND IMAGERY HELPS

Dr. Lieberman said to me, "You're a classic forefoot striker."

I replied, "No, I'm a forefoot *lander*."

He looked at me and smiled, the internationally renowned researcher from one of the world's most illustrious academic institutions, amused that a barefoot computer technician from Cal State Long Beach had the temerity to suggest he'd used incorrect terminology.

But language is important. I go more into this in the next chapter, but the gist of it is this: If you think "jogging," a common synonym for running, it's easy to accept bouncing, jarring, pounding, jogging sensations as normal, and perhaps even necessary, aspects of running. If you say foot "strike" or foot "striker," as Lieberman did, you'll have more of a tendency to slam your forefoot into the ground and try to push off harder.

I say we should ban "strike" and choose different imagery: gently *hover* the feet above the ground, then *lift* them off (one at a time, of course).

It's common practice to use imagery in our training, and it can be very important in determining the way we do things. Language is a way we communicate imagery to others, and to ourselves.

Try this experiment during a few steps of your next run: think of yourself "striking" the ground with your feet. Now try thinking of yourself "floating" slightly above the ground, pulling your feet up, and just "letting" your feet touch the ground. (Don't forget to bend your knees.) See what a difference it makes in how smoothly you run.

Using inappropriate terminology may be merely annoying in some cases, like calling the "accelerator" in an electric car the "gas" pedal. But when running barefoot or otherwise, inappropriate terminology can be hazardous to our health!

Runners must forget the words "toe-off" and "push-off." These terms are harsh, aggressive, and, worse, incorrect. Ban them forever, except when describing *undesirable* running technique, because they do not apply to the spring theory. If you land correctly, you don't need to make any conscious effort to push off, because you activate the springs the right way: relaxing them, allowing them to alternately return the energy.

To close out this important point, try this analogy: You won't drive any faster by pushing the needle of your speedometer, rather than the accelerator pedal. The speedometer, like our bare soles, is an indicator of the vehicle's proper function, not the cause of what we are doing.

I like indicators that let me know what I'm doing, rather than telling me what to do. So if you allow the foot to land correctly, it will, but only as a result of a cascade of proper form that begins far up the body.

Try this: throw a ball into the air, really hard; it takes a while for it to return to the earth. Now throw the ball up just a bit, and see how long you have to wait for it to return. We can throw the ball up into the air more frequently when we don't throw it very high.

Finally, there's yet another way to look at the difference. Rather than to trying to launch the entire mass of our huge body high up into the air, it's a lot easier, and quicker, to use the huge muscles of our legs and body to lift our tiny little foot. This results in much gentler landings, too.

So lifting the foot early and often reduces impact, makes our landing more gentle and smooth, and creates less abrasion. Ultimately, the question comes up, "How do we 'push' our body off the ground?" The short answer is, "We don't—at least, not with a conscious effort."

9 SOLES: MASTER THE "1-2-3 LANDING," CURVING UP THE TOES

Some minimalist-footwear runners (a.k.a. fake barefoot runners) often talk about the joy of running up on their "toes" (after all, they don't feel pain because they can't feel the gravel digging into their un-bare soles—but that is *not* an advantage). Soon, many of these fake barefooters complain of aching calves and sharp pains on the top of the feet. Other barefooters, both fake and real, think that they should always land flat-footed to spread the load. But they wonder how they can stop the constant blistering.

Both of these techniques cause pain—but not because they are wrong. Pain is the warning that these techniques are wrong because they can injure you in the long run!

Yes, we land on the balls of our feet first. But why work to stay there?

And yes, your toes and heels should touch the ground while running barefoot. Most of the time your foot is in contact with the ground, your weight should be distributed evenly across the whole foot to spread the load. But—and this is important—that contact happens in a sequence.

Confused? As I came to discover, years after I started running barefoot, the ideal barefoot landing is a bit more complicated than it might initially seem. I call it the "1-2-3 landing."

The 1-2-3 landing is easy. It's a three-step technique with three sequential landing points. And the cool thing is, if we are doing steps 1 through 8 right, the 1-2-3 landing happens naturally.

Remember, the soles of our feet have an orgy of nerve endings, so although the landing will happen when we are doing everything else correctly, paying attention to our landing is a great indicator of whether we are doing everything else correctly (or not).

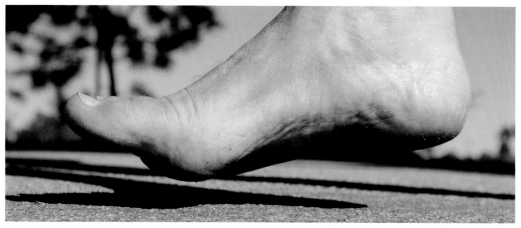

1: The ball of your foot touches first because your toes are curved up and your knee is bent. With the ball of foot landing first, the skin on your sole is already "spread" ready for a smooth landing.

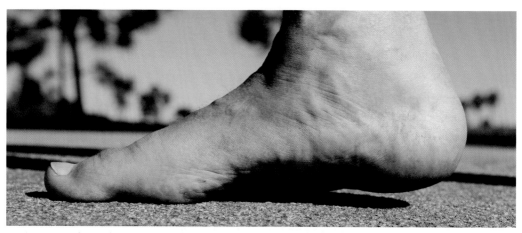

2: Next your toes (or heel) land. You already stretched the skin between your toes and the ball of your foot by gently curving the toes up before landing, so the toes don't slide forward on loading and there is no excess abrasion.

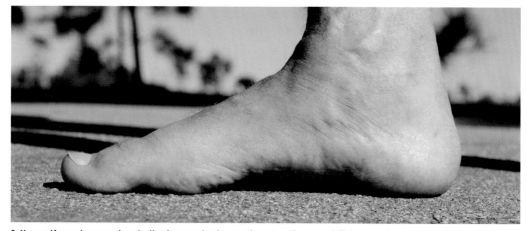

3: Your calf muscles are relaxed, allowing your heel to gently rest on the ground. This prevents strain over the length of your foot, calf, and all tendons that are tightened when you excessively strain your calves to stay up on your forefoot. Because the arch is already loaded (stretched out) before the heel comes down, the heel doesn't slide backwards across the ground away from the ball of your foot.

Overview of the 1-2-3 Landing

The bent knee puts your foot in a position to land on the forefoot, including the ball of the foot and the toes. The burly ball is designed to handle the impact; the tiny toes aren't. (Think about it: You break a fall with your palms, not with your fingers.)

For that reason, your instinct upon approaching the ground is to protect the toes from the initial impact by curving them up slightly. This also prevents them from getting scratched up by the "suction cup effect" (see "The Epiphany of the Curved-up Toes" on page 100). That's why the ball of the foot touches the ground before the toes do. Then, to spread the load over the entire sole, the rest of the foot lands milliseconds later.

To the human eye watching a video of the running barefoot technique, it might look like the entire foot comes down at once. But it's really a 1-2-3 landing—either ball-toes-heel or ball-heel-toes, depending on the terrain. After the ball lands, the heel and curved-up toes simply follow.

This raises the big question: Is it 1-2-3 or 1-3-2? Ball-heel-toes or ball-toes-heel? While writing this book, looking at countless pictures and videos of myself running, and assuming that the toes were shorter and therefore closer to the ground, I had incorrectly assumed that I was landing ball-toes-heel. It was difficult to see, even in videos at sixty frames per second (which was the fastest I could get out of my video cameras). But fortunately, my recent summer road trip gave me the opportunity to run on a treadmill in Dr. Lieberman's Skeletal Biology Lab at Harvard. There, with a high-speed video camera recording at incredible frame rates, I could see that my heels actually landed before my toes!

So, as for the question of 1-2-3 or 1-3-2, the answer obviously is . . . drum roll, please . . . *it's not really important.*

Depending on just how high your heel is, how bent your knees are, how relaxed your calves and toes are, all of which may vary depending on the terrain, then *either* the toes or the heel will land after the ball, followed by the other. Landings are also affected by anatomical differences, such as being bowlegged or knock-kneed. Ultimately, it comes down to this: "Does it *feel* comfortable?" A 1-2-3 or a 1-3-2 is up to you. You probably won't even know which you're doing until you're recorded at 500 frames per second.

The fact that the heel touches the ground at all may surprise many barefooting newbies who are under the impression that's a no-no. But as many have already painfully discovered, straining to keep the heel from touching the ground puts them at risk of huge strain on the Achilles tendons, calves, and metatarsals. By letting the heel down in a calm, low-impact manner after the ball of the foot, we complete a "bed of nails" effect, where your body weight and impact forces are distributed over many points with relatively minor stress on any of them. (See the section on gravel in chapter 4.)

Try to keep the heel down until liftoff. This has the dual benefit of loading the calf for the "spring" effect, and discouraging a forced push-off/toe-off. That's a good thing, because the toes and metatarsals simply are not designed to handle heavy, repetitive loads for long distances. Although running on your toes can seem fun and exhilarating for a while, it can lead to stubbed toes, blisters, and metatarsal stress fractures (a too common malady particularly striking in beginning Vibram/minimalist-footwear runners (see chapter 6.) According to some podiatrists, a jump in the number of metatarsal stress fractures with Vibram FiveFingers has led some running stores to require buyers to sign waivers that they've been warned of the dangers. We haven't been able to verify that, but, judging by comments on my website, stress fractures are a real risk. Sadly, barefoot running is often blamed for these types of injuries because the shoes are frequently advertised as "barefoot" running shoes.

The tensed-up calves of the elevated heel are also an indication that you're not bending your knees enough. If you bend your knees properly, your calves naturally go limp. That means that an exclusive forefoot landing slows you down; you're only using the spring in the arch of your foot, not the much bigger spring—your leg.

Given the inefficiency of staying up on the toes or forefoot alone for more than a millisecond, why the complexity of the sequential 1-2-3 landing? Why not just make it a "1"— and land with a flat foot? The problem is what I call the "suction cup effect."

How to Fight the Suction Cup Effect

Think of sticking a plunger or suction cup on any smooth surface. All the edges of the plunger contact the surface simultaneously. When pressure is applied, the edges slide outward.

Try this experiment with the palm of your hand on a smooth tabletop: arch your hand like a suction cup. When you place your arched hand on the tabletop, the fingertips and heel of your palm will be touching the surface. Now, maintaining contact, flatten your hand, and you'll feel your fingers spreading in one direction, while the heel of your palm slides in the opposite direction.

Your bare foot, built atop an arch linking the ball and the heel that is designed to flatten like a spring to absorb impact (an amazing feature that the arch supports in running shoes prevent), also slides like a suction cup—on the road. The ball of the foot moves horizontally away from the heel; it's like you're sandpapering your soles against the asphalt. It not only is an inefficient use of your arch "spring," which functions better when you land ball first, but also it is almost certain to cause blisters if you run far enough.

A little friction isn't a problem for a few steps, perhaps even a few miles for someone with tough soles. But it was a problem one year for Barefoot Jon Gissberg of Seattle, a part-time barefooter who worked long hours, lived in cold, rainy weather not conducive to winter running, and could log only a few hundred barefoot miles a year. Even worse, he landed flat-footed. He ran unscathed most of the time. But by the end of the 2002 San Diego Marathon, at age fifty-nine, in the worse case of suction cup friction I've ever seen, there were huge slabs of skin separating from his soles.

Many accomplished part-time barefooters, including my Orange County buddy Dave Parsel, who ran a 5-minute mile at age fifty-five in 2010 (see his profile in chapter 7), limit their barefoot mileage because they believe it wears their soles down. I say the problem is not the mileage, but the landing. I solved my excess wear problem a few years earlier by changing my technique.

Just remember to avoid the suction cup by using the 1-2-3 sequence: ball first, then heel or toes. Another way to look at it, according to Ozzie Gontang, is "ball/heel/ball,"—the ball touches down first, then the heel; the heel then comes up first and the ball is the last part of the foot to lift off the ground.

Most of the foot's complexity takes care of itself, if we allow it to. Landing ball first solves the problem of the heel and ball moving apart, because it gives the arch a moment to flatten out under the load before the heel touches. Because the two have already moved apart before landing, there is no sliding apart on the ground.

As you can see, the "instinctive" barefoot landing is a lot more complex than you might have thought. But it's very easy to master (you can practice it running in place while watching TV), and the payoff in safety and performance is great, especially when paired with the focus on lifting early and often.

Curve Up the Toes

To protect the toes from blisters and repetitive impact stress during a 2003 marathon (see "The Epiphany of the Curved-up Toes" on page 100), I learned to curve my toes up on the landing. Here's why this technique, which allows the toes to land a millisecond later than the ball of the foot, works to avoid a suction cup effect similar to that described above.

There is a little arch between the toes and the ball of the foot. Unlike the arch between the heel and the ball, the tiny arch behind our toes isn't really designed, nor is it in the right place, to absorb impact. But it does present a problem nearly identical to the simultaneous ball-heel landing in that the toes and the ball slide away from each other if they land at the same time, creating friction that can lead to blisters.

Curving the toes up gently, though not loading that arch, stretches out the skin between the toes and ball of the foot and stops them from sliding apart. That little trick got me through my nineteenth barefoot marathon, and about fifty-seven more marathons since.

Curving the toes upward isn't difficult to do, and may even be instinctive. That could explain why I didn't have problems in my first eighteen barefoot marathons; I wasn't too tired to instinctively lift my toes. Ironically, the instinct to raise them might exacerbate a shod runner's heel strike. Stuck inside stiff shoes, the toes can't really curve up, encouraging the entire foot to angle up in an exaggerated way that makes the heel strike more pronounced. Ouch.

THE EPIPHANY OF THE CURVED-UP TOES

I've often said that marathons are like my graduate school. They give you the intensive, specialized, in-depth training that you didn't get during the course of your normal four-year degree. That's because they're long enough and challenging enough that the slightest imperfections and inefficiencies—the ones that you might never notice in your daily run, yet cause the cumulative damage over the years that can wreck your running career—eventually come out. It may take one marathon or it may take a hundred, from running in rain to running in 100°F (38°C) heat to running completely de-trained due to too much travel or a long illness, but the marathon will reveal the truth. That's usually, in my experience, by the "Wall"—mile 20.

Case in point: the 2003 Bayshore Marathon in the place I grew up, Traverse City, Michigan, where listening to race results on the radio four decades earlier had inspired me to set the goal of running one marathon in my life. It wouldn't be my first—in fact, it was my nineteenth barefoot marathon—but it was inevitable. And it turned out to be very important, because it was the race where I learned an essential rule that many barefooters have never heard of, but it makes running barefoot so much more comfortable and efficient: *Curve up thy toes.*

I wasn't expecting much at Bayshore, maybe a four-hour time at best. I had the flu the week before and hadn't run much. My body was sluggish and fatigued from doing little but sitting, as I'd taken a bus from Orange County to Denver, then carpooled with my brother Pat to Michigan. I even put a list of all my excuses at the beginning of my race report on the Web.

But I felt good come race day, when I arrived late and was one of the last of the 700 racers to head out into the misty, cold morning on the rough road surface. I ran amazingly well despite my long list of excuses, and the first 15 miles (24 km) flew by. Then, between mile 18 and 19 (29 and 30 km), both of my little toes began to sting. All I could think was, "Dang this rough road, and the flu, and the sitting around for days. It obviously left me with wimpy, untoughened soles just when I didn't need it."

Soon, the only thing on my mind was my stinging toes. Trying everything I could think of to avoid it, I played around with all the variables: the bend in the knees, the posture, the cadence. I made sure I was properly lifting my foot straight up, not toeing off. Nothing worked. I was getting dejected. I started slowing down and thought I might have to walk this one in due to blisters—something I hadn't suffered during a race since the first and only marathon I did with shoes, in 1987.

At mile 20 (32 km), I called my sister Adreah on my cell phone. The Bayshore Marathon route goes out a peninsula and loops back, and she, her son, and my brother were driving the course and shooting pictures and video at prearranged spots. My nephew Oryon answered.

"I'm slowing down," I told him. "My toes are a mess. It's going to be at least an hour before I get to the finish line. Maybe more. I'll just try to survive the last 6 miles (9.6 km)."

After we hung up, I went back to my painful pinkies and my checklist. After a couple of miles of trying the same thing, I just curved my toes up to avoid further abrasion.

So I angled my toes up slightly, not too much, like I was barely raising the drawbridge up from across a moat. It was nearly impossible to keep them entirely off the ground, but just lifting them gently seemed to work. At that moment, the pain disappeared—and was soon replaced by a completely new mind-set of boundless, endless, can-do energy. This wasn't just a second wind; it was wind to the second power, wind squared. Suddenly, running was fun again. And as you know, fun often translates to fast.

At mile 23 (36.8 km), literally feeling no pain after I experimented with raising my toes to different heights (and worked out my new rule: no strain, just a little bit curved up, touching down after the ball of the foot makes ground contact), I called my nephew again. "On second thought, I'm running pretty well. You better get to the finish line quick, because I'm going to be there in about 20 minutes."

With the blisters silenced, the legs fresh due to the cool, misty, drizzly day, and the attitude so wildly positive that Tony Robbins surely would have high-fived me at the finish line if he'd been in the Great Lakes region, I surfed to the finish line on a wave of exhilaration. When I crossed the line in 3:29, I was so stunned that I couldn't speak. It wasn't a PR—that was a 3:18, still my best, done at Pacific Shoreline in Huntington Beach in 2000. But it was light-years ahead of where I thought I'd finish back at mile 20 (32 km). In fact, it was fast enough to qualify me for the Boston Marathon, although I wasn't planning on running it yet.

I didn't bother to tell my brother about my curved-toed epiphany as we drove over to our parents' house. It may have been a huge, monumental day in advancing the science of barefooting, but he wasn't a runner and I was more concerned about eating and napping, anyway. Still, before we raided the refrigerator, we went out to the back porch to take pictures of the blisters on the bottoms of my feet, one of the few notable injuries I'd had in all my years of barefoot running and racing.

I hadn't stopped to look at my blisters during or immediately after the race, and I was expecting nasty, open, raw wounds. Instead, there were two tiny, barely perceivable red dots—blood blisters, one on each little toe less than a ¼ inch (6 mm) in diameter. One was so faint that it barely showed up in the photos.

Yet from the point of view of someone who hates pain, it *was* a big deal. Runners who are less sensitive than I, or more macho, or simply better able to tolerate pain, might have laughed at my tiny blisters, but the fact is that these little problems are indicators of bigger problems with our technique. They are canaries in the coal mine—signs of impending back pain, knee pain, foot pain, and other big issues destined to come back to haunt you in the long run.

All this begs a couple of questions: Is curving up the toes something that ancient barefoot men and women runners did naturally? I don't know, but I do know that it helps prevent you from stubbing your bare toes, and that you cannot do it while wearing shoes. And is curving the toes a performance enhancer? I don't know that, either. But I do know for certain that it is a pain and abrasion avoider. "Enduring" pain or injury while barefoot or shod defeats the purpose of our senses. Besides, pain drains energy—that's why, once I had eliminated the cause of the pain, I had a second wind.

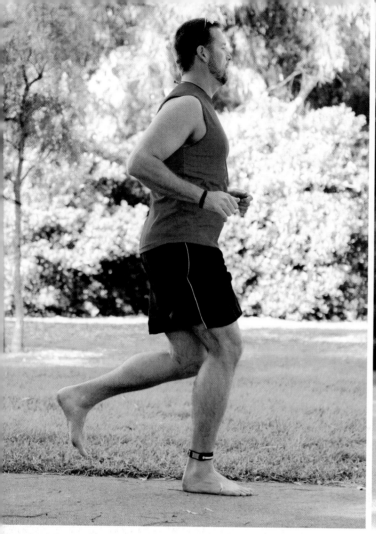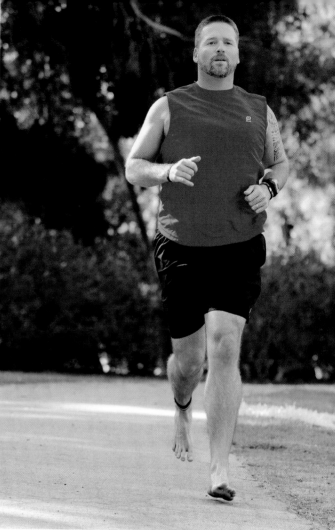

WHAT TO DO: Maintain a vertical posture of the torso, relax your calves, and allow your hips to fall forward. Each foot lands below your torso, not ahead of it. This means you will avoid the braking effect that results from over-striding, providing for a much smoother forward flow—no interruption of our forward momentum.

10 OVERALL BODY MOVEMENT: INITIATE MOVEMENT BY LETTING THE HIPS FALL FORWARD

If there is no push-off, and we lift our feet straight up and down and don't lean our body forward by bending at the waist, how do we propel ourselves forward?

Answer: We simply *fall* forward. Just move the entire torso—still vertical—in front of the feet by relaxing the calves and allowing the *hips* to fall forward. You need to move the feet quickly under the hips to catch yourself. Each foot lands below the vertical torso, not ahead of it. (By contrast, a foot-forward landing effectively puts on the brakes with each step, encourages a heel strike, and ratchets up shock and eventual damage to the knees and hips.)

For those of you familiar with the pronounced forward-body lean of the Pose and Chi methods of running, what I advocate is not less lean, just less of the body (only the legs) leaning. Yes, you need to lean to throw your body slightly "off balance" in the direction you want to run to feel like you're falling forward. Maintaining vertical posture of the torso (more accurately, a posture that *feels* vertical to us) and keeping the forward lean below the hips will make you feel like you're falling *forward* rather than falling *down*. It's a big difference, on which I'll elaborate in chapter 4.

TAKING YOUR SHOES OFF IS JUST THE FIRST STEP

While running barefoot may initially seem as simple as just taking off your shoes and running, there is a definite technique that can help you maximize benefits and minimize drawbacks. The entire body is involved to run in a gentle, efficient manner that turns your legs and feet into springs that move you forward, with little or no shock and injury. While there are two key elements—the bent knees/squatted running position and a ball-first forefoot landing that then touches down on toes and heel—there are important supporting roles for all body parts from head to toe. Several extremely beneficial things happen when we adapt this gentle running technique:

THE RUNNING BAREFOOT TROUBLESHOOTING CHECKLIST

- If the bill on your baseball cap is bobbing up and down as you run, that indicates too much bouncing up and down. Remember that the goal of running is to move forward; it is counterproductive to try to launch your body up—lift, lift, lift your foot.
- If you feel your heels pounding, don't tense the calves; instead, relax and bend your knees, and let your torso pull you forward.
- If your heels are not touching at all, you are asking for problems. Relax your calves, letting the heels come down to the ground instantly after the landing of the ball of the foot. The toes should be slightly curved up so they don't land first, but allowed to land just after the ball of the foot lands.
- If your feet are slapping, try a faster cadence, i.e., lifting your feet earlier and/or quicker.
- If your feet never touch the ground, you are lifting your feet too early. And you should be writing your own book.

- We're using muscles to cushion our landing.
- We strengthen the muscles that help support our joints (allowing some runners to discard their knee braces and other support devices).
- By allowing our joints to bend, energy is stored like a spring. When our body moves in front of our foot, the spring expands, pushing us forward without a conscious effort to push off.
- The lack of a pronounced push-off is much gentler on the body. In fact, when we put the foot ahead of the body and push it into the ground hard and early, we generally lose all of the above benefits—the knee can't bend naturally and the heel gets pounded into the ground, rattling our joints and effectively hitting the brakes. And why would we want to do that?

SEVEN STEPS TO PERFECT BAREFOOTING

Let's look at this another way. You've already got the ten-point plan. Maybe this condensed version, in seven steps, will help the technique sink in.

1 DON'T BE LAZY; USE A FAST CADENCE.

Get your feet moving. Practice lifting your feet 180 times a minute, preferably faster, while running in place, to start. The longer time you are in the air with each stride, the longer you will be falling back toward the ground. If your steps are quick and short (in time, not necessarily distance), you will spend less time accelerating toward the ground, and will reduce impact.

2 *DO* BE LAZY. DON'T PUSH OFF; LIFTING IS EASIER.

Don't focus on landing. Focus on lifting your feet *before* landing. Don't worry, gravity will ensure that you land, but, by starting to lift your foot *before* you land, you will be decelerating its fall toward the ground. It's like when you drive your car. Most of us don't wait until after hitting the car in front of us to slow down! Likewise, we don't want to wait for the ground to decelerate our footfall.

3 RELAX; LET YOUR BODY BEND.

The largest natural springs we have are our ankles, knees, and hips. But they have almost no shock-absorbing capability when straightened out like a pogo stick. Their real advantage is in the ability to bend. Too many people run with these joints "locked" or rigid, because they are convinced that their shoes will protect them.

4 STRAIGHTEN YOUR POSTURE.

The human body is designed to stand at rest in such a way that every body part is stacked vertically on top of another with no help from muscular tension. In order to do this, you must be balanced. Grab the top of a broomstick and hold it upside down. If the broomstick is not balanced vertically in your hand, it takes more work to hold it in position. So, make sure that your posture is vertical, with your head erect on top of your shoulders and your body erect on top of your hips. The big mistakes many people make are leaning their head and torso forward and sticking their butt out in back. This has the added drawback of straightening the legs, which should be bent to absorb shock (see step 3).

5 LEAN YOUR HIPS FORWARD.

To start moving forward, you lean—but not the head and torso (see step 4). You lean from the ankles up to the hips, which creates an imbalance that makes you fall forward. To avoid falling down, you should already be moving your feet quickly. Lean is your accelerator. Increase forward lean and you will run faster. Decrease forward lean and you will slow down.

6 BE AWARE.

Listen to your feet. If they're in pain, it's time to stop, or slow down and try to figure out how to move without pain. If we go beyond what our bare feet are ready for, chances are other parts of our body are already overworked or misused.

7 DON'T REACH.

You know those magazine shots of those long, luscious strides that reach out in front of your body? Forget about them! Running fast does not come from lengthening your stride. Long strides come from the body moving forward fast. Again, too many people stretching a stiff leg lazily out in front, waiting for gravity to do its worst, end up with a slow, plodding, *jogging*, injurious stride. It's much easier to simply fall forward. If you land with your foot out in front of your body, you are hitting the brakes. Your foot just got in the way of moving your body forward.

On the other hand, if you're running really fast, you'll need to lengthen your stride to get your feet under your torso for the next step—but don't just throw it out in front and wait for the crash. Start pulling your foot up and back *before* landing, so that the speed and direction of your foot travel matches that of the ground.

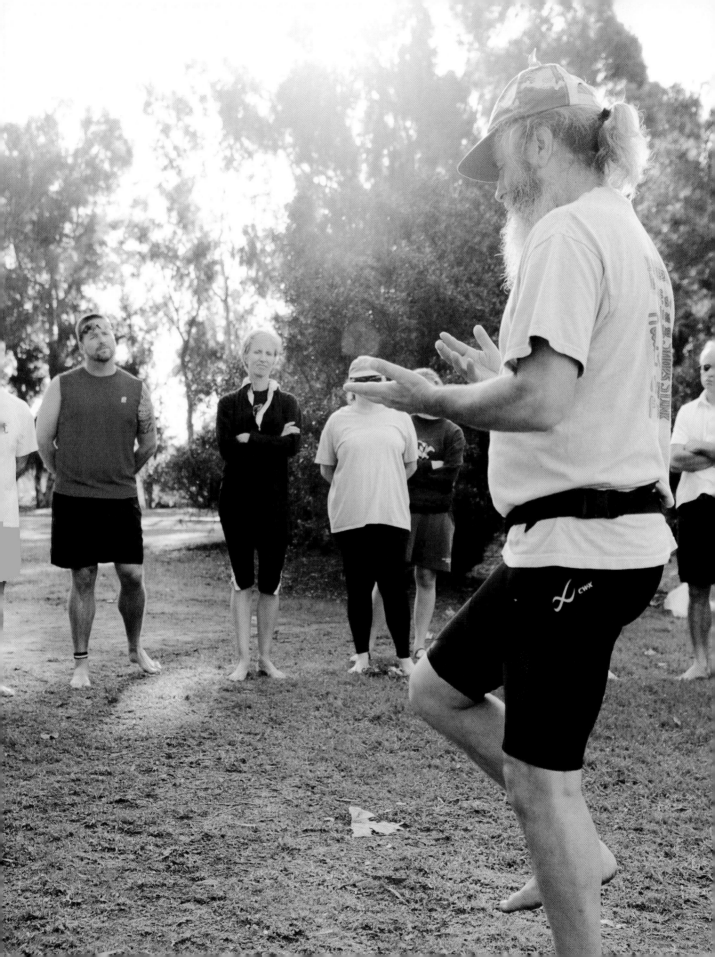

CHAPTER 4

BAREFOOT PLAY
IMPROVE YOUR TECHNIQUE, REDUCE INJURIES, RUN EASY, AND HAVE FUN

Drills and IDEAS (imagery, deep conjecture, essential concepts, and advice) will help you lock in barefoot technique

> YOU WANT TO KNOW THE SECRET TO SURVIVING AIR TRAVEL?" SAYS A FELLOW AIRLINE PASSENGER TO OFFICER JOHN MCCLANE. "AFTER YOU GET WHERE YOU'RE GOING, TAKE OFF YOUR SHOES AND YOUR SOCKS. THEN WALK AROUND AND MAKE FISTS WITH YOUR TOES. I KNOW IT SOUNDS CRAZY. TRUST ME, I'VE BEEN DOING IT FOR NINE YEARS. YES SIR, BETTER THAN A SHOWER AND A HOT CUP OF COFFEE.
>
> —*DIE HARD*, 1988

Hearing that line spoken to Bruce Willis's character just a few months after I got rid of my running shoes over two decades ago gave me a nice jolt of validation: yes, I must be on to something if Hollywood's already got a hold of it.

I love the movies, TV, and popular culture. That's where I get a lot of my inspiration, philosophy, and imagery for running barefoot and other things in my life—just as many children of the '60s probably would. I grew up on John Wayne, Julie Andrews, and James Bond movies and classic TV sitcoms like *My Mother the Car*, *I Dream of Jeannie*, *Bewitched*, *Get Smart*, *Andy Griffith*, *Gomer Pyle USMC*, *Petticoat Junction*, *Hogan's Heroes*, *Batman*, *All in the Family*, *The Jeffersons*, *Sanford and Son*, and *Gilligan's Island*. So it's only natural, when I think of running-related issues such as the heel strike—the evil spawn of running shoes that barefooting will help you avoid—that I think of *Rowan and Martin's Laugh-In*. After all, if the heel could talk, it surely would be saying, "Don't *sock it to me!*"

I particularly liked shows that took people out of their normal environment and put them in a strange new world, like when New York banker Eddie Albert and his socialite wife Eva Gabor went to live on the farm in *Green Acres*, and when Robin Williams's man from Ork came to live on Earth in *Mork and Mindy*. Given that, it makes perfect sense to me to reference TV and the movies when we take you out of your normal environment—shoes—and put you in a strange, new (yet completely natural) one—bare feet. It's not just a fun hook. Hollywood images have spurred ideas and analogies and helped me remember things easier. Especially things I don't like doing—like practicing drills.

I hate drills; they seem a lot like homework—and I generally hate work. As Ryan Whitaker recently told a beginner on one of our forums, "have fun, explore, experiment, dance, hop, skip, jump, and smile, and splash in puddles." That's what "drills" should be—play! The idea is to get you out of the rut that you've probably been running in with shoes and get you to play, to discover that barefoot running isn't the same running you did in shoes. . .unless you frequently ran around barefoot as a child. Many of these "drills" I've been doing all along and didn't realize they were drills until I started doing workshops. More crop up all the time, often when a newbie barefooter writes in with a new question or revelation.

Since I often relate to the world through a 1960s sitcom prism, consider this drills- and advice-filled chapter to be the second half of the book's *Odd Couple*–like pair of "technique" chapters—the loose, fun-loving, Jack Klugman–type counterpart to the straight-laced and organized Tony Randall of chapter 3. To turn the forthcoming visualizations and exaggerated motions into a good time, each of the ten drills in the first half of the chapter draws on some of my favorite TV and movie heroes—from Groucho Marx's squatted walking to Red Skelton's drunken staggering. Hopefully, they'll turn this mandatory homework into a fun game that'll help you understand, practice, and continuously improve your barefoot running.

BEGINNER DRILLS

DRILL 1: THE STAGGERING DRUNK

Inspired by the teeter-tottering drunk boxer, Cauliflower McPugg, played by legendary comedian Red Skelton on his popular show on CBS throughout the '60s, this drill should help with the concept of "falling" forward, as well as relaxing while running. It's okay to practice this on a barefoot-friendly surface like soft sand or grass.

Here's the gist: stand and relax—extremely relax, as if you're drunk (being literally drunk probably will not help). Keep your torso vertical, unlock your knees, and rather than leading with your foot, let your balance shift over your toes until you're moving forward. If you don't want to fall, you'd better get your feet moving under your torso.

Practice slowly, inch by inch, step by step (okay, I did steal that from Lucille Ball, who stole it from Abbot and Costello, who stole it from the Three Stooges, who stole it from Harry Steppe). The moment that you start to get the idea of "falling" forward, you can make it a more continuous movement (without the staggering). The big difference between actually being drunk and running is that our legs should end up moving much more smoothly and gracefully (see chapter 3, steps 7 and 8).

→ DRILL 1: The Staggering Drunk. Keep your torso vertical, your knees unlocked, your posture relaxed, and your balance shifted over your toes. You should feel a falling sensation, but keep your torso vertical and quickly move your trailing foot under your torso to prevent yourself from actually falling. Repeat until you see a cop approaching. This drill helps you get used to the forward falling sensation that keeps you running forward.

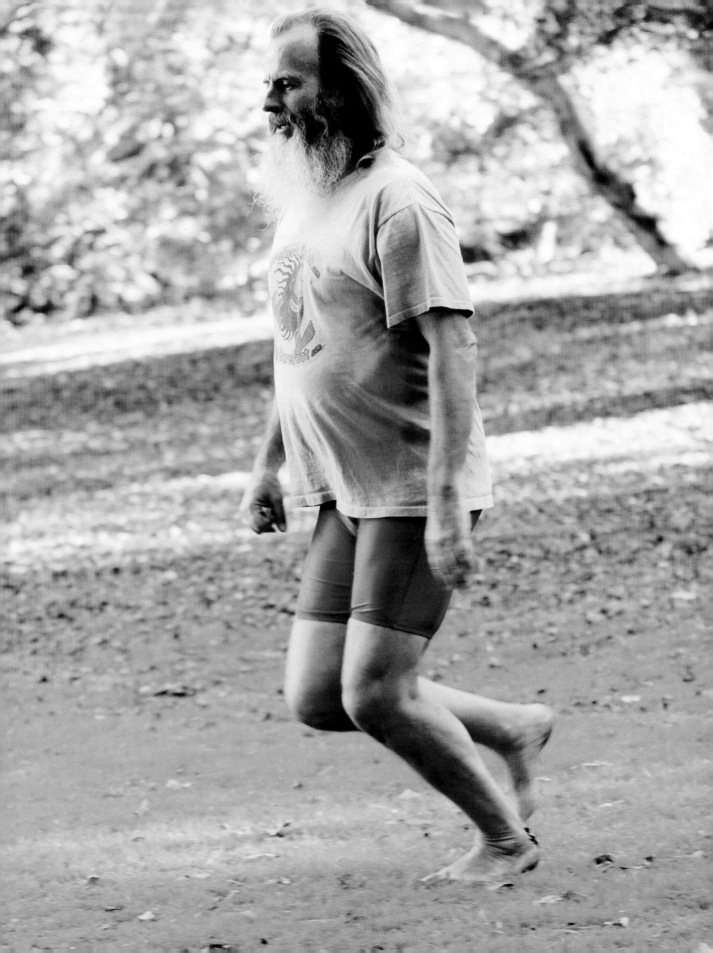

DRILL 2: THE GROUCHO CROUCHO

Derived from the comedic genius of Groucho Marx, this drill should help emphasize the concept of bent knees by simply exaggerating the bent-knee depth. I've never seen anyone run with his or her knees too bent, although chances are you won't get any lower than Groucho managed to; his famous crouched run/walk actually does work very well.

Crouch down low, almost like you're sitting (albeit without a chair), keep your torso vertical, and try walking. Focus on keeping your torso low but straight up; the lowness comes from the bent knees, not from bending over at the waist. Your torso should be vertical as you "roll" along smoothly, as if crouched on a skateboard or roller skates.

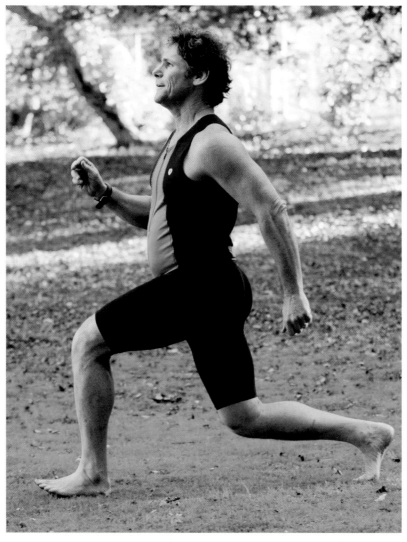

DRILL 2: Groucho Croucho. Bend your knees to crouch down low, keep your torso vertical, and walk like the legendary comedian Groucho Marx. Cigar is optional. Bending your knees to excess in this drill helps you get used to bending your knees more than you're used to, and helps you find that sweet spot where your legs return the maximum forward spring.

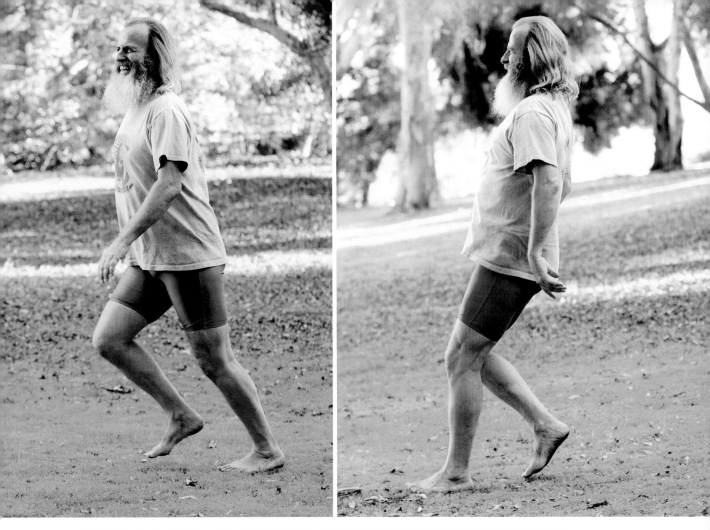

DRILL 3: The Brooks Bell. Run in place, bending your knees and lifting your feet quickly. Then shift your balance forward, then back, as pictured, and repeat as often as you like. This helps you get used to the feeling of falling in the direction you want to run and teaches you how to control your direction through lean, not pushing your feet into the ground. Note the full-body lean in this case, because I am accelerating, not running a steady pace.

DRILL 3: THE BROOKS BELL

This a controlled, smoother version of the Staggering Drunk that is inspired by either comedian Foster Brooks, who made a standup career out of looking and sounding like he was about to fall over, or the Tarahumara Indians featured in *Born to Run*, whose spare time is filled with dancing while inebriated from corn beer.

Unlike the Staggering Drunk, the Brooks Bell focuses on the concept of using lean (in this case full body lean, as we will be accelerating back and forth) to control both speed and direction. To do it, start by running in place, with a vertical torso and bent knees, lifting your feet quickly (all of the first nine rules in chapter 3). Then, shift your balance forward, then back, then forward, then back. When you get it, you'll be running forward and backward alternately, like a bell swinging back and forth.

For a variation, you can also try running side to side by shifting your balance from side to side. Experienced runners may find this helps on switchbacks.

For some alternative imagery, think of the direction you want to travel, and notice that your legs will be on the opposing side of your body. For example, if you want to run to the right, your legs should be trailing on your left side. When you think about it, this makes perfect sense—our body leads our legs and feet, because our legs are pushing us in the direction we're running even though we're not making an effort to push off (see Drill 4: Lucy, Don't Be Pushy).

DRILL 4: LUCY, DON'T BE PUSHY

Who was more conniving and pushy than Lucille Ball's character Lucy Ricardo on *I Love Lucy*? To great comic effect, she grated on everybody—much like pushy feet will grate on your skin.

To stop blisters on any surface, you need to learn to lift the foot rather than push off. This will not be easy, as the terms "push-off" and "toe-off" are so embedded in the running lexicon. Well, when you're barefoot, that's a prescription for blisters, metatarsal strains, and stress fractures. The only "off" you need to worry about is the one they do at Cape Canaveral: liftoff.

Unlike a rocket, however, barefooters don't blast their foot up from the bottom, but lift it from above. Think about it: it's a lot of work trying to push your massive (relatively speaking) body with your tiny (relatively speaking) foot. But, it's really not much work for your massive body to pull up your tiny little foot; all you need to do is bend your knee. Note: It doesn't matter if your foot is a size 13, triple E. Your body is usually bigger than your foot.

Lifting the foot is easy: simply *lift* the foot off the surface when it has finished traveling backward behind your body. (To the outside observer, your body is traveling forward in front of your foot.) Do *not* try to push off, or do anything else that causes the foot to slip on the surface.

No matter how smooth or soft the surface, do *not* do anything that would cause undue pain or injury on a rough, hard, pointy surface. If you can't resist, go back to practicing on gravel, even after you have it down; think of it as a refresher class. I look for the opportunity to practice running barefoot on sharp gravel wherever I run. As I like to say, *running barefoot on a little gravel each day keeps the pounding away!* If you get sloppy with your running barefoot technique on sharp gravel, it is immediately, and painfully, apparent—a good thing for the learning process.

No matter how rough the surface, imagine it as being a smooth surface covered with wet paint, and you don't want to slip, slide, or twist in the paint. Don't leave skid marks! If there were wet paint on our soles, the only images we would paint with our feet while running barefoot would be nice, clear, smudge-free footprints.

Now, curve your toes slightly, gently upward, so that your foot lands a bit more like a ball, rather than a suction cup. This will allow the foot to spread as it lands, instead of landing, and then spreading. (See chapter 3 sidebar, "The Epiphany of the Curved-Up Toes" on page 100.)

And lift the entire foot. Most people lift only the heel, and let the toe or ball of the foot push down into the ground, causing unnecessary abrasion. So put a little effort into lifting the front of the foot as well as the heel, so it feels as if the heel is lifting with the toes. Note:

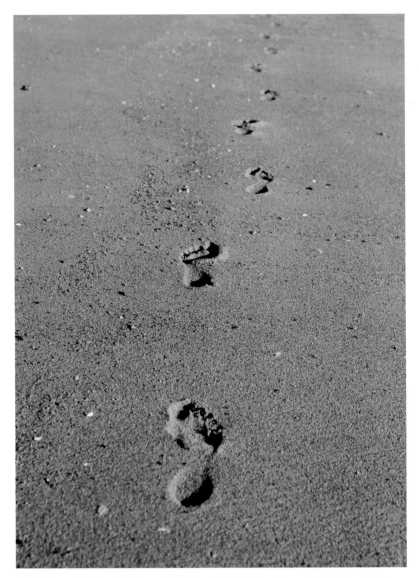

DRILL 4: Lucy, Don't be Pushy. Learn to lift the whole foot rather than push off with your toes. Practice lifting the foot once it has finished travelling backward behind your body. To test if you're doing it correctly, run on sand or mud and try to make your footprints clear and even depth.

Remember that a full-foot liftoff is how it feels to the runner, not how it looks to an outside viewer. If you actually do manage to lift your entire sole off the ground at precisely the same time, you'll be lucky if you manage to not fall down! The feeling you're looking for is a little bit of effort to lift the forefoot (with toes curved up), mostly just to avoid pushing down with the forefoot or toes.

And finally, at least for now, no matter how soft the surface, distribute your weight across the entire sole of your foot (see Drill 5: Romancing the Stones).

DRILL 5: ROMANCING THE STONES

The 1984 Michael Douglas–Kathleen Turner romantic comedy *Romancing the Stone* focused on the hunt for an emerald. In that spirit, this drill encourages you to do something that might seem rather counterintuitive for a barefoot runner: seek out rocks.

Many "experts" (who are not named Ken Bob) routinely advise new barefooters to head for "barefoot-friendly" terrain like grass or sand, so that you don't feel any pain. Unfortunately, these "easy transition surfaces" do not teach you how to run barefoot very well, if at all. In fact, because the surfaces are comfortable and forgiving (they move out of the way of your foot, instead of the other way around), they can leave you with the same bad habits you started with. Fact: If you want to learn how to run barefoot correctly in a way that will then transfer to any surface, you need to learn how to handle the rough stuff first. That's why, in my travels around the country, I make a concerted attempt to start my clinics off with gravel. And I'm not talking just any gravel. Forget about smooth, polished, round stones. I look for the stuff that's been recently crushed, with sharp edges—lots of them!

I'm no sadist. Yes, I love seeing people cringe at first. But even more, I love seeing them learn to handle it, learn to relax the calves and bend the knees, become "one with the gravel," and understand that the gravel isn't going to push up into their feet any harder than they push down into it. I love seeing them realize that gravel is not their enemy, and then go fearlessly on to easier surfaces—like run-of-the-mill rough concrete—as if it were as smooth as a baby's behind.

The method for handling gravel is really just an extension of what I talked about in Drill 4: Don't Be Pushy. An appropriate visualization is the "bed of nails" analogy, wherein you distribute your weight over as many points as possible. Think of the holy men of India or Nepal, wearing nothing but loincloths, lying on a rectangle studded with a thousand nails— and not even drawing a drop of blood. How do they do it? The trick is physics: they evenly distribute their weight across as many points as possible, so that not one of them bears a heavy load. If a 200-pound (91 kg) man lays his body evenly atop 800 nails, then each nail only supports ¼ pound (100 g). Yes, each nail is sharp, and can puncture the skin if enough weight is put on it. But it doesn't because each nail point is supporting a small fraction of the yogi's body weight.

Therefore, your job on any surface—not only rough surfaces—is simple: spread the load, your body weight, evenly across it. Of course, an irregular ground surface studded with rocks and twigs is different from a bed of uniform-height nails in that you literally need to mold your soles to a different surface with every step, sort of letting the sole go limp and draping it over the terrain. As corny as it may sound, you need to let your feet become "one with the earth" in a shape-shifting flow over the rocks. It may be intimidating at first, but actually not difficult if you relax the feet certainly, but also the calves and ankles, bend the knees, relax the shoulders, and resist the urge to tense up and push off. Pain is your guide; it will instantly tell you not to skid, shuffle, grind, or push your feet down on sharp gravel.

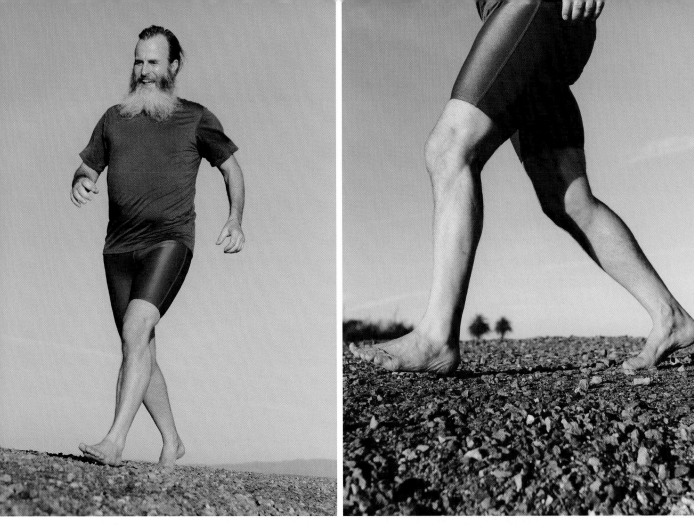

DRILL 5: Romancing the Stones. Learn to run on a rough surface by spreading your body weight evenly across your sole. Remember to relax your calves and ankles, bend your knees, relax your shoulders, and don't tense up or push off. Anytime you feel yourself pushing up away from the stones, you're actually pushing your feet harder *into* the stones.

To start, practice standing on the gravel, relaxing and shape-shifting your soles as you spread your body weight gently and evenly from heel to toe. When you get comfortable with that, lift one leg at a time—remember to lift, not push. Finally, slowly run across the gravel. Remember to relax the shoulders; raising your shoulders won't make you lighter and, in fact, will push your toes even harder into the gravel.

Once you can handle running on gravel, everything else is easy. That's because the gravel gives you a ton of information. And that's the idea here: Get the maximum amount of stimulation you can handle. If you respond to the stimulation by complaining or screaming in pain or anger, it only gets worse. If you respond by relaxing, the formerly forbidding, ever-changing gravel surface now becomes interesting, educational, and oddly, almost comfortably, stimulating. If you feel pain, relax and spread the load until it goes away.

It might seem strangely contradictory that I enjoy running barefoot on rough gravel surfaces, given that I've made it so clear that I'm quite sensitive to pain. And yet that is the strange truth. That's because learning to handle the gravel teaches me how to minimize pain—that if I'm gentle with the surface, it'll be gentle on my soles.

I also like to think that the gravel offers philosophical benefits: in the journey of life, every road has its bumps and rough patches. Since we can't repave or re-sod every path we encounter, it's better to understand and live with the diversity of terrains and surfaces, no matter how strange, foreign, and perhaps even unbearable they may seem. If we want to enjoy the journey toward our destination, we must deal with the trials and tribulations along the way. They just might have something to teach us.

SHOCK TREATMENT

"It's generally our reaction that causes injury" were the wise words of my first-term electronics teacher back in my community college in Michigan in 1977. Before I started working on computers for a living, and before there were personal computers (that you didn't need to build yourself), I was an electronics technician. I was working on televisions back when many of them were filled with vacuum tubes. It takes a bunch of voltage to get current to flow across a vacuum, so these old televisions had more than their share of high voltages. One of the first things our instructor taught us was that the electric shock may cause pain, but most injuries to electric shock victims are the result of the victim's reaction to the shock, not the electric current going through the body. For example, pulling the hand suddenly away from the bare wires we just touched might result in breaking the back of the cathode ray tube and slicing our hand open on the sharp edges.

And so it is with running barefoot on rough surfaces. While the initial pain we feel when our bare soles press into the sharp edges of rough gravel may not be as comfortable as a feather bed, it is only a bit of discomfort. It isn't injury . . . yet! The injury generally comes when we try pushing down on our feet even harder. "Why would we do that?" you might naturally ask. Well, when we're standing, walking, or running on sharp gravel, and feel like we're trying to pull our body up and raise our shoulders, that is when we are pushing our feet harder into the ground.

So, relax and let your body sink low (which helps pull your feet away from the sharp edges). Think of how your leg collapses to a "limp" when unexpected pain hits your foot. Now limp on both sides, and it won't be a "limp."

DRILL 6: BOTTOMING OUT THE SPRINGS

Timothy Bottoms is a prolific veteran actor a few years older than me who stooped hilariously low while portraying President George W. Bush on the 2001 Comedy Central show *That's My Bush.* His good name can be a useful instrument for remembering proper downhill technique, in which the bent knee, stooping to an extreme form as you keep a vertical back, turns your whole leg into a superb shock-absorbing spring on the steepest of hills.

I found a good place to practice this in the short hills of Peter's Canyon in nearby Tustin, which features a 6-mile (9.6 km) loop all the way around a lake with a variety of trails for shortcuts and multiple loops.

One of the steepest hills, short but studded and furrowed with stones, loose gravel, and ruts in a hard-packed clay base (except during the rainy season), was a great joy for me to practice my favorite downhill technique: "letting go." Since the hill wasn't long, I didn't have to maintain this all-out speed for very long, and at the bottom it had a natural braking surface in a pit of soft sand kicked down the hill by bicycles, horses, and runners climbing and descending the trail. I loved that nearly out-of-control feeling, and I learned a lot about running softly from both doing it and watching others try it.

On this hill, being barefoot turned out to be an advantage to letting go. Hitting the brakes on hard rocks or while stepping in a deep rut would literally be a pain in my bottom . . . er, not that bottom . . . my soles. To glide over the various obstacles fast but gently, to maintain a vertical posture, I just sort of let myself fall forward and down the hill. While I had to bend my knees to lower my body for the next step, the ground was falling out from under me, so even with an extreme knee bend, my next step started with my knee barely bent. It was all I could do to lift my feet fast enough to keep up with my body going down the hill. When I hit the big sand pit at the bottom of the hill, where the trail leveled out, my knees collapsed fully, heels into butt!

But I was still upright and on my feet. I hadn't fallen down, skidded to a halt, or anything nasty like that. My springs simply bottomed out at the bottom of the hill. I felt wonderful. I'd used my "springs" to their fullest extent, and they worked.

I watched the rest of the group, all shod, as they pounded their way down the hill, and wasn't surprised. Extending straight legs to control their speed, they'd inadvertently launch themselves up, and away from the hill, as if pole-vaulting (with the stiff leg acting like the pole). It was horrible. I could see the future: pulverized knees that, a decade later, would not be running—and I was right. Many of those pole-vaulting knees are retired, the fight against gravity won in the short term and lost in the long term.

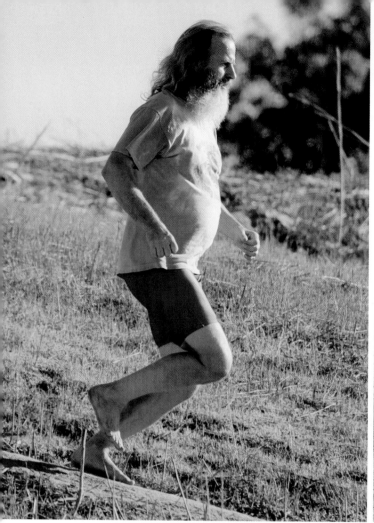

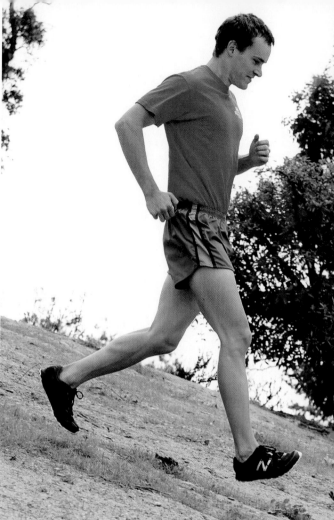

WHAT TO DO: Keep your head facing the direction you're running (parallel with the slope). Relax and let yourself fall forward down the hill. Lift your feet early and quickly, and let your knees collapse under your weight. This reduces the knee-pounding braking effect of trying to slow yourself when running downhill. (Note: Practice on gentle inclines before advancing to steeper hills.)

WHAT NOT TO DO: Don't push your body up away from the hill, don't land stiff-legged, don't hunch over, and don't tilt your head down. Launching yourself away from the hill results in injurious impact. Because you tend to run in the direction you are facing, facing the ground tempts the chances that you will fall face-first into the ground.

Here's how to try proper bottoming out without actually running down a steep hill: Relax and keep your torso vertical. Now, keeping your heels on the ground, squat as low as you can. Then squat more, and you'll feel your heels come off the ground.

Ultimately, the more we bend our knees, the more we make it unlikely to strike the heel into the ground. However, I did meet one person at one of my Running Barefoot Workshops in Texas who had extremely flexible calves, and could do a full squat with heels still touching the ground. My friend, Tina Thomas (author of the book *A Gentle Path: A Guide to Peace, Passion, and Power*), said, "Too much flexibility, not enough power." But most Americans probably have the opposite problem: too much power, not enough flexibility.

Now try walking while in this extreme squat. You're almost doing the next drill, the Pirate Walk.

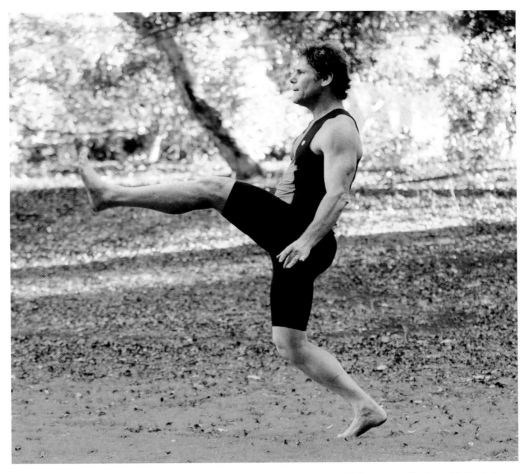

DRILL 7: The Pirate Walk. Standing on one leg, with your knee bent in a near-crouch, throw your other leg out in front of you. Just before it lands, quickly bend your knee, bringing your foot back so it lands underneath you. The leg you were standing on will trail behind you. Relax your calves and try not to push off with your toes.

DRILL 7: THE PIRATE WALK

Inspired by Kevin Kline's "With a Cat-Like Tread" dance in the *Pirates of Penzance* (1980), this drill utilizes extreme bent knees, a trailing foot, and a great stretch. It illustrates the barefoot running concept of lifting the foot up and back before landing.

Standing on one leg, with your knee bent in a near crouch, throw the other leg out in front. But before it lands, quickly bend your knee, bringing your foot back, so it lands underneath you as your body moves forward. Your previous supporting foot should be trailing far behind you. Repeat with the other foot. Extra credit: Do all this while repeating the words "Aye, me matey" in a throaty Scottish brogue.

DRILL 8: ENTER THE DARK SIDE

Tales from the Darkside (1990), starring Deborah Harry, one of my all-time favorite rockers, is an anthology of horror stories a child tells to keep from being eaten by a witch. This drill is designed to keep you from being consumed by fear of dangers lurking afoot when the sun is down. It's quite valuable for teaching you how to trust your senses, run light, and "flow" your foot over objects.

Running at night is beneficial precisely because you *can't* see the rocks. Here's why: beginner barefooters are often afraid of stepping on unseen objects, so they are initially preoccupied with looking at the ground. This isn't good, as it causes them to tense up and run with an unbalanced, unnatural forward hunch. Even after they have trained on gravel, practiced lifting the feet quickly, and geared up to run longer distances, there is often a fear of the *one* stone—the one sitting at the edge of the road waiting patiently, silently, to jump out into your path and bruise your sole.

The tension caused by this fear is often as bad as striking the rock itself—maybe worse. That's because when you tense up, it is that *tension* that causes pain. To absorb the rock and flow around it, your foot muscles need to be relaxed and flexible.

One way to keep them loose is to not see the rock. Here's what I mean: when you run at night, you are forced to de-focus from the details, and by extension, the tension. You can't see small rocks as you scan ahead to avoid the big obstacles that really can injure you. Because you can't see small details, even on most full moon nights, you are forced to react by feel, to rely on your increasingly sensitive soles to land, flow, and adjust over small objects. Instead of focusing on the ground and stones in your path and tensing up in anticipation, not seeing stones can make it simpler to relax and allow your foot to mold around any stones your soles touch.

Running at night isn't for beginners, and it isn't for whiners—this is only for those who are ready to take a proverbial leap of faith, who believe that running barefoot is really a gentler way to run. If you don't believe it, you'll tense up, and you won't be able to do it!

This drill will also let you know if you've fully bought into the whole concept of relaxing, of running so gently that you aren't pushing your feet into sharp objects.

So, if you aren't going to sue us for any injuries you do get while doing it in the dark (see the sidebar "Glass, Thorns, and Nails—Oh, My!"), be ready to take your barefoot running to a relaxing new level.

GLASS, THORNS, AND NAILS—OH, MY!

Over the years, I have only had a few splinters of glass, thorns, and one stainless steel screw puncture my soles. It's quite simple to deal with: stop and pull the offending object out of your foot. If it's a screw, unscrew it. And, in most cases, continue running. (Nails have never punctured my soles while running barefoot, but it happened twice while wearing shoes. Because I didn't feel the points of the nails until there was enough pressure to pierce the sole of the shoe, and my sole, the nail went in deep. By contrast, when I once struck a nail while breaking up some old boards with my bare feet—something I no longer recommend unless you're certain they're nail-free and you have adequate instruction in kick-boxing—it barely punctured my sole before my reflexes pulled my foot away.)

The real problem is when you continue running with an object embedded in your foot. It just moves deeper and deeper into the skin. So, remove it as soon as you feel it. There's no more reason for a barefoot runner to be embarrassed about stopping to pull a splinter of glass out of her foot than for a shod runner to bandage up a blister! After all, if you can't accept occasional minor cuts and abrasions, and deal with them in the process of having a really great time running barefoot, then you certainly shouldn't accept blisters from your running shoes, either!

Ultimately, the quantity and depth of objects sticking into our feet is limited by how gently we land. And that's what this book—along with all those nerve endings on the soles of our feet—is about: teaching us to run more gently.

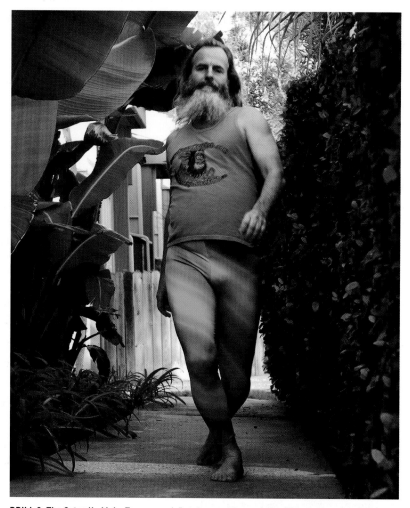

DRILL 9: The Catwalk. Make Tyra pround. Rotate your hips and shoulders in opposite directions. Let your arms move with your shoulders, but do not try to swing them. Place one foot in front of the other. Keep your knees bent.

DRILL 9: THE CAT WALK

Inspired by my cowriter Roy's favorite reality TV show, Tyra Banks's *America's Next Top Model*, this drill emphasizes barefooting's bent knees and opposite-rotating shoulders and hips. For those of you who read books about running, this was referred to as the "Double Spiral" by Balk and Shields in their book *The Art of Running with the Alexander Technique* (2000).

Start with knees bent, keep your torso vertical, and twist your hips one way and your shoulders another. Move your hips forward in front of your feet. Your feet will need to follow your hips. If your left arm was forward, then you should be twisting your torso so that your right arm moves forward, and your left leg should follow your hip.

IMAGERY, DEEP CONJECTURE, ESSENTIAL CONCEPTS, AND ADVICE (IDEAS)

In addition to the aforementioned drills, many good learning tools about running barefoot come in the form of visualizations, analogies, and conceptual approaches. Here are some of the most effective.

IDEA 1: RELAX. NO, *REALLY* RELAX

I can't say it enough: relax, relax, relax. Allow the ankles to go kind of limp, so that the heels touch (gently). If they're "touching" too hard (hitting, striking, jolting, jogging), then it's time to relax more, and allow the knees and hips to bend more. Push those hips down and forward, ahead of your feet. Think of running as a race, with your feet chasing as your hips fall forward.

Slowing Down Will Help Perfect Your Form

Things straighten out when you go fast. It's when you go slowly that things get sloppy. That's why you need to practice running slowly. When you go fast it is more difficult to really analyze what you are doing. To internalize these lessons quicker, you need to think about them, not just react to circumstances. *You* should be in control—not your speed, not the terrain, not your orthotic shoe inserts.

So relax a little. No, on second thought, *relax a lot*. And over time, you'll be able to relax going really fast. That's what happened to me.

My fastest 5K was a 3:33 minute/km pace, at age forty-four, on a very flat course, and it was one of the most relaxed races I've ever run (I was also in excellent condition, just previously having trained for and completed the mostly downhill St. George Marathon in 3:20—50 minutes faster than my previous best marathon).

If we don't relax, we have a tendency to keep running *up*, taller, and taller, until we end up running tippy-toed, with straight, rigid legs, until we have no natural springiness in our step at all. I've seen it thousands of times, the "Frankenstein run," where someone is running as if his knees don't exist (and probably no longer do, in the way they should). One time I watched as an elderly woman, running like the Frankenstein monster to the start line of a 5K race, was using her legs like pogo sticks. There was no discernible bend at all, as if her knees had been welded straight. She was wearing knee braces and a pair of Nike Shox, which have visible springs in the heels. If only she would let her knees bend naturally she wouldn't need springs in her heels, I thought. But as her running partner explained to me later, "She no longer can bend her knees." It's the old "use it or lose it" principle. If we don't let our knees bend sooner, then we might not be able to bend them later.

Running tall is fine—when it's from the hips to the top of our head. Keeping the torso vertical is great. Some of my running partners and I like to imagine a string attached to the top of our heads, with our bodies dangling from the string. But that string isn't pulling us up higher and higher. Instead, it is suspending us "too" low, so that we have to bend our knees and lift our feet to avoid tripping over the ground.

Springs in the top of your body wouldn't help much. That'd be like the old farm tractors in the early 1900s, which had springs in the seat for the comfort of the driver. But the whole tractor was vibrating, shaking, and bouncing with every rev of the engine, and every variation in the surface. Likewise, bending at the waist may cushion some shock to your head, but, besides being a lot of extra work, it doesn't provide any protection for your knees and back.

Bend the Knees

The knees need to bend in order to be all they can be: cushions and batteries, absorbing and storing energy and returning it as we move forward. The ankles should be relaxed, and you should be pulling your foot off the ground (beginning before the foot lands) rather than driving it into the ground, which results if you incorrectly try to push *up* on your toes or the balls of your feet, trying to keep the heels off the ground.

Whether the heels touch or not (during a 3:33/km pace or any other pace, even when walking slowly) is not really the right question to ask. You should be asking whether you are relaxed enough to take advantage of the natural springiness in your calves and quads. And the only way to do that is to experiment. In fifty years of experimenting, this is what I've discovered: If my heels never touch, then I'm not taking full advantage of my natural cushioning, and more important, of the energy these springs store and return naturally with each step (which allows me to move forward more quickly and with less effort).

But if you are doing everything else correctly, this bottoming out of the heels on the ground isn't like a slamming. It should ideally be a continuation of your muscles being activated to start lifting your feet *before* they land. So even when the heels touch, and even though your ankles are relaxed, your knees are continuing to bend as your body moves forward over the foot, which creates a kind of balance that prevents any slamming of the heel (see Drill 6: Bottoming Out the Springs) as your Achilles tendon and calf naturally pull the heel up. At some point, this pulling your foot off the ground will pass the point of decelerating toward the ground, as the foot touches and rests on the ground, and will allow your hips to continue "falling" toward the ground.

Remember the goal of running is to move the body forward, not up and down. So, as you run, you should check the horizon ahead and see if it is bouncing. If it is bouncing, then you can probably pull your feet up sooner and more often (quicker cadence), and relax by letting your hips "fall" down and forward a bit more, which is done by relaxing and allowing the knees to bend. Wear a baseball hat or a sun visor, and try to keep the end of the bill reasonably steady in comparison with the horizon. (Unless there's an earthquake, in which case, just wait for the horizon to steady.)

To find the balance or "sweet" spot, you first have to experiment with going too far (relaxing, and sinking too low) beyond that sweet spot. Learning to run gently is a game; it is play—which is to say, a time of learning and discovery, which we should continue until the end of time (or at least the end of our time).

IDEA 2: THE SWEET SOUND OF YOUR FEET

Lose the iPod and make your own music—you might even scare a dog.

I like atmospheric music, but not headphones. They disconnect me from my running. Many people like to get away from the "drudgery" of running as they try to whittle themselves down to a size 6. But they are missing a symphony: the crunching of the leaves underfoot, the whistle of the wind, the rhythmic in-and-out of your own breathing, the seamless shuffle of your soles lightly touching terra firma. Don't escape running by blocking it out; enjoy it. Even more important, learn from it. If running isn't enjoyable for you, then you haven't figured out how to do it right yet.

In the fifty-some years that I've been running barefoot, analyzing what works and what doesn't, I've come to look at my seventy-six marathons as graduate school. In a marathon, I notice that I start getting tired and floppy after 20 miles (32 km), and that's when I really need to pay attention. It's good to practice running slow (see "Slowing Down Will Help Perfect Your Form" on page 123). And that's also why sound is key.

"Listen closely," advises my good friend Barefoot Julian Romero, Ph.D., who has become a master of making sweet music without shoes, without a shirt, and without an iPod. "Find a perfect, smooth sidewalk on a quiet Sunday morning—and listen to your feet. Pay attention to the noise, like slapping or heel striking. It takes energy to make noise. The more noise your feet make, the more energy you're wasting.

"When I'm smooth and efficient, I can hear the sound of other runners' shoes pounding on the other side of the street," says Julian. "You know you're a good barefoot runner when you scare other runners because they don't hear you when you come up from behind them. When you can scare a dog, you know that you are really good. That really puts a smile on my face."

I don't encourage scaring dogs—that can lead to serious retribution, like the dog scaring you back, or worse. My tactic is both to acknowledge and alert dogs that I am approaching—usually a "Hi, puppy," in a higher-pitched, nonthreatening voice, does the trick. But don't stare at or approach the dog head on. Let her approach you if she's ready. And often, if the dog wants to be my friend (with the owner's approval, of course), I'll stop and give her a little back scratch, which, like running, can be a great stress reliever.

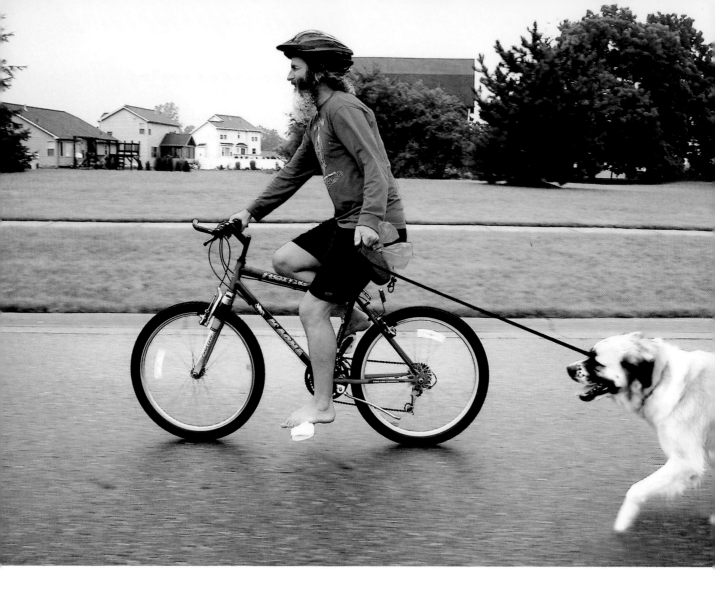

IDEA 3: BETTER BAREFOOTING THROUGH BIKING

Feel. Respond. Adjust. Repeat. Yes, you need to learn "the right way" to do something like running barefoot to replace dangerous movements with safer movements. But you also want to be flexible and responsive to varying conditions, both in the terrain and within your own body. I never had a way to explain this dichotomy until one day I bicycled to work and started playing around with a couple of different ways to pedal:

1. Just push the pedal down and let the circular motion of the pedals control the movement of the feet. It seems like an occasional or inexperienced cyclist would do this.
2. Take control of the motion of the feet by moving them in a circular motion *with* the pedals, as an experienced cyclist would.

The first method results in a rather jerky, uneven, let's say "forced" pedaling motion. The second results in a smoother, more fluid, graceful pedaling motion.

The goal of this drill is not to memorize these motions, but rather to be responsive to the motion of the pedals. That's actually pretty easy, since the pedals always move in precise circles, but you can also play with bending your ankles, changing the angle of your foot as the pedals turn.

How do we apply this lesson to running?

In running, there are no pedals, no crankshaft keeping the pedals (and our feet) in a precise circular motion. But there is the ground, and we definitely do (especially when barefoot) want our feet to land on the ground at precisely the speed and direction the surface is traveling underneath us. Otherwise, there'll be impact and friction between our soles and the ground surface. (Note that the ground is moving backward relative to the runner.)

Like Barefoot Julian says, it's often pretty easy to hear shod runners, especially when they're scuffing their shoes against the roadway. "You wouldn't be wasting energy scuffing your feet like that if you were barefoot," I often tell them as I pass.

So, to land without skidding or sliding, you must take control and responsibility for the motion of your foot. And the best way to accomplish this is to move it in a smooth curve—not really a circle, but more of a flat-bottom oval shape. At the bottom of this oval, the foot should be traveling at precisely the speed and direction the surface is traveling beneath us. When it's done right, it will feel a lot like you're bicycling.

When it's time to lift the foot, we can avoid pushing it back or dragging it along the ground by lifting straight up. As it elevates, the foot's relative backward momentum (in relation to your body) should start to slow, and then start to accelerate as it is automatically pulled foward by your body and leg.

Now, while swinging your leg forward, it is time to do something that seems counter-intuitive: start lifting the foot before it lands. It's easy enough—just bend the knee. Since your body is still falling, it takes time to reverse the direction of the foot, which continues to travel down toward the ground. But in relation to your body, the foot is actually beginning to move up. This relative rise also starts your foot moving backward—the direction the running surface is traveling beneath us. Like an airplane landing, your sole should gently and gracefully touch down; unlike an airplane, however, it won't roll forward on the surface, but stays in one place on the ground and moves backward relative to your forward-moving body. And there you are, back to the same position where you began, except that you're two steps forward.

Again, the goal here is not to try to rigidly or robotically drill the above-described motion into your running, but rather to *feel* how you are moving, and respond by making adjustments and fine-tuning. Ideally, within several steps you'll have progressed to a much smoother, less jerky, more "curvy" motion. Whenever you need to be responsive to unknown terrain, your bare soles give you the cues instantly, so that you can respond appropriately.

IDEA 4: LEARN LIKE A CHILD

A barefoot child learns good running technique without "working" at it. Children naturally respond to the senses in their bodies by playing and experimenting until they find the best technique, just like they learn language: by listening and playing with sounds, so that, eventually, they can imitate the sounds they hear, and later the words of the language in their environment.

But they aren't thinking, "Gee, I have to learn this language so that I can tell my parents what I want for dinner," or "so I can recite Homer's *Iliad* to my luncheon club." They're just being curious children. And from the child's point of view, they have all the time in the world. That is, they aren't so impatient that they want to go out and give an hour-long speech within the first week they begin talking. From a child's point of view, it's all about listening, experimenting, and discovering (between eating, sleeping, and going to the bathroom). When a child is born deaf, however, like my wife was, then learning to speak does require intensive training and conscious effort.

If we have no sensation in the soles of our feet or constantly wear shoes while learning to stand, walk, and later run, we have blocked the nerves in our soles, thus making the process of learning to stand, walk, and run more of a chore, and often requiring some external coaching (much like trying to teach a congenitally deaf child to speak). Since we are not as able to feel the way we are running, someone may need to watch us run and explain to us what should be changed. Otherwise, unless we just happen to get it right, which a few out of the millions of shod children do, the rest of us will probably grow up running rather awkwardly and, at some point in our lives, probably just decide that we weren't "born to run." That's something our friendly neighborhood shoe and orthotic salesperson will be happy to confirm.

It's easy to tell by the sound of the voice whether someone was born deaf and has never been able to hear or accurately imitate the sound of human speech. Likewise, there are plenty of runners who have clearly never run barefoot, especially on rough, hard surfaces. And it's obvious, because they run as if they expect their shoes, or the running surface, to protect them from impact and abrasion.

But most of us have a choice, and once we remove our shoes it often takes a bit of time to figure out how to interpret what our soles are telling us. Our habit, from years of wearing shoes, is to try to ignore the pain, so that we can continue running the way we learned (with the senses in our soles muffled by shoes).

Alternatively, we can take the time to relearn, and pay attention to what our soles are telling us. As I've said many times, this could be a short or long time, but it is the most important time, and it is the reason I encourage folks to start with short, slow distances, even just standing and walking at first, on hard, rough, uncomfortable surfaces. The idea is to "think" like a child who is learning to run barefoot. It is not to think, "How will I ever be able to finish a 26.2-mile (42 km) marathon running barefoot by next month?"

It is when we can get in the frame of mind of ourselves as children (some of us never left) that we are most open to learning. At that stage, it isn't "work" and doesn't require "thinking." It's all about curiosity, experimenting, and of course, fun!

With your mind in a childlike state, running barefoot on rough surfaces will teach so much more about technique, because a child pays attention now, instead of thinking about how far he'll be running next week. The adult in us is often reluctant to abandon all those sloppy techniques we learned after decades in shoes. We're thinking, "I've invested so much time running this way, all I need is the 'right' pair of shoes so I can continue." But it isn't about the shoes; it's about the technique.

Shoes don't damage your body; they simply mask the sensations from your soles that would tell you when you are running destructively. Think of shoes like a silk blindfold. It's very comfortable. And it prevents us from seeing where we're going, so we can drive in ignorant bliss. But we should be seeing where we're heading, especially if it looks like we're heading for a collision! And that's exactly why, whenever practical, we should be running barefoot.

I give advice on technique because, after some fifty years of running barefoot (at least part of the time), twenty of those mostly barefoot, and twelve years of intensive running nearly exclusively barefoot* more than most people run in shoes, I'm still learning and hopefully improving.

The technique tips in this chapter are for those who perhaps are a bit less intuitive or just less patient, or don't have a good hard, rough surface to run on, or don't want to take the time a child does to learn. A shortcut, yes—like taking any class. You still need to study, but you start with some direction. Why spend fifty years of your life reinventing the wheel (as I have)? Besides, it's better than the shortcut of blocking the sensation from your soles with shoes or drugs to avoid the learning process altogether and ending up unable to run later due to chronic injuries.

Anyway, as I've said, the best way to learn *how* to run barefoot is to *run barefoot*, especially on surfaces that wake up the nerves in your soles, and the child in your brain, so that learning to run barefoot becomes a game where the goal is to adapt to the surface, and make those adaptations habit, so that when you get on a smooth, comfortable surface, you "instinctively" run without pounding or skidding. But the instinct isn't really an instinct for running; just as humans do not have an instinct to not stick our hand in a flame, the true instinct is simple: to avoid pain. Our instinct teaches us many things, like not sticking your hand in a flame, and that running gently is the safest way to run!

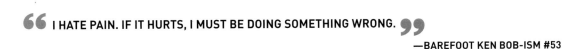

I HATE PAIN. IF IT HURTS, I MUST BE DOING SOMETHING WRONG.

—BAREFOOT KEN BOB-ISM #53

*I ran a total of nearly 30 miles [48 km] in shoes since 1998—about 28 [45 km] of that in 1998.

IDEA 5: WATCH YOUR LANGUAGE

Before you start running barefoot, you should understand that a lot of the language you learned from running in shoes perpetuates bad running. If you don't eliminate some questionable words, they have too much power to conjure up the wrong images, the wrong impression of what running barefoot is about. Examples:

Foot strike: If you like your feet and the earth, you won't "strike" them against each other. Let your foot "touch" or "kiss" or "land on" the ground gently.

Endurance: Running barefoot isn't something that you should "endure." Running barefoot, once you start listening to your feet, should be enjoyable.

Jogging: The only term I hate more then "jogging" is the new marketing deception, "barefoot shoes!" To jog something, according to *Webster's*, is to "jar," to "pound," to "strike," to "hit," to "upset." Running barefoot will naturally be a smoother, more graceful motion than jogging, because your soles will complain immediately when you are *jogging*!

Language is a reflection of our thinking, and often guides our thinking. The words we use to describe our actions affect the way we think about the things we do—and the way we do them. So when we use seemingly innocent words and phrases like "pounding the pavement" or "hammering out a few miles," it is no wonder that we so readily accept the misconception that running is a high-impact activity. That's why it's important to carefully choose the words we use to describe running barefoot.

"Pounding" and "impact" are so ingrained in our vocabulary about running that it is difficult to separate them from any discussion about running. This is my recollection of a conversation I have had many times with runners.

Curious runner: "How can you run barefoot? I mean, what about the pounding?"

Ken Bob: "I avoid pounding because my bare soles teach me to run gently."

Curious runner: "I understand that, but what about the impact?"

Shoe companies aren't about to discourage this misconception, often touting figures like "the average runner strikes the ground with several times his or her body weight and pushes off with two to three times his or her body weight." (I even found seven or eight times the body weight cited in an article at www.ehow.com/how_2034732_reduce-impact-running.html, along with other misleading phrases like "hit the trails" and "hinge forward at the hip.") My "foot landing/push-off" was measured in Dr. Daniel Lieberman's lab as less than twice my body weight, but that peak pressure isn't even the real problem; it's how quickly that pressure is loaded—the difference between a gentle nudge and a collision.

The Myth of Jogging

Let's examine "jogging" a little more. Older runners remember the start of the "jogging" craze back in the early 1970s. The word *jogging* has been so overused since then to simply describe slow running that many have forgotten the criticisms and why it was called "jogging" in the first place. I have nothing against running slowly; a lot of long slow miles are great. But to do that safely and enjoyably, we must learn how to run without pounding, without the sensation of jogging.

From the time jogging first became a synonym for running, experts were warning us that we were bouncing and that our internal organs were being "jogged" up and down with each impact. As it turns out, it's worse than they thought: our joints are getting "jogged" (and jolted, hammered, and beaten up), too. Knee and back injuries are rampant among runners today—and strangely accepted. We are more likely to accept the idea that most runners will eventually require knee surgery than the idea that we are simply running badly and should change the way we run. And many ex-runners might still be happily running today if not for chronic knee or back pain and injuries acquired while running—or in these cases, let's do say "jogging!"

So I suggest we start a new definition to replace *jogging*. Perhaps the term *jogging* should be avoided for a generation. Most people probably won't notice the not-so-subtle difference until the usage of "jogging" as a synonym for running has faded and people have accepted that running isn't bad. Jogging is!

Instead of jogging, say "running slowly" or "running easily." There's nothing wrong with including slow or easy running in the definition of running. But there is something wrong with assuming slow running is "jogging."

Instead of foot "strike," maybe we could use words like "landing" or "touching" or "caressing," none of which legitimize the debilitating "pounding," "hammering," or "striking," and all of which encourage a smooth interaction with the ground.

As I mentioned, hearing barefoot runners describing their foot landing to others as a "ball-of-foot strike" rather than a "heel strike" drives me up the wall. As with jogging, "strike" assumes that impact is a natural part of running, like it is in, say, boxing. Runners who have never run barefoot on a hard surface frequently assume there ought to be a huge impact while running barefoot. Let's go to *Webster's* again:

> *striking; noun, adjective, verb (used with object)*
> *to deal a blow or stroke to, as with the fist, a weapon, or a hammer*
> *to drive so as to cause impact*
> *to thrust forcibly*

Yikes! It's pretty clear that "striking" the ground is going to hurt too much while running barefoot, and in the long term it's likely to cause injury, even in shoes. The problem here is that even if you have been running with shoes for decades, running barefoot really is a new activity. And as with most new activities, it has a new vocabulary to learn. More importantly, running barefoot requires us to start thinking about running in a whole new way. After all, we might talk about the slow, plodding, jarring, heel-striking strides of joggers in heavily cushioned shoes, but jogging would be very uncomfortable while running barefoot.

The images we paint with our words, especially with the Internet available to so many people, can be seen by millions, perhaps billions, of people, and these people will carry those images away from their computers, or this book, on their next run. So, by calling a gentle foot landing a "foot strike," many people curious to try running barefoot will get the wrong idea about it. They might go out for a barefoot run, slam their bare feet into the ground just as they did in cushioned shoes, get the idea that they're not tough enough to endure the pain of running barefoot, and give it up. Running barefoot might have saved that guy's running career if he'd used the right words to describe it.

Or worse, he might have continued, as many do, believing the pain is something he's supposed to get used to, or block with drugs, in order to run.

Two Coaches: One Left, One Right, Both Correct

One day I was running—barefoot, naturally—down the Santa Ana River bike path in Newport Beach, when I passed an elderly fellow walking along. He yelled at me, "You'd better not do that, I blew my knees out running barefoot on the beach. I thought the soft sand was protecting me from the impact, but it wasn't!"

He was right. The soft beach sand didn't protect him from impact any more than soft running shoes do. They just make us less aware of the impact, so we don't feel or respond to it immediately, allowing us to run ignorantly and blissfully until our knees give out. But if our sensitive bare soles aren't allowed to alert us about impact, the impact just moves on up, and our knees let us know later.

By then, we've so habitually ingrained our running technique that it's really difficult to change. If only we could find and afford a coach who could follow us around every time we ran, and tell us when we need to correct our technique. The cool thing is that most of us came with *two* such coaches.

Contrary to popular opinion, I am not "tough," nor do I need to be tough to run barefoot. I'm actually a wimp! I run barefoot because I find I'm not tough enough, or callused enough, to run any kind of distance with shoes torturing my feet. It is the great deal of natural sensitivity in my soles (my two coaches) that encourages me to run very lightly, gently, softly, smoothly, and efficiently. It is the light, gentle, soft, smooth, efficient running, which I learned while barefoot, that allows me to run barefoot faster and farther and longer than the average shod runner can. I was running much longer and faster in my forties than when I was pushing insensitive rubber soles into the ground while occasionally running in shoes into my mid-thirties. Which brings me to the topic of "push-off."

Don't Be a "Push-Off"

There really is no need to consciously push our bodies up into the air while running. It's mostly a waste of effort, and results in greater impact upon landing, as the push against the ground to launch your body is precisely the same push into the ground as the foot strikes (and in this case, the foot actually is "striking" the ground). But, many of us, through ChiRunning, Pose Method, or Evolution Running, or simply by listening to our own bare feet, have discovered that it's so much easier (which means we can actually run faster and farther on less energy) to simply lift the feet, rather than attempt to launch the body into the air.

After all, the direction we want to travel while running is forward. Any unnecessary up and down (or side to side) movement of the body (or one might say, diversion of our "center of balance" from its desired forward path) is counterproductive to our goal (forward movement). So think of the body moving forward, horizontally, rather than "jogging" up and down, and simply lift your feet and continue traveling forward.

"Joggers" need to launch their body forward with each step because they reach out in front and wait for their foot to crash into the ground, hitting the brakes at the beginning of each step. "Jogging" is like a series of broad jumps—leaping up and forward, with a jolting landing disrupting forward momentum, again and again, rather than a smooth continuous forward motion.

The trick besides faster cadence is to use your forward momentum by leading with our body, rather than interrupting your forward momentum by leading with your foot.

So, I don't want to hear any more talk about the foot "strike" or "pounding" or "impact" of running, at least not from any barefoot runners. The words we choose are important. When we think about our feet "touching" the ground, instead of "hitting" the ground, it becomes much easier to run gracefully. When we think of ourselves as "running smoothly, efficiently, and gently," instead of "jogging," that relentless jarring feeling in our ankles, knees, back, and head that used to accompany every run will quickly recede into distant memory, where it belongs.

IDEA 6: IMAGERY: TRAIN PISTONS, FAIRY FEET, AND FAT TODDLERS

You may have heard barefoot runners talk about analogies like running on hot coals, running down stairs, and prancing like a ballerina on your toes. Well, imagery definitely helps people "get" running barefoot, and the more the better. Three of the best images I've ever heard of came to me in this email.

I have noticed that the movement of my feet feel rather like the pistons of a train, and then my arms start to make the same kind of piston movement. So I imagine that my feet are just spinning around in little circles, hardly touching the ground ("fairy feet" as one of my friends recently called it).

When I really got into this image I was able to kick up the speed a little. (I am not, by nature, a speedy runner.) And I wasn't "trying" to run faster—it just happened. (Oh, there was some mention recently of running faster by pushing the hips forward. You can also go faster by engaging your arms more; when you consciously pump your arms/shoulders, that translates into more rotational movement of your spine/pelvis and increased speed results without having to work your legs more.)

This train image then translated into the image of a toddler with little legs just going nineteen to the dozen, and we all know how fast toddlers can run!

During the times when this imagery stayed with me, my steps felt lighter, less contact with the ground. There was also a moment when I thought my calf was going to tighten, and I imagined the back of my leg was a material that could soften and lengthen (taffy is a good image) so that my heel could then "soften" into the ground. That worked too, and the potential tightness went away.

We all have to find language and ideas and images that work for us: "doing," "not-doing," "feeling," "sensing," "creating pictures," "hearing."

Thanks for all the continued information and sharing. And I have to admit that I am feeling a joy in this running that I never felt before. I was never a "lover" of running (even though I have enjoyed partaking in races and doing marathons). I have been in the shower after a VFF (Vibram FiveFingers) or BF (barefoot) run and want to go straight out again (though, of course, shouldn't—not yet, anyway). And while I still have a-ways to go getting my feet conditioned, I am loving the feeling of my bare feet on the ground!

—feldyjan, January 7, 2010

IDEA 7: FINALLY, CLEANSE THY SOLES

The first question many people ask me, "Can I see the bottoms of your feet?" is often followed by the more urgent question, especially among people who plan to start running, walking, or just standing around barefoot outside the house: "How do you clean those things?"

Keep in mind that your shoes may also be dirty, but this book isn't about running in shoes, or the etiquette of keeping your shoes clean. That would be far too daunting a task to take on in a book of this scope.

But there are some important tricks to cleaning your soles, which may help keep your spouse, parents, or kids from wanting to kill you!

Much of this is just about being considerate. Example: Let's say a friend has adapted the custom of requiring guests to remove their shoes before entering her home, which is totally carpeted in white. In this case, at the entryway, when everyone else is removing their shoes, I put my socks *on*. If my soles are especially dirty or black, I put on thick, clean socks of natural fibers like cotton or wool, which absorb dirt and odor better. Dirt can easily work its way through thin socks.

At home, to keep your floors reasonably clean, the ideal would be to have a little footbath at your front door. But this is rare, even when practical. So, below you'll find some practical advice to help preserve your household's sanity, keep your floors relatively unsmudged, and maybe even keep your feet cleaner. (Notice I said "cleaner," not "clean." You will probably not be able to keep your feet clean. Even wearing shoes, our feet get "dirty," given that the inside of a shoe is ideal for incubating fungus and many kinds of bacteria. So, even if your feet appear clean, they probably aren't.)

Most of us will want to wash our feet, at least occasionally, and especially after running on asphalt, trails, or anywhere in a large city. So let's start before we enter the abode, then work our way inside.

1 **RUN IN THE WET.**
One of the best ways to get your feet clean, when circumstances are right, is to run a few miles, barefoot, on a wet surface (rainy street or sidewalk or low tide at the beach). Once, I ran a marathon on rough roads in the rain; a picture of me a few miles into the race, from behind, showed that my soles were sparkling clean.

2 **BE A PUDDLE JUMPER.**
If there is a hose, a nice puddle of water, or even a wet or damp lawn a short distance before you get to your door, then take advantage of it. Stand in the puddle. Soak your feet. Be sure to lift your feet (one at a time) to let the water get under your feet and to gently "scrub" your soles (not by rubbing, just by lifting and setting your feet down). Hopefully this puddle is on a relatively clean concrete, asphalt, or other hard, non-dirt, surface.

3 **GET IMMEDIATE SHOWER ACCESS.**

It would also be great if you have a shower or bath near your front door, before you get to the carpet. Whenever you come in from a barefoot outing, instead of taking off your shoes, head for the bathroom and wash your feet. We have a bathroom with a shower right next to our front door.

4 **SCRUB YOUR FEET CORRECTLY.**

The only problem with my shower is that it's made of plastic, not porcelain. Plastic bathtubs and showers, which dirt can easily be ground into simply by twisting a dirty heel while standing in the tub, require a bit of special care, although the same technique can be used in porcelain or ceramic tubs and showers, too.

- It's a good idea to keep a scrub sponge (the kind with a scrubbing surface on one side) in your bath or shower. This also makes a good soap holder, and after each shower, the wet bar of soap soaks into the sponge and this keeps the sponge saturated with soap. Liquid soap could be squirted onto the sponge as an alternative or supplement.
- Get the shower or tub floor wet, before stepping in.
- Step carefully; don't twist or slide your feet (pretend you're standing on a cheese grater and don't want to remove the skin from your soles). By the way, this is good practice in the course of your barefoot outings, to help avoid blisters.
- Now, you're standing in the tub or shower on a wet floor, and, as with the puddle outside, you should be lifting and setting your feet down gently, and remember, if you don't want to grind dirt into your tub or shower, no skidding, scuffing, twisting, or grinding.
- Now, take the soap-soaked scrub sponge, and use it to apply soap to your soles. Do *not* scrub vigorously: you want to save your skin for running barefoot, so scrub very gently, and let the soap and water do the work.
- Scrub your toenails gently, too.
- Repeat with the other foot.
- Rinse and dry, and be sure to dry between the toes, too.
- Basically, we should treat our feet with the same respect we treat our hands. Wash them gently, but regularly.

5 **CLEAN THE HOUSE BAREFOOT.**
Another way to clean your feet is to clean your bathtub, mop your floors, and steam clean your carpet, all while barefoot. Besides, we really should do more than our share of keeping the house clean in order to eliminate the least bit of argument that going barefoot contributes to a dirty home, at least among members and guests of your household.

6 **BE A BETTER BATHER.**
We should treat our personal hygiene well, showering and/or bathing often. Barefoot runners should smell better than nearly anyone who wears shoes, and it's really not very difficult, considering how much shoes stink!

Videos or links to videos illustrating some of these drills, dances, play, and concepts can be found at BarefootRunningStepbyStep.com, along with new ones as we discover or make them up.

SAXEY IMAGES

Some of the most helpful running barefoot imagery we've come across was sent to us by Robert Saxe, Ph.D., a sixty-six-year-old retired marketing research consultant and father of two from La Cañada Flintridge, California. After running for three decades, Saxe developed knee pain in 2005 and did not run from 2008 to 2010. Then, he read about Daniel Lieberman's persistence-hunting research, came across Ken Bob's site, and tried barefoot running. His knee pain instantly disappeared, and he is back to running and racing regularly. Here are some of the imaginative visualizations that ran through his mind in the early days of transitioning from a total beginner to an advanced beginner.

1. SPARE THE ANTS: Run gently, so that you won't hurt ants if you step on them.

2. GO EASY ON MOM: Run as if you were running on someone's skin. Perhaps on Mother Nature's back, or on the palm of her hand.

3. TURN FEET INTO HANDS, NOT SHOES: At first, I thought that as I ran more I would make my feet like shoes, by toughening the skin on the soles of the feet. Then I thought that was wrong, that the idea was to make the feet like hands—sensitive and intelligently linked to the brain. After all, the more intelligent the feet become, the less tough they need to be. But now I realize that both of these are needed—the feet need to be toughened but also to be used sensitively and intelligently. It's similar to the way guitarists need to have callused yet sensitive fingers.

4. GET TO KNOW YOUR TOES: As I gained more experience, I began to understand the function of the toes—for balance, for feeling the ground, for adjusting the landing, for gripping like fingers. Before, I felt like they had no real function; in fact, when they're inside shoes, they don't seem to have much of a function. This also might relate to my arches getting stronger and deeper from barefooting; flat, weakened arches would seem to put less pressure on the toes.

5. THINK "DANCE": I like the idea of dancing around obstacles rather than always having a regular, mechanical stride. It's also nice to think of running as producing a gentle, harmonious, relaxed, rhythmic yet varied form, like a dance.

6. A FAMILIAR OLD CROUCH: The bent-knee stance of barefoot running reminds me a bit of the crouch used in many other sports, such as wrestling, basketball, and racquetball.

7. IT'S LIKE LEARNING PIANO: Learning to run barefoot reminds me of learning how to type, or play an instrument, or get into a new sport—every few days or weeks there is a new plateau to break through, new learning to build on what you've learned before. Sometimes I think I've got it, and stop concentrating on technique for a while, and then I realize I've got a lot more to learn, and go back to trying to improve my form.

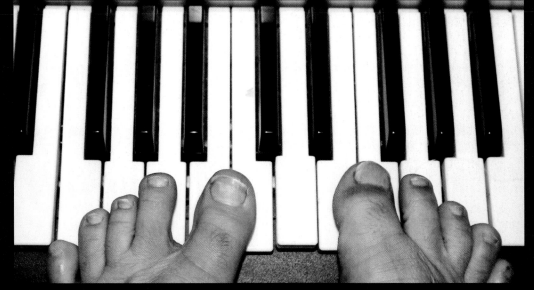

Key point: Barefoot running is a skill that you continually refine and develop. You won't play Beethoven from the beginning, but in time, your running will be a beautiful symphony of coordination, efficiency, and grace.

8. BE ONE WITH THE ROCKS: When first running on trails and roads, I would watch carefully to see rocks and other road hazards, and carefully avoid running on them. Recently, however, I sometimes experiment with deliberately running over various size rocks, on various parts of my feet, to see how it feels. Often they do not hurt. I am trying to learn how to land on obstacles safely, to learn which ones I can run on and which ones I need to avoid.

9. BE A HUMAN WASHING MACHINE: I found that running "relaxed" while running with short, quick steps at 180+ steps per minute, both of which Ken Bob emphasizes, can be difficult to do at the same time. For practice, I've found that it helps me to learn his mantra of "relax, relax, relax" by concentrating on a very gentle footfall, while moving at a very slow, sub-180-step pace. I think of it like the "delicate" cycle on a washing machine—gentle/slow. Then I try to increase the steps per minute while maintaining the relaxed feeling. Summary: Relax first, then up the cadence.

10. FINALLY, ENJOY THE FEELING: Barefoot running gives you a new start, so you can be happy just being able to run and do something difficult without being concerned with setting personal bests.

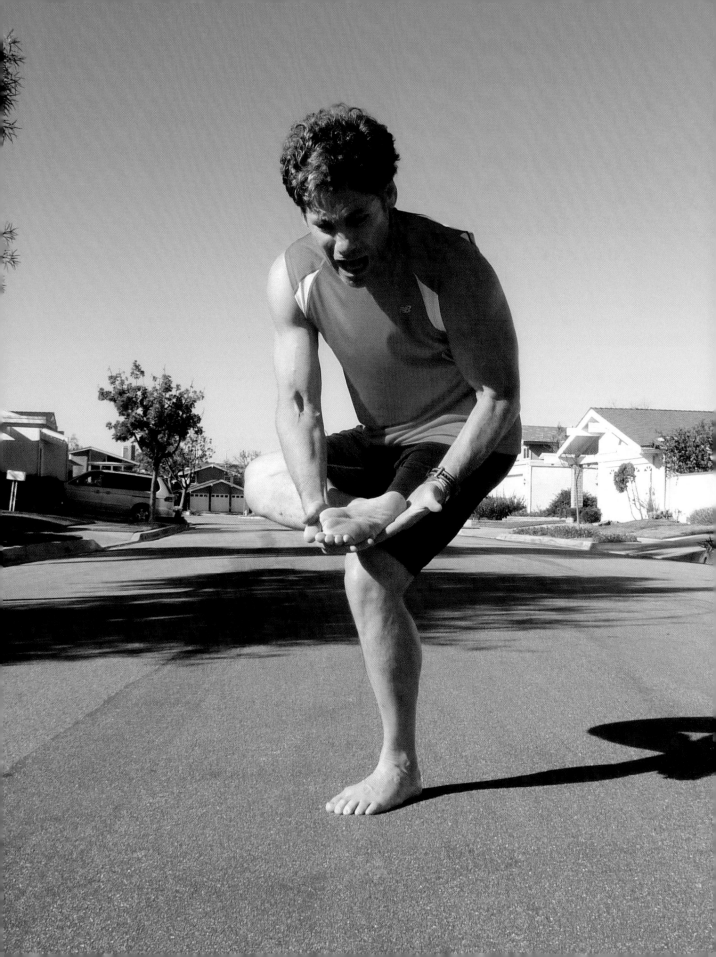

CHAPTER 5

BEWARE OF BAREFOOT RUNNING EXUBERANCE SYNDROME
TOO MUCH TOO SOON CAN DERAIL YOUR PROGRESS

Yes, running barefoot is addictive and exhilarating the moment you try it. But the new biomechanics will make you pay if you don't take it slow. Here's a plan.

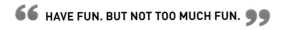 **HAVE FUN. BUT NOT TOO MUCH FUN.**

—KEN BOB-ISM #67

"The first thing I noticed on my first barefoot run was the change in my running stride—no more heel-to-toe foot strike," said Eric Vouga of Ingleside, Illinois. "The second thing I noticed was that I felt light and fast—gazellelike—total exhilaration. The third thing I noticed was that my feet were beginning to feel like they were on fire. I wanted to keep running, but I couldn't. My feet were screaming at me. My calves were screaming at me." It took three months, with several bouts of foot and calf soreness, and a couple of blisters, before he could build back up to his previous shod mileage.

Vouga's experience is typical of new barefooters: They get so excited that they do too much too soon. And why wouldn't they? When you run barefoot, your toes spread wide and airy, your unleashed sensors fire with thousands of dazzling new inputs each second, your mind floods with sensations of wonder and happiness, and you tend to run much lighter. People often say they feel like a child, or a wild animal, or connected to the earth—free, exhilarated, empowered, more alive than they've ever felt. In a word, running barefoot is incredibly fun. It makes you feel exuberant. It feels so good that you want to do more and more of it. You don't want it to stop. And you won't—until your body hurts so bad that it will make you stop. For some people—maybe most people, like Vouga—this situation occurs on their very first barefoot run.

Do you know how many times I've heard stories like Vouga's—stories of wild exuberance gone bad? So many that I made up a name for it: B.R.E.S., the Barefoot Running Exuberance Syndrome. (Note: The "E" in B.R.E.S. could also stand for eagerness, ebullience, ecstasy, effervescence, elation, electrification, elevation, enchantment, enhancement, enthusiasm, enjoyment, euphoria, exaltation, excessiveness, excitement, or exhilaration.)

B.R.E.S. is a very real threat to new barefooters. They go from a giddy high to a pain-wracked crash. The new biomechanics giveth, and the new biomechanics taketh away— often within the same run. Body parts that have been unused or underused for years while performing the heel strike of shod running—the calves and other muscles, which I'll detail later—are knocked for a loop. Even people who sort of know they have to take it gradually, like supposedly analytical journalists, get caught up in B.R.E.S. It happened to my cowriter Roy when he first ran on the beach bike path for 3 miles (4.8 km) with me in 2004; he was thrilled that day, but his calves and Achilles tendons were crying the next.

What's that calf pain feel like? I don't know because I never really had it (just a little soreness once when I stayed way up on the balls of my feet for a couple of miles straight after bruising my heel on a rock), but I've heard descriptions like "a thousand needles piercing my soleus" and "brutalized slabs of muscle being crowbarred off my tibias." One of the most vivid descriptions I've seen of the hellish morning after came from writer Bill Gifford in a June 2010 story in *Men's Journal*. He reported that the day after his first barefoot run, a hilly 3½-miler (5.6 km) with *Born to Run* author Christopher McDougall, "I woke up feeling like someone had driven six-inch nails through each of my calf muscles."

Yikes. No wonder Robert Forster, a well-known Santa Monica physical therapist, was quoted as saying that he loves people to take up barefoot running "because it gets me more clients."

I could have very well addressed B.R.E.S. and the advice about how to fight it in chapter 4, rather than make it the sole subject of a separate chapter. But as someone who hopes to see all runners take advantage of the great benefits of running barefoot, I am genuinely alarmed by B.R.E.S.'s potential to turn thousands of people away from barefooting before they have a chance to find out how good it is.

When people get injured quickly, many won't follow Eric Vouga's example and figure out what they're doing wrong. Instead they give up or go to a doctor or physical therapist who encourages them to stop. Soon, they're back in shoes, back to the same problems, or out of running forever. South African exercise physiologist Ross Tucker, Ph.D., coauthor of *The Runner's Body*, estimates, that out of a hundred rookie barefooters, at least thirty people will pick up an injury that forces a long layoff or a return to shoes. Though we're skeptical of Tucker's estimates, we do suspect that most such cases are due to B.R.E.S.

So, to help you temper your exuberance about running barefoot before you end up abandoning it, we've underscored the danger of B.R.E.S. by giving it its own chapter. The B.R.E.S. message is twofold: Learn the proper technique, and don't go too far, too fast, too soon. Or, as I also like to say, "Have fun, but not too much fun."

That means keep it in perspective. The first time you do any new physical activity or any old physical activity you haven't done in years, you hurt like crazy the next day. That applies across the board, whether it's hiking up a mountain, digging a ditch, shoveling snow, or riding a mountain bike. You haven't played tennis in fifteen years? You're gonna feel it the next day. But running barefoot presents a particularly unique problem for most beginners: Because they've already been running for many years, they think they already know how to run barefoot. They think that they don't have to learn anything.

Well, that's baloney. Barefoot running is so different from shod running that it's practically a new sport. To enjoy it injury free at the beginning, you need a new technique—and a new attitude.

A HARD LESSON TO LEARN

All this won't be easy. Experienced runners who've been hammering 5 miles (8 km) a day in shoes for years will naturally think they can instantly keep hammering 5 miles (8 km) a day barefoot. In fact, it feels so darn good, so exhuberating, they might want to do even more. On their maiden barefoot voyage, the last thing a newbie wants to do is throttle back, ease into it, go slow, and gradually learn the nuances of the new technique. Then comes the evil morning after . . .

This is why, incidentally, I've often found that the easiest people to teach barefoot running to are non-runners. They don't have any bad habits to break or an unreasonable expectation to bolt out of the gate and do 25 miles (40 km) a week. They're happy doing maybe 200 yards (182 m) at first, then ease up to 1 mile (1.6 km) while learning to run more gently, all pain free. After a month, they're up to a 3-mile (4.8 km) run.

Longtime shod runners, by contrast, usually don't have the patience and don't have the right emphasis. Many of them tend to erroneously assume that the main issue involved in the barefoot transition is toughening up their soles. It's not. Yes, your soles are pale and weak and thoroughly wimpy after years cloistered in shoes, but they are surprisingly resilient and learn fast. Teaching the soles proper barefoot running is easy: Just listen to the pain. Pain teaches you to pull your hands out of the fire. In barefooting, it teaches you that a rock hurts when you tense up as you land on it and that you need to distribute your weight across as many points of the soles as possible to lessen the sting. And guess what? You *will* do this successfully almost instantly if you relax.

If you're lucky, you will have unusually sensitive soles that will tell you when to stop before anything is injured. If you aren't so lucky, you'll go too far and maybe end up with blisters. In either case, the soles are not the big problem area with B.R.E.S..

Biomechanics is. Relearning your long-forgotten natural physiology is. Fixing up what the past twenty years in running shoes with 1½ inches (3.8 cm) of heel padding that encouraged you to heel strike is.

Overcoming ingrained and improper biomechanics is not hard in itself. One barefoot landing on your heel on asphalt, concrete, or a pointy rock goes a long way toward curing you of heel striking forever; you'll naturally want to switch to a ball-of-the-foot landing. Unfortunately, it won't be perfect. Your body and its muscles have spent decades adapting to the function of an unnatural heel landing in a shoe with an unnaturally elevated heel cushion. They've spent years overdeveloping the quads and underdeveloping the calves and Achilles tendons, leaving them shorter and weaker than they would be barefoot. So they certainly won't be familiar with barefoot biomechanics, in which the knees bend more, changing the angle of the foot at contact with the ground, the calves and Achilles are finally allowed to flex and work, and potentially more leverage is placed on the metatarsals (especially when not following my advice to relax the calves).

You might not notice these stresses at first, unless you're taking my advice to play on rough or gravel surfaces. Stressed-out calves often will not scream with acute pain unlike the soles do when you step on a sharp rock—that is, until later in the day, after you've run too many miles, or the next day, when you cannot get up out of your chair and walk without gasping and whimpering.

As Dr. Timothy Noakes, author of *Lore of Running*, found out in his 2003 study of Pose/barefoot runners (which found up to 50 percent less shock to the knees; see chapter 2), the bent knee and forefoot landing decrease the eccentric loading on the knee joint and the quads, and increase it on the ankle, calves, and Achilles tendons. This change in muscle activity so frequently results in injury that warnings are now routinely issued about it.

In fact, Dr. Daniel Lieberman's research group put the following go-slow warning on the front page of its pro-barefoot running website after his 2004 article in *Nature*, about how humans evolved as a long distance runner, was published: *"Please note that we present no data on how people should run, whether shoes cause some injuries, or whether barefoot running causes other kinds of injuries."*

On the other hand, thousands of barefoot runners, sharing our experiences through The Running Barefoot website and forums for more than a decade, have figured out how to avoid these pains and injuries. These concepts, reviewed, analyzed, and tested by me personally, are what we are sharing with you in the pages of this book, so that your transition need not be injurious or painful—well, except for those short bits of "learning" pain in your soles reminding you that you aren't finished yet!

THE ANTI-B.R.E.S. TRAINING PLAN

Many of the attendees of my workshops told me that the reason they showed up was not necessarily to meet me (oh, well), but to figure out how to avoid the calf and Achilles pain and metatarsal stress fractures that accompanied their earlier attempts at barefooting or running in Vibrams. (I have my own opinion about the dangers of Vibrams, which far exceed those of barefooting; see chapter 6.)

Many also ask me for a training plan that will help smooth their transition into running barefoot. They often ask about doing blended, part-barefoot/part-shod workouts, which I personally would never do and am against from an ideological and practical point of view. However, while I believe that any shod running somewhat corrupts the barefoot transition, the reality is that some people do not want to give up their mileage. For those lucky few who don't get injured from running in shoes and don't wish to make use of cross-training to fill in the fitness gap (a strong recommendation of my friend Preston Curtis; see chapter 10), we have provided a blended program below.

Your first step is to identify which one of three categories of runner you are. After that, go to step 2 and find the plan that fits you.

STEP 1: WHAT CATEGORY OF RUNNER ARE YOU?

1. A veteran shod runner sick of getting injured.

2. A first-time runner intrigued by running barefoot.

3. A veteran runner with no history of injuries, who is just curious about running barefoot or improving technique.

1 INJURED VETERAN SHOD RUNNERS

If you're one of the many who is constantly getting injured from running, with regular knee, back, and other pain, I advise you to throw away your shoes for good and exclusively run barefoot. You might start with about 300 yards (273 m) of barefooting and work up from there, depending on how your body adapts, and fill in your exercise needs with cross-training activities until your barefoot mileage rises.

After all, why continue running in shoes if it injures you and could leave you permanently disabled? If you do a blended barefoot/shod workout and remain injured, you'll never know whether the barefoot portion is actually helping or not.

2 NEW RUNNERS

If you've never run before, you're in luck! You never need to buy a pair of running shoes. You can start on the same gradual barefoot program as the injured runners do, but will probably have an easier time of it, since you have no bad habits to unlearn and should have no unreasonable cravings to immediately do big miles. You have a natural limit on B.R.E.S.

3 CURIOUS, NONINJURED VETERAN SHOD RUNNERS

If you're one of the few who never get injured running in shoes ("yet," as my friend Dr. Irene Davis likes to add), but have the foresight to plan for an uninjured future, you can stay in shape while you learn to run barefoot by employing a blended program. (Again, I want to be on record as being in favor of pure barefooting for *everyone*, injury prone or not, during the transition, with cross-training filling in the fitness gaps rather than shod running. But if you insist . . .) This plan will start with 5 minutes of before-and-after barefooting, sandwiching your normal shod running workout, and gradually increase. This allows you to dial in the forefoot-first landing before you put on your shoes, and ratchet up your percentage of barefooting over the weeks and months until you can go 100 percent. Even when not running, you should play with technique—practice relaxing your calves, standing with your torso vertical, unlocking your knees, reviewing the concepts in this book, etc.

STEP 2: FIND THE SAMPLE TRAINING PLAN THAT FITS YOU

For Injured Runners and Rookie Barefooters

	WEEK 1	WEEK 2	WEEK 3	WEEK 4
MON	5 min barefoot run	10 min barefoot run	15 min barefoot run	20 min barefoot run
WED	5 min barefoot run	15 min barefoot run	15 min barefoot run	20 min barefoot run
FRI	10 min barefoot run	15 min barefoot run	20 min barefoot run	25 min barefoot run

For Noninjured Veteran Runners

	WEEK 1	WEEK 2	WEEK 3	WEEK 4
MON	3 min barefoot/30 min regular shod run/3 min barefoot	7 min barefoot/22 min regular shod run/7 min barefoot	8 min barefoot/20 min regular shod run/8 min barefoot	15 min barefoot/11 min regular shod run/10 min barefoot
WED	5 min barefoot/26 min regular shod run/5 min barefoot	7 min barefoot/22 min regular shod run/7 min barefoot	10 min barefoot/16 min regular shod run/10 min barefoot	15 min barefoot/11 min regular shod run/10 min barefoot
FRI	5 min barefoot/26 min regular shod run/5 min barefoot	8 min barefoot/20 min regular shod run/8 min barefoot	10 min barefoot/16 min regular shod run/10 min barefoot	30 min barefoot

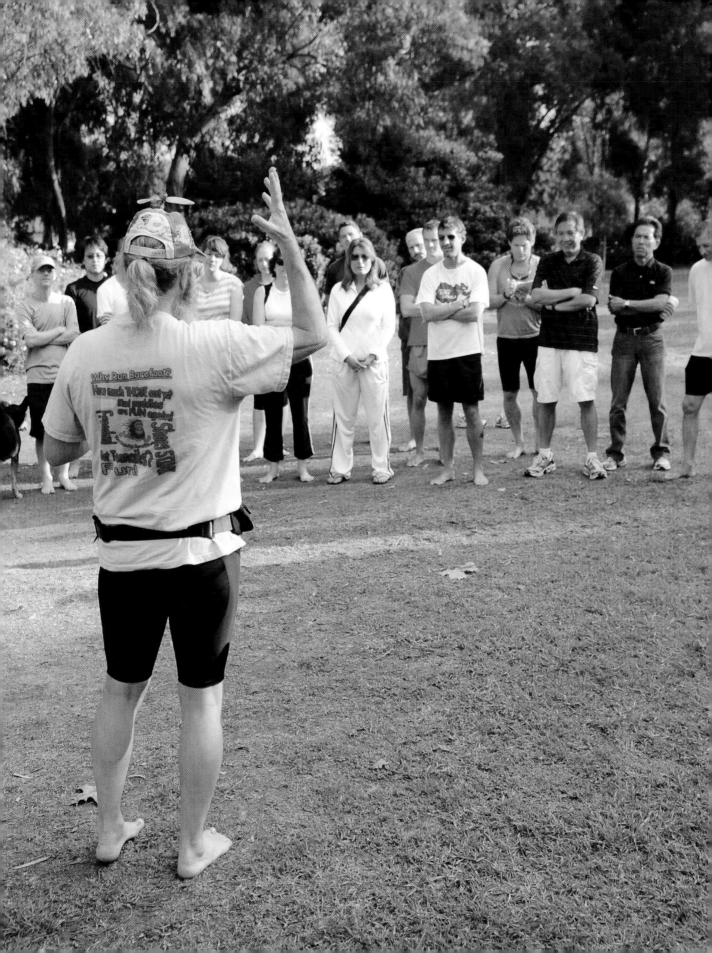

GUIDELINES FOR EVERYONE

No matter what training plan works for you, these four tips apply:

1. DON'T RUN TWO DAYS IN A ROW. While running gently is very easy, learning to run gently can be hard on the body. It is while resting that your body has a chance to rebuild and your mind has a chance to review what you've experienced. If running two days in a row is not fun and comfortable, then your mind and body are not ready for that much play.

2. RUN SLOW, AT A CONVERSATIONAL PACE. It's easier to pay attention to proper barefoot form at slow speeds, and if you master it slow, you can run it fast. Whenever you fail the talk test (find it hard to speak complete sentences), slow down, because you are going too fast.

3. REMEMBER THAT TRAINING PLANS ARE JUST EXAMPLES, NOT THE BIBLE. I am not a big fan of training plans. While hard numerical goals can prevent you from doing too much and succumbing to B.R.E.S., they can also pressure you to do more than you might want to or are capable of. It's especially difficult to set numbers in stone, not only because stones are really hard, but also because every body has a different fitness level and will react differently to the new barefoot biomechanics. Your body may tolerate more running or less. So only use the above numbers as a rough example of a progression that could take someone up to a 25- or 30-minute barefoot run within a month. If you're ever feeling acute pain, slow down or add more rest days.

4. FINALLY, IT'S ALL ABOUT FUN. It's important to start your barefoot journey with a change of mind-set: barefoot running is not about performance (at least at first); it's all about *fun*. That is the primary reason I run, and precisely why I run barefoot. Why run if it isn't going to be enjoyable? If it's going to be torture, there's no reason to stick with it. And if barefoot running is fun, learning how to do it should be too.

RULES FOR KEEPING IT FUN

RULE 1: INCREASE MILEAGE INCREMENTALLY.

Don't even think about setting a goal to race or to increase your distance until you have run 80 to 90 percent of that goal distance comfortably—before, during, and after.

RULE 2: THINK OF BAREFOOT RUNNING AS PLAYING, NOT RUNNING.

Think of your newly unshod feet as newborn barefoot babies—and a baby doesn't learn to walk, or run, in a day. Forget the miles and forget the speed for a long time. To transition gradually, and to enjoy it, focus on playing, learning, and keeping it fun. I was ready to run my first barefoot marathon because running had become fun, not because I needed to work at it.

RULE 3: DEPUTIZE YOUR SOLES BY STARTING ON STIMULATING SURFACES.

How do you protect yourself from B.R.E.S. until the various parts of your body that were underworked get strengthened and adapted to the new biomechanics? Answer: Get a warning from your soles.

Just as the eyes are the windows of the soul, the soles are the windows of the barefoot runner. Trouble is, most concrete, asphalt, and other modern surfaces (and, of course, grass and sand) are too easy on the soles to make them complain much, which is why I recommended starting on a rougher surface. You need to put your soles in a situation where they'll let you know when you've done enough, and before you do too much. Then you should listen closely to them.

RULE 4: PAIN IS YOUR FRIEND.

In the last couple of chapters, I've suggested that you start running barefoot on gravel, first standing on it, then shifting weight back and forth and side to side on it, then eventually running. If that's too forbidding for you, amend that to "rough pavement"—just make sure there is at least slight discomfort. Then *play* with your technique until you get reasonably comfortable. Before considering easier surfaces, keep in mind that the more stimulating the surface, the more information you get from the start, and the sooner you will be running gently enough to run farther and faster on any terrain.

Pain lets you know when to change the way you're standing, walking, running, and moving. Pain protects us; it's our first line of defense against doing stupid things, like running too far on newbie bare feet on our first several outings. So listen to your body and soles. If you feel pain while running, it's a cue to adjust your technique to avoid future injury.

Sometimes, you need a little pain to get it right. Yes, the goal here is to avoid calf pain. However, it is in figuring out *how* to avoid calf pain that leads to correct techniques, such as allowing your heels to touch the ground after the ball-of-the-foot landing and not to run up on your toes; it will remind you not to force the forefoot landing, but to bend the knees more. The only way that you can force the forefoot down is to actively contract the calf, which will result in four or five times your body weight smashing down on a contracted soleus. It can't handle that for too long. The calf already has enough work in store for it with the change to your natural barefoot biomechanics; don't give it more.

RULE 5: WALK WHEN YOU FEEL LIKE IT.

There are some runners who refuse to walk. They'll stop and stand around, but you'll never catch them walking during a "run." Mistake! Walking is a good thing. It gives your running muscles, especially new stressed-out barefoot muscles, a rest from running itself while continuing to move you forward. Former Olympic marathoner Jeff Galloway has made a career out of getting people to do his run/walk/run training and racing method for a good reason: it works.

As for walking technique, I recommend that people simply practice the standard barefoot running technique, as detailed in chapter 3, *while walking*. The only difference is that you are going slower (much less than 180 steps per minute) and *not* flying through the air. (That's why slower steps are okay.) One foot is always on the ground while walking, while both are in the air at some point of your stride in running. If you like, think of walking as the slow end of the running spectrum, while sprinting would be the fast end. By definition, the only difference between walking and running is flight.

So, when you walk, unlock and bend your knees, relax your hips, keep a vertical torso, and so on—all the same stuff you'd do in normal barefoot running. Just do it slower and maybe a little less intensity.

RULE 6: RUN HALF YOUR PREVIOUS "SUCCESSFUL" RUN.

People do stupid things when they try to follow a schedule. They might miss a run one day, then try doubling the distance the next day to make it up. Not smart. If anything, we should run *half* our previous successful outing!

Let me explain. A successful run is without injury and with little or no pain after the run. Therefore, if you ran 200 yards (182 m) last time with no blisters, no sores, no aches, no pains, etc., then your goal for the next run should be 100 yards (91 m). Or, if you're running for time, your goal would be 2 minutes if your last successful run was 4 minutes.

I can see your heads shaking. "What? We'll never increase our distance with that plan!"

I know. This is simply a goal to begin your run; it isn't written in stone. If you feel good, make a quick check of your body (see below) at 100 yards (91 m), and then go longer—to 200, 300, or 400 yards (182, 273, or 364 m). The beauty of this system is that if you don't feel like running (or walking) anymore and only do the 100 yards (91 m), you aren't a failure. You've still met your goal.

RULE 7: STOP AND EVALUATE WHEN YOU ARE AT YOUR GOAL.

A corollary to rule 6, rule 7 simply asks that you stop for a few moments to evaluate whenever you reach a goal. Ask yourself questions: How do you and your feet feel? Are they getting sensitive, achy? Inspect your soles thoroughly. Feel them, massage them. If everything checks out and feels good, go ahead and run farther if you want.

Important: Every time you complete your goal that day, take a break. So if your beginning goal was 100 yards (91 m), stop every 100 yards (91 m)—at 200, 300, 400 yards (182, 273, 364 m) —and do an evaluation. Here's why this is necessary.

Oftentimes, such as in an intense race, I've noticed that my feet will let me run as far as I like—until *after* I stop. Within a few minutes, my soles become supersensitive. They didn't say a word to me while I was running, but finally told me "it's time to stop" when I paused and gave them a chance to talk.

I think this system evolved as a survival mechanism: If you're running away from danger, a fierce creature, a flood, or a girlfriend's angry father, you're going to need to continue running on adrenaline until you're safe. When you stop, you realize that you're worn out. Our feet understand the urgent need to continue at such times, and they have no way of knowing that most of our runs aren't urgent, so they don't complain until after we stop. "Okay, you're safe now," they say. "And by the way, your Achilles is a mess. Better pack it in for today."

That's why it's so important to stop and wait a few moments when you attain your goal. You need to let your feet and body figure out whether they are really ready to continue comfortably. It's like eating; we don't feel overstuffed until later. That's why it's good to wait several minutes between courses of a big meal.

Remember, if we're in pain *after* we stop running, then we probably went farther or faster than we were ready for. In which case, it's time to take a day off.

RULE 8: TAKE A DAY OFF.

Taking a day off between runs, especially at the beginning, is at least as important as the running itself. Many starter running programs, like the C25K (couch-to-5-kilometer), advocate running only three days a week at first. Just because some elite athletes run five or six days a week and several times a day doesn't mean that all runners should run that much, and certainly not at the beginning.

So honor the rest day. Soak in a hot tub and get a massage, read a book, read this book *again*! But don't run. You should not be in pain after you're done running, except on the rare occasion when you've pushed yourself, which should be rare. Most of the time, you should feel refreshed after a run—like you could run more.

Of course, as your feet get fitter, and more important, you learn how to run more gently, you might run on a normal rest day, following the old Forrest Gump adage, "I just felt like runnin'." That's okay. But beware of running too many days in a row. If you do that, you'll soon require the next rule.

RULE 9: TAKE A WEEK OR TWO OFF.

When I first upped my mileage with long Sunday runs in the hills, a couple of 11-milers (17.6 km) to and from work every week (sometimes both directions in the same day), and running in the evening with one of the local running clubs, I'd occasionally log more than 80 or 90 miles (128 or 144 km) a week. For me, that's a lot. So the next week, when I didn't feel like running at all, I didn't.

Likewise, I think everyone could benefit from taking a week or two off from running, at least once a year. If you greatly exceed your average mileage one week, the next week would be a great time to take a rest. The week after you take off, you may just find that you feel like running more than ever!

In which case, be wary of the dreaded B.R.E.S.!

RULE 10: POOPING OUT IS OKAY SOMETIMES.

Sometimes it's okay to not finish a run, or even a marathon. It happened to me at the Long Beach Marathon in 2000 due to under-training, an intestinal bug, and too many dates (the fruit; I'm happily married).

Because I'd been hitting the wall by around mile 16 of my long fun runs, I lined up for the start at Long Beach with a secret weapon: a bag of dates, I figured I'd eat one date each couple miles to keep my energy up. Unfortunately, I didn't really feel like carrying the bag, so I ate them all just before the marathon started.

Initially, I seemed to be running pretty well, keeping up with some friends who were aiming for a 3:30 marathon. That would be another Boston qualifier if I could keep the pace.

But suddenly I needed to go to the bathroom . . . bad! I'd skipped the first restrooms at mile 1 and mile 2—far too many people waiting in line. Ah, mile 3, a porta-potty with no line. Just in time. I jumped in.

I felt good. I ran on, and caught up with and passed my friends again. They were still on a steady pace for 3:30, maybe 3:35.

I stopped again at the next porta-john at mile 4. Back on the run, I caught and passed my friends, again. I was doing pretty well, considering I had to stop at the next restroom . . . and the next one . . . and the next one. Perhaps I should have walked a bit.

I ended up stopping at a restroom every mile, running pretty well in between, and catching and passing the same group of friends who were still pacing for a 3:35, 3:40, maybe 3:45 finish.

But as I left the outhouse at mile 18, it was clear that I was running out of "gas" (both kinds). I was "pooped" out, literally and metaphorically.

At the next aid station, I stopped for a rest. According to my GPS watch, I'd finished about 19.5 miles, but I knew I had nothing left to carry me the remaining 6-odd miles. It was time to walk away, but I didn't have the energy to walk—away or anywhere. So I let the volunteers know I would need a ride back to the finish area.

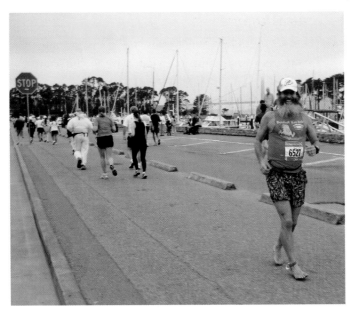

It's okay to walk, or even take a nap, even in a race, if that's what your body needs. And sometimes you need to know when to stop, even if it's before you finish.

Waiting on the side of the road, I could barely stand. I laid down, then eventually sat up to cheer for the other runners, including my wife (who seemed a bit confused that I was not at the finish line already).

Eventually the road was clear enough for the rescue van (a.k.a. the "dead meat" wagon) to start making rounds and picking up the dead meat like me. I was feeling pretty good, a bit "flushed," so to speak, but all the toxins had left my body by then and I couldn't understand why everyone else in the van was looking so dejected. You'd have thought they just attempted running a marathon and couldn't finish.

Then I passed out. In my sleep I heard the girl sitting next to me, whose shoulder my head had fallen against, saying, "I think he passed out" . . . and I woke up.

"I'm fine," I announced. And I really was. This would turn out to be the only marathon in my life (so far) I did not finish, but it doesn't bother me that I now have 76 marathon finishes on my resume instead of 77. I don't know what physical and/or mental damage I avoided by stopping that day, but I do know that the last mile six (10 km) would have been terrible—and that I had nothing to prove. I'd started and finished a dozen marathons already, including the first one in 1987, which of course was my only one in shoes. That day, chasing my lifelong dream to run a marathon, I was so blistered and beat up that I had to walk the last six miles (10 km). After all, at that time, I DID have something to prove.

But that day in Long Beach in 2000, with lots of marathons under my belt and many more to come, I recognized that I'd simply been dealt some bad cards. I was pooped out, and I wasn't going to worry about it. I knew I'd be back the next year.

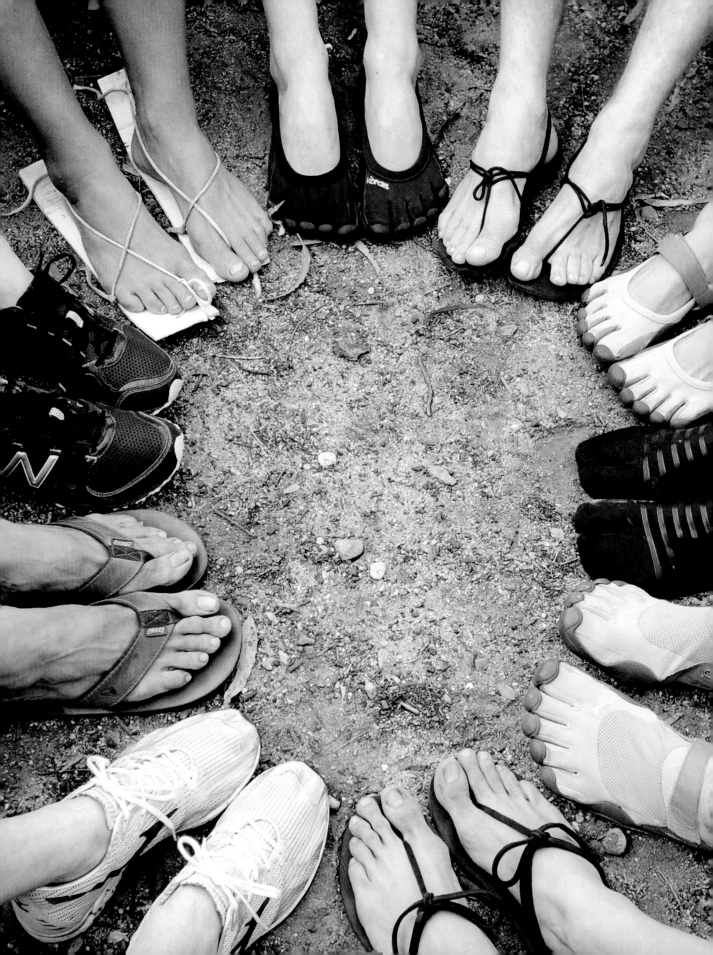

CHAPTER 6

VIBRAMS AND OTHER HALFWAY SOLUTIONS
WHY YOU STILL NEED TO LEARN BAREFOOTING FIRST

Anything between you and the ground interrupts the feedback that your bare feet need to help you run impact and injury free.

> **IF CONVENTIONAL, HEAVILY CUSHIONED RUNNING SHOES ARE LIKE BOXING GLOVES FOR YOUR FEET, MINIMALIST FOOTWEAR ARE LIKE GARDENING GLOVES: YES, YOU CAN NOW HIT THE PIANO KEYS, BUT YOU STILL CAN'T PLAY BEETHOVEN VERY WELL.**
>
> **—KEN BOB-ISM #98**

Okay, maybe that's not one of my most clever aphorisms, but the mixed metaphor does clearly underline the point I want to make in this chapter: that the interaction of earth and sole while running barefoot creates a symphony of sensation, an explosion of vivid feedback that amplifies every instrument in your physiological orchestra. Put any barrier between you and the ground—no matter how "minimal" it is or how "soft" you try to land—and that beautiful music is muffled and off-key, often resulting in incorrect technique and greater injury potential. Of course, this may come as no surprise to anyone reading this book, as I've been repeating that message over and over. But it might surprise you when I say, for those trying to learn to run more gently and protect themselves from injury, that using the Vibram FiveFingers may be one of the *worst* things you can do.

THE FOOTWEAR ANTI-INJURY EFFECTIVENESS SPECTRUM

In my hierarchy of feedback-friendly footwear, the popular Vibram FiveFingers are far better than regular shoes, but far behind the runners-up to naked feet, socks and paper booties.

The Pose and Chi techniques, which largely emulate the barefoot biomechanics, can greatly lessen the injury potential from running but might not eliminate it, for one obvious reason: They are performed while you are wearing shoes. When you leave your expensive running technique class, you leave your coach behind. When you leave your shoes behind, you take your coaches with you everywhere!

Best	10	BAREFOOT
	9	THIN PAPER MEDICAL BOOTIES (WITHOUT SHOES)
	8.5	THIN SOCKS
	7.5	THICK SOCKS
	7	POSE AND CHIRUNNING TECHNIQUES IN VIBRAMS
	6	POSE AND CHIRUNNING TECHNIQUES IN SHOES
	5	PLASTI-DIP SOCKS
	4	VIBRAMS, FEELMAX, SKORA, OTHER MINIMALIST FOOTWEAR
	3.5	VIBRAMS WITH INJINJI TOESOCKS
	3	RACING FLATS
	2	NIKE FREE
	1	CUSHIONED RUNNING SHOES
Worst	0	ARMY BOOTS

THE PROBLEM WITH VIBRAMS

Vibrams FiveFingers, the "foot gloves" with the 2-mm-thick rubber soles that are often mistakenly referred to as "barefoot shoes," can be dangerous if not used properly. Many news reports and websites are filled with stories of injured Vibrams wearers. I am not totally against Vibrams, especially for those who can't handle cold weather. But *beginner barefoot runners should simply not use them*, except for walking around where you aren't allowed to go barefoot. Those who advocate using Vibrams as a "transition shoe" to running barefoot have it backward; you should run barefoot as a transition to wearing Vibrams!

That's because you can really only run with true barefoot form in Vibrams *after* you've learned how to properly run barefoot, and that's hard to do with 2 mm of rubber blocking your sensors. Even then, you need regular booster shots of barefooting to maintain injury-free form. And instead of Vibrams, you might be better off in something more minimal, like socks. (See page 164.)

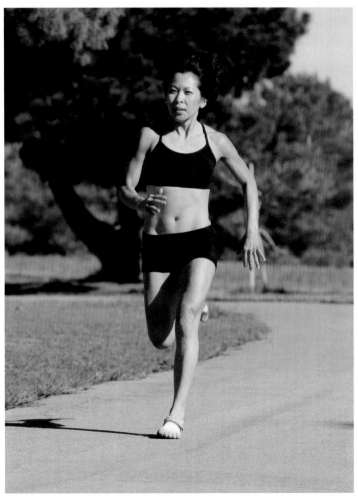

Even in Vibrams FiveFingers it is far too comfortable to land with the leg outstretched and the "brakes" on to discourage runners from pounding the pavement.

The problem with Vibrams is a false sense of security. The 2 mm of rubber protection and near weightlessness (less than 6 ounces [170 g]) unleash a wave of hyper-barefoot euphoria that makes the Barefoot Running Exuberance Syndrome (chapter 5's B.R.E.S.) feel like a sedative. Vibrams beg you to run too far, too fast, too soon in poor form because they take away the artificial support of shod running without the quality control of a bare sole to ensure you to run safely. The result is a mutant, exaggerated version of B.R.E.S.—V.F.F.E.S., if you will—that slams your body with enhanced, barefootlike stress on calves, Achilles tendons, and metatarsals, but blunts true barefoot feedback that teaches your body good technique and reminds you when to stop, resulting in injuries typical of "barefoot shoes," for which true barefoot running often gets blamed. So beginners initially get out of control, and injured worse than they ever would barefoot.

While B.R.E.S. is like learning to drive in a sports car with a huge engine and bad brakes, VFFES is that same too-fast car with no brakes at all, no lights, bad suspension, a broken steering column, and no user's manual.

Bottom line: You simply should not try to get away with the inherent sloppiness of Vibrams to start off your barefoot-running career; and, once you have learned how to correctly run barefoot, you probably still cannot use Vibrams for long, unbroken periods of time without getting sloppy. Dr. Kevin Kirby, the "Angry Podiatrist," told us that metatarsal stress fractures had become so common in Vibrams that he'd heard that "some running shoe stores were making buyers sign disclaimers when they buy them." We weren't able to verify that, but found the following comment, dated May 4, 2010, from "Adrian" on one Vibram FiveFingers sales site, birthdayshoes.com:

> "I took a break over the winter months. Back out for the past few weeks, I got impatient . . .
> So, I 'pushed it' one day, and ran twice my usual distance in the Vibram FiveFingers KSO
> . . . A day or two later, I was nursing a dull, aching tightness just below and behind my inner
> ankles (medial malleoli). Anyway, I've self-diagnosed myself with posterior tibial tendonitis
> and have forced myself to avoid running for the past two weeks. Lesson learned. There really
> should be a disclaimer on these things . . . If you can't run the distance barefoot (and your
> skin will let you know . . .) . . . then you can't run it in a pair of FiveFinger shoes."

Most people don't heel strike in Vibrams, and this lack of what is known as an "impact peak" makes VFFs unquestionably better for your joints than regular cushioned trainers. And they do provide almost the same foot, arch, and leg strengthening opportunities of barefooting. But as her example illustrates, those advantages can easily become disadvantages, because you can simply get away with too much sloppiness in VFFs. They don't teach you as well as true barefooting. So all that foot and calf strength you develop in Vibrams? If you're still running incorrectly, which is easy to do in Vibrams, you'll need all that strength and more—or you'll most certainly injure yourself!

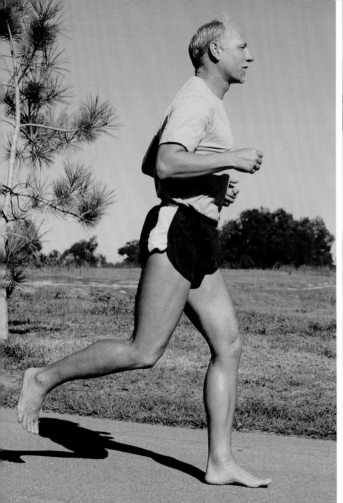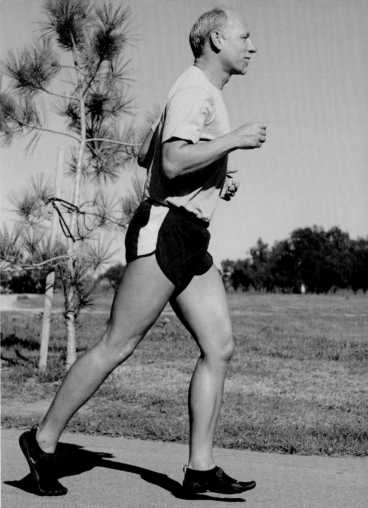

Many people believe it feels the same to run in Vibrams as it does barefoot. However, your bare soles tell you exactly how your weight is distributed so you can make precise adjustments or corrections. Vibrams don't—after all, they are still shoes. (Doh!)

So why waste time injuring yourself? Learn to run barefoot correctly and more quickly by starting off barefoot. Then, if you later run in minimalist or even regular shoes, you'll at least start with the right technique. Going barefoot first has precedents: My buddy Barefoot Ted runs ultra marathons in Vibrams, but he learned barefoot first. Kenyans run great in shoes because they often run barefoot as kids.

Christopher McDougall began running barefoot while writing his book. He began with Vibrams, thanks to Barefoot Ted. But after hurting his toe kicking the table leg one night, he couldn't get the Vibrams on his foot, so he tried running barefoot. "It was like a whole other world," he told me. "My soles were flooded with all the subtle information that you can't get through the Vibrams." Now he almost always runs barefoot.

HOW VIBRAMS HELP AND HURT

I could share hundreds of comments and posts about the problems and even a few about the benefits people are experiencing with Vibrams. Here are a few representative examples from my website that illustrate both the bad and the good.

SLOPPY, BUT HELPFUL IN WINTER
Posted by: Doug
November 7, 2009
Categories: Testimonials, Vibram FFs

I was having pain in my feet and heels and wanting to know why. After reading Chris McDougall's book *Born to Run* (and finding this site), I decided to just chuck the shoes and start running barefoot. For the first time in years, I started to enjoy running to run and not just forcing myself to exercise.

I was slated to run my first 5K this weekend. The temperature has been dropping and the race was scheduled for fairly early in the morning. I really wanted to do well, particularly since several of my friends knew I had been running barefoot and I felt pressure to represent. On Friday morning, the day before the race, I got up to run and it was 31°F (-0.5°C). The ground was *cold*. I was so distracted by the cold that my foot placement was all wrong and after just a few miles my feet were hurting pretty bad from hot spots. Despite the warnings about putting stuff between my feet and the ground, I felt like I needed something for the cold.

So I went and bought a pair of Vibram FiveFinger Sprints. The good news is the race went very well. I ran faster than I've ever done on any of my daily runs by several minutes (32 minutes for my first 5K, down from my usual pace of about 38 minutes). When I got home from the race, I still hadn't run the dog so I did another 4½ miles (7.2 km) with her for a big 7½ miles (12 km) for the day. Without the VFF there's no way I could have run that far or that fast. So it sounds like a win, right?

I'm not so sure. First, I could tell that my running was sloppy. I just didn't have the feedback I needed to make sure my feet were landing right or that I was picking them up right. My form was okay, certainly better than anything I could have done in "shoes." I don't know if it was really the lack of immediate feedback or just that the VFFs kept me from having tight control over my feet. Second, having the Vibram protection on my feet was also a bit disturbing. After just a month of running barefoot, I had gotten used to feeling the ground—more than I thought. It was actually a bit disconcerting to not feel the ground. I felt like I was just plowing through whatever was on the ground without a second thought. A couple of times I looked down to see I was standing/running through some pretty trashy stuff—and I hadn't noticed. That may be a good thing, but I don't think so. I think it's probably better to know where your feet are.

The moral of the story is that I'll keep wearing the VFFs through the winter. I live in Ohio and I really do think I need something to protect my feet from the cold. I don't have the luxury of running year-round in mild climates. Having the VFFs takes the apprehension out of getting up in the morning to run. It also gives my wife some peace of mind as well. She's a little freaked by my running barefoot. However, I feel like come spring I'll take the VFFs off and run as God intended: skin on the earth.

2009 NOVEMBER 10, 2009, ALSO FROM DOUG

So I've gotten a few more runs in with the VFFs. My reaction is still mixed. My runs are "easier" (and by easier I mean I come home with less direct pain in my feet) and thus it's easier to motivate myself to get out of bed early and go run. However, I think I've pinpointed what bothers me about running in the VFFs.

First, it's easier to push off with your toes. As we know, when running barefoot you're supposed to lift your foot. With the VFFs there's no real pain from pushing off. Second, it's hard to know if I'm landing on the ball of my foot with my toes lifted or if they are just flat. The Vibram sole is flat and wants to stay that way. Lifting your toes in the VFFs takes a tad more energy than doing so barefoot.

These two aspects of the VFFs are the two leading causes I've found of blisters when running barefoot. So, I think switching back to barefoot will be tricky after running in these for a while. Also, I can really see why BKB says these aren't a good transition tool from shod to barefoot. The VFFs don't really help you run correctly. On the plus side, I can run in the VFFs (even if a little wrong) and come home without any foot pain—and I can run in the winter. With it getting cold out in the mornings I was dreading running more and more. Now with my VFFs I don't dread running in the cold. To me there are a couple of important goals: 1) run and 2) enjoy running. Prior to the VFFs, being barefoot in the cold was causing me to miss both goals. Maybe that's all that matters in the end.

TRY WATER SOCKS INSTEAD

Posted by: "Grumpy"
November 12, 2009
Categories: Testimonials, Vibram FFs

I looked at the VFFs at REI. I found they are hard to put on and restrict my toe movement. And . . . they're expensive. Instead, I went to Sports Authority and bought a pair of water socks for $10. I bought them a little big so my feet and toes have plenty of room to move and flex. They work great on the treadmill at the gym (the gym won't let me run barefoot). But more important, they work great outside. I did a 4-mile (6.4 km) run in them (outdoors) yesterday, all on concrete. Then I did a fifth mile barefoot. My feet are only a little sore, but I've only been at the barefoot running thing for two months. If you have to wear some footwear due to gym regulations or the cold, I highly recommend cheap water socks over the more expensive and restrictive VFFs.

A FOND LOOK AT POSE AND CHI RUNNING TECHNIQUES

I have tremendous respect for the Pose Method and ChiRunning, which are similar methods for teaching anti-injury running techniques, invented respectively by Dr. Nicholas Romanov and Danny Dreyer, that have taught thousands of runners how to run softly, barefootlike, in shoes. They work. In fact, Romanov is, in a way, responsible for this book; Roy met me when, in the course of writing a story about the Pose Method for *Runner's World*, he called Romanov and said, "This seems a lot like barefoot running." When Romanov agreed, and mentioned that he devoted a chapter to it in his book, Roy Googled "barefoot running" and found yours truly. An hour later I had him running barefoot on the asphalt beach bike path.

While I have never been a fan of charging a fee to teach people how to run, which is what Romanov and Dreyer do, I love that they teach you many good things. Rather than buying a pair of Vibrams for $85, I'd certainly recommend that you spend $15 or $20 for one of their books. I did, and it saved me in the 2004 Big Sur Marathon.

Six days earlier, I'd finished the Boston Marathon and was pretty worn out. I was also in a months-long slow-running slump. Fortunately, at the expo a couple of days before Big Sur, I bought Danny's book and learned two mainstays of both Chi and Pose: the 180+ cadence and "falling forward," the idea of leaning so that gravity helps pull you along. Although I must have been using the faster cadence during my shorter, faster races, it hadn't occurred to me to do it while running a slower marathon pace. The concepts clicked for me and I tested them in the race. Without a doubt, they helped me get over those daunting Big Sur hills. By increasing my cadence and simply shifting my body weight—especially my hips—in front of my feet, I could feel gravity pulling me forward. Despite being exhausted and aching, I finished nearly an hour faster than I had six days earlier in Boston!

KEY DIFFERENCES FROM RUNNING BAREFOOT

That said, although I like the Pose and Chi methods and what they do for people, I don't think you need more than one hour-long lesson, and Chi and Pose teachers make you sign up for all-day and all-weekend clinics. Running barefoot is cheaper, and your coaches are with you every step of the way. They're also slighly different in terms of technique.

One key difference is that in Chi/Pose, you lean your whole body like the Leaning Tower of Pisa. Barefooters, at least this barefooter, don't. When Roy and I looked at videos of one another we'd shot on the beach that day, we were leaning forward from the hips down, but our torsos were straight up, the same rule discussed in chapter 3. The full-body lean, after initial acceleration, is extra work. You do too much work and overdo it. It's also more stress on the toes (which may not be a big deal in shoes). I have no laboratory research to prove my way is better, just observations of hundreds of barefoot runners and thousands of shod runners in the front, middle, and the back of the pack, at everything from world-record races to casual runs on the local bike path.

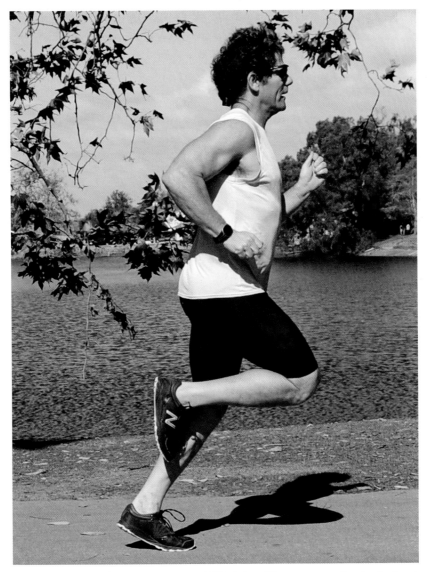

A runner using The Chi/Pose method. Note the full body lean. When you are running at a steady pace, a full-body lean tends to be counterproductive. Having your shoulders out in front of your hips means that the upper torso isn't going to be loading your "springs" (bent legs) fully, which reduces your ability to spring forward. Also, because you are not accelerating, the full-body lean requires your back muscles to work more than if your torso were balanced upright on top of your hips.

Then there's also simple logic: If Pose and Chi are modeled on barefooting, then why not do exactly what a barefooter does naturally, rather than change it a bit? That may somehow be related to the key difference between barefooting and Pose/Chi: shoes. Pose and Chi teach you in shoes, so getting feedback is difficult and imprecise; by definition, doing barefoot technique just right in shoes is impossible. So as perfectly as you may learn the Pose/Chi rules, which are very similar to running barefoot, just wearing shoes almost begs you to slip back into your old bad habits.

DO-IT-YOURSELF MINIMALISM

WHY PAY $90 FOR TOESOCKS? TRY $5 PLASTI-DIP SOCKS.

Many people call me a zealot, and I wouldn't disagree. I run barefoot, period. Nike gave me a pair of Frees, and after evaluating them I gave them away. Footwear for running is definitely not for me. But that doesn't mean I haven't thought about it.

When I could see worn spots on the balls of my feet in the weeks before my first road marathon in January 1999, the idea of wearing minimalist shoes or socks—or even painting rubber cement on my soles—did cross my mind. But since I'm such a procrastinator, I didn't really do anything about it—other than run more gently. That worked.

But Dave Wright and Michae Legault (pronounced "Mee-shay") are different. They had similar issues, and actually did take concrete action. I don't hold it against them at all.

When Dave pulled out a pair of special socks he'd dipped in liquid rubber at mile 13 (20.8 km) of the 2005 Boston Marathon and said to me, "Go ahead, Ken, I've got to put these on," I wished him well. I knew he was in pain and couldn't finish 26.2 miles (42 km) barefoot today. I wouldn't find out if he finished or not until after sundown.

Dave, a New Orleans architect, started running at age thirty-three in 1998, built up quickly, and did a couple of marathons. But by 2003, wracked by a painful iliotibial band, he started doing some research. "I saw that the fast guys were using racing flats," he says, "so I dumped my big cushions, did New York pain free that fall, and qualified for Boston at Chicago at 3:14 in 2004. But by then I developed a bad case of plantar fasciitis. That was the last straw. I decided to go full-time barefoot."

Trouble is, Dave was living in North Carolina, where it gets to 24°F (-4°C) in winter. "I'm not the tough guy that Barefoot Rick (known to run barefoot to near-frostbite levels in Missouri) is," he says. "There were no Vibrams yet. So I tried duct tape on the bottom of socks. When that didn't work, I came across Plasti Dip, a flexible, waterproof polyurethane paint used for coating metal tool handles."

To get a proper shape, he had to paint it on the sock while wearing it, which required sitting outside for 45 minutes and trying not to breathe the fumes. He experimented with different types—cotton, nylon, polyester—before settling on a superthin, skintight model that didn't shift around on his foot. He made four pairs of gray socks with black Plasti Dip, all washable and recoatable.

"It wasn't exactly barefoot, but still way thinner than Vibrams are," he says. "I'd still feel it when I'd step on a pebble. And the reaction from other runners was almost the same as being barefoot." He used them until the weather warmed, then switched to barefoot.

Five weeks before the Boston Marathon, Dave got a metatarsal stress fracture. Training stopped. He flew to Boston undertrained, lined up at the start with Ken Bob and Rick while carrying his socks as backup, and ran with his buddies until the stress fracture started acting up around mile 13 (20.8 km).

"The pain altered my stride," he says. "I wanted to finish, and knew I needed more protection. But I didn't want to embarrass the barefooters, so I let them go. Then I put a crumbled-up paper cup around my foot and put the sock on over it to hold it on. It was a bit lumpy. The crowd reaction was funny: 'You're in socks!' they screamed." He trudged to the finish in 5:58.

(continued on page 166)

Roy attended a Pose clinic one weekend, thinks Romanov is a genius, and has fond memories of his wife Svetlana encouraging him, "lift your feet up!" But he told me that his group spent hours learning and relearning how *not* to heel strike. On a hard surface, that takes about 2 seconds in bare feet! Our "clinic" on the bike path only took about 45 minutes, including warmup and cooldown, versus the entire weekend he spent with the Romanovs.

So why waste time learning barefoot running in shoes, from Nike to Vibram, especially when they are clearly inferior to the real thing? Remember, no matter what the shoe companies say, anything between your sole and the ground does not function as "transition" footwear, but as a harmful muffle. It's like trying to appreciate the subtle smile of the *Mona Lisa* in a dark room with sunglasses on. It's like eating spicy chili with a clip on your nose (smell being a key element in taste). It's like seeing the Eiffel Tower by going to the Paris casino in Las Vegas. It's like (I'm told) phone sex is to real sex. Go ahead and think of your own analogy. When you try to run "barefoot in shoes," you're still in shoes—smothering the army of sensors on your soles, weakening your foot muscles, putting the quality-control inspectors in the closet, and waiting for the pain that tells you you're already injured. The bare foot, by contrast, gives you constant biofeedback *right now*, with no distortion or delay. If you feel the slightest discomfort, your feet and body will try to fix it before it leads to injury. Our feet aren't out to protect just themselves, but our whole body. They are our first-alert system, our first line of defense against . . . ourselves.

Yes, you can run Pose-like and Chi-like in shoes *after* you learn how to run barefoot first (you'll actually run better if you use a more vertical back). But you won't have to pay Romanov or Dreyer to teach you. You'll have two enthusiastic instructors any time you're barefoot for the rest of your life who won't charge you a dime.

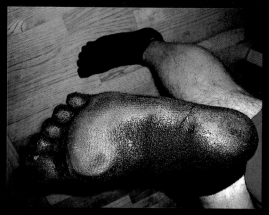

David Wright's plasti-dip socks helped get him through Boston Marathon when he was under-trained. Advantages: custom fit and cheap!

When Vibrams came on the market, Dave ordered a pair right away, but found them too warm and too thick to feel the ground. He went back to his coated socks, upgraded by now to Injinji toesocks and patched with moleskin when necessary.

"I've never seen anyone else do it," says Dave. "I mentioned it on a barefoot forum, and after a bit of discussion no one paid much attention."

Too bad. The cost for a pair of regular socks is about $5; Injinjis, $12. "And it's way better than Vibrams—better fit, cooler, less sweaty," Dave says. "And why spend all that money?"

Dave hasn't run as much in recent times but is usually barefoot when he does, convinced that it has kept him injury free the past five years. But the crumbling, rock-strewn streets of New Orleans scared him into wearing Nike Frees at the Mardi Gras Half Marathon in February 2010—and wishing he had brought his Plasti Dips in his fanny pack.

"I came across a barefoot runner struggling with the bad roads. He was so beat up by mile 9 (14.4 km) that he stopped and decided to do the half. He could've finished it in my socks."

Plasti Dip sells for $7.60 on Amazon.com. The nonslip, nonskid, moisture-resistant rubber coating will coat twenty pairs of pliers with eight to ten coats each and probably four or five pairs of socks. A foam paintbrush is recommended to daub it on the soles. Reviewers generally liked the product but criticized the loose plastic lid.

PLAIN OLD SOCKS SAVED THE DAY

In another corner of the barefoot running universe, Michae Legault, a fifty-year-old housing contractor and running coach from Pleasant Hill, California, says you've truly arrived not when you can run in plain old, unplasticized socks but can run in the same pair of socks *forever.*

A lifelong runner who peaked with a 3:26 in the 1,320-yard (1,201 m) run in eighth grade, then got into triathlons and cycling after college and gave up running for a decade, Michae has always done his own thing—odd jobs, dumpster diving, eating only apples for weeks at a time, and, by his mid-thirties, farming blueberries in Oregon. He started running 6 miles (9.6 km) a day so that he could buy a newspaper in the closest town, 3 miles (4.8 km) away. At thirty-six, after finishing the Portland Marathon in a hobbled, broken-down 4:10 that left him limping for a week and angry at himself, he got serious. He bought a book on LSD (long slow distance) training, ran over 100 miles (160 km) every week for the next seven years, scored a 3:10 personal record (PR) in the San Francisco Marathon, became a high school cross-country and track coach, and started paying attention to his form after he almost keeled over from dehydration on a 105°F (40.6°C) day on mile 41 (65.6 km) of the Rio del Lago Ultra in California.

"To stop what I called my 'energy constipation'—leg fatigue, aching back—I started pushing my pelvis down to the earth and lifting my crown to the heavens to stretch my spine," he said. "It was like an imaginary rack. With meditation—I'd go on ten-day yoga retreats that would teach me to be aware of my breathing, posture, and the heat in my pelvic girdle—I developed a straight posture that forced me to land on the balls of my feet." Craving flatter shoes, he cut the sole off his New Balances, ran on his toes, and got extreme calf pain that wrecked his streak of 100-mile (160 km) weeks. Then, on January 21, 2001, he noticed Barefoot Ken Bob at a 5K race in Huntington Beach, California.

"Can I fondle your feet?" Michae asked—and he was astounded by the lack of calluses. It was the beginning of a long friendship and an epiphany that led him to barefoot running—and socks.

In December 2003, in a deep, meditative trance at a winter solstice festival, Michae responded to the question "What do you want to get rid of?" with one word: "shoes." A month later, 2 miles (3.2 km) from the finish line of the 2004 Phoenix Marathon, his feet mysteriously wracked by his first-ever case of Purple Toe Syndrome, he took off his shoes for the first time and ran in socks. "People yelled out 'Hey, barefoot dude!' even though I wasn't barefoot," Michae said. "It was awesome." He went home and bought a 12-pack of the ankle-highs.

Switching between socks, bare feet, and homemade shoes cobbled out of yoga mats, Michae dumped shoes for good that summer when he couldn't find them minutes before the Bay to Breakers. "People called me 'Ken' as I ran by—because I'm a white guy with a beard and long hair and bald in the same spot," he said. "It was awesome."

At the 2005 Lake Tahoe Marathon, running alongside Ken Bob, Michae put on socks to handle the rough road at mile 20 (32 km), and was stunned at the finish line. His socks, which were usually scuffed and torn with every run, were unmarked at the finish. It had taken eighteen months, but he had finally learned how to run gently.

Michae doesn't wear the socks anymore and only runs once a week on average, "even though I can still do a 20-minute 5K—always had natural speed," he says. "But in the spirit of David Carradine, who started every episode of *Kung Fu* by saying to his students, 'When you can walk across the rice paper without tearing it, that is when you know you are ready,' I say this:

"Go buy a 12-pack of the cheapest socks you can find to train in. Work on your form. And someday, if you can run a marathon in socks without wearing a hole in them, then you will know that you have truly arrived at the level of barefoot mastery."

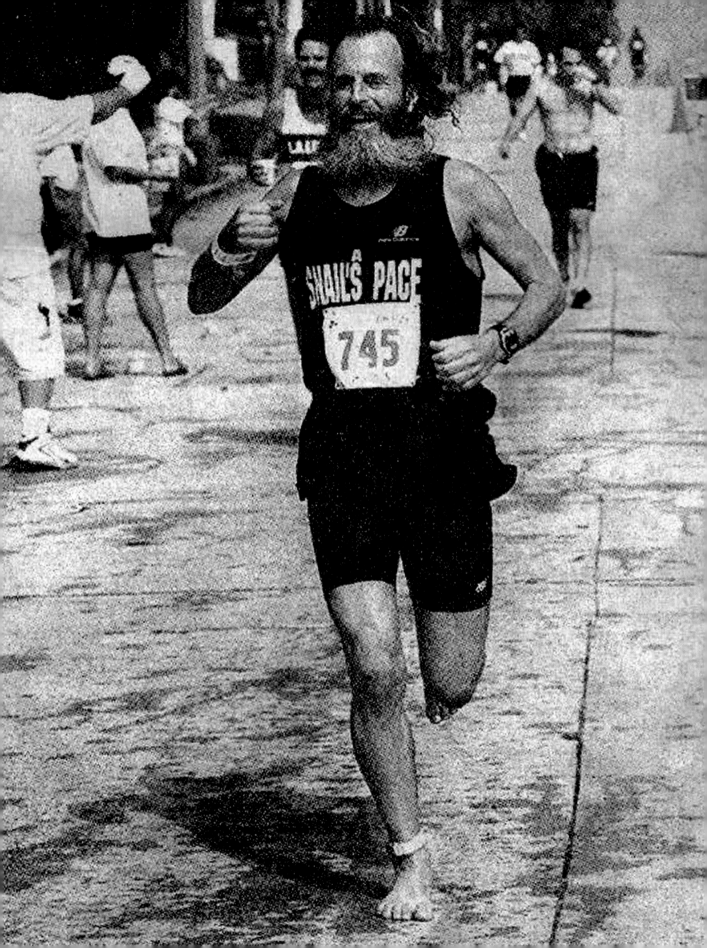

SECTION III:

WHY BAREFOOTING
WILL MAKE YOU FASTER

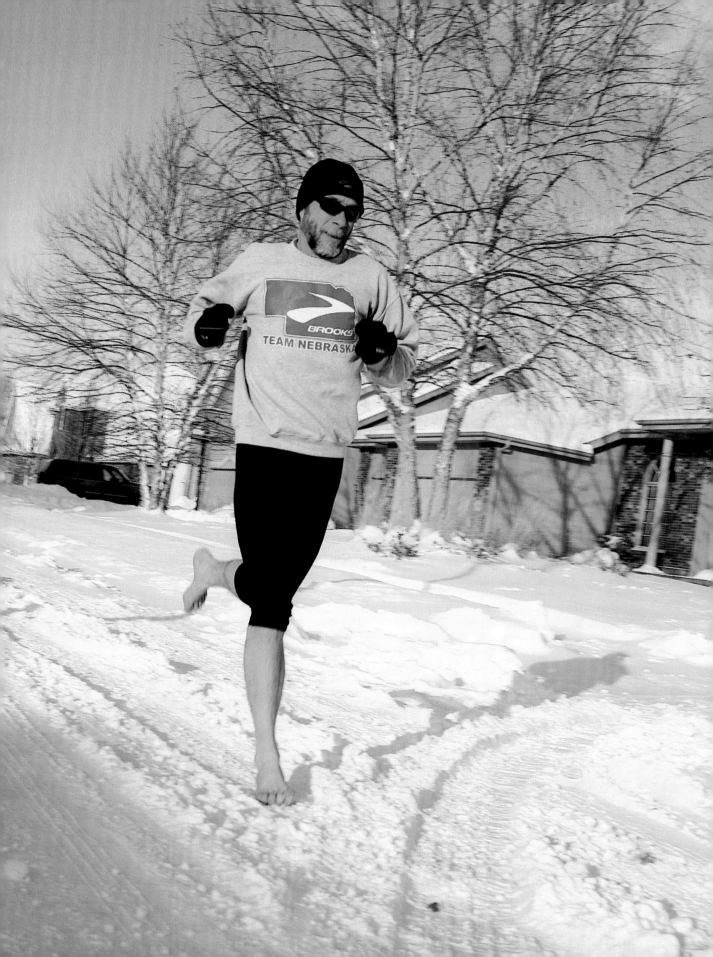

CHAPTER 7

FAST TIMES IN NEBRASKA
HOW BAREFOOTING TURBOCHARGES YOU FOR RACING

A landmark study proves that running barefoot can speed you up, strengthen your feet, and fix your form. And the best part: you don't have to commit 100 percent. A little bit of barefooting—like 25 percent—can even make you faster *in shoes*.

> **THREE BUDDIES GO RAFTING ON AN OREGON RIVER IN SEARCH OF LOST TREASURE. WHEN THEY ARE CONFRONTED BY A BEAR, ONE OF THE FRIENDS STARTS TO TAKE OFF HIS SHOES.**
>
> **'WHY ARE YOU TAKING OFF YOUR SHOES?' SAYS DAN.**
>
> **''CAUSE I RUN FASTER WITH NO SHOES,' REPLIES JERRY.**
>
> **'BUT YOU CAN'T OUTRUN THAT BEAR,' SAYS DAN.**
>
> **'I DON'T HAVE TO OUTRUN THE BEAR,' REPLIES JERRY, AS HE WATCHES DAN TAKE A HIT OFF HIS INHALER. 'I JUST HAVE TO OUTRUN YOU.'**
>
> —*WITHOUT A PADDLE*, 2004

"Yeah, yeah, so it stops injuries. But what about performance? I heard it makes you slower. Why bother doing it if it doesn't make you faster?"

I get this all the time. Tradition-bound runners (and that's most of them), even when presented with reams of anecdotal and empirical evidence about how running barefoot strengthens, rehabs, and rejuvenates feet, knees, and running careers, cannot shake this obsession with velocity. The need for speed trumps safety and fogs rationality. If it won't lower their PR, they won't do it. So when shod runners, already leery of barefooting, hear stories, some true, about barefooters who never run as fast barefoot as they did in their shod glory days, or can't plow through road gunk like they can in shoes, it causes them to discount all evidence to the contrary. Shoe-centric running historians love to point out that two-time Olympic gold medalist Abebe Bikila, who won the marathon without shoes in 1960 in Rome, had a faster winning time by three minutes in Tokyo in 1964 in shoes. They point to Zola Budd, the barefoot South African teenage sensation of the 1980s, and note that the middle-age mama now runs in shoes. They write off the barefoot Romero brothers, Alex and Julian, who finished first and second at the 2008 Albuquerque Marathon (see below), as freaks.

←Will Lindgren "warming" up before heading indoors to run on the treadmill. Previous page: It may not make you faster, but in races, try to look fast and happy for the cameras. If your pictures gets in the local paper the next day, as mine did after the Long Beach Marathon in 2002, you may be congratulated on "winning" the race!

When I quietly mention, in my modest, deferential way, that I qualified five times for the Boston Marathon (marathon PR 3:18.58) and have a fairly decent 10K PR of 37:02, all barefoot, and that my buddy Dave Parsel, who trains barefoot, has (while racing in shoes) beaten the legendary Steve Scott on the Carlsbad 500-meter course, on which Scott had set the world record in 1986 (13:32) and 1988 (13:30), and ran a mile barefoot in 5:04.8 at age fifty-five (see below), they shrug. Anti-barefoot bias even downplays stories about how coaches at all levels, including Olympic coaching legends like Brooks Johnson and Joe Vigil, used running barefoot drills for decades to make their national and world-class runners stronger and faster. "So what?" they'll say. "Where's the proof—where are the studies, the published scientific-journal, peer-reviewed, shod-versus-unshod tests showing that barefooting can make you faster?" Furthermore, they'll add, where's a big-time, national- and world-class runner who can show results in real competitions from running barefoot?

The answer: Nebraska.

Now it's a fact: Running barefoot *can* make you faster—*absolutely* faster, not just *relatively* faster as your ever-injured shod age-group peers self-destruct. It can even make you faster *in shoes*, even if you just run barefoot during a fraction of your workouts. And, not surprisingly, the proof does not come out of the ivy-bedecked buildings containing the hallowed research labs of Harvard University or the trail-running hot spots of Colorado, but from a place that has quietly emerged as a mecca of barefooting: the first place in the world to start a barefoot marathon division (Omaha in 2006; ten barefooters ran it in 2009), the great cornhusker state of Nebraska.

A landmark study by a University of Nebraska at Omaha (UNO) researcher that debuts in this book (see below) proves that running barefoot is not just a little more efficient than shod running, but *a lot more efficient.* In Nebraska, a runner in her mid-thirties came back after a ten-year layoff to post national championship times in the 400 m and 800 m (in shoes) due to doing nearly all of her training barefoot or in Vibram FiveFingers. In Nebraska, a fifty-three-year-old running coach who'd been knocked out of the sport by injuries used barefooting to run more than 2,700 miles (4,320 km) one year, 500 miles (800 km) *more* than any other in his life, even though he only ran 25 percent of the time barefoot. In Nebraska, an elite international pro miler and 1,500 m runner who grew up running barefoot uses it a couple of times a week to stay fast and injury free. There are more examples of great barefoot successes below, some of them not even from Nebraska. Some run barefoot all the time, some do it once in a while, and some never touch pavement. But all agree that, with enough patience and planning, reawakening and resensitizing your naked soles can speed you up as well as fix you up.

A LANDMARK STUDY

Running barefoot was briefly big in the mid-1980s, probably due to the Zola Budd effect, and there have been many barefoot running studies since then. "I know that because I cited them in mine," says Nick Hanson, a twenty-eight-year-old doctoral student in exercise physiology at Ohio State who runs 50 miles (80 km) a week, one-third of it barefoot, and ran the 2010 Boston Marathon in Vibram FiveFingers in 3:06. "But they always studied biomechanics—and concluded that the decreased impact forces of running barefoot should lessen the frequency of injury (see chapter 2 for more details on this). But I wanted to come at it from a performance perspective—running economy." Was barefoot running more economical—that is, did it burn less oxygen (VO_2)—than shod running? Could barefooters go the same speed with less effort, or go faster speeds with less effort, than they could with shoes on?

Hanson already knew that the answer was yes, but not a convincing one. Back in 1985, a study by Burkett, Kohrt, and Buchbinder found that barefooters had slightly better running economy, but the researchers were unsure as to whether it was due to the weight of the shoe, a change in form, or both. In 2007, a study by Divert et al. concluded it was the decrease of mass on the feet that led to a higher economy, not barefoot form. However, it should be noted that this, and many other such studies, did *not* look at experienced barefoot runners who have had time to refine their barefoot running techniques. A study at the Université de Valenciennes in France in June 2008 agreed, but also speculated that the damping (shock absorbing) characteristics of the shoe may lead to a decrease in the storage and restitution of elastic energy capacity, which could contribute to the lower net efficiency of shod running. Although these were interesting studies, Hanson felt he could study barefooting more thoroughly, in a more real-world fashion, given that the other studies used treadmills, not outdoor running. ("A treadmill is comparatively lazy," he explains. "Pulling yourself through space is much harder." Using a 1 percent grade on the tread equalizes its VO_2 max values with flat outdoor running.)

Hanson's study, conducted in 2009 for his UNO master's thesis, proved him right. He not only showed that running barefoot was *far more economical* than shod running in outdoor conditions, but he was also the first to measure performance in three important ways: oxygen uptake, heart rate, and rate of perceived exertion.

The study included ten subjects who ranged in age from nineteen to twenty-nine (five men, average age of twenty-four, and five women, average age of twenty-three) who were healthy, reported no previous lower limb injuries, and ran at least 10 miles (16 km) per week for six months prior to the study. Two of the subjects were barefooters, two others had tried it, and six had never done it before. Each participant ran both barefoot and shod on tread and track at 70 percent of their VO_2 max (measured before the testing began), getting four scores. The findings, published in the *International Journal of Sports Medicine* and debuting in this book, are eye-opening.

Compared to shod running, running barefoot has:

Less oxygen uptake: Barefoot runners on a track used 5.7 percent less oxygen than they did while running shod, compared to just 2 percent less oxygen when running on a treadmill.

Lower heart rate: Barefoot runners had 2 percent lower heart rates on both track and treadmill.

Reduced RPE (rating of perceived exertion): On this subjective measure of how much work they were doing, shod runners thought that they were working 7.5 percent harder on the track and 6 percent harder on a treadmill than they did while running barefoot.

The study is a considered landmark because the 3.7 percent difference in oxygen usage found between treadmill and track/shod versus unshod (5.7 - 2 percent) is huge.

Bottom line: Thanks to Hanson, we know that barefoot running is not just more efficient than shod, but *way more efficient.*

It was nice to hear from Hanson that TheRunningBarefoot.com website helped motivate him to do the study. "I started running (in shoes) after college, then overdid it and got hurt—my IT band flared up," Hansen explains. "I'd heard about barefoot running, and stumbled on Ken Bob's site. Barefooting fascinated me—maybe because one of my parents was a hippie. Seeing it as a good supplement to training, I started taking my shoes off for the last mile and finishing my runs barefoot. I loved it; it was very freeing. As I ran barefoot and in Vibrams more and more, my feet and calves strengthened, and my IT band injury disappeared."

Soon Hanson was a daily runner, racking up 50 miles (80 km) a week; by mid-2010, he'd done three marathons and a 50K. He got hooked on Vibrams in 1998; he now wears shoes occasionally on rough trails and tries to do 5 to 10 miles (8 to 16 km) barefoot to maintain his sensitivity and proper gait. "I don't pay attention to form when running in the FiveFingers, which is why you need to run barefoot," he says. Barefooting has been good to Hanson: he hasn't been injured since he started it, qualified for Boston with a 3:06 in Omaha in September 2009, and, of course, found a dissertation topic he could sink his teeth into.

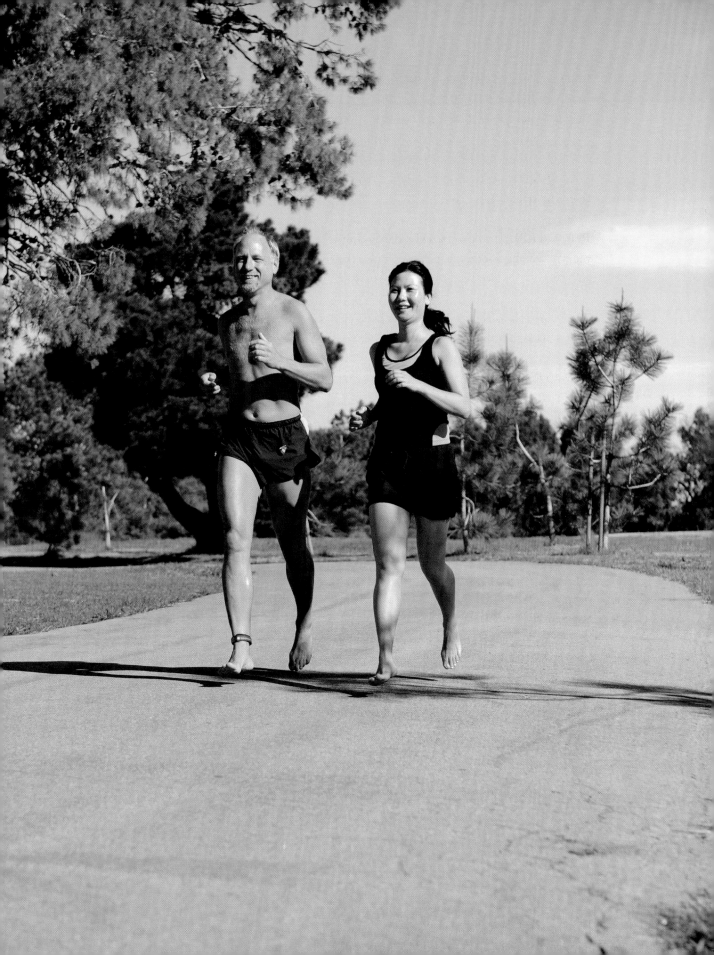

THE ACCIDENTAL EVANGELIST

A couple of years before Hanson began his master's thesis, Omaha Marathon race director Susie Smisek took a phone call from Barefoot Sanjay Goel, who'd done the 2005 race barefoot. "Okay, let's do it," she agreed. "We'll start a barefoot division in 2007."

That decision would ultimately turn Nebraska into a barefoot running hotbed and help prove that even minor unshod training can make anyone—middle-age marathoners to national-class half-milers—healthier and faster. The unlikely messenger was a bearded, barefoot, pack-a-day smoker often seen leading a giant Great Dane named Duder while pushing a toddler in a jogging stroller. His name is Benny Foltz.

An occasionally homeless jack-of–all-trades who's been a pharmacy technician, fireman, and microbrewery salesman, Foltz is a divorced Omaha father of one who started barefooting out of simply curiousity. He doesn't have any grand personal epiphanies about how it saved his running career from injuries (he never had any), turned him into a world-class runner (he's not), or even got him a membership in the Society for Barefoot Living (they rejected him). He just likes how it makes him feel. But his ability to convey that made him a key player in the barefoot revolution.

In love with running for as long as he can remember, Foltz ran cross-country and track in high school, ran on his own in college, and racked up tons of 5Ks and 10Ks, five marathons, and a 50-mile (80 km) ultra by age twenty-six, all in shoes with no injuries. "I had no interest in changing my running style or going barefoot," he says. That changed when he noticed that the 2007 Omaha Marathon had a barefoot division.

"I thought, 'This is a joke—barefoot division? Come on—who would be dumb enough to run a marathon barefoot?' So I signed up for it."

Driven by his wacky new commitment, Foltz found Ken Bob's website and some journal articles. "Going back to what's more natural made sense," he said. "So I started running barefoot, just like that. Never had a problem with it, other than stepping on a bee once."

To prepare for the marathon, Foltz ran the Omaha Corporate Cup 10K, where he was swamped by questions. "I'm not sure if that was due to running barefoot or pushing a stroller with a two-year-old crying the last three miles," he says. He successfully did the Sioux City Half Marathon, then the Omaha Marathon. Although too slow (over five hours) to see Ken Bob or the other barefooters who showed up, he was thrilled, finishing with perfectly unblistered soles.

"After that, I became a barefoot diehard, trying to live barefoot," he says. "That first winter, I tried to run barefoot in a blizzard—only made it ¼ mile (400 m). I soon was getting kicked out of restaurants and clubs. One night, security kicked me out of a Widespread Panic concert before it started. I got back in when I bought a pair of bright pink flip-flops off a homeless woman for five bucks. Now I carry sandals with me in public—just in case."

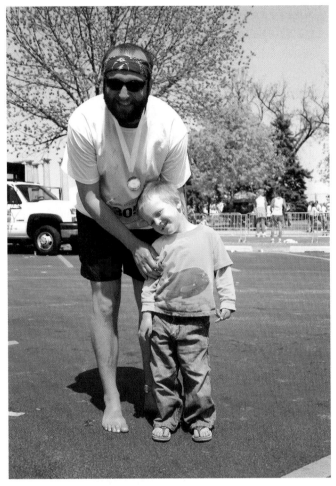

Barefoot Benny Foltz, shown here with son and frequent running companion Breken, unwittingly helped make Nebraska a barefoot hotbed.

As Foltz raced three barefoot marathons over the next few years, his influence grew. Four buddies picked up barefooting; one, previously injured all the time, ran Sioux City barefoot and qualified for Boston. Foltz participated in Nick Hanson's study proving that barefooters use less oxygen. He also spread the shoeless gospel to coach Will Lindgren (see next page) and his elite athletes, who illustrate barefooting's power to resuscitate injury-racked careers, upgrade mileage, and even increase speed.

Ironically, none of this impressed the Society for Barefoot Living. They turned down his application because he only wrote 30 words on a required 100-word entry form.

Foltz demurs at suggestions that he put Nebraska on the barefoot running map. "Nebraska changed me into a barefooter," he says. "Through luck, I just helped return the favor."

THE REBORN, REVVED-UP, MEGA-MILE COACH

"I'm fifty-three, a historian of the sport, with one of the biggest running memorabilia collections you'll ever see," says Will Lindgren, who's logged 2,000 miles (3,200 km) a year for the past three decades. "Barefooting has always popped in and out of the historical context of running, and it always intrigued me. But I never did anything about it until two years ago, the summer of '08, when I saw Benny running with his dog Duder at one of my races. That day changed my running career—and is changing others', too."

As president of Team Nebraska Brooks, an elite development club, Lindgren is a key link in a chain of competitive running in the state, staging races and searching for talent that he can coach and nurture to the next level. From 2002 to 2009, he was the chairman of the women's long distance national championship. Internationally connected, he's responsible for bringing legendary Kenyan running star Henry Rono out of retirement. So at fifty-one, when Lindgren hadn't run in fourteen weeks due to acute deep calf injuries that didn't allow him to take one step without stabbing pain, he was in a true crisis that looked like it could destroy his world.

"It wasn't due to the shoes," asserts the father of three, as any good sponsoree of a big shoe company like Brooks might. "I traced it to the natural age- and mileage-related muscle weakness and breakdown of my stride. I could foresee an escalating series of injuries continuing, and my running career ending, if I didn't strengthen my lower extremities and correct my form. So I decided I was gonna reinvent myself from the ground up. I had to do something drastic."

So he called Barefoot Benny. Then, to be sure, he called his buddy Henry Rono. "He told me that running barefoot is why Kenyan runners were so strong and don't get injured—that it *wasn't* the altitude." So he went out for his first barefoot run—and came home electrified.

"I immediately had sensations I'd never felt before, lines of communication with the ground that had all my receptors humming with feedback. I flashed back to when I was ten years old in Illinois running along a fenceline. I was up on my toes—no longer a heel striker. It was like I was flying—without a care in the world. I knew right then that this would allow me to sense the weak areas in my legs instead of compensate for them, to strengthen them naturally. I studied Tibetan Buddhism and Lakota Sioux philosophy, and I live on the Zarinsky Prairie Preserve, so I'm out in the woods meditating a lot, but barefoot running brought me a sensitivity I'd never experienced before."

Rebuilding his running base, Lindgren started warming up and cooling down unshod, doing the first ¾ mile (1.2 km) barefoot, the next 3 miles (4.8 km) in Brooks, and the final ¾ mile (1.2 km) bare. When he complained of tender skin, Benny told him about Vibram FiveFingers. Soon, he was doing 25 percent of his runs barefoot. "Within six months," he says, "I was seeing profound results: sustained mileage, gradual weekly increases, and more mileage than I'd ever run in thirty years of running—all without any injuries." After ten months of mixed barefoot and shod training, he ran his first marathon in thirteen years (in 3:32).

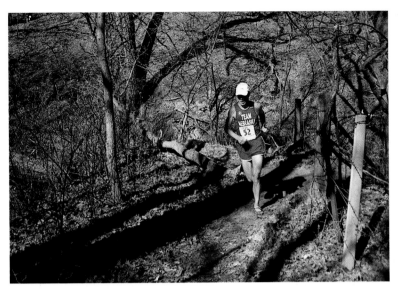

It's okay to run in minimalist footwear, or shoes, *after* you have learned to run barefoot. Will Lindgren running a trail race in Vibrams.

In 2009, the numbers were astounding: "I was fifty-two, so I wanted to do 52 miles (83.2 km) a week for fifty-two weeks. When the year was up, I had done 2,734 miles (4,374 km)—the most I've ever done by 500 miles (800 km)! People were asking, 'How can you do that at your age?'" He'd kick off a shoe and point to a bare foot.

Lindgren was also getting faster, pulling 10-mile (16 km) training runs at a sub-7-minute pace. He ran a 1:30 half marathon in September 2009 and a 1:32 at the 2010 USA half marathon nationals, both very close to his age-graded PR. Both, as in all his races, were done in shoes.

"That is a message that I am now spreading to all my runners: that barefooting can help shod runners go faster," he says. His club members got the message. Half of the twenty-five marathoners that he concentrates on now incorporate running barefoot and Vibrams into their training regimens. And barefoot training isn't limited to marathon distances. Four national or world-class middle distance Nebraska men (Shannon Stenger, Paul Wilson, Mike Beatie, and Peter van der Westhuizen, profiled below) use it enough to dub themselves "The Barefoot Striders," and budding 800-meter superstar Angee Henry, also profiled, likewise has had great success bare.

"A good thing about running barefoot is that a little of it goes a long way," says Lindgren. Because a ratio of 25 percent bare/75 percent shod initially worked so well for him, he stuck with it. Lindgren uses Vibrams for a quarter of his barefoot runs—mainly those on concrete and trails with high prairie grass; on more forgiving dirt trails, he does pure barefooting. The only reason that he doesn't run barefoot more is his sponsorship. "My loyalty compels me to run in Brooks, which is very good to me and my club, and makes it possible for me to support my athletes. Otherwise, I could very well see working up to 100 percent barefoot."

A LATE BLOOMING OLYMPIC HOPEFUL

First came knee surgery, then a child, then a decade out of competition. Then, a comeback—a 3-second improvement in one year. Finally, a national championship at age thirty-four, a decade older than most of her competitors.

You don't often hear stories like this in big-time, high-level sports. But Angee Henry, the 2010 Club National Champion in the 800 meters, says she's improving so much that she's set her sights on the 2012 Olympics—and she owes most of it to running barefoot.

A ten-time All-American, 1996 NCAA indoor and outdoor long jump champion at the University of Nebraska at Lincoln, and former Nebraska high school record holder in the 200 and 400 meters (at Belleview West High), Henry lived in France and competed as a long jumper on the European track and field circuit in the late 1990s before dropping out. Her comeback in 2008 went moderately well, with an 800-meter time of 2:06 indoors and 2:04 outdoors (the smaller indoor tracks are slower due to more curves), but was stunted by worrisome late-season quadriceps weakness, imbalance, and pain that forced her to figure out her own body and ultimately rethink her footwear.

"Looking in the mirror one day, I noticed that one quad—the right—was smaller than the other," she says. "That's when I realized that's why I hurt my knee in 2000: I've always run on the side of my right foot and worn out the right shoe. A massage therapist told me that I wasn't activating the muscles on the right side."

Henry began going to the gym to strengthen her right quad. She also started looking into running barefoot, which her club's long distance coach Will Lindgren was raving about. "I'd never heard of people using barefooting in track, but I thought it might make me more aware of what my body was doing," she says. The off-season of 2009 was a good time to try something new, so she got on the Internet, Googled running barefoot, and started walking barefoot. By July, she was "pounding out the miles" in Vibrams on a treadmill and wearing them 24-7, both in the gym and around town.

Despite a slightly strained calf from doing too much too quickly, the benefits were clear and came quickly. "I had almost no break-in period. I felt stuff activating—hips, glutes, calves, quads. No pain," she says. "I loved it right away."

Within a month, she saw the results: her right quad expanded. Her calves got bigger. "Suddenly, parts of my body started waking up. I was using muscles I didn't use before," she says. "My legs just felt stronger and more balanced."

Henry began formal track training again in August and September. At a Christmas preview meet, her performance shocked her coach, Sarah Domeier. "She was thinking I'd do 55, 56 seconds in the 400, because I'd done a 54-something at the 2009 Nationals. Well, I ran 53. She was so surprised that she literally screamed!" Henry wore Brooks racing spikes for the meet, but the Vibram/barefoot training got her there.

On April 26, 2010, at the Drake Relays in Des Moines, Iowa, Henry ran a 51.89 in the 400 meters, just behind winner Shareefa Lloyd of Jamaica (51.84) to earn an IAAF (International Association of Athletics Federations) top-40 ranking. It was 3 seconds faster than she'd run the year before—a quantum leap. "If you can run a 50, you go for a spot on the Olympic relay team," she says. "I was focusing on my love, the 800, and doing the 400 just for fun. But the 400 Olympic relay is my goal now."

Of course, Henry's no slouch in the 800. At the 2010 USA Track & Field Club National Championships in June in San Francisco, hers was named Most Outstanding Performance of the meet when she won both the 800 and the 400 and finished third in the 200. Setting a new PR by 2 seconds, she won the 800 in 2:01.81, a meet record time that beat a two-time Olympian from Guyana.

"I feel pretty good that I figured it out," says Henry, who's typical fall workout includes a 1-mile (1.6 km) barefoot warmup with sprints and plyometrics followed by a 7-mile (11.2 km) outdoor or treadmill run in Vibrams. "Shoes exaggerate your imbalances and adjust to it. If you don't step right, the shoes compensate for you." As the track coach at her old high school, she has her kids take off their spikes and warm up/cool down barefoot two or three times a week. "In high school, they all try to walk cool," she says. "Going barefoot fixes their form."

The bottom line: By kicking off her shoes, Angee Henry went from national class to world class. "I say that 80 percent of my improvement last year was due to running barefoot. It got me back to where I needed to be. First, it rehabbed me. Now it's improving me, teaching me to push through my arches." And it's also pushing her toward London, 2012.

A WORLD-CLASS RACER

Peter van der Westhuizen doesn't necessarily think barefooting itself makes him faster, but it does help ensure that he keeps getting better. That's why the 2008 University of Nebraska at Lincoln alum, who grew up running barefoot and now is a rising pro star on the international circuit (12th in the 1,500 meters at the 2009 IAAF World Championships, in 3:35.33, and 13th at the mile at the 2010 Worlds, in 3:54.9), is going to keep doing it at least a couple of times a week, as he has been ever since he was a kid.

"It's a maintenance thing," says van der Westhuizen of the regular 1-mile (1.6 km) barefoot cooldowns he does at the end of his training sessions. "Barefooting plays a key role in keeping the foot muscles strong and injury free. I've never had a serious injury, which was especially important during my developing years."

Raised in South Africa and trained mostly on grass tracks, van der Westhuizen ran almost exclusively barefoot through high school. As in Kenya, India, and other less developed countries, it is not uncommon for South African kids of all races to train and race barefoot.

"My dad (well-known coach Glen van der Westhuizen) didn't want to put lads in spikes until tenth grade, so that we would strengthen our feet during the growing years," says Peter. "Having gotten the benefits of running barefoot in my foundation, I now don't need to do it more than a couple of days a week to keep my feet strong. That's why, when I got a scholarship to go to the United States, I remained a strong barefoot advocate at Team Nebraska."

Unlike Zola Budd, the South African barefoot sensation of the 1980s, van der Westhuizen has not and will not race barefoot. "I love the feeling of nothing on my feet, but spikes are faster on the track," he says. During a race, he tries to get as close to barefoot as possible with 4-ounce (113 g) track spikes from his sponsor, Saucony. During his regular non-barefoot training, he uses a 7-ounce (198 g) spike, which lets him pursue a train-heavy/race-light workout regimen popular among top racers.

Unlike many barefoot 10K runners and marathoners, van der Westhuizen says he has never run barefoot on a paved surface—and never will. "It's dangerous and stupid to go out and run on concrete," he says. "We weren't designed for that. Yes, we were designed to run long distances barefoot on softer surfaces in warm weather—like the Bushmen (primitive tribes in South Africa's Kalahari Desert). I plan on getting a pair of Vibrams for longer runs, and would run barefoot a lot more on golf courses—3, 4 miles (4.8, 6.4 km)—if I had the time. I will definitely implement barefoot drills when I coach someday."

THE BLAZING, BAREFOOT ROMERO BROTHERS

The first running of the Omaha Marathon's Barefoot Division in 2007 created a buzz in the barefoot community that drew several of the country's best-known barefooters, including Missouri's Barefoot Rick, Ken Bob, and Tiger Paw. The biggest impact, however, was made by a newcomer on the barefoot scene: Julian Romero from Los Angeles, who took fourth place overall in 3:10. But a 3-hour barefoot marathon was just a warm-up for Barefoot Julian, who, along with his younger brother Alex, would go on to dazzle the running world—not just the barefoot world—two years later in their hometown of Albuquerque, New Mexico, in October 2008.

Rick Wright, a reporter for the *Albuquerque Journal*, explained why in the first lines of his article about the race: "The Romero brothers, Alex and Julian, run barefoot. Judging from their performance in the 25th annual Duke City Marathon, perhaps everyone should.

"Sunday morning, displaying lots of heart and plenty of sole, the two Albuquerque High graduates finished first and second. Alex Romero, 23, the 2002 New Mexico big-school state cross-country champion, won in 2:40:23. Julian Romero, 25, was the runner-up in 2:47.10."

The Romeros aren't the first barefooters to win a marathon (Bikila, anyone?) and Duke City is not the hot marathon destination for the sub-2:07 Kenyan and Ethiopian elite. But a 1-2 finish in a tough, mile-high marathon in bare feet was enough to make the front page of the popular LetsRun.com website, stoke a serious discussion in online forums across the running world, and make it clear that "speed" and "barefooter" can comfortably coexist in the same sentence.

The brothers, both studying for their Ph.D.s at the California Institute of Technology (CalTech) in Pasadena, California, at the time of their Duke City dominance, have become the ambassadors of high-performance barefooting at marathons all over the West.

"Barefooting does not compromise performance," says Barefoot Julian, who parlayed his Ph.D. in macroeconomic game theory into an assistant professorship at Purdue University in Indiana in 2010. "There's less weight—no shoes—less friction, better heat management, and automatically better form."

HE AIN'T HEAVY, HE'S MY BROTHER

Ironically, the 200-pound (91 kg) Julian, a thickly muscled former collegiate baseball player, was the family's barefoot guinea pig, not the sleeker 6-foot-1, 170-pound (77.3 kg) Alex, a longtime runner. Julian came to running barefoot out of intellectual curiosity, not injury. "In 2004, Alex read the profile of Ken Bob in *Runner's World* and told me about it," says Julian. "He couldn't try it yet because he was running track and cross-country at Duke University. I was just getting into running and was intrigued. I'd just been up in San Francisco doing my first marathon (in shoes, in 2:52.30), and heard a lot people say that marathons were bad for your knees, especially for heavier people. Hearing running barefoot had less impact, I decided to give it a try."

His first barefoot run in August 2006 in San Marino was a mixed bag. "I saw that I immediately had to change my form—no heel striking, clapping my feet on the ground, landing on the outside of my feet. I had to stop and stretch my Achilles. My feet were very tender. It was clearly going to be a difficult adjustment. I was not convinced running barefoot made sense. Luckily, I ran 10 miles (16 km) the next day in shoes—and got really sore. That was my last run in shoes."

The transition wasn't pain free. "The muscles of my feet—which I'd never felt before—got pretty sore," he says. "At times I'd think, 'What am I doing?'" After just three months of running unshod, an unusually rapid adaptation period for artificially shortened calves and Achilles tendons, barefoot Julian lined up at the 2006 Las Vegas Marathon. Expectations were low; in training, he was doing 10-minute miles, far slower than in shoes. So he was shocked to run a 2:55.

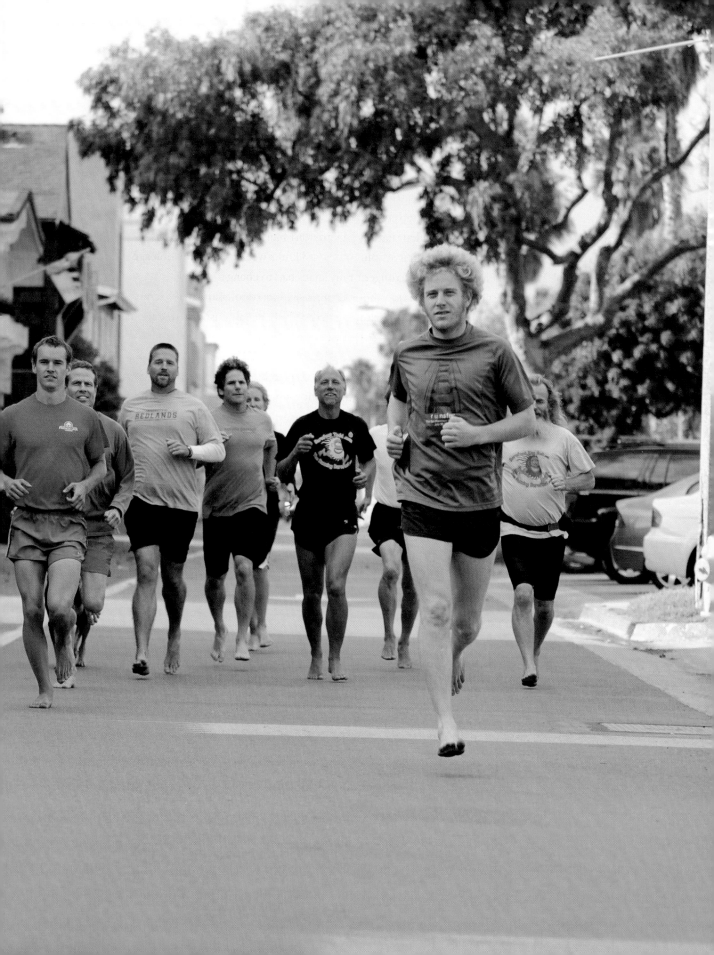

"The most difficult part about running barefoot in Vegas that day was all the attention; I didn't like it," he says. "People saw the no shoes and no shirt and 40°F (4.4°C) starting temperature and looked at me like I was crazy. But on the plus side, I didn't have any problems at all, and I met Barefoot Ken Bob at the finish. I was already on his email list."

As Julian was racking up his first of fifteen unshod marathons and 8,000 barefoot miles (12,800 km, by September 2010), his little brother Alex back at Duke was chomping at the bit to go barefoot. "Starting with a stress fracture in my tibia during freshman year, I was injured all the time—bursitis in my hips, knee problems, back problems, you name it. I wanted to know why," he recalls. "I finally concluded that my legs couldn't handle my aerobic fitness— that I *was too fit for my feet*! I was running 80-plus miles (128 km) a week, double my mileage in high school. Either my feet had to get stronger or my shoes had to change."

In high school, running in what he calls "crappy Etonics, with hard soles and barely any cushioning," Alex was never injured. At Duke, running in the plush, deeply cushioned Asics Kayanos provided free to the team in a typical collegiate sponsorship agreement, he was always injured. Barefooting seemed like the answer. "I'd always intended to get into it; as an evolutionary biologist I was convinced that we humans were optimized by evolution to run barefoot over millions and millions of years. But I thought it would take years [to make the switch from shoes]. Well, it doesn't! Julian proved it."

FIRST, WALK THE LINE

Nonetheless, Alex began his barefoot odyssey slowly. The gravel track that the team worked out on was too rough and painful for running barefoot, so he started by walking barefoot everywhere around the Duke campus—until the cafeteria workers told him that he couldn't dine unshod. One time, seeing that shoes were required in a grocery store, he fashioned impromptu slippers out of newspaper and duct tape—and was kicked out by a security guard. "It was crazy," he says, looking back. "I was trying to argue with the guard that my 'shoes' were more substantial than the flip-flips most students wore."

When he started running barefoot after graduation, the aches and pains quickly disappeared—and neglected body parts began to reappear. "I started feeling muscles I hadn't felt before—on my feet, calves, thighs," he says. "It made me think, 'Hey, your calves are big, strong muscles—why aren't we using them? It turns out that the entire lower leg gets underused when you run in shoes, which force you to emphasize the upper leg's glute and hamstrings. It's like if you'd been in a wheelchair all your life and started walking. The strength and coordination of the lower legs must catch up to that of the upper legs."

One of the most exciting aspects of running barefoot to Alex was the feedback. "The feedback from your soles tells you when to speed up, when to run softer, when to cool it," he says. "I started feeling like an efficient animal rather than a clumsy human being." In shoes,

←Alex Romero (front) won the 2008 Duke City Marathon while running barefoot.

Alex could run 15 miles (24 km), but usually felt fatigued during the second half. At the end of 15 barefoot miles (24 km), he felt balanced and fresh. The barefooting also taught him how to run correctly in shoes. On rough trails, while wearing his old Asics cross-country shoes, he could feel that his form was better.

When Alex joined Julian at CalTech, the brothers turned it on, running 35 miles (56 km) from Pasadena to Long Beach on Thanksgiving. When they did the San Francisco Marathon in the summer of 2008, Alex's 2:42—a new PR—was 10 minutes faster than his shod time there in 2006. Then came the trip home to Albuquerque for the 2008 Duke City Marathon.

"I was surprised to win," says Alex. "I wasn't feeling that good in the morning, and had strong intentions to drop out at 7 to 10 miles (11.2 to 16 km). But everything clicked."

His 2:40:23 time is still his PR, as the rigors of Ph.D. studies and founding a rock band, People of Animal Town (he sings and plays guitar, keyboards, and ukulele), cut into his running time. "But watch me at L.A. next year (2011)," he says. "I'm training for a 2:30. Bikila can rest easy with his 2:15 in Rome, but if there's a domestic barefoot record, I will break it someday."

Like pied pipers, the Romero brothers spread the word whenever they run. At the 2010 L.A. Marathon, a racer with bib number #25363 was seen crossing the finish line barefoot while holding his shoes in his hands. When he began cramping about mile 18 (28.8 km), he told a reporter that he had had a brief conversation with a barefooter who turned out to be Julian, who finished in 2:56. "He told me how good and natural it felt, so at mile 20 (32 km), I kicked off my shoes and ran the last 6 miles (9.6 km) barefoot. It feels weird at first, but you adapt. My cramps went away. I'm sold on barefoot running. I'm going to start training without shoes and will try to do my next one barefoot."

THE FIFTY-FIVE-YEAR-OLD 5-MINUTE MILER

It makes me feel good that so many people—as everyone mentioned so far in this chapter—first heard about running barefoot by reading an article about me, by Googling "barefoot running" and finding TheRunningBarefoot.com, or by meeting someone who'd done that. But running barefoot was around long before me and my website, and long before Nebraska became such a hotbed—and I don't just mean Bikila and Phidippides. In fact, when I first joined the Snail's Pace Running Club, I was its *second* barefooter. The first turned out to be one of the finest age-group runners in the world, and today remains a phenomenal athlete, more proof of barefooting's power to protect and preserve your running performance. Meet my friend Dave Parsel, age fifty-five, skin cancer survivor, California state indoor 20K record holder in the 45–49 age group, and one of the rare fifty-five-year-olds who has run a 5:04.8 mile (at the Southern California Road Runners 1-Mile on August 9, 2010).

→ Dave Parsel leading the pack, as usual

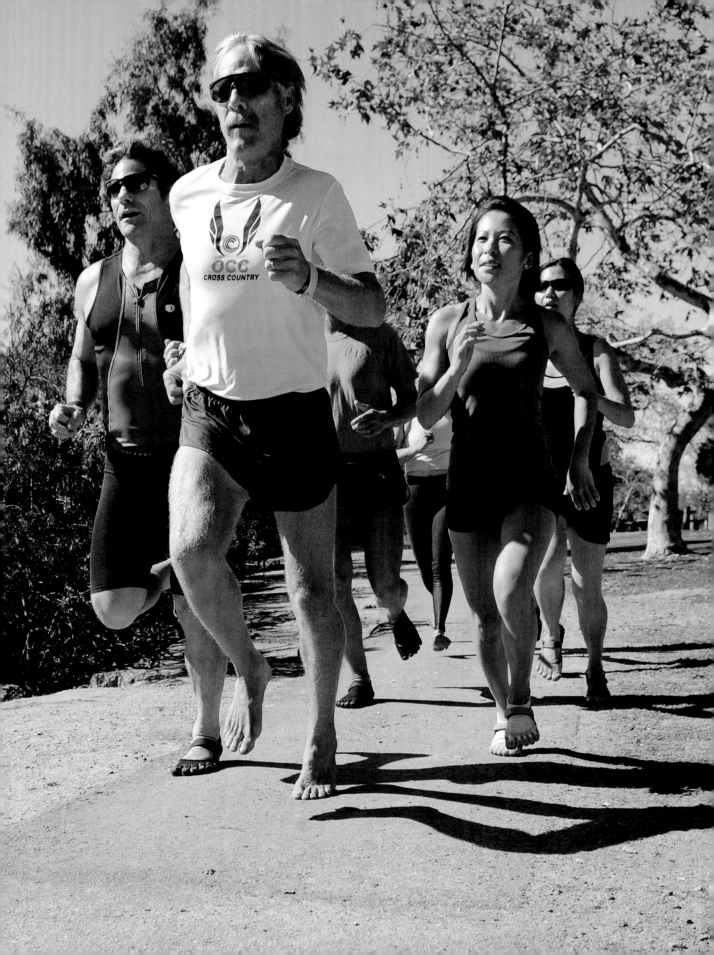

The son of a Newport Beach doctor, Parsel grew up barefoot on the sands of Lido Island, a tony enclave of yachts and million-dollar homes. "At school, we were barefoot at recess because we were on the beach, playing Frisbee and watching gray whales migrating every spring and winter," he recalls. "Other than wearing cleats in Pop Warner football, I was barefoot all year." In high school, Parsel was a wide receiver on the football team and a sprinter on the track team, doing the 100 m, 220 m, long jump, and relay—"all for fun." Fast, with good hands, he later ran track and played football at Orange Coast College, and had a scholarship offer to play small-college football at Redlands. Then, in a game in the fall of 1977, he got stuck in clay mud while catching a pass, took a hard hit, broke his fibula—and began to reevaluate his future.

"I realized that I wanted to be healthy as I got older," he says. "Football was over; the pros don't want a guy only 5'9". So I saw that running was something that I could do for the rest of my life." Always a big fan who admired Frank Shorter and Steve Prefontaine, he'd never run over 5 miles (8 km) at a time and was "never one of these super-skinny guys who do cross-country." But he set a goal to break 45 minutes in a 10K, and in a "fantastic day" in the summer of '78 ran a 43:30. Thrilled, he began to run on his commute to work when he moved to Aspen to ski for a couple of years. Soon, he was heavily into triathlons, doing many half Ironmans and a near-full Ironman in Nice, France, while working variously as an athletic club manager, a prefab electrical technician, a machine operator, and a deliveryman/courier. All the while, he ran barefoot on the beaches and in the parks, remembering from his childhood that he could always run the sprints faster barefoot.

At age thirty-one, after showing some speed in some local races and mentioning to the coach that he still had two years of college eligibility remaining, Parsel was invited to join the track and cross-country teams back at OCC, his junior college alma mater. "It sounded like fun. So I took fifteen units—first aid, weight lifting, swimming, and light academics," he says. "And I ended up doing the 4 mile in 19:52 and becoming the cross-country conference champion in the fall of '86. In the spring, at age thirty-two, I won the 10K state championship in 30:47, and took second in the 5K." Rumor abounded that the blond, long-haired Parsel, a dozen years older than everyone else, was a retired pro surfer who'd discovered running. After his eligibility ran out, he stayed around for ten years as a coach, and currently still volunteers.

In the decades since, Parsel has run twelve marathons, with a PR of 2:33 at age forty-four, and hundreds of 5Ks, his favorite distance. "They're fast—and you can do a lot of them because you can recover by the next week." He set his 5K and 10K PRs of 14:29 and 30:37 at age thirty-two, ran a 15:17 at age forty-five, and at fifty-two did 5Ks in 16:35 barefoot and 16:31 in shoes, and ran a 10K in 34:22. He can still push it into the high 16s, but says a 17:45 is usually enough to win his age group as long as his pal Richard Burns isn't in the race.

Although Parsel starts most workouts barefooted at an easy 8- to 9-minute pace, does sprints on grass or a rubberized track, and did a few 5Ks on the track unshod (spikes weren't allowed), he's always run the road in shoes. "I'm into performance, not pain, not into running hours a day on thorns and gravel," he says. "Ken Bob will run on lava fields in Hawaii barefoot, but not me." Just once, in 2007, he barefooted a road race, the local Pacific Shoreline 5K (16:45, fifth place overall, first in the 50–55 year old male division), "because Ken Bob gave me a free entry. But I checked out the streets first."

Parsel doesn't know for sure whether the barefooting makes him stronger, but he likes the feeling and the simplicity. "If my feet could handle it, or if I had a problem with shoes—I haven't—I'd go barefoot all the time," he says. "I'm no zealot. I'm not crowing from the top of the world about running barefoot. It's simply fun and enjoyable for me. Everyone can remember running barefoot in the park, so why not do it as an adult? But my rule is: don't push it. Everyone's different. I'm still running at fifty—most aren't. I have my kids at OCC do barefoot drills, but only if they want to."

Never much for material things—he lives in a small house, married late in life, and has no kids—Parsel likes the economics of running barefoot. "It's saved me thousands of dollars in shoes," he says. "I'd never use Vibrams unless they gave 'em to me; why spend the $80? I'd rather step in dog doo barefoot than in $100 shoes." Fortunately, his running club gives him New Balance shoes, which he wears when he isn't in his favorites: knock-off Crocs. A few years ago, he bought five pairs for $1.99 each. "They're as light as racing flats. I use them when it's cold and the surfaces are rough. It's better to pull a sticker out of a Croc than out of bare feet."

Parsel averages more than 60 miles (96 km) of running a week. Fifteen to 20 miles (24 to 32 km) are in his fake Crocs, 20 to 30 miles (32 to 48 km) are barefoot, including most of his interval training, and the remaining 10 or 20 miles (16 or 32 km) are in New Balance. "I've never liked to wear just one pair of shoes," he says. "My advice is to stay out of a rut. Mix it up. The barefooting keeps you strong, but don't go overboard. There's nothing better than running 6 miles (9.6 km) on the beach barefooted, but 600 feet (183 m) works, too. Above all, make sense: if the route's got rocks, wear shoes. Do what works. If it adds to your enjoyment, I'm all for it."

FAST TIMES ON AS LITTLE AS 25 PERCENT

Running barefoot, as you have seen by Nick Hanson's landmark study and the various athletes profiled in this chapter, can make you faster. The elimination of shoe weight, combined with the natural foot strengthening and form restructuring, yields an economical, fast-turnover, soft-landing stride that safeguards your training against injury and leaves you faster—*even if you run in shoes most of the time*. The amount of barefooting practiced by the people profiled in this chapter varies from 100 percent to a couple of warmups a week. The people range from kids just out of college to baby boomers, and from barefooting diehards who absolutely won't do anything else to those who run mostly in Vibrams.

Personally, except during winter in Michigan, I can not conceive of running in shoes 75 percent of the time—and for the past thirteen years I've rarely worn shoes at all. It is nearly true, as my buddy Barefoot Ted was once quoted in a Los Angeles Times article, that I am a "zealot" who won't even touch "minimalist shoes," much less cushioned trainers. I say *nearly* because I have touched them. Ted once offered me a free pair of Vibrams. I figured they'd be good for whenever I want to go into a store guarded by "shoe police," but while Ted and I were being interviewed for a running documentary, all the samples were grabbed up by his running-club friends except for a size 11. I'm an 8. And back in 2005, at Nike's request, I did do a couple of evaluation runs in the new Nike Free; it felt weird, like my soles were being deprived of their sense of touch. I told them that they were "just shoes." After all, I equate shoes with discomfort, and as I made clear in chapter 1, I like comfort. But that does not stop me from being ecstatic over these emerging stories from the running world that show that even a little bit of running barefoot can go a long way for people who run shod most of the time.

As Peter van der Westhuizen demonstrates, it is clear that once you learn how to run correctly—i.e., barefoot, as he did while growing up—you can transfer that form to shod running in minimalist shoes or racing flats *as long as you occasionally refresh and revisit your pure barefoot technique*. If you don't, as I elaborated on in chapter 6, which took a hard look at Vibrams, you'll get sloppier and sloppier until eventually your sloppy technique gets you injured again.

You never really get running barefoot technique locked down, partly because it's a matter of responding to so many variations in terrain and in your own body, as well as continuous improvement from experimenting, getting feedback from your quality control inspectors (the soles of your feet), and playing. But I am not uncomfortable advocating the "25 percent Nebraska rule": do a quarter of your runs barefoot. If you're competing on the track, emulate Angee Henry and warm up and cool down barefoot. I've come to realize that running barefoot is a lot like any task at my work: Once I've learned how to do it, there's still room for improvement and, of course, experimenting—playing around trying to figure out a better or easier way to do it. Running barefoot occasionally is more than simply a refresher course to keep yourself on track—it lets you know when the track changes! That's why almost every shod runner should run barefoot, at least occasionally, to avoid getting sloppy.

I thought of another analogy while driving on the freeway one day after discussing this chapter with Roy, my cowriter. Watching a car ahead of me weave back and forth in his lane, as the driver adjusts his radio, read a text message on his phone, or something, self-correcting when his wheels hit the disclike "Bots Dots" that mark the lane dividers, it hit me that you can run or drive along a path for a while with your eyes closed, as long as you open them once in a while. Occasionally opening our eyes—i.e., "baring your soles"—will allow you to make the adjustments you need to keep yourself in the center of the path (i.e., ideal running technique).

To stay in your correct biomechanical "lane," do you need a 5-minute barefoot warmup and cooldown before and after a shod run, a once-a-week 5-miler (8 km), a barefoot run every other day, a half-barefoot/half-Vibrams regimen, or pure daily barefooting? The answer, to continue with the car analogy, depends on many individual factors: How familiar are you with the road? Do you drive this way every day? Could you, in fact, drive it blindfolded? How familiar are you with your vehicle (are your tires aligned, is your frame bent)? How attentive are you—do you pay more attention to the way you are running, or just kind of zone out? The latter might be okay—as long as good running technique is so ingrained in your body that you couldn't run badly if you tried. Some people have never run barefoot and have never had injuries. Some people need to run barefoot every day to prevent injuries.

So how much should you run barefoot after you've learned to run barefoot? A baseline, like the 25 percent Nebraska rule, may be enough for some. To be as fair as possible to all the benefits shoes provide, I would say "run barefoot as much as possible." It's sensible that if you are starting to get injured, it is a sign that you should run barefoot more often. And when you do, don't be surprised if you start running faster.

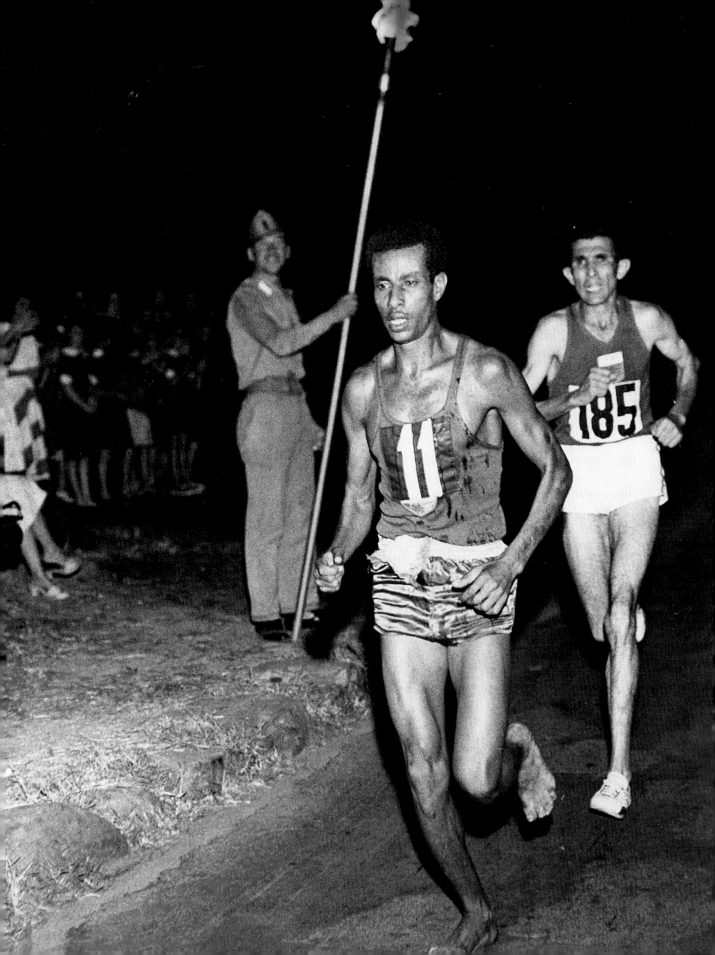

CHAPTER 8

MORE THAN BIKILA
PROFILES OF THE GREAT UNSHOD

Ten of history's greatest barefoot running stories prove that barefoot-bred speed is the real deal at the highest levels.

Skeptics who are convinced that rumors of elites running barefoot are a myth roll their eyes every time a barefoot advocate immediately mentions Abebe Bikila or Zola Budd whenever he needs proof of a fast barefoot runner. "Him again? Her again? Aren't there any more than those two?" they squawk. Well, they're right to ask. There are plenty of other notable examples of unshod feet producing world- and national-class performances, such as the people profiled in this chapter. And keep in mind that these are surely the tip of the iceberg, as there are untold hundreds or thousands of great Olympians and world champions, particularly Africans, who spent years living, walking to school, and training in bare feet.

So why don't you see unshod toes on the Olympic telecasts every four years? The answer has nothing to do with simply running economically; it is simple economics: Money talks. Shoe company contracts require the athletes to lace up on the big stage. There's no other reason to sponsor them. The takeaway here: A history of running barefoot and continual shoeless training helps many athletes "get away" with the inefficiencies of shoes. And fear not if you were unfortunate enough to grow up with modern conveniences like shoes; one English barefoot star profiled below, Bruce Tulloh, didn't do his best until he dumped his shoes at age twenty-four.

Here's a brief roundup of some of the standout feet—and feats—of modern barefoot running history.

←Abebe Bikila running the 1960 Rome Olympic marathon barefoot

ABEBE BIKILA: THE BAREFOOT ICON

The only man to win the Olympic marathon twice, Ethiopia's Abebe Bikila did it both barefoot and shod, setting world records each time. A son of a shepherd, the twenty-eight-year-old soldier arrived at the 1960 Rome Olympics with a secret that his coach had deliberately kept hidden: He'd won his county's Olympic trials a month earlier—in shoes—in 2 hours 23 minutes—2 minutes faster than the winning time at the 1956 Games in Melbourne. No one knew it, but he arrived at the starting line on September 10, 1960, as a favorite for the gold medal. Yet he surely was not anonymous; he'd created a minor sensation by being the only one of the sixty-nine competitors to show up without shoes. Many of his amused rivals flatly predicted that Bikila would not finish the marathon, much less have a chance to win.

According to the book *Triumph and Tragedy: A History of Abebe Bikila and His Marathon Career*, by his daughter Tsige Abebe, Bikila did not plan on running barefoot in Rome. "The sneakers he brought with him were worn out," he writes, so Bikila went shopping, bought a new pair, and wore them around for a few days to break them in. "However, his pointed, slender feet could not adapt to the sneakers; instead, he developed painful blisters. No solution seemed to be in sight. There was only one thing to do: Run barefoot." He had not run barefoot in nine years.

What followed after the gun sounded at 5:30 p.m. that day would amaze onlookers and competitors alike. With spectators pointing at his feet and reporters scratching their heads, Bikila seemed to fly over the huge, rounded cobblestones of the city's Via Appia Antica, which intimidated the other runners. Staying with the leaders to the 18K (11 mile) mark, he was the only one to hang on when Rhadi Ben Abdesselam of Morocco surged. Dropping about 70 meters (76.7 yd) back of his fellow African, Bikila slowly began pushing the pace, and ran side by side with his fellow African until they reentered the center city of Rome. Then, with the last 500 meters (547 yd) to go, Bikila surged. The barefoot runner crossed the line 26 seconds ahead of Rhadi in a new world record time of 2:15:16.2.

A national hero in Ethiopia, Bikila, who was promoted to the rank of corporal by Emperor Haile Selassie and awarded the Star of Ethiopia medal, was aggressively pursued by the shoe companies and never raced barefoot again. He won shod marathons in Greece, Japan, and Czechoslovakia in 1961; took fifth in the Boston Marathon in 1963; and won the Addis Ababa Marathon in 1964 as a tune-up for that year's Tokyo Olympics. Although not expected to compete forty days after having his appendix removed, he appeared at the start line in either Pumas or Asics (depending on the source), dropped Aussie Ron Clarke and Ireland's Jim Hogan by the 30K (19 mile) mark, and won the Olympic marathon by 4 minutes over Britain's Basil Heatley in a new world record of 2:12:11.2. And this time he did it in shoes. The emperor again promoted him, and he received his own car, a white Volkswagen Beetle.

A favorite for the 1968 Mexico City Olympic Marathon, Bikila had to leave the race after 10½ miles (17 km) due to an injured right knee, leaving the victory to his friend, countryman, and longtime running partner Mamo Wolde. A year later, swerving his VW to avoid student protests during civil unrest in Ethiopia, he crashed and was left a paraplegic. But being wheelchair-bound didn't stop him. In 1970, he participated in a 25K cross-country sledge competition in Norway and won the gold medal. In 1973, at forty-one, he died in Addis Ababa from a cerebral hemorrhage, a complication related to the accident. His funeral was attended by 75,000 people, and Emperor Selassie proclaimed a national day of mourning.

GARRY BJORKLUND: MY LEFT (BARE) FOOT

When twenty-five-year-old University of Minnesota grad Garry Bjorklund took his place on the starting line of the 10,000 meters at the 1976 Olympic trials, held July 22 at Hayward Field in Eugene, Oregon, he was not a barefooter. That changed—partially—about halfway through the race, ensuring his place forever in the barefoot hall of fame.

By the 4-mile (6.4 km) mark, the race for third place at the U.S. Olympic team's 10,000-meter qualifier race for the Montreal Olympics looked about over. Frank Shorter and Craig Virgin had sewn up the 1-2 spots. With a lap to go, third placer Bill Rodgers was 25 yards (22.7 m) ahead of Bjorklund, whose left shoe had fallen off at the 3-mile (4.8 km) mark. Rodgers's lead seemed insurmountable, especially against a man clumping along imbalanced on one shoe and one bare foot. But having missed the 1972 trials due to an operation on the same foot, Bjorklund, the 1969 AAU 15K champion, heard the bell lap sound and shoved it into overdrive like he'd never done before. After all, this was probably his last shot at the Olympics. Saying later that he was motivated by the chant of "BJ! BJ! BJ!" from his supporters in the East Grandstand pulsating through his head, he pulled even and passed Rodgers with 50 yards (45.5 m) remaining, finishing in third place by less than a second in 28:03.74, his PR.

He'd just made the Olympic team on one shoe. And one bare foot.

In two shoes, Bjorklund went on to finish 13th in the 10,000-meter final in Montreal in 28:38.08. Lasse Virén of Finland won in 27:40.38. After that, Bjorklund went on to win the 1977 and 1980 editions of Grandma's Marathon in his hometown area of Duluth, Minnesota, setting a PR of 2:10.20. He set his 10K PR of 27:46.9 in 1984. In 1991, the Garry Bjorklund Half Marathon, which starts an hour before Grandma's, was created to recognize his contributions to long-distance running in Minnesota.

ZOLA BUDD: THE BAREFOOT PRODIGY

Nobody had seen anyone like Zola Budd. The broken records, the controversy, the picture-perfect form, the almost total barefoot training and racing. In less than three years, from 1984 to 1987, the young unshod South African twice broke the 5000-meter world record and twice won the World Cross Country Championships.

Budd burst onto the international scene in 1984 at age seventeen when she set her first 5,000 m record of 15:01.83, more than 6 seconds under Mary Decker's current mark. The time was not ratified by the IAAF due to South Africa's Apartheid-based sanctions, but a couple of years later, she cut 12 seconds off that while running under the British flag. Although the controversy over her conveniently changed nationality threatened to overshadow her participation in the 1984 Los Angeles Olympics, that was soon overshadowed by a bigger controversy: a brief collision in the final of the Olympic 3,000 m between Budd and American icon Mary Decker, who was sent sprawling into the grass. The unnerved Budd finished a disappointing seventh place, but recovered in grand style in 1985, winning the World Cross Country Championship and breaking the UK and Commonwealth records for the 1,500 m (3:59.96), the mile (4:17.57), the 3,000 m (8:28.83), and the 5,000 m (14:48.07)—the latter time setting a new world record by a whopping 10 seconds. In 1986, she repeated as World Cross Country champion and set an indoor world mark of 8:39.79 in the 3,000 m.

That year, ironically, injuries not directly related to running barefoot led to poor results and forced Budd to begin racing in shoes. A chronic hamstring injury, ultimately tied to leg-length differences, led to a stress fracture where the hamstring joins the pelvis. In 1987, a kinesiologist relieved the pain by placing wedges made of cut-up phone book pages in her shoes, which she had to wear in races 3,000 m and longer to avoid pain. She still ran barefoot in short races and training.

Budd's plans for competing for Britain in the 1988 Seoul Olympics were ended by a one-year IAAF suspension, punishment for competing in one race in her home country. Out of shape and 30 pounds (13.6 kg) over her 1984 Olympic weight of 89 pounds (40.5 kg), Budd began training again in mid-1989 and gradually won her form back by 1991, posting the world's second-fastest 3,000 m time (8:35.72). She competed in the 3,000 m for newly unsanctioned South Africa in the 1992 Barcelona Olympics, but, afflicted with tick-bite fever, was eliminated in a qualifying heat. In 1993, she took fourth at the World Cross Country Championships, and then settled into married life. In August 2008, she and her family moved to Myrtle Beach, South Carolina, on a visa that allows her to compete on the U.S. masters' circuit. In recent reports she was volunteering as a college coach and racing, including a win in the women's division of the Dasani Half Marathon during BI-LO Myrtle Beach Marathon on February 14, 2009, in 1:20.41—in shoes.

MICHELLE DEKKERS: BAREFOOT PEDAL TO THE METAL

A barefoot sensation in the mold of her countrywoman Budd, Cape Town native Dekkers not only was undefeated in 1988, but also joined Indiana University teammate Bob Kennedy that season to become the first runners from the same college to win individual NCAA Cross Country Championships in the same year. That day, in 28°F (-2.2°C) temperatures in Granger, Iowa, Dekkers did what she did in every single race that year: Bolt from the pack and never look back. After leading the 3-miler (4.8 km) from the start to her 16:30 finish, she explained that barefooting gave her a special motivation. "I prefer running without shoes. My toes didn't get cold. Besides, if I am in front from the start, no one can step on them."

Although that was her only NCAA championship, Dekkers remained strong through her graduation in 1990, winning the Big 10 title for the third time and the NCAA District IV. On July 12, 2000, Dekkers sent a quick update in response to her name appearing on my website. "All of my children love to run around barefoot. My oldest boy (eight-year-old Michael) seems to be under the impression that shoes will only slow you down, especially running through the mud and sand. I can't wait to get back into running after this baby is born. My dream would be for all my children to enjoy the freedom of running barefoot over open grass fields or along the beach! Since I just turned 32, I hope I still get into racing shape and be an inspiration to all my children. We currently live in Fort Lauderdale, Florida, and I have been married to Jim Maton (NCAA indoor 800-m champion) for ten years."

HERB ELLIOTT: DR. FRANKENSTEIN'S BAREFOOT MONSTER

Herb Elliott, one of history's great middle distance runners, was the 1,500 m gold medal winner at the 1960 Olympic Games in Rome; ran seventeen sub-4-minute miles; and as a senior runner, was undefeated at both the 1,500 m and the mile. In 1958, the Australian set new world records in both the 1,500 m (3:36.0) and the mile (3:54.5), the latter broken by a tenth of a second four years later by Peter Snell. Elliott's 500 m win in Rome was by the largest margin ever recorded in Olympic history.

Although none of the above races were performed barefoot, serious barefoot training helped make them possible. Under the tutelage of coach Percy Cerutty—a renaissance man, yoga proponent, barefoot believer, and health food nut regarded as an eccentric genius—Elliott made extensive use of barefoot running in training, running unshod on all surfaces, including famously sprinting up sand dunes until he dropped at his Port Sea training camp on the Victorian coast. Photographs of Elliott during barefoot training runs twice graced the cover of *Sports Illustrated*—on a sand path (November 10, 1958, issue) and on a road (May 30, 1960, issue).

A link to a French-made late-1950s film of a white-haired Cerutty demonstrating barefooting can be found by going to BarefootRunningStepbyStep.com and clicking on the "videos" tab.

After capping off his three-year unbeaten span by winning the gold in Rome in 1960, Elliott retired at the age of twenty-two, on April 19, 1962. He went on to an extremely successful business career as chairman of the board of Fortescue Metals Group and CEO of Puma North America.

RON HILL: MINIMAL FOOTWEAR, MAXIMAL LIFE

Barefoot Olympian. World record holder. Boston Marathon winner. One hundred and fifteen marathon finisher. Running shoe and clothing manufacturer. Racer in a hundred countries. Proud owner of "The Streak"—a daily run of at least 1 mile (1.6 km) in length since December 20, 1964; as of 2010, that's about 154,000 miles (246,4000 km) over forty-six years and about 17,000 days in a row. Ron Hill, a superstar on the British and world running stage in the 1960s and '70s, known for his boundless energy, stellar performances, and relentless innovation, is a force of nature.

A committed "minimalist" who pioneered the use of lightweight shoes and synthetic clothing, including a near-naked mesh running vest, Hill set records in the 10-mile (46:44.0 in 1968), the 15-mile (1:12:48.2), and the 25K (1:15.22) in 1964—over a minute faster than Emil Zátopek's previous mark); in 1970 he was the first marathoner to break 2:10 on a disputed course; and he raced barefoot frequently in the 1960s, including an unshod win at the English Cross Country National Championship and at one of his three Olympic Games (1964, 1968, and 1972). Despite a closet full of Commonwealth Games medals, he never brought Olympic metal home in the 5,000 m, 10,000 m, or marathon. But he did draw "some gasps" (as he put it) from the Mexico City crowds in 1968 when he stepped on the tartan track for the 10,000-meter final while barefoot, ultimately taking seventh place in 29:53.2.

After shattering the course record by 3 minutes at the 1970 Boston Marathon (in 2:10.30), and clocking the first undisputed sub-2:10 (2:09.28) at Edinburgh that summer, both in minimalist shoes he designed, Hill set his sights on running the 1972 Olympic Marathon in Munich barefoot. "I meant to put everything on the line that day," he told Amby Burfoot, editor of *Runner's World* magazine. "But as it turned out, the Germans resurfaced some of the park pathways with these fresh, sharp stone clippings. It made going barefoot impossible." Instead, he wore ultra-light shoes—and again didn't medal. I'm not saying Hill would have won that day barefoot, but using my technique and with the additional stimulation of the rough pathways, who knows—he might have run even faster!

Although he ran in an era of minimally cushioned shoes (compared to today's shoes), Hill was always worried about the "wobble" of bigger shoes, which he said increased strain on the ankles, knees, and hips. Convinced evolution designed us to run barefoot, he felt modern materials made it possible to give the foot adequate cushioning in an almost-barefoot shoe. Ironically, Hill says he did a lot of his road training in heavier shoes. "That way, when I raced barefoot or in my light shoes, I felt like I was floating."

ELIUD KIPCHOGE: NANDI DIRT POWER

It seems almost cliché to assume that every great East African runner grew up barefoot and trains barefoot, but a fact's a fact—that's what you see at the Junior races at the cross-country championships in Kenya and Ethiopia. Young up-and-comers run them in bare feet because they have no other choice; they're unknown and have no shoe sponsors. As they mature, win internationally, and attract sponsors, they'll often race in shoes but maintain barefooting at home.

Example: One of the last decade's fastest 5,000-m runners, Kenyan's Eliud Kipchoge. The 2003 world champion (in 12:52.79), 2004 Athens Olympics bronze medalist, 2007 world's runner-up, and 2008 Beijing Olympics silver medalist is a member of the renowned Nandi, the "running tribe" of the high-elevation hills rising from the Rift Valley. The sweeping dirt roads that curve into the horizon are perfect for running barefoot, which Kipchoge does every day, according to the Fat Kenyan Runner, a Nandi blogger living in England. Kipchoge's 2003 world championship win over Ethiopian 5,000 m and 10,000 m world record holder Kenenisa Bekele (12:37.35 and 26:17.53, respectively) was a David-versus-Goliath slaying that had everyone scrambling for answers. "He won it by training completely barefoot along those hills by my grandfather's farm," writes the Fat one.

Unfortunately, winning giveth and taketh away. In the years since, Kipchoge has seen less success against the Ethiopian superman. Could the problem be shoes? "He felt his stride became less powerful after he won the world 5K championship and was given lots of shoes to train in," reported an observer. Joseph Ebuya, the 2010 world cross-country champion who has beaten both Kipchoge and Bekele, has a similar story: he was given shoes after his coach "discovered" him running barefoot—and almost immediately wound up injured. A good example of how to avoid the problem may be Christopher Kosgei, a Kenyan 3,000 m steeplechase specialist of the 1990s who became known for winning the silver medal at the 1995 World Championship in 8:06.86 while running barefoot. Four years later, he became world champion in his distance with an 8:05.43. He kept barefooting in training and continued to run many Grand Prix meets in Europe without shoes.

DR. CHARLIE ROBBINS, THE BAREFOOT PIONEER

The godfather of American barefoot running, Robbins won two U.S. national marathon championships in 1944 and '45 while running barefoot, which he did for sixty-eight years. A legend in the Northeast, the man known as Doc won a variety of Amateur Athletic Union titles at 20K, 25K, and 30K; completed twenty Boston Marathons, finishing third in 1944; and ran fifty-seven Thanksgiving Day Manchester Road Races near his childhood hometown of Manchester, Connecticut, including a streak of fifty straight that ended in 2001. Most of the 5-mile (8 km) runs were unshod, though he'd put on a pair of socks if the temperature dipped below 20°F (-6.7°C). His death in August 2006 at age eighty-five was noted by runners, barefoot and non-barefoot, all over the country.

"In 1947, when I ran in Central Park, a policeman asked what I was doing," Robbins had said. "I said, 'Running.' 'Nobody does that in the city,' he said, 'and you'd better put your shirt on.'" That exchange, reported by George P. Blumberg in a 2002 *New York Times* story, illustrates how far ahead of his time he was.

As a teenager, Robbins caught the barefoot running bug by running 4 miles (6.4 km) home at midnight from clandestine meetings with his girlfriend and future wife Doris at her grandfather's farm. A star runner in high school and the University of Connecticut, he saw no reason to stop after he began his medical practice. In fact, because he found that he needed the physical activity of running, he integrated it into his career and family (the Manchester Road Race was a Thanksgiving morning family tradition) and became one of the first doctors to advocate running and fitness. While other doctors played golf on Wednesdays, Robbins was joining cross-country practices with undergrads like Amby Burfoot. Active to the end of his life, he typically did several a hours a day of sawing and splitting wood and breaking up rocks with a sledgehammer, then 30 minutes of running "to take the soreness away." Adhering to a simple diet and lifestyle, he was slim as a rail throughout his life, 5'7" and just over 100 pounds (45.5 kg).

"Running barefoot seemed natural," Robbins once told the *New York Times*. "Five million years of evolution didn't include shoes. I run the same or a little better speed than with shoes. Sometimes I race halfway with and halfway without shoes. The change feels good. When you run barefoot, you don't pound," he said. "When I don't feel well, I go out and run and things seem better."

Just before Robbins died, Ken Bob visited Connecticut to make "Doc" Robbins the first inductee into TheRunningBarefoot.com Hall of Fame. To honor the memory of his old running partner before the 2006 Manchester Road Race, Amby Burfoot organized and led the Charlie "Doc" Robbins Memorial Barefoot Warmup, a 15-minute barefoot run up Main Street to the start line.

DALE STORY: GONE BAREFOOT

On a cold afternoon on November 27, 1961, Dale Story, a junior at Oregon State, won the NCAA Cross Country Championship at East Lansing, Michigan. By defeating future Tokyo Olympics 10,000-meter gold medalist Billy Mills, and Australian Olympians Pat Clohessy and Al Lawrence, he helped the Beavers to their first (and fifty years later, only) national team title. The temperature that day was 30°F (-1°C), and it was snowing. Story was barefoot.

Then he disappeared, literally, into the woods. A diehard outdoorsman and naturalist who liked hunting, fishing, and hiking and disliked the city life associated with college, Story did not make running his priority post-graduation.

Growing up shoeless as a kid in Orange, California, Story ran a 4:32 mile as a barefoot sophomore in high school and set a national high school mile record of 4:11 as a senior, wearing spikes. Mostly, he ran barefoot.

"I just liked the feel of running barefoot, of being free," he told Kerry Eggers of the *Portland Tribune*. He never wore shoes in high school meets until the California Interscholastic Federation made uniforms mandatory. "Because there was a bit of slippage on the track, I started wearing spikes for some track meets my junior year. But I always ran cross-country barefoot."

Story trained for a short time after his graduation in 1965 with the idea of taking part in the 1968 Olympic trials, but his discomfort with urban life got in the way. Soon he got married and gave up the dream. "My heart just wasn't in it," he says. "I struggled with that for the next twelve years or so. I felt like a failure. Then finally, I realized I did what I wanted to do; I didn't achieve all my goals, but who does?"

Story never competed again, but he continued to make his mark, coaching track and field for twenty-nine years and cross-country for twenty-five at Wallowa High. His boy's teams won seven state championships in track and two in cross-country, and his cross-country teams finished among the top five in the state eight other times.

Now retired, Story is quite active. He hikes the nearby hills, often without shoes. Long one of the Northwest's premier bow hunters, he has bagged thirty-one big-game animals, including black bear, moose, and a bull elk with antlers big enough to stretch across two counties.

"Sometimes when I'm moving in for the stalk, I will take off my shoes," he told Eggers. "It is quieter. You can feel the ground with your feet. I have been doing it for so many years, it is kind of a like a good-luck charm."

BRUCE TULLOH: IT'S NEVER TOO LATE TO GO BAREFOOT

Unlike most good barefoot runners, Bruce Tulloh of Great Britain did not take up running barefoot until he was an adult, at age twenty-four. But so many good things happened so fast that he has gone down as one of the most successful barefooters in history, most notably winning gold at the 1962 European 5000 Championship in Belgrade without shoes. He also won a bunch of British distance titles and records, mostly without shoes.

A late starter to running, Tulloh didn't seriously take up the sport until he was twenty, while doing his National Service in Hong Kong in 1955. Convinced shoes were impeding his performance, he began competing without them in 1959. "I ran a bad time for the 3 miles (4.8 km) and I decided to try it without shoes on," he told Amby Burfoot. "It worked and a few months later, I won my first British Amateur Athletic Association 3-mile title (in 13:31.2)." He dropped that to 13:17.2 and 13:12.0 in the next couple of years, but withered in the severe heat in Rome and did not make the Olympic 5,000 m final. In 1962, he set a new UK 2-mile (3.2 km) record of 8:34.0, ran what many think was the world's first sub-4 mile, then made his historic trip to Belgrade for his greatest moment, the European 5,000 m Championship.

With 700 m (765 yd) to go in a slow, tactical race with the Russians Bolotnikov and Zimny, he kicked. On the second lap, the barefooter broke it wide open, winning in 14:00.6.

Moving to longer distances, in 1966 he set a UK 6-mile (9.6 km) record of 27:23.8 on a cinder track, and took sixth in the 10,000 meter at the European Championships in Budapest in a PR of 28:50.4 before retiring the next year.

Later, Tulloh taught in Africa, coached, wrote books, ran solo across America (2,876 miles [4,602 km], albeit in shoes), and kept running barefoot.

"The only reason that more people don't run barefoot is that they're afraid to be unconventional," he says. "On the right surface, barefoot is the best way to run. It was really a matter of convincing myself that I could do it in a major event," he told BBC Sport Online.

"It depended on the track. If it was gritty enough, then running barefoot was the most efficient way. It's the lightest running shoe ever."

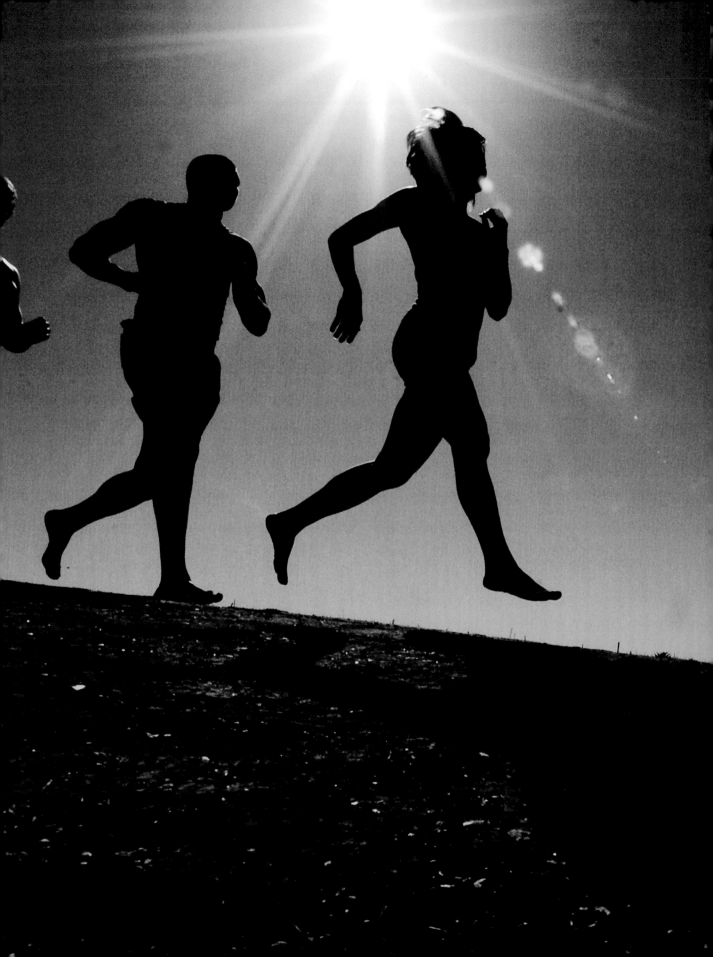

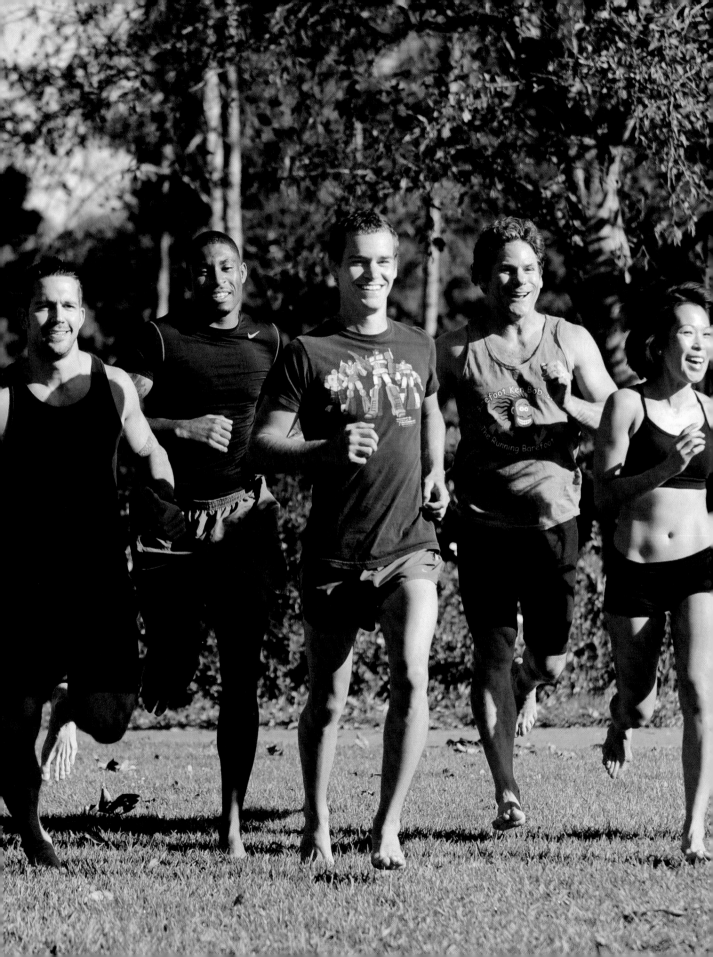

SECTION IV:

REAL-WORLD BAREFOOTING

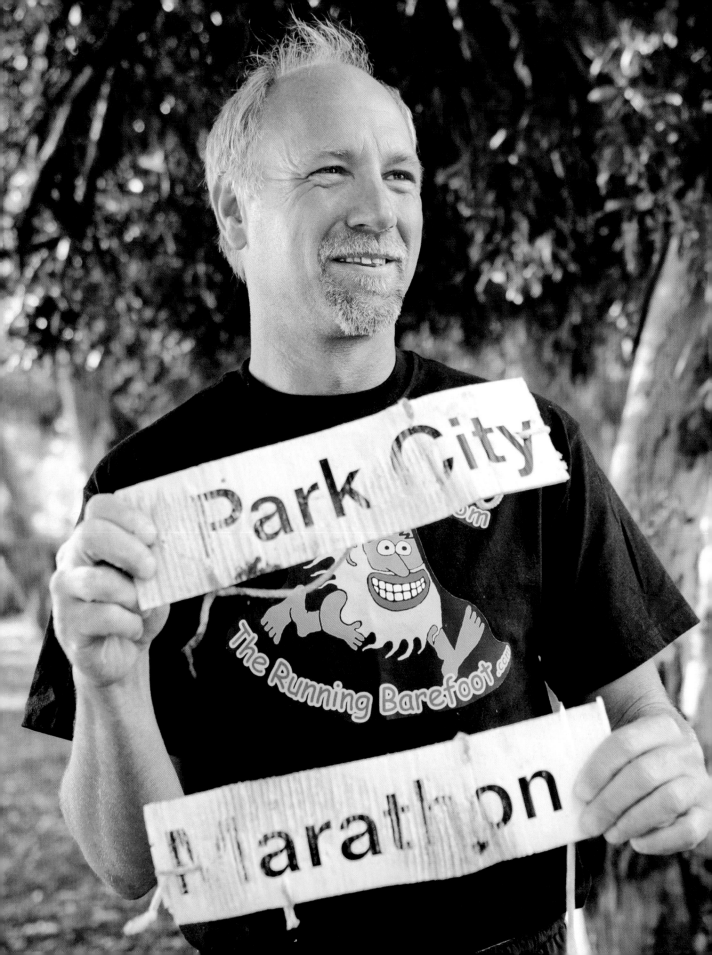

CHAPTER 9

THE BAREFOOT RACING LIFE
RUNNERS TELL IT LIKE IT IS

Barefooting is not mainly about PRs and how many miles per week you do. Here, in their own words (and mine), meet an 8-hour marathoner, a totally bare 5K runner, and other unique, unshod tales of comedy, triumph, and fun.

> 66 RUNNING BAREFOOT IS TO RUNNING IN SHOES AS MOUNTAIN BIKING IS TO ROAD BIKING: INSTEAD OF THE NUMBERS, THE SPEED, THE PLACING, IT'S THE VIEW, THE FEELING, AND THE EXPERIENCE THAT MATTERS MOST. 99
>
> — BAREFOOT KEN BOB-ISM #104

Yes, I've been mildly obsessed with numbers, not unlike any shoe-wearing runner. I've got my marathon-a-month streak (in 2004) and my year of excess (fourteen marathons in 2006, including four in a fifteen-day period). I've got my various PRs and respectable age-group finishes.

But when I look back on the moments that really stand out in my decades as a barefoot runner, they focus more on once-in-a-lifetime tales of camaraderie, struggle, and triumph that have little to do with numerical accomplishments and more to do with the unique sensations and vantage points offered by a couple of bare feet interacting with the environment.

Some people, like my friend Owen McCall (author of one of the stories below that make up this chapter), say that they happily lose their desire to race when they get into running barefoot, but not me. I love racing. I love the buzz of hundreds or thousands or even just a couple dozen runners coming together, congregating in a new city or an old one, and experiencing the course together. But by doing it barefoot, the racing is even better, the experience heightened; you "feel" the course on several new levels and get a satisfaction that—for me, anyway—makes the importance of the numbers fade.

I've got dozens of stories I'd share if this book had a couple hundred more pages (see BarefootKenBob.com), but there's no better example of my most cherished experiences as a runner and as a human than the 2007 Park City Marathon with my buddy Barefoot Todd. We like to call it . . .

THE LOST BOYS

Could this be the longest marathon run in history?
by Barefoot Ken Bob

In the summer of 2007, I got a call from Barefoot Todd Byers, who was doing a marathon a month that year. I had met Todd, a former officer of the Seattle Marathon and now one of my best friends, during a barefoot run that my running club did for a *Los Angeles Times* photo shoot and story about me in January 2000. Already a dedicated marathoner with 140 finishes (in shoes), this aerospace engineer, Team in Training coach, and race-course certifier started running barefoot that day and never stopped, completing over 140 more marathons since—the majority barefoot. He racked up his 100th barefoot marathon on January 15, 2011. (Incidentally, he's never had any injuries in or out of shoes, but stuck to barefooting so that he could swim with me during the San Diego Marathon. For details on that, see the sidebar.)

Anyhow, Todd loves traveling all over the world to compete in marathons, including New York City (ten times), London, the Great Wall of China, and Antarctica (this one done in 422 laps on deck 6 of a ship anchored offshore because a snowstorm made it too difficult to land). Now, he was calling to say that he wanted me to join him at the Green River Run with the Horses Marathon in Green River, Wyoming. I wasn't planning on running any marathon that August, but it's always fun to hang out with Todd, and this would be a quick two-day trip. The plan was that we'd fly to Salt Lake City, then drive two and a half hours north. But after we booked the flights, I found something more interesting and convenient that same day, just thirty minutes outside of Salt Lake City in the resort town of Park City.

The course description of the Park City Marathon told us to expect mostly paved roads and paved bike trails, with a 7-mile (11.2 km) stretch of "smooth" gravel trails along a rails-to-trails path. The rest of the marathon was on paved roads, with the last 5 miles (8 km) on a paved bike path.

It turned out to be our first—and last—8-hour marathon.

Concerned about the "smooth gravel" trail section in the description, Todd was unsure whether to run in shoes or go barefoot. So we drove up to the course the day before to check it out, getting woefully lost in the process and driving out of our way for a couple of hours. Finally, we came across a small rail-to-trail path that turned into very rough gravel at about mile 5 (8 km). "I can't run on this!" Todd exclaimed, pointing to sharp rocks everywhere. I didn't say a word. I had run and raced barefoot many times on rougher gravel; however, this was the kind of rough stuff that Todd usually avoided, sticking to smooth roads and sidewalks. So we planted his shoes behind a green roadside utility box near the beginning of the gravel and returned the next day for one of the weirdest odysseys of our running lives.

The first 5 miles (8 km) of the marathon was an uneventful cruise on creamy smooth asphalt, as expected. Taking it slow, we hung near the back of about 400 racers and entertained ourselves by watching hot air balloons high above our heads and trying to get pictures of each other standing close to the cows along the route. The cows ran off whenever Todd got close. Yes, ladies, Todd is still available (BarefootTodd.com)!

Todd retrieved his shoes from behind the utility box and we polished off the next 7 miles (11.2 km) of gravel easily, which brought us to a smooth asphalt bike path. Todd kept his shoes on for a couple of miles, waiting for a good spot to stash them where we could drive back and pick them up later. I amused myself by sharing pictures of my dog with other dog owners alongside the course and updating my website from my new phone. As we headed into upper Park City, Todd quizzed some fire personnel volunteers near a bike shop about the extent of gravel trails further on. Some said they didn't think there were any, but one guy was certain there was several more miles of gravel starting at the big white barn, a featured landmark of this course.

Todd, feeling strong that day, decided to stash the shoes anyway, and chance either not running into gravel or being able to tough it out. So we continued on, both barefoot, running uphill, circling around the Deer Valley ski area, past some of the 2002 Olympic ski runs. Then looping back down the hill toward the bike shop again, we caught up with a walker named Dale, who had started early. By then, since we were back at the bike shop, we realized we'd missed a turn somewhere. The volunteers had already left, so we asked one of the bike shop employees to look up the course map online.

The three of us backtracked together at walking pace up the paved bike path, and just before mile 14 (22.4 km) saw a dim faded line of green chalk on the pavement, pointing the way. Back on course, we waved goodbye to Dale and ran through a fancy play area, with a large chess set and an amazing skate park. We were behind schedule, having done 4 extra miles (6.4 km), but at least we were running again. We figured that we could still finish before the 6½-hour cutoff time.

SKILL-BUILDING ON THE ROCKY ROAD

About mile 21 (33.6 km), we saw the big white barn. I remembered the course description stated that it would be 5 miles (8 km) from here to the finish on a "paved" bike path. I may have remembered badly. As we approached the barn, we saw the worst kind of gravel there is to run on: big white stones with sharp edges, the kind often used in railroad beds. Todd wasn't too happy about having left his shoes behind.

Although I could have run ahead, I would have needed a 10-minute pace to finish before the cutoff, and at this altitude with no training, I just didn't feel like it. And it wouldn't have been nearly as much fun as teasing Todd for the next six miles. After finishing more than 200 marathons, many of them barefoot, the gravel seemed to be his kryptonite! Besides, I didn't feel right leaving Todd out here alone on the trail, without shoes, and uncomfortable running

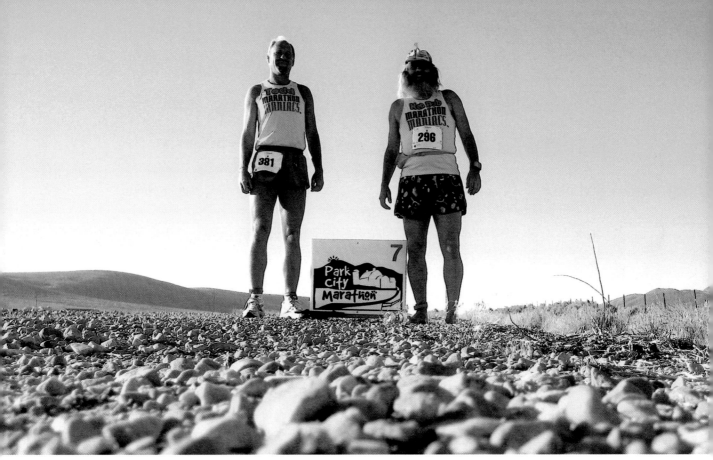

Barefoot Ken Bob is pictured here with Barefoot Todd Byers, who mixed it up in the Park City Marathon by running barefoot on the road, then with modern running shoes across the first 8-mile (13 km) stretch of gravel.

barefoot on this exceptionally stimulating gravel. After all, I was only here in Park City because of Todd. Yes, I could have finished, then run back with his shoes. But, because we already got lost once, I would already have covered more than 30 miles (48 km) by the time I finished, 12 to 13 miles (19.2 to 20.8 km) of that on gravel trails (plus a few more if I ran back to Todd after finishing), and might have required a MedEvac helicopter to get me home. So I did what I went there to do: run with Todd.

We ran on the road parallel to the bike path for a ½ mile (0.8 km), then got back on the trail when it veered away to continue the marathon. The gravel wasn't as bad as it was by the white barn, but Todd was practically limping and talking about giving up. To buoy his spirits, I told him that he was making good progress with his technique, since limping is really just bending your knees more—a good thing. Once you balance out your limp with both legs equally, it's no longer a limp.

Within a mile, Todd gave up, and then started again. It looked like we'd be out there all night when we saw the plastic 22-mile (35.2 km) marker sign. On the back was a smaller 24- by 4-inch (61 by 10 cm) piece of sign material with the words "Park City Marathon" printed on it. It was about the size of two shoe bottoms. Suddenly, we seemed to be thinking the same thought: Make sandals out of it!

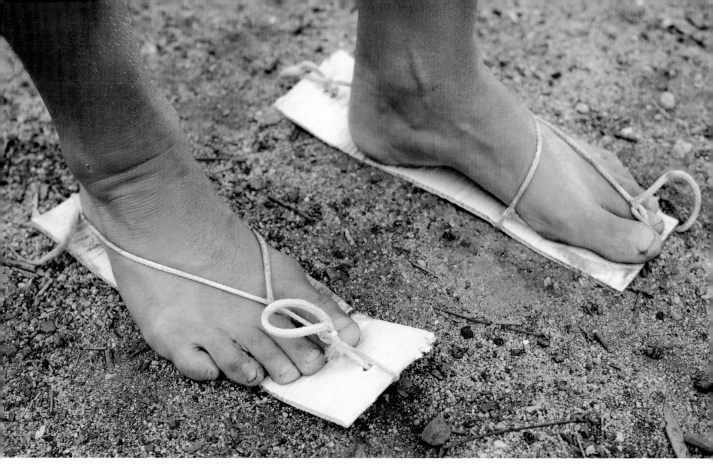

Sandals were improvised from a Park City Marathon mile-marker sign, and strings from our running shorts, to help Todd cope with the last few miles of gravel trails in the Park City Marathon.

Todd tore the plastic off the back of the sign. After breaking the sign in half, we used some sharp rocks to drill holes. We both removed the strings from our shorts for makeshift laces. It was a wonderfully strange and primal feeling, using sticks and stones as tools, to transform the raw materials from our nearby surroundings to create a practical solution to the problem. What do you expect when a former aerospace engineer and a technician are stuck in the woods?

Todd ran the strings through the holes, and tied the sandals to his feet. Just as we were finishing the manufacturing process, Dale caught up with us.

Soon, Todd was happily walking along in his new sandals, and the three of us started walking the final 4 miles (6.4 km) toward the finish. We ran into a man named Rich, whose backyard bordered on the bike path, and he and his family offered us glasses of cool, refreshing water, which we enjoyed immensely before continuing on our way.

A few places along the gravel path, there were some nice little cow paths, which were a relief for me, now that I was the only one barefoot. Dale chatted on his phone with his wife, and she asked the race organizers to set aside three shirts and three medals for us before most of them left for the day.

Eight hours and 11 minutes and 16 seconds after we started, we straggled across the finish line into a pleasant grass park, numbers 384 and 385 out of 386 finishers, to find that a couple of the organizers had decided to wait and see these crazy "barefoot runners" finish. I enjoyed showing them that my feet had indeed survived intact on the second-most challenging gravel I've ever run or walked on (number 1 is the last 15 miles [24 km] of the Shadow of the Giants 50K), and one of the longest *times* I had spent barefoot on gravel.

I rarely, if ever, want to discourage people from going barefoot most places. The Park City Marathon is a beautiful course. I strongly recommend you ride your mountain bike or cross-country ski on it. Because no matter how stimulating or invigorating running barefoot on gravel is, half a marathon's worth can clearly push the envelope. If you only run barefoot on golf courses or sand, and want to very quickly understand the importance of bent knees and relaxing to running gently, try the last section of the Park City Marathon for 5 or 10 minutes. Eight hours may be a bit much.

THE MARATHON AS A DUATHLON

In 2003, Barefoot Todd and I ran the San Diego Marathon together, neither of us pushing too hard. I was running it as a training run for the Pacific Shoreline Marathon in Huntington Beach the following week. He had only been doing shorter distances barefoot, so he ran San Diego in shoes. We ran a lot and walked a little until mile 23 or 24 (36.8 or 38.4 km), where the course goes along the ocean. I immediately ran into the water for a quick dip to cool off, while Todd lagged behind as he took off his shoes. When we came out of the water, I then had to wait for him to clean off his feet to put his socks and shoes back on. "What's taking you so long?" I joked. "If you didn't have shoes, that wouldn't be a problem!"

In 2004, Todd decided he didn't want to make me wait again, so he bit the bullet and ran San Diego barefoot—his first-ever unshod marathon. Ironically, over the past year I had taken to carrying a fanny pack with a cell phone during my races, so when we came out of the water he now had to wait for me as I retrieved my pack. "Come on, Ken, we have a marathon to finish!" he said.

Todd went on to do seventeen more marathons that year, eight of them barefoot. He began using some barefoot techniques, such as not skidding the feet, to successfully teach his Team in Training runners to run gently and blister free. As of late November 2010, of his 280 career marathons, 97 have been done barefoot.

Of course, if any of those courses skirt the water, Todd jumps in. "Now, I don't call them marathons," he says. "They are actually duathlons."

THE ONLY NUDE BAREFOOT RUNNER

First, he took off his shoes. Then he went all the way.

by Hank Greer

I filled out the registration form and reached the part where it said, "Indicate if you will be running nude. You may change your mind later if you wish."

Oh, I'll be nude, I thought, and then some.

I had recently taken up barefoot running and thought this would be the consummate race for running with bare feet.

I circled "yes," completed the rest of the form, and mailed it in with a check for the registration fee. Then I asked myself: *do I have the cojones to run in the nude?* I still had a month and a half to decide. For the time being, though, I felt pretty confident about wearing my birthday suit in the 2009 Bare Buns Fun Run, held for the 25th straight year at the Kaniksu Ranch, north of my home in Spokane, Washington.

I wasn't familiar with the roads to Kaniksu, so I left home early on the morning of the race. After driving 30 miles (48 km), I ended up on a long, dusty road passing through some beautiful woods and pastures. In the distance, two hazy clouds told me I was following a couple of other vehicles. Another car caught up and closed in behind me. Waiting at the gate to the ranch was a man sitting on an ATV and wearing goggles to protect his eyes from the dust. He waved us through.

I slowly continued along the road for another mile or so, and reached what looked like a water station. A fire truck was parked nearby and a few people milled about a table holding a couple of watercoolers. A man in an orange vest pointed, directing me to make a left turn into the woods. I noticed the road was mostly packed dirt and that it had been hosed down that morning, probably to keep the dust down.

After about a half mile (0.8 km), I came upon a most unusual sight standing at the side of the road: a nude potbellied man with very long gray hair streaming down between his shoulder blades.

A table on the other side of the road held a couple of watercoolers and a package of cups, indicating another water station. The man smiled, waved, and said hi as I drove by. I couldn't help but think of him as a very large, nude, beardless gnome standing in the woods.

Arriving at the main compound, I found tents filling a grassy area surrounded by cabins. Plastic yellow tape and orange cones marked the race path going through the compound. Kiosks selling food, drinks, jewelry, and other goods were set up near the finish line. A tranquil pond behind the kiosks reflected the gray sky. Another man—this one wearing clothes and an orange vest—told me to continue up the road and park anywhere I could find a spot.

I parked my van, stuck the key in the tiny pocket of my running shorts, and walked back to the compound. A few clothed and a lot of unclothed people were present, which is to be expected at a nudist ranch. But several people were wearing shirts and nothing else down below, apparently because it was a cool morning. I found the combination of covered torsos and exposed lower bodies—especially the men—very disconcerting. It was like a number of people had started to dress or undress, forgot what they were doing, and continued on their day completely oblivious of their half-dressed state.

But what really struck me was the lack of what would generally be considered beautiful bodies. You know those images epitomizing health and beauty that are fed to us by the fashion and entertainment magazines in supermarket checkout lines, the ones that remind us of our many imperfections and implore us to firm up or lose weight in ten days? They were not present this day. There were people of every conceivable shape and size here with absolutely nothing to hide and not trying to. Nobody was Photoshopped and everyone was pretty casual and indifferent about it.

At the registration desk, I picked up my race number and a piece of yarn to tie it around my neck with. A Velcro band containing a chip to time my run went around my left ankle. I also received a commemorative pin marking the 25th anniversary of the Bare Buns Fun Run. How funny to hand out pins to a bunch of nudists. I managed to shove the pin into the pocket holding my key. I asked a man at the desk if it was okay if I just set my clothes off to the side at the start of the race. He said, "Sure. Nobody around here wants any clothes anyway." Good point.

I walked over to the start area near the field of tents and patiently waited. A few minutes later, there was a bit of excitement. I saw smoke rising about 200 feet (60 m) away. A kiosk blocked my view so I couldn't see what was on fire, but I thought it odd that there was a fire. As the smoke thickened and the rising flames were now visible from my viewpoint, a few people closer than me started yelling, "Fire!"

Remarkably, most people seemed unconcerned. I moved to the side until I had a clear view of a propane-fed cooker engulfed in flames. Two propane tanks sat at the base. My imagination instantly created newspaper headlines announcing hundreds of nude people horribly burned by exploding fuel tanks and I started backing away. Then a man with a large fire extinguisher—and I don't mean in a figurative sense—put the fire out. With the short-lived but potentially devastating emergency over, I walked back to where I was before. A race official dressed only in an orange safety vest and carrying a bullhorn walked by me, tugged on my shirtsleeve, and said, "You can take those off at any time, you know."

"I plan to," I said.

I found it interesting that although I wasn't ready to take my clothes off yet, I really wasn't that concerned about running nude. My mind was on something apparently no one else had considered: running barefoot.

FIRST SHOES, THEN CLOTHES

Two months earlier, I had read about the benefits of running barefoot and decided to give it a try. It turned out to be more involved than I could have guessed. Besides the obvious need for thick calluses, I had to change my running style and strengthen some muscles in my lower legs. There were some painful times for my shins and soles, but I was now at a point where I could comfortably run barefoot for 3 miles (4.8 km) on a mix of asphalt, cement, and grass. Yet even with my thickened soles it still hurt to step on rocks, so I had to pay attention to the running surface, keeping a careful eye out to avoid landing on stones and debris. And yet, even though my feet needed to toughen up some more, there was one benefit to barefoot running I did not expect.

Running was no longer a chore I did to stay fit. The change in my running form was taking less of a physical toll on my joints and muscles. I felt like I was gliding along and using my body more efficiently. Running was now fun.

As the start time neared, runners were directed up one road and walkers to another. Now I started to feel a little self-conscious, since I was one of the few people wearing clothing. One nude man wore a knee brace and a couple of men and women were wearing only heart monitors. You have to be a serious runner to be wearing a heart monitor on a nude run. I didn't see many people wearing clothes. And why would I?

I was thinking about running barefoot again and asked a man next to me about the surface of the route. He said most of it is packed dirt but there was a rocky area near the turnaround point. With that, I decided to go for it.

After all, my whole reason for doing this was to run the Bare Buns Fun Run completely bare. I removed my shoes and socks and set them on top of a nearby stone wall. I pulled my shirt off and shucked my shorts, folded them up, and set them on top of my shoes. I decided not to stretch for two reasons. One, I didn't need to. It was only 3.1 miles (5 km) and I wasn't racing. Second, I noticed several men—and it was mostly men in the runners group—who were stretching. The human body may be beautiful, but not from all viewpoints. Certain stretches being done by nude men and viewed from certain angles just makes you turn away with an "I don't even need to see that." I thought it considerate of me not to put the others through that.

I returned to the group and became disconcertingly preoccupied with where to put my hands.

Funny how being completely uncovered can make you feel so perplexed. Should I cross my arms? Maybe put my hands behind my back? Let them hang straight down?

While I periodically changed hand positions, unlike everybody else, and tried to look casual, like everybody else, I noticed there were very few people in my skin tone category. Many were tan all over and some were pale all over.

I'm an avid cyclist, and thanks to the cycling shorts and jerseys, I am tan from the bottom third of my thighs down to my feet, from mid-biceps to my hands, and on my face and neck. Pasty white in the middle and brown on the ends, I likened myself to an undercooked gingerbread man.

Since I could not remember being nude outside ever in my lifetime, I'm guessing this was the first time my butt had seen sunshine since I was two or three years old, if at all. But the nonchalant attitude that surrounded me actually made me very comfortable and I gradually relaxed. Nobody was pointing or staring. Until . . .

"Now there's a bare runner," said a man pointing at my feet.

"That's hard-core," said another.

I didn't respond. I didn't know what to say, and besides, they weren't asking me a question. In a self-conscious reaction I did glance down at my bare feet and spied a quarter lying on the ground. Normally I would pick that up, I thought, but I don't have anywhere to put it.

EVERYTHING'S OFF—AND THEY'RE OFF

Unexpectedly, a cannon boomed to start the race. The cannon was so loud and surprising that had I not gone to the bathroom beforehand I surely would have made an embarrassing wet spot on the ground.

The crowd of runners started down the road ahead of the walkers and passed by the cheering spectators at the starting line who would also be there when we finished, since the line served a dual purpose. The sensor dutifully marked the passage of the chips on our ankles. Wearing a race bib, timing chip, glasses, wedding ring—yes, this (c)hunk is happily spoken for—and hearing aids, I was off on my first and probably only nude run.

As I mentioned before, an important aspect of running barefoot is that I need to see the ground ahead of me so I can avoid stepping on hurtful objects. I was in a large crowd of people going down a single-lane dirt road, so it was difficult for me to see. I would slow down a bit to create some space ahead of me and someone behind me would pass me by and fill it in. Consequently, my first mile was rife with uncomfortable stabbing pains from landing on the occasional small stone. Just past the 1-mile (1.6 km) mark, the gnomelike man I drove past earlier—now wearing the orange vest of a race official—was handing out cups of water to anyone who wanted one. I pressed on.

As the group of runners stretched out I was able to pick out my path and speed up my pace. Then suddenly I was boxed in. A young woman was right in front of me, and there were people to her left and right. As with any race, random people converge and match pace for a bit and you have to wait for the group to break up so you can move ahead. I was looking down at this woman's butt, which under other circumstances would not have been an unpleasant sight, but I wanted to see the path.

I nailed a couple more rocks before the other runners separated from her and I was able to get by. This was an out-and-back race, so as the faster runners came back up the road, they forced us to stay to the right and I had to be more careful to avoid getting blocked in again.

Nearing the turnaround point, I was greeted by the water station I saw when I first drove in and a roadbed of fist-size rocks. I put the brakes on and carefully walked across the rocks while the shod runners I had just passed now returned the favor. I ran to the turnaround point and returned to pick my way across the rocks again.

"Where are your shoes?" asked a woman at the water station as I gingerly stepped by.

"Up at the start," I replied. Leaving the rocks behind, I took off. Being familiar with what was ahead and having a very clear view, I could pick up the pace and had a much more pleasant return trip. Along the way, a few more people commented about my bare feet. The potbellied man smiled at me as I zipped by.

After crossing the finish line in my birthday suit, a race official stopped me and asked if I ran the whole course barefoot. He said he'd never seen that before.

I walked over to the T-shirt table and traded my bib tag for a shirt, one I probably won't be wearing in mixed company. The design is a nude woman sitting on a bear leading a lot of nude people on a run. And it includes the words "Nude Finisher" to indicate the wearer did in fact cross the finish line nude. I grabbed a cup of water and walked back to the start area where my clothes sat undisturbed.

I put them back on and picked up the quarter I spied earlier. My feet were a little sore and it felt good to have shoes back on. Because the road to the ranch was also the race route, I couldn't leave yet, so I watched the remainder of the finishers come in, all of them unconcerned about their various floppy body parts slapping time with each step as they ran down the hill to the finish. Some of the people wearing clothes would strip down just before the end and then cross the finish line nude, thus meeting the minimum requirement for receiving a nude finisher shirt.

As I watched and waited, a number of finishers walked by. One of them asked, "Hey, aren't you the guy who ran barefoot?"

"Yes," I answered.

"That was pretty cool."

So there's the answer to the question at the beginning of this story. I do have the cojones to run the Bare Buns Fun Run in the nude—but you had to be there to see them. And having seen my fifty-two-year-old body in the mirror, I'm betting my run down the hill to the finish line was not the most attractive sight. I'm also sure that nobody cared. No, the only thing remarkable about me running nude for a little over 3 miles (5 km) was that I wasn't wearing shoes. And like all my barefoot runs, it was fun.

Hank Greer is a computer programmer in Spokane, Washington. A longtime runner, cyclist, and exerciser, he expects to keep barefoot running forever but has no plans to do the Bare Buns Fun Run again. "Been there, done that, and moved on to the next thing," he says.

TEN MONTHS TO THE TRIPLE CROWN

Big Damon dumped his shoes, zapped his injuries, had more fun, and scored his big dream.

by Damon Hendricks

The weekend of August 15, 2010, was a good one for me. I completed the America's Finest City Half Marathon (AFC) in San Diego, reached my 500th barefoot mile, and *finally* conquered the Southern California Half Marathon Triple Crown (Carlsbad, La Jolla, and AFC all in the same year). And I couldn't have done it without going barefoot.

The Triple Crown had been a goal of mine for the past four years, but I kept getting hurt. I have been running consistently for about twenty years, averaging about 25 to 30 miles (40 to 48 km) per week, and participated in dozens of half marathons and a couple of full marathons. I have had a litany of injuries, everything from a pulled calf muscle, to stress fractures, to sprained ankles, and other various strains and pains. I even required major ankle surgery a couple of years ago from a softball injury. But my primary injury was plantar fasciitis, which I could not shake at all for about three years. I tried everything to get rid of it—rest, ice, stretches, exercises, massages, shoes, insoles, custom orthotics—and nothing worked.

Last year I read *Born to Run*, did all the research, found Ken Bob's website, blah, blah, blah . . . the same thing that most of his readers have probably done. I also am fortunate enough to live in Southern California and attended a few of Ken Bob's workshops in Huntington Beach.

After October 11, 2009, when I ran the Long Beach Half Marathon, I decided to transition to barefoot running and start at square one: no phasing it in, just stop wearing shoes completely on my runs. I started with walks and gradually began running and increasing my mileage carefully.

Within thirty days of my transition, my plantar fasciitis was completely *gone*! I noticed my feet getting stronger and tougher, and my new barefoot running style was leaving me feeling refreshed and satisfied after my runs rather than tired and achy. (By the way, I'm forty-one, 6'1", 215 pounds [98 kg].)

My initial goal was to complete the Carlsbad Half Marathon barefoot on January 21, 2010—and I did it. That's basically zero to 13.1 miles (21 km) in four months. I think I was the only other barefooter there (not including at least one other person in Vibrams). The reactions I got from other runners and spectators along the course were fantastic, and I had so much conversation during the race that time flew by. The only downsides are that I did get blood blisters on each big toe (I still need to work on my downhill form), and I was about

30 minutes slower than my shod times. In this race last year I ran at an 8:36 pace, which was a PR for me. This year barefoot I ran it at a 10:51 pace. Admittedly, I was apprehensive and nervous about my first barefoot race and the fact that I had not gone 13.1 miles (21 km) barefoot yet. I purposely took it easy to make sure I would finish. However, I started to notice a change quickly, as I began getting more comfortable and saw my times coming down. Two weeks after Carlsbad, I ran the Surf City Half Marathon in Huntington Beach, and knocked my time down to 10:29 per mile. And my body felt way better than it did after Carlsbad.

Overall, the blood blisters and slower times of Carlsbad were a small price to pay for the way I felt both mentally and physically after the race.

I then went on to finish the La Jolla Half Marathon, leaving only San Diego to go for the Triple Crown. That day, by the end of the big race, my feet felt fantastic. Not a cut, scrape, or blister anywhere, only a little street grime. By the way, AFC is a beautiful run, barefoot friendly, and I definitely recommend it. Miles 2 through 5 are all downhill, so your downhill form will definitely get challenged.

As I mentioned, a very cool side effect for me is how fast the races seem to go by now. That's because I spend so much time talking to other runners along the way, most of whom have heard of running barefoot and have read *Born to Run*, and a few who want to transition themselves.

About 99 percent of the response is very positive, but you always get that one guy. This race I had a guy come up to me and told me to meet him after the race so he could give me his card. As he pulled ahead of me, his wife pointed to the logo on his back and laughingly said, "He's a sports medicine doctor!" My reply was, "Sorry, dude. I used to see you guys on a regular basis, but since I ditched the shoes, I don't need you anymore."

For those of you who are questioning whether or not you can do this, trust me: You can! Even with my linebacker size and history of injuries, including ankle surgery two and a half years ago as well as the plantar fasciitis, the transition to my first half marathon was just ninety days. My advice: Start slow, and listen to your feet.

I have run in my VFFs a couple of times but I just didn't like them as much as running barefoot. As Ken Bob has mentioned, you think you can run harder/farther than your body is ready for when wearing the VFFs, and I did have some pains in my foot after wearing them. Now I only wear them if I have to run on a treadmill.

Trust me, it hasn't all been a bed of roses; at times I found myself questioning whether I could go on. I've had my share of bad runs and bad experiences barefoot running, and I still do. Just fewer of them. It does get frustrating at times. But I figure it is all part of unlearning the bad habits and relearning the good. Then, when you have that one great breakthrough run,

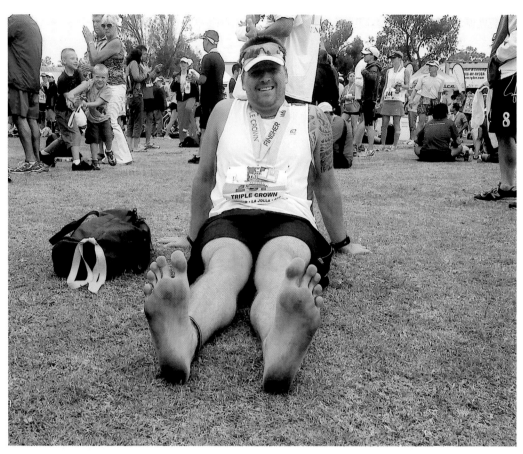

Big Damon dumped his shoes, lost his pain, and achieved his goal.

where you feel amazing when it's done, you forget about all the bad runs and focus on what you just did right and try to carry that over to the next run. For me, the good has far outweighed the bad. I'm currently about 90 seconds slower per mile than I used to be shod, but I'm not tearing my body up in the process. And besides, I was never that fast to begin with. When my feet say I'm done or take a day off, I do.

As of late October 2010, I've been injury free for 650 barefoot miles (1,040 km) over a year's time. Running is fun again, and I am able to do it consistently, which keeps me happy. To me, that's what it's all about. Who knew all I had to do was to take off my shoes?

Damon Hendricks is a forty-two-year-old Boeing engineer from Placentia, California.

TRYING TO MAN-UP AT THE CHICAGO MARATHON

A hard-core trainer battles "pussification" by barefooting at fifty.

by Eric Vouga

When I read *Born to Run* in the winter of 2009–10, it really struck a chord with this armchair naturalist and wannabe tree-hugger. It didn't require any sacrifice or money (no more buying $100 running shoes every three months); it is very natural, good for my feet, and something very few people ever considering doing. Plus, as a personal trainer, I knew that a lot of knee and back issues could be traced back to the feet, and I understood the importance of exercising them and keeping them healthy.

I immediately wanted to go outside and run wild and free, but because it was about 10°F (-12°C) outside, it was out of the question. Instead, I did the next best thing and hopped on the treadmill to give my very white feet a test run.

It was amazing. First, the immediate change of stride, the elimination of the heel-to-toe foot strike. Second, a light and fast, gazellelike feeling—not confirmed by my speed, but I sure felt that way. Then the third: my feet were beginning to feel like they were on fire. After not stepping outside without some form of protection for at least thirty years, it was amazing how soft and wimpy they had become. I wanted to keep running, but couldn't. My feet were screaming at me, my calves were screaming at me. Eventually, I was forced to listen to them and cut my run short.

But that was okay. In fact, that was good. When you run barefoot you *have* to listen to your feet, which can eliminate a lot of injuries. McDougall writes, "If you do anything wrong, the foot will tell you, 'uh uh, don't do that.'" It only took me about 5 minutes running in my bare feet to find this to be very true. But I was hooked and couldn't wait to do it again.

It took three months, several bouts of foot and calf soreness, and a couple of blisters, but eventually I was able to build up to running 8 miles (12.8 km) on the treadmill in my bare feet. On Monday, March 29, 2010, it was 50°F (10°C) and finally warm enough to run outside unshod without fear of frostbite. I took a few timid jogging strides outside on my driveway and felt the cool asphalt underneath my feet. It felt rough and foreign. It also felt like it could be painful. I promptly went back inside and got on the treadmill.

Why was I so afraid? I am no Indiana Jones, but I have climbed Mt. Rainier, rock climbed the Devil's Tower, run the Chicago Marathon five times, gone three days without showering while camped out in the backwoods, and gone canoeing up in Canada for two weeks without a cell phone. Not exactly living on the edge, but certainly more challenging than taking a short jog outside in my bare feet.

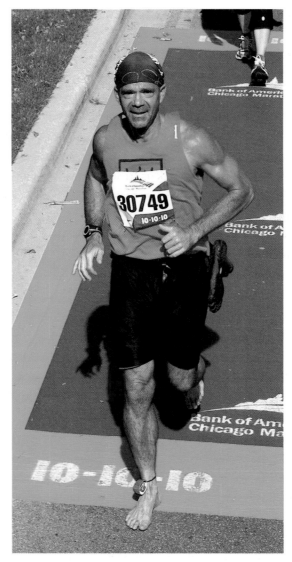

Eric Vouga "mans up" by finishing (although not starting) the
Chicago Marathon barefoot.

In the prologue to one of his books, travel writer Chuck Thompson writes, "We've done a lot to eliminate trouble and physical pain in this country. Like yours, my life is and largely has been too easy . . . We've become soft. Like Jell-O. You. Me. Everyone. America. Americans." Thompson calls this the "pussification of America." Why couldn't I take off my shoes? Was I too delicate to run in bare feet?

Wednesday, March 31, 2010, was clear, breezy, and 80°F (26.7°C). The time had come. I had already picked the Volo Bog State Natural Area, a 1,150-acre park 3 minutes from my house, as the safest and best place to test out my new and improved feet. Besides being so close to home, the natural, ungroomed trail offered a wide variety of running conditions—woods, wetlands, fields, prairies, and most important, long stretches of grassy running surfaces. I stood on the concrete walk in my bare feet and stared at the dirt path that wound through the bog. Was I crazy for doing this? Perhaps so, but I had told enough people (with a touch of braggadocio, I might add) that I was going to run outside in my bare feet, that backing out was not an option. So with a slightly elevated heart rate and glow-in-the-dark white feet, I moved into a slow trot down the warm concrete sidewalk toward the woods. The closer I got to the dirt trail the more of a fearful wussy I became.

What if I puncture a foot on a sharp rock or stick? What if I step in dog or coyote poo? What about a snake? What if? But it was too late to keep what-iffing . . . I was already off the concrete and on the dirt.

How nice it felt! When was the last time my feet touched Mother Earth out in the woods without being securely wrapped up in cotton, rubber, and canvas? When I was twelve? It was way too long ago for me to remember any sensations, pleasant or unpleasant. This was something new that I immediately liked. Instant feedback!

I quickly found out that running barefoot on a treadmill is not anything like running outside. On the rapidly changing terrain of a trail you cannot simply zone out. A nice, grassy, debris-free stretch of flat ground can quickly become a rocky decline of pure pain—which led to my second observation. Barefoot trail running is like interval speed work. Nice, grassy, debris-free stretch of flat ground? Take off. Rocky decline of pure pain? Slow down and take it easy.

Whatever the conditions, you have to be acutely aware of where you place your feet. I learned this the hard way. My confidence picked up, as did my speed, especially after I noticed that I'd run almost 3 miles (4.8 km) in the woods and nothing bad had happened. My legs and lungs were working in unison, my feet felt great, and the heat from the sun felt fantastic after a long, cold winter. Ahead of me lay a stretch of the trail that was cool, hard-packed mud, and I took off down the path like Geronimo. In fact, in my mind I had become Geronimo, running—no, gliding through the woods like a fleeting shadow—from the White Man.

As I floated over the trail dodging bullets and losing my pursuers, I heard a young girl screaming in the background—softly at first, then suddenly quite loudly. It took about three seconds for me to realize that I was not Geronimo but was now in fact a young schoolgirl screaming in pain. Apparently, Geronimo had forgotten the first and most important rule of running barefoot—always watch where you put your feet. While I was eluding my captors I had inadvertently stepped on a very sharp rock protruding from the dirt path. From the amount of pain that had shot up my foot through my leg and out my kneecap, I was certain that my first foray into the woods without shoes had suddenly come to a bloody end.

But I was wrong. My treadmill-hardened feet had withstood the rock's assault and had left only a slight indentation. I was fine, and after looking around to make sure no one else was witness to my bout of "pussification," I continued on with my run. But I was no longer

Geronimo. I was just me again—a somewhat humbled first-time barefoot runner—and I resumed my run on high alert and with a bit of trepidation.

As I began jogging down the last ½-mile (0.8 km) stretch of trail, I passed a family out on the paths enjoying the spring sun and warm temperatures. Sadly, like a lot of people I pass on the streets, the adults avoided eye contact and barely acknowledged my greeting. But as I rounded the last bend that led back to the parking lot, I heard one of the kids say to his parents, "Did you see that guy? He was a barefoot runner!"

I have to admit: it felt pretty good to hear those words *and* survive 6 miles (9.6 km) in my bare feet. Maybe I wasn't such a wuss after all.

That first run convinced me that running shoes, which were an integral part of my life for so many years, were no longer necessary. Running those trails unshod made me feel closer to nature . . . almost part of it. So many things in our lives separate us from the world we live in—from air conditioning in our cars and homes to wearing shoes almost 24 hours a day—that actually feeling the earth with my feet was a renewing and invigorating experience. Will I have that same experience every time I run? Probably not. Will I ever hurt or cut up my feet so I can't run for a few days? Probably. But that's not such a bad thing. Everyone needs a few days of rest once in a while.

After that day, everyone started asking me The Question: Will running without shoes make you faster? That planted the idea in my head of running the Chicago Marathon barefoot on October 10. After all, I ran my first marathon when I turned forty. How fitting it would be to run my first barefoot marathon the year I turn fifty. And what better way to prove that I'm not a wussy, after all.

Eric Vouga is a personal trainer in Ingleside, Illinois.

EPILOGUE

After sticking to running barefoot on dirt trails because, "I swear I smelled burning flesh on my first midday run on scalding-hot Chicago pavement," Vouga always used Vibram FiveFingers on the road. However, convinced that running trails unshod did not adequately prepare him for barefooting 26.2 miles (42 km) of rough Chicago asphalt, and feeling the pressure from a *Chicago Tribune* reporter following his quest, he compromised: start out in the VFFs and kick them off at some point. He'd planned on switching at mile 13 (21 km) but instead ended up waiting until mile 20 (32 km) to go barefoot. Proud to finish the last 6.2 miles (10 km) unshod ("only one other runner ran barefoot, out of 38,000 runners," he says), he's convinced that one more year of running barefoot will harden his feet enough to handle a full 26.2 miles (42 km).

OBLIVIOUS TO GLASS IN THE FRENCH QUARTER

There's more to life than races for an unshod, lifelong racer.
by Owen McCall

I used to be a race maniac—a 5K or 10K every weekend for thirty-five years. One of the strangest things about barefoot running is that I gave up the desire to run competitively. I stopped subscribing to *Runner's World*; they had nothing to tell me. I still do 4 to 8 miles (6.4 to 12.8 km) every other day. At over fifty, I think it's probably not a good idea to run every day. There's nothing to prove. But now, I don't even care about running fast—even though, oddly enough, I run as fast as I ever did.

At the beginning, I was very slow while barefooting, but over time, I got faster and faster. I didn't even know it, because I never timed myself anymore. My mind-set had shifted to "having fun," not speed. You just feel happier running in bare feet than in shoes. There are two reasons for that: it feels better physically and it feels better mentally.

Compared to shod jogging, where you finish feeling like you've been punished and mugged due to the endless crashing down on your heel, barefooting is silky smooth and leaves you relaxed. Mentally, it reminds me a lot of reflexology: it's so stimulating. For 24 hours after a run, I'm mellower, calmer. Yes, you get some of this from shod running, too, due to the calming neurological effect of the repetitive motion—the runner's high—but barefooting adds a whole new level of stimulation. It's like coming out of a dark room into the light. It's like you're drinking orange juice instead of Tang, the real thing instead of artificial ingredients.

I first went barefoot in 2002, at age forty-nine. For six months, I had been having various foot problems, so when I heard about barefoot running, I tried it on my own before seeing Ken Bob's website.

That first day you take off your shoes is like getting a cast off and touching skin that has been so starved of tactile input that it's hypersensitive. Unused to having your arch touch the ground, the barefoot sensation overloads you at first. It shocks you almost in the way that pain shocks you, but you quickly learn to enjoy the feeling for what it actually is: extra stimulation, the kind that barefoot people around the world get every day.

Unfortunately, I got a metatarsal stress fracture after a month and a half, then got two more on other toes when that one healed. Three in a row in six months! But I didn't give up. Thank God for the Internet. I discovered Ken Bob, and that you had to transition to barefooting slowly. I'd been trying to run like a sprinter, on my toes and on the ball of my foot.

When you run balanced, not up on your toes, you spread the load over the whole foot. Combine that with a toughened-up sole, and you can handle almost anything. I was in New Orleans recently for a meeting, staying at a hotel in the French Quarter. About 10 or 11 p.m. one night, I finally got away for a run and was a little worried. I remembered that back in college, the French Quarter was always filled with a bunch of yahoos and broken glass. But I didn't see one piece my whole run. In the morning, however, I noticed that that whole street looked liked it was paved in diamonds. I'd been running on broken glass all night! I couldn't even feel it because my feet were so tough. Humans evolved running on the soft African savanna, like Lucy did, but modern concrete is a breeze, and you can eventually handle much rougher stuff.

It's like the analogy of the guy lying on a bed of nails, and not feeling anything because his weight is so evenly distributed. I can run barefoot on the roughest trails. I've gashed my foot and not even known it. I've gotten to the point where if I feel something stick into my foot, I just brush it off. Once in a year, I brush it off and it feels wet with blood, so I know I have a cut. But later, when I stop, I cannot locate the cut—it's healed!

What's amazing is that every month or so, I get some new little insight about how to improve, how to do it better. Example: quietness. Three or four months ago, I couldn't sneak up on people. Now I can. I bend my knees a little more—doing the "retrorocket" before you touch down on the moon, you don't heel strike or toe strike or any strike at all. You aren't striking or sliding or twisting on every landing; you're just touching. So you don't wear out your feet (or shoes when you wear them).

Take bouncing. One of my students was bouncing like a pogo stick. It took him every ounce of effort not to bounce, just like me at the beginning. At first, my calves were screaming. It's a lot of work, and you're also stressed thinking you'll step on something.

I love Vibrams for sailing, which is what they are actually made for. They have siped soles like a deck shoe, so you don't feel like you'll twist an ankle. I don't like them for running, unless it's gnarly, gnarly trails. And I don't wear them in the cold because, as anyone from Chicago will tell you, in the deep winter you wear mittens, not gloves. So I just use aqua socks—$35 at most, maybe $10 at WalMart. Anything more than aqua socks is *less* functional, not more functional.

Thank God for Christopher McDougall. *Born to Run* caught so many people's imaginations that it changed everything. It turned me from lunatic to luminary. One time a cop yelled at me, "Sir, sir, sir—somehow, I had this idea that you were running away from an insane asylum. We got a report that a drunk guy was running on the streets." People would yell, "Where're your shoes?" when they saw me. When the book came out, that all changed. So thank God for McDougall. And, oh yeah, Ken Bob, too.

Owen McCall is a retired Highland Park, Illinois, molecular biologist who's been running since 1975.

> **YOU CAN HAVE FUN RACING IN MANY WAYS. IT'S FUN WINNING, BEING IN THE MIDDLE, AND EVEN LOSING. BUT WHEN YOUR SHOES ARE HURTING YOUR FEET, IT'S NO FUN AT ALL.**
>
> —BAREFOOT KEN BOB-ISM #105

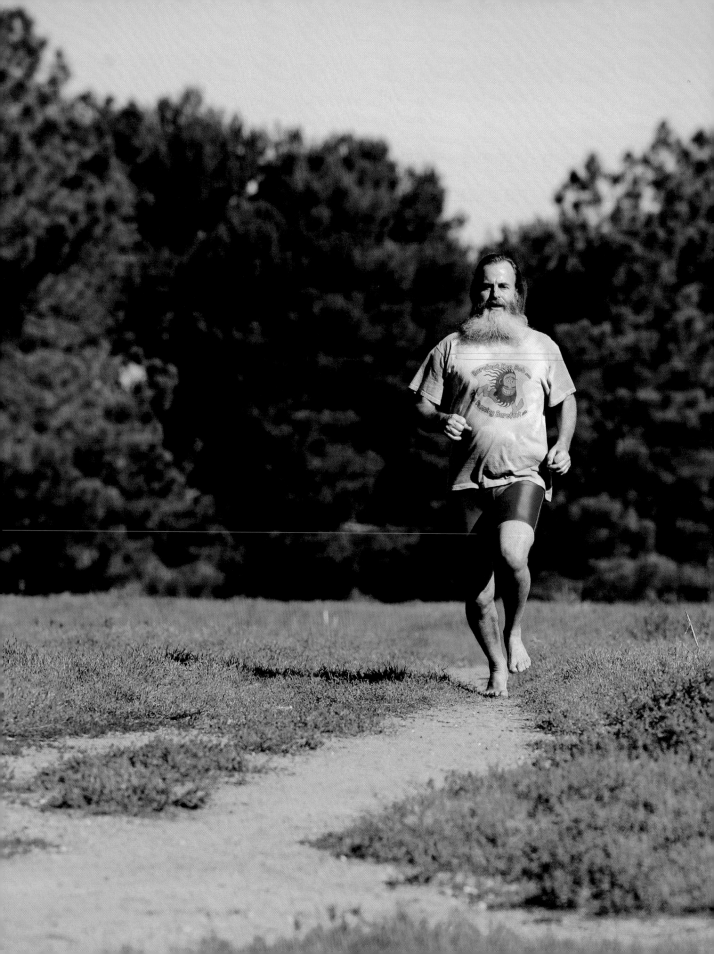

CHAPTER 10

IS BAREFOOTING A FAD?
OR IS IT THE NEW DIRECTION OF RUNNING?

Barefooting won't fade away if you follow Preston Curtis's "anti-flash-in-the-pan" plan.

> I DO THINK IT'S A FAD. IN FACT, I DON'T THINK IT EXISTS; NO ONE IN MY UNIVERSE IN EASTERN PENNSYLVANIA RUNS BAREFOOT. IN TERMS OF MINIMALIST SHOES AND VIBRAMS— YES, POSSIBLY A TECTONIC SHIFT THERE. BUT IN TERMS OF RUNNING WITHOUT SHOES, I DON'T SEE IT.

—AMBY BURFOOT, LONGTIME EDITOR OF *RUNNER'S WORLD* MAGAZINE, WINNER OF THE 1968 BOSTON MARATHON, AND FREQUENT WRITER ABOUT BAREFOOT RUNNING

> TO ME, RUNNING SHOES ARE THE FAD. IN OUR LIFETIME, THEY ARE THE NEW THING. AND UNFORTUNATELY, THEY ARE BEING TESTED NOT BY RATS, BUT BY REAL PEOPLE—WHO ARE BEING INJURED. AS FOR EASTERN PENNSYLVANIA, WHERE I GAVE A WORKSHOP IN LANCASTER ON JUNE 4, 2010, I DIDN'T SEE AMBY THERE. STILL, I WOULDN'T GO SO FAR AS TO SAY, 'AMBY BURFOOT DOESN'T EXIST.'

—BAREFOOT KEN BOB

> BEFORE *BORN TO RUN* CAME OUT, I FIGURED MAYBE 1 PERCENT OF THE RUNNING POPULATION WOULD BE GOING BAREFOOT. EVERYONE WOULD STILL BE HUNG UP ON, 'AREN'T YOU AFRAID OF STEPPING ON GLASS?' NOW, I WOULDN'T BE SURPRISED SOMEDAY TO SEE 50 PERCENT OF RUNNERS GOING BAREFOOT OR IN MINIMALIST SHOES.

—BAREFOOT JULIAN

> IF BAREFOOT RUNNING IS A FAD, THEN IT'S A 2 MILLION-YEAR-OLD FAD. FROM THE PERSPECTIVE OF EVOLUTIONARY BIOLOGY, I CAN ASSURE YOU THAT RUNNING IN CUSHIONED, HIGH-HEELED, MOTION CONTROL SHOES IS THE REAL FAD.

—DANIEL LIEBERMAN, PH.D., PROFESSOR OF HUMAN EVOLUTIONARY BIOLOGY, HARVARD UNIVERSITY

> **THERE'S A LOT MORE TALK ABOUT BAREFOOTING THAN PEOPLE ACTUALLY DOING IT. I CALL IT A PASSING FAD. IT'LL FADE. IN FIVE YEARS, THEY'LL BE SAYING, 'REMEMBER THOSE CRAZY BAREFOOTERS?' SAME THING FOR VIBRAMS.**
>
> —KEVIN "THE ANGRY PODIATRIST" KIRBY

> **LOTTA LOOKY-LOOS RIGHT NOW. BUT BAREFOOT RUNNING IS HERE TO STAY AS A TOOL. IT'S A LONG PROCESS AND REQUIRES A CHANGE TO A NEW MIND-SET—FROM A SHOD RUNNER'S PRS AND MILEAGE TO A BAREFOOTER'S 'HOW MUCH FUN ARE YOU HAVING, AND HOW LITTLE HAVE YOU BEEN INJURED?' REAL RUNNERS ARE INTERESTED. A HARDCORE WILL STICK WITH IT.**
>
> —FRED VAN PATTEN, MASSILLON, OHIO, BAREFOOT RUNNER

Notice how all the people who say that running barefoot is a fad are people who don't do it?

I must admit that I get a little defensive and overprotective when people I know, respect, and consider friends, like Amby Burfoot and Kevin Kirby, say running barefoot will turn out to be a fad, a flash in the pan. To me, them's fightin' words. Because the way I and thousands of others see it, barefooting is definitely here to stay.

First of all, I like to point out that *fad*, as defined by *Webster's* dictionary, is "a temporary fashion, notion, manner of conduct, especially one followed enthusiastically by a group," and that once you learn the how-tos of running barefoot, it is the opposite of "temporary"; it is a permanent solution to running injuries that can extend your running career by decades.

Next, keep in mind that running barefoot is both too old and too new to qualify as a fad—too old in that the human race has done it from the beginning, and too new in that most modern people haven't really done it in significant numbers until the last year or two. It's too soon to call it a fad; in the summer of 2009, an ESPN poll of 6,000 runners around the country found that 34 percent of all runners were considering giving barefooting a try; who knows—a year later, it might be double that. Running barefoot has never gone away: in the modern age, it was championed in 1935 in the book *Running* by Arthur Newton, whose ideas influenced the great Australian runner and barefooter Herb Elliott. A survey of three decades of research by Dr. Craig Richards in 2008 couldn't find one study proving that running shoes reduced injury. I love to ask barefoot detractors, "How many millions of years have Nike, New Balance, Asics, Adidas, and Puma been around?"

It's clear to many of us that the tide of running-footwear history is changing, that there's a new paradigm. Today, barefooting is out of the bag, and shoes are coming off the feet—some full time, some part time. It's a movement—not a fad.

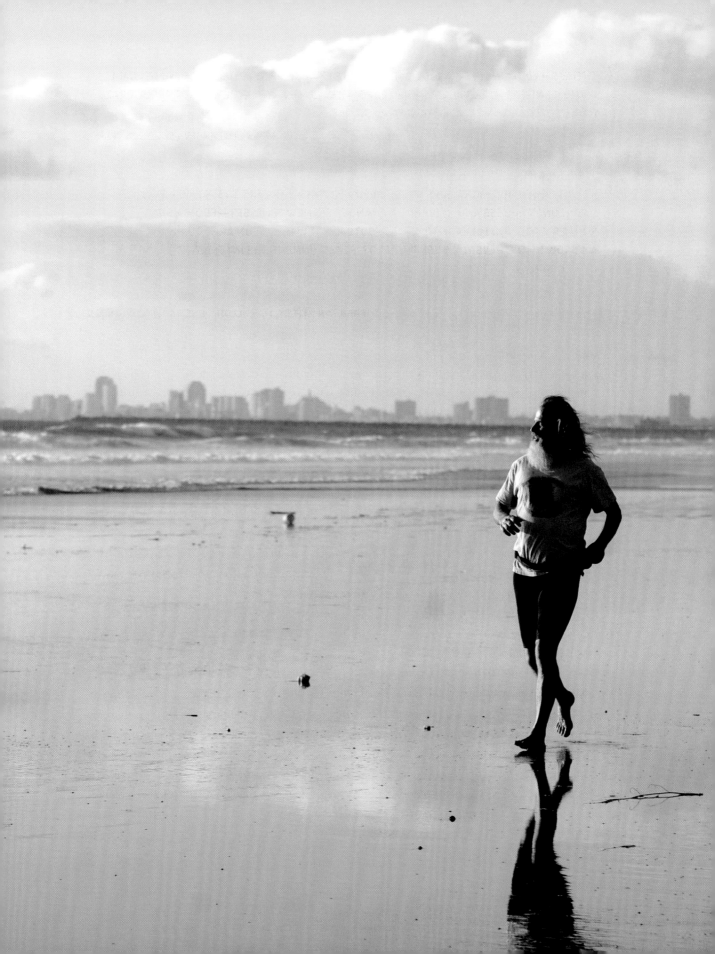

However, I must stress, as we have throughout this book, that there is a real danger of barefooting being less used than it ought to be, unless we get it right. Burfoot told us he believes that it appeals mostly to two highly motivated groups: the chronically injured, who have nothing to lose, and the young and ambitious, who will try anything to get faster. I agree, but I don't think that this *limits* the numbers of potential barefooters. On the contrary, "chronically injured" ultimately includes almost *every* runner—making running barefoot a viable option for the vast majority of runners. So just due to sheer numbers of potential users, barefooting will never just be a minor fad. But it is being radically underutilized right now because it isn't being taught and emphasized correctly.

No one I know (besides me) is more alarmed by this issue and has spent more time analyzing whether running barefoot could flame out than one of the early pioneers of barefoot running, my friend Preston Curtis. One of the most thoughtful theorists on the barefoot scene, Curtis dumped his shoes before we met, and has always impressed me with the lessons he's learned during his barefoot journey as a participant and teacher. For several years the only other barefooter in my neck of the woods, he has served as my brainstorming partner, critic, and guinea pig for testing new techniques.

When Curtis tells me that he sees a lot of interest in barefooting, yet only a tiny percentage of newcomers sticking with it unless he repeatedly emphasizes some concepts similar to those discussed in this book, it becomes quite clear that we've reached a tipping point: the biggest issue is no longer convincing people that barefooting is good for them—they know that now—but preaching that they approach it with patience. The key is adapting their feet and bodies (and minds) slowly and methodically so that they avoid the new injuries that cause many to flee back to shoes or out of running altogether.

Will barefooting, after the mad rush of attention in recent years, become a footnote of history? Not for those who have paid attention to recurrent calls in this book to take it slow, listen to your body, and beware B.R.E.S. (Barefoot Running Exuberance Syndrome), and now heed some of the sage advice offered below by Curtis. Here's the story of how he learned what he knows.

PATIENT PERSISTENCE PAYS OFF

In August 1992, things weren't going so well for Preston Curtis at the America's Finest Half Marathon in San Diego. Then twenty-nine, the Massachusetts native had just started running the year before, and loved it, but his right knee always bothered him on long runs. Sure enough, at mile 6 (9.6 km), it started hurting so much that he had to walk. On top of that, it was hot that day—so hot that it felt like his feet were burning up. "All I could think was, 'I have to take my shoes off,'" he said. And that's what he did, when, after another 5 miles (8 km) of walking and running, he saw someone with a hose, removed his shoes, and doused his feet.

"It felt great to be barefoot," he says. "And at that moment I had an epiphany: Why not just run to the finish this way? It was only another mile." So he did, and surprisingly, his knee didn't hurt a bit.

Despite the epiphany, Curtis didn't run barefoot again for years. "There was a line drawn in my mind. Even though I wanted to run barefoot, and instinctively knew it'd be better for my knee, the weight of society weighed me down. I lived at the beach and lots of people walked around barefoot, but I'd never seen anyone actually *run* barefoot." The next year, while he was back home running the famous Around the Cape 25K on Cape Cod, his knees actually buckled in pain. But instead of taking off his shoes, he gave up running for the next five years, in-line skating to stay fit.

In 1997, Curtis moved to Newport Beach, California, and felt the knee pain again when he tried to run. Then he remembered that one pain-free mile he'd run barefoot in San Diego years before. "This is my last chance to stay a runner," he thought. "Otherwise, if this doesn't work, it's back to Rollerblading." He ran 10 minutes on the beach barefoot—pain free! Then he rested three days, and repeated the process, slowly increasing his barefoot time. After two months, he ran 40 minutes barefoot with no pain.

"There's something here," he thought. "It's either the beach, the barefooting, the gradual buildup, or a combination of everything." To know for sure, he knew he'd have to test barefooting on the place he feared to tread: the street.

"It wasn't that I was worried about stepping on anything, because I walked barefoot all the time," he says. "My only fear was about being seen—a social, self-conscious fear of people seeing me run barefoot."

After weeks of delay, Curtis summoned the courage to execute his plan. "I ran on the beach as usual, then quickly cut back into the alleyway, so no one would see me," he says. "And if they did, I could just cut back to the beach."

Curtis ran barefoot for 30 minutes, mostly on the streets. No one seemed to care. When he was done, he took a deep breath. Then his head exploded with joy.

"This is incredible!" his synapses screamed. "I've hit the jackpot! This is the way we were designed. This is it! This is perfect. Your gait feels so natural, your body feels so coordinated, in tune and in touch with yourself and the ground. It feels so good, so wonderful, like you're on sensory overload. And my knee is feeling no pain!"

Suddenly, Curtis was doing all of his every-other-day 3-mile (4.8 km) runs barefoot. "I felt like a born-again runner," he says. "I'd broken all these preconceived notions. You *could* run barefoot on asphalt—and it felt great. And no one cared!" He only told his girlfriend and a few friends about his epiphany, because he knew no other runners, but he wanted to shout it to the world. So he joined the Society of Barefoot Living—and out of the blue got an email from Ken Bob.

"I thought, 'You gotta be kidding. This is a dream: I've had all these social hang-ups about running barefoot, and here's a guy one town over from me who's been doing the same thing?" he remembers. After he ran a couple of times with Ken and other barefooters, and saw that he wasn't all that unusual, his barefoot social anxiety was gone forever.

Today, after thirteen years of 10 or 15 miles (16 or 24 km) a week of pain-free barefoot running, Curtis is back in his home state of Massachusetts, working as a real estate appraiser and teaching barefoot running workshops. He talks a lot about the physical, mental, and social barriers of barefoot running, and emphasizes the importance of group runs. "In my first class, a woman attendee looked out the window before she started running to see if anyone was watching. So the social fear of running barefoot is real. And that's why doing it in a group to start with is so important to keeping newbies in the game."

And a lot of newbies are sticking their toes in the barefoot waters right now—and, to Curtis's dismay, not jumping in. "We had a perfect storm of barefoot running in 2009 and 2010, with *Born to Run*, Vibrams going mainstream, Dr. Lieberman's research, all the magazine and newspaper articles, and the base created by Ken Bob and added to by Barefoot Rick, Barefoot Ted, and others," says Curtis. "Now we have to keep people doing it. Of the first 200 people I taught, only three or four are still running barefoot. Barefooting could be a massive flash in the pan. It bums me out."

He sees two reasons for the attrition rate: the social fear and impatience.

"It's not fear of stepping on something," he says. "Maybe 90 percent of them say that, but I don't believe it; that's just a smokescreen for their subconscious social worries, because once you run barefoot you know the ground feels great. Networking with other barefooters will address that. But the problem that ultimately kills barefoot careers in their infancy is that it feels so good that people overdo it without the base or the technique."

Curtis sees stress fractures. He sees feet battered by overdone forefoot landings. He sees people running too much in Vibrams before they learn how to run barefoot. "Vibrams are creating a backlash. They are not an $85 panacea. I'd say 75 percent of Vibram wearers have problems. Even when I use them in the winter, I can feel my knee pain coming back. They are going to help barefoot running flame out unless we get people educated fast!

"I was successful with barefoot running because I took it slow and ran purely barefoot," he says. "I ran 10 minutes unshod every three days at first to let my feet strengthen and body adapt. You can't push it. If you condition your feet for barefooting before you do lots of barefooting, you'll be in this for the long run."

And you'll be proof that barefoot running isn't a fad.

PRESTON CURTIS'S FAD-FIGHTING BAREFOOT RUNNING PLAN

1 READ BAREFOOT
Take off your slippers before going out to get the morning newspaper off the driveway.

2 PAWS ON PAVEMENT
Walk your dog barefoot to get your feet ready to run.

3 GET SOCIAL
Ask a partner to run barefoot with you so you don't feel like a freak. For barefoot running groups to run with, visit BarefootRunningStepbyStep.com.

4 START SLOWLY
Don't run more than 10 minutes barefoot every third day for the first couple of weeks.

5 THIRTY-DAY DELAY
Wait a month to do your first 20- or 30-minute barefoot run.

6 DON'T MIX; DO CROSS-TRAIN
Don't alternate barefooting and shod running. "That's a catch-22," Curtis says. "It's like trying to learn tennis and squash at the same time. It's confusing. If you need to stay in shape at the beginning, ride a bike, swim, or Rollerblade, but do not run in shoes. And that includes minimalist shoes, too. Anything on your feet clouds the perfection of running barefoot."

7 DON'T EQUATE VIBRAMS WITH BAREFOOTING
VFFs are an $85 quick fix that gets you a lot of attention, makes you feel cool, and inevitably cajoles you into overdoing it. Don't use them at all if possible, especially at the beginning. You must run barefoot to learn how to run barefoot. Your bare feet will tell you to start slowly and when to stop. Vibrams cannot.

8 OBSERVE NINETY DAYS OF PURITY
Give yourself three solid months of barefoot running before you put on Vibrams or regular running shoes again. For most people, three months will be enough time to get rid of bad habits and learn the new biomechanics.

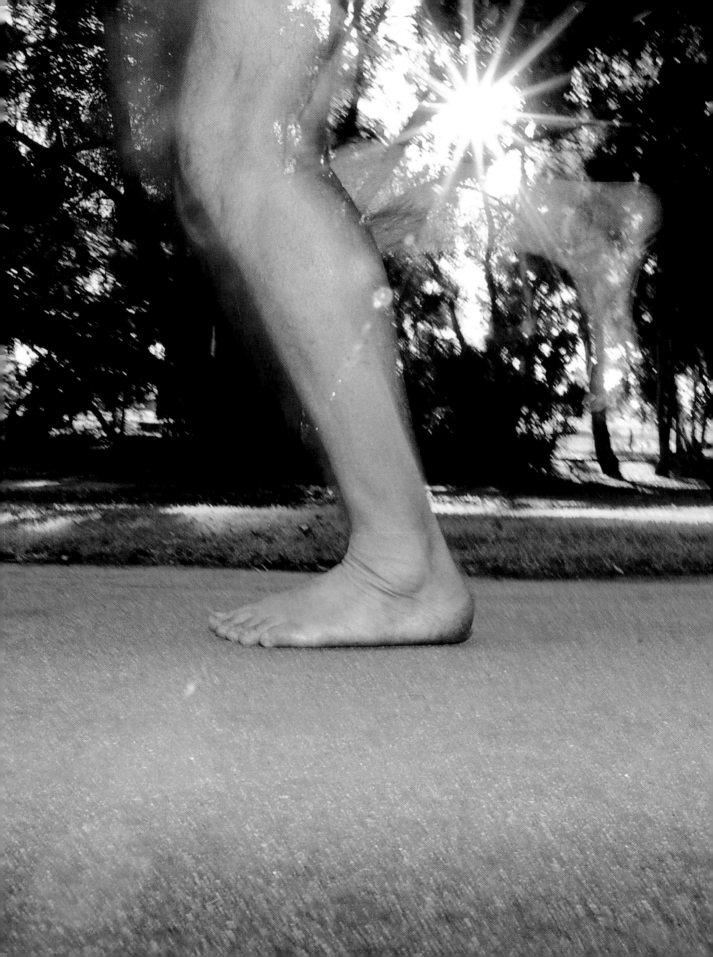

Curtis sees a lot of different motivations among beginner barefooters—the faddists who want to do the new, cool thing; the good runners looking for a new, magic ingredient that will improve their running ("although, realistically, most runners won't fix it if it isn't broken," he says); the "IRA" runners—planners who prepare early for a healthy future, in the same way that they would put money into an IRA for retirement; the injured and desperate, who see barefooting, as Curtis did, as a last chance to stay in the sport of running; and brand-new runners—those who are just off the couch.

The latter are invariably the best students. "The newbies don't know anything or have any regular speed or mileage goals to keep, so they listen," says Curtis. "If everyone could do that, we'll have millions of happy barefoot runners in a few years."

BAREFOOT SUCCESS REQUIRES SMALL STEPS, NOT A GIANT LEAP

A couple of decades from now—or maybe even just a couple of years—will we look back on barefoot running as a fad or a revolution?

That depends on how good Curtis, I, and other committed-for-life barefooters are at teaching the new recruits to take it slow and listen to the wisdom of their bodies. Certainly, the wide exposure barefooting has gained recently will bring hundreds of thousands of runners to try it. While many will stick with it, greatly multiplying the barefoot ranks, it will be a shame if it shrivels back to being practiced by a relatively small core group. Barefooting has so many great benefits to offer all runners—ending injuries, strengthening your feet and posture, potentially adding decades to a running career, and restoring a simple, carefree joy to an activity we were all born to do. But it won't come easy or overnight for most people, because we've been in shoes so long that it has corrupted our natural form. Barefoot running is gratifying the first second you try it, but to get your body through the critical first weeks of readjustment you have to be smart and cautious, take your time, and maintain the right attitude. That means enjoying the step-by-step increments and suppressing the urges of an instant-gratification world to do it all in one day.

In 2000, the Los Angeles Marathon had one barefooter: me. In 2010, the L. A. Marathon set an unofficial world record when twelve completed the entire 26.2 miles [42 km] barefoot—out of a total of 22,403 finishers. Some more (like the runner with bib number #25363, who removed his shoes the last 6 miles [10 km]—see chapter 7) ran barefoot part of the way. Some barefoot pessimists, like Dr. Kevin Kirby, dismissively write off the dozen finishers as a mere 0.06 percent of the total and say that's proof that barefooting is a fad. But optimists like me, Curtis, Julian Romero, and thousands of other barefooters, whose lives have been changed for the better by running without our shoes, see it another way: The word is out, the revolution is here, and we only have another 22,391 more marathoners in Los Angeles to convince.

ABOUT THE AUTHORS

Ken Bob Saxton is the guru of running barefoot, the world's leading instructor and proponent of the unshod art. One of the most recognized runners in the world, with his dense beard, long hair, and of course, bare feet, he's been featured in *Runner's World*, the *New York Times*, hundreds of other periodicals, and the best seller *Born to Run*. Ken Bob has trained thousands of people across the country in person at his free workshops and through his popular website TheRunningBarefoot.com, where he and thousands of other barefooters worldwide have been sharing their experiences since it (and its precursors) were founded in 1997. He has completed one marathon in shoes and seventy-seven marathons barefoot (as of January 2011), with no plans to do any more of the former. He began his barefoot odyssey when he stopped running in shoes after incurring bad blisters in 1987, and says if he couldn't run barefoot, he probably wouldn't be a runner. Although Ken Bob claims to have no exceptional athletic ability, he has racked up quite respectable PRs of 17:43 in the 5K, 37:02 in the 10K, and 3:18 in the marathon. He has qualified for and run the Boston Marathon several times, survived an astounding marathon-a-month challenge in 2004, and topped that with sixteen marathons in 2006, including four in a fifteen-day period—all barefoot. Most important, he is the type of person who frequently wonders "How?" as in, "How does that work?" and "Why?" as in, "Why do we do need shoes for running?"

Roy M. Wallack wants to be fit forever. A Southern California writer, editor, and author who specializes in running, cycling, triathlon, fitness training, gear, and adventure travel, he has competed in some of the world's toughest cycling, running, and multisport events, and has no plans to stop. A longtime fitness-gear columnist and feature writer for the *Los Angeles Times*, he is the former editor of *Triathlete, Bicycle Guide*, and *California Bicyclist* magazines, and a contributor to a variety of magazines, including *Outside, Men's Journal, Runner's World, Muscle & Fitness, Bicycling, Mountain Bike, Playboy, Competitor, Consumer's Digest*, and others. Convinced that staying fit is one of the keys to happiness and that we all can be lifelong athletes, Roy has authored and coauthored several books that lay out plans for high-level, long-term fitness: *Be a Better Runner* (2011), *Run for Life: The Breakthrough Plan for Fast Times, Fewer Injuries, and Spectacular Lifelong Fitness* (2009), *Bike for Life: How to Ride to 100* (2005), and *The Traveling Cyclist: 20 Worldwide Tours of Discovery* (1991), which describes

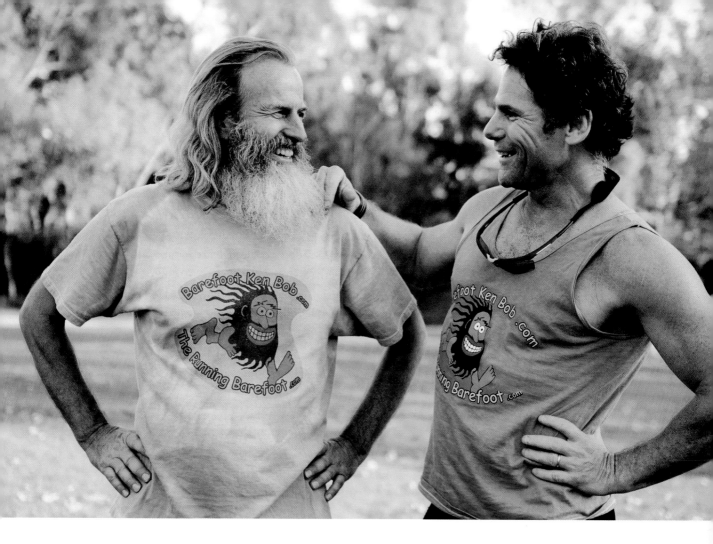

his thousands of miles of bike trips around the world, including the first one into the Soviet Union, in 1988. A former collegiate wrestler, Roy has done hundreds of running, cycling, and triathlon races and has participated in some of the world's toughest endurance events, such as the Badwater Ultramarathon; the weeklong Eco-Challenge and Primal Quest adventure races; the 750-mile (1,200 km) Paris-Brest-Paris randonée; and epic multiday mountain-bike stage races, including TransAlp and TransRockies Challenges, La Ruta de los Conquistadores, BC Bike Race, and the Breck Epic. He was inducted into the 24 Hours of Adrenalin Solo Hall of Fame in 2008 and finished second in the World Fitness Championship in 2004.

2005 Edition

ANSI/AF&PA NDS-2005

Approval Date: January 6, 2005

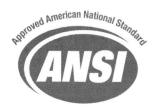

ASD/LRFD

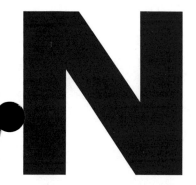 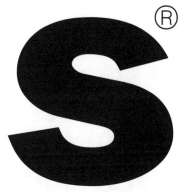

N D S®

NATIONAL DESIGN SPECIFICATION®

FOR WOOD CONSTRUCTION

WITH COMMENTARY AND
SUPPLEMENT: DESIGN VALUES FOR WOOD CONSTRUCTION

National Design Specification (NDS) for Wood Construction with Commentary and Supplement: Design Values for Wood Construction 2005 Edition

Third Printing: August 2006
Fourth Printing: February 2007
Fifth Printing: February 2008

ISBN 0-9625985-9-3 (Volume 1)
ISBN 0-9625985-8-5 (4 Volume Set)

Copyright Permission
AF&PA American Wood Council
1111 Nineteenth St., NW, Suite 800
Washington, DC 20036
email: awcinfo@afandpa.org

Printed in the United States of America

FOREWORD

The *National Design Specification® (NDS®) for Wood Construction* was first issued by the National Lumber Manufacturers Association (now the American Forest & Paper Association) (AF&PA) in 1944, under the title *National Design Specification for Stress-Grade Lumber and Its Fastenings*. By 1971 the scope of the Specification had broadened to include additional wood products. In 1977 the title was changed to reflect the new nature of the Specification, and the content was rearranged to simplify its use. The 1991 edition was reorganized in an easier to use "equation format," and many sections were rewritten to provide greater clarity.

In 1992, AF&PA (formerly the National Forest Products Association) was accredited by the American National Standards Institute (ANSI). The Specification subsequently gained approval as an American National Standard designated ANSI/NFoPA NDS-1991 with an approval date of October 16, 1992. The current edition of the Standard is designated ANSI/AF&PA NDS-2005 with an approval date of January 06, 2005.

In developing the provisions of this Specification, the most reliable data available from laboratory tests and experience with structures in service have been carefully analyzed and evaluated for the purpose of providing, in convenient form, a national standard of practice.

Since the first edition of the National Design Specification in 1944, the Association's Technical Advisory Committee has continued to study and evaluate new data and developments in wood design. Subsequent editions of the Specification have included appropriate revisions

to provide for use of such new information. This edition incorporated numerous changes considered by AF&PA's Wood Design Standards Committee. The contributions of the members of this Committee to improvement of the Specification as a national design standard for wood construction are especially recognized.

Acknowledgement is made to the Forest Products Laboratory, U.S. Department of Agriculture, for data and publications generously made available, and to the engineers, scientists, and other users who have suggested changes in the content of the Specification. The Association invites and welcomes comments, inquiries, suggestions, and new data relative to the provisions of this document.

It is intended that this Specification be used in conjunction with competent engineering design, accurate fabrication, and adequate supervision of construction. AF&PA does not assume any responsibility for errors or omissions in the document, nor for engineering designs, plans, or construction prepared from it. Particular attention is directed to Section 2.1.2, relating to the designer's responsibility to make adjustments for particular end uses of structures.

Those using this standard assume all liability arising from its use. The design of engineered structures is within the scope of expertise of licensed engineers, architects, or other licensed professionals for applications to a particular structure.

American Forest & Paper Association

TABLE OF CONTENTS FOR THE NDS

TABLE OF CONTENTS FOR THE NDS COMMENTARY

LIST OF TABLES IN THE NDS

LIST OF TABLES IN THE NDS SUPPLEMENT

LIST OF TABLES IN THE NDS COMMENTARY

LIST OF FIGURES IN THE NDS

LIST OF FIGURES IN THE NDS COMMENTARY

GENERAL REQUIREMENTS FOR STRUCTURAL DESIGN

AMERICAN FOREST & PAPER ASSOCIATION

1.1 Scope

1.1.1 Practice Defined

1.1.1.1 This Specification defines the method to be followed in structural design with the following wood products:
- visually graded lumber
- mechanically graded lumber
- structural glued laminated timber
- timber piles
- timber poles
- prefabricated wood I-joists
- structural composite lumber
- wood structural panels

It also defines the practice to be followed in the design and fabrication of single and multiple fastener connections using the fasteners described herein.

1.1.1.2 Structural assemblies utilizing panel products shall be designed in accordance with principles of engineering mechanics (see References 32, 33, 34, and 53 for design provisions for commonly used panel products).

1.1.1.3 This Specification is not intended to preclude the use of materials, assemblies, structures or designs not meeting the criteria herein, where it is demonstrated by analysis based on recognized theory, full scale or prototype loading tests, studies of model analogues or extensive experience in use that the material, assembly, structure or design will perform satisfactorily in its intended end use.

1.1.2 Competent Supervision

The reference design values, design value adjustments, and structural design provisions in this Specification are for designs made and carried out under competent supervision.

1.2 General Requirements

1.2.1 Conformance with Standards

The quality of wood products and fasteners, and the design of load-supporting members and connections, shall conform to the standards specified herein.

1.2.2 Framing and Bracing

All members shall be so framed, anchored, tied, and braced that they have the required strength and rigidity. Adequate bracing and bridging to resist wind and other lateral forces shall be provided.

1.3 Standard as a Whole

The various Chapters, Sections, Subsections and Articles of this Specification are interdependent and, except as otherwise provided, the pertinent provisions of each Chapter, Section, Subsection, and Article shall apply to every other Chapter, Section, Subsection, and Article.

1.4 Design Procedures

This Specification provides requirements for the design of wood products specified herein by the following methods:
(a) Allowable Stress Design (ASD)
(b) Load and Resistance Factor Design (LRFD)

Designs shall be made according to the provisions for Allowable Stress Design (ASD) or Load and Resistance Factor Design (LRFD).

1.4.1 Loading Assumptions

Wood buildings or other wood structures, and their structural members, shall be designed and constructed to safely support all anticipated loads. This Specification is predicated on the principle that the loading assumed in the design represents actual conditions.

1.4.2 Governed by Codes

Minimum design loads shall be in accordance with the building code under which the structure is designed, or where applicable, other recognized minimum design load standards.

1.4.3 Loads Included

Design loads include any or all of the following loads or forces: dead, live, snow, wind, earthquake, erection, and other static and dynamic forces.

1.4.4 Load Combinations

Combinations of design loads and forces, and load combination factors, shall be in accordance with the building code under which the structure is designed, or where applicable, other recognized minimum design load standards (see Reference 5 for additional information). The governing building code shall be permitted to be consulted for load combination factors. Load combinations and associated time effect factors, λ, for use in LRFD are provided in Appendix N.

1.5 Specifications and Plans

1.5.1 Sizes

The plans or specifications, or both, shall indicate whether wood products sizes are stated in terms of standard nominal, standard net or special sizes, as specified for the respective wood products in Chapters 4, 5, 6, 7, 8, and 9.

1.6 Notation

Except where otherwise noted, the symbols used in this Specification have the following meanings:

A = area of cross section, in.^{2}

A_m = gross cross-sectional area of main wood member(s), in.^{2}

A_n = cross-sectional area of notched member, in.^{2}

A_s = sum of gross cross-sectional areas of side member(s), in.^{2}

C_D = load duration factor

C_F = size factor for sawn lumber

C_L = beam stability factor

C_M = wet service factor

C_P = column stability factor

C_T = buckling stiffness factor for dimension lumber

C_V = volume factor for structural glued laminated timber or structural composite lumber

C_b = bearing area factor

C_c = curvature factor for structural glued laminated timber

C_{cs} = critical section factor for round timber piles

C_d = penetration depth factor for connections

C_{di} = diaphragm factor for nailed connections

C_{eg} = end grain factor for connections

C_{fu} = flat use factor

C_g = group action factor for connections

C_i = incising factor for dimension lumber

C_r = repetitive member factor for dimension lumber, prefabricated wood I-joists, and structural composite lumber

C_{sp} = single pile factor for timber piles

C_{st} = metal side plate factor for 4" shear plate connections

C_t = temperature factor

C_{tn} = toe-nail factor for nailed connections

C_u = untreated factor for timber poles and piles

C_Δ = geometry factor for connections

COV_E = coefficient of variation for modulus of elasticity

D = diameter, in.

D_r = root diameter, in.

E, E' = reference and adjusted modulus of elasticity, psi

E_{min}, E_{min}' = reference and adjusted modulus of elasticity for beam stability and column stability calculations, psi

$(EI)_{min}, (EI)_{min}'$ = reference and adjusted EI for beam stability and column stability calculations, psi

E_m = modulus of elasticity of main member, psi

E_s = modulus of elasticity of side member, psi

F_b, F_b' = reference and adjusted bending design value, psi

F_b^* = reference bending design value multiplied by all applicable adjustment factors except C_L, psi

F_{b1}' = adjusted edgewise bending design value, psi

F_{b2}' = adjusted flatwise bending design value, psi

F_{bE} = critical buckling design value for bending members, psi

F_c, F_c' = reference and adjusted compression design value parallel to grain, psi

F_c^* = reference compression design value parallel to grain multiplied by all applicable adjustment factors except C_p, psi

F_{cE} = critical buckling design value for compression members, psi

F_{cE1}, F_{cE2} = critical buckling design value for compression member in planes of lateral support, psi

$F_{c\perp}, F_{c\perp}'$ = reference and adjusted compression design value perpendicular to grain, psi

F_e = dowel bearing strength, psi

F_{em} = dowel bearing strength of main member, psi

F_{es} = dowel bearing strength of side member, psi

$F_{e\parallel}$ = dowel bearing strength parallel to grain, psi

$F_{e\perp}$ = dowel bearing strength perpendicular to grain, psi

$F_{e\theta}$ = dowel bearing strength at an angle to grain, psi

F_{rt}' = adjusted radial tension design value perpendicular to grain, psi

F_t, F_t' = reference and adjusted tension design value parallel to grain, psi

F_v, F_v' = reference and adjusted shear design value parallel to grain (horizontal shear), psi

F_{yb} = bending yield strength of fastener, psi

F_θ' = adjusted bearing design value at an angle to grain, psi

G = specific gravity

I = moment of inertia, in.^{4}

K = shear stiffness coefficient

K_D = diameter coefficient for dowel-type fastener connections with $D < 0.25$ in.

K_F = format conversion factor

K_M = moisture content coefficient for sawn lumber truss compression chords

K_T = truss compression chord coefficient for sawn lumber

K_{bE} = Euler buckling coefficient for beams

K_{cE} = Euler buckling coefficient for columns

K_e = buckling length coefficient for compression members

K_f = column stability coefficient for bolted and nailed built-up columns

K_r = radial stress coefficient

K_t = temperature coefficient

K_v = shear coefficient

K_x = spaced column fixity coefficient

K_θ = angle to grain coefficient for dowel-type fastener connections with $D < 0.25$ in.

L = span length of bending member, ft

L = distance between points of lateral support of compression member, ft

L_c = length from tip of pile to critical section, ft

M = maximum bending moment, in.-lbs

M_r, M_r' = reference and adjusted design moment, in.-lbs

N, N' = reference and adjusted lateral design value at an angle to grain for a single split ring connector unit or shear plate connector unit, lbs

P = total concentrated load or total axial load, lbs

P, P' = reference and adjusted lateral design value parallel to grain for a single split ring connector unit or shear plate connector unit, lbs

P_r = parallel to grain reference rivet capacity, lbs

P_w = parallel to grain reference wood capacity for timber rivets, lbs

Q = statical moment of an area about the neutral axis, in.^{3}

Q, Q' = reference and adjusted lateral design value perpendicular to grain for a single split ring connector unit or shear plate connector unit, lbs

Q_r = perpendicular to grain reference rivet capacity, lbs

Q_w = perpendicular to grain reference wood capacity for timber rivets, lbs

R = radius of curvature, in.

R_B = slenderness ratio of bending member

R_d = reduction term for dowel-type fastener connections

R_r, R_r' = reference and adjusted design reaction, lbs

S = section modulus, in.^{3}

T = temperature, °F

V = shear force, lbs

V_r, V_r' = reference and adjusted design shear, lbs

W, W' = reference and adjusted withdrawal design value for fastener, lbs per inch of penetration

Z, Z' = reference and adjusted lateral design value for a single fastener connection, lbs

$Z_{\parallel}$ = reference lateral design value for a single dowel-type fastener connection with all wood members loaded parallel to grain, lbs

$Z_{m\perp}$ = reference lateral design value for a single dowel-type fastener wood-to-wood connection with main member loaded perpendicular to grain and side member loaded parallel to grain, lbs

$Z_{s\perp}$ = reference lateral design value for a single dowel-type fastener wood-to-wood connection with main member loaded parallel to grain and side member loaded perpendicular to grain, lbs

$Z_{\perp}$ = reference lateral design value for a single dowel-type fastener wood-to-wood, wood-to-metal, or wood-to-concrete connection with wood member(s) loaded perpendicular to grain, lbs

a_p = minimum end distance load parallel to grain, in.

a_q = minimum end distance load perpendicular to grain, in.

b = breadth (thickness) of rectangular bending member, in.

c = distance from neutral axis to extreme fiber, in.

d = depth (width) of bending member, in.

d = least dimension of rectangular compression member, in.

d = pennyweight of nail or spike

d_e = effective depth of member at a connection, in.

d_n = depth of member remaining at a notch, in.

d_1, d_2 = cross-sectional dimensions of rectangular compression member in planes of lateral support, in.

e = eccentricity, in.

e_p = minimum edge distance unloaded edge, in.

e_q = minimum edge distance loaded edge, in.

f_b = actual bending stress, psi

f_{b1} = actual edgewise bending stress, psi

f_{b2} = actual flatwise bending stress, psi

f_c = actual compression stress parallel to grain, psi

f_c' = concrete compressive strength, psi

$f_{c\perp}$ = actual compression stress perpendicular to grain, psi

f_r = actual radial stress in curved bending member, psi

f_t = actual tension stress parallel to grain, psi

f_v = actual shear stress parallel to grain, psi

g = gauge of screw

ℓ = span length of bending member, in.

ℓ = distance between points of lateral support of compression member, in.

ℓ_b = bearing length, in.

ℓ_c = clear span, in.

ℓ_e = effective span length of bending member, in.

ℓ_e = effective length of compression member, in.

ℓ_{e1}, ℓ_{e2} = effective length of compression member in planes of lateral support, in.

ℓ_e/d = slenderness ratio of compression member

ℓ_m = length of dowel bearing in wood main member, in.

ℓ_n = length of notch, in.

ℓ_s = length of dowel bearing in wood side member, in.

ℓ_u = laterally unsupported span length of bending member, in.

ℓ_1, ℓ_2 = distances between points of lateral support of compression member in planes 1 and 2, in.

ℓ_3 = distance from center of spacer block to centroid of group of split ring or shear plate connectors in end block for a spaced column, in.

m.c. = moisture content based on oven-dry weight of wood, %

n = number of fasteners in a row

n_c = number of rivets per row

n_R = number of rivet rows

p = depth of fastener penetration into wood member, in.

r = radius of gyration, in.

s = center-to-center spacing between adjacent fasteners in a row, in.

s_p = spacing between rivets parallel to grain, in.

s_q = spacing between rivets perpendicular to grain, in.

t = thickness, in.

t = exposure time, hrs.

t_m = thickness of main member, in.

t_s = thickness of side member, in.

x = distance from beam support face to load, in.

α = angle between direction of load and direction of grain (longitudinal axis of member), degrees

β_{eff} = effective char rate (in./hr.) adjusted for exposure time, t

β_n = nominal char rate (in./hr.), linear char rate based on 1-hour exposure

γ = load/slip modulus for a connection, lbs/in.

λ = Time effect factor

ϕ = Resistance factor

DESIGN VALUES FOR STRUCTURAL MEMBERS

2

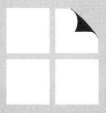

2.1 General

2.1.1 General Requirement

Each wood structural member or connection shall be of sufficient size and capacity to carry the applied loads without exceeding the adjusted design values specified herein.

2.1.1.1 For ASD, calculation of adjusted design values shall be determined using applicable ASD adjustment factors specified herein.

2.1.1.2 For LRFD, calculation of adjusted design values shall be determined using applicable LRFD adjustment factors specified herein.

2.1.2 Responsibility of Designer to Adjust for Conditions of Use

Adjusted design values for wood members and connections in particular end uses shall be appropriate for the conditions under which the wood is used, taking into account the differences in wood strength properties with different moisture contents, load durations, and types of treatment. Common end use conditions are addressed in this Specification. It shall be the final responsibility of the designer to relate design assumptions and reference design values, and to make design value adjustments appropriate to the end use.

2.2 Reference Design Values

Reference design values and design value adjustments for wood products in 1.1.1.1 are based on methods specified in each of the wood product chapters. Chapters 4 through 9 contain design provisions for sawn lumber, glued laminated timber, poles and piles, prefabricated wood I-joists, structural composite lumber, and wood structural panels, respectively. Chapters 10 through 13 contain design provisions for connections. Reference design values are for normal load duration under the moisture service conditions specified.

2.3 Adjustment of Reference Design Values

2.3.1 Applicability of Adjustment Factors

Reference design values shall be multiplied by all applicable adjustment factors to determine adjusted design values. The applicability of adjustment factors to sawn lumber, structural glued laminated timber, poles and piles, prefabricated wood I-joists, structural composite lumber, wood structural panels, and connection design values is defined in 4.3, 5.3, 6.3, 7.3, 8.3, 9.3, and 10.3, respectively.

2.3.2 Load Duration Factor, C_D (ASD only)

2.3.2.1 Wood has the property of carrying substantially greater maximum loads for short durations than for long durations of loading. Reference design values apply to normal load duration. Normal load duration represents a load that fully stresses a member to its allowable design value by the application of the full de-

sign load for a cumulative duration of approximately ten years. When the cumulative duration of the full maximum load does not exceed the specified time period, all reference design values except modulus of elasticity, E, modulus of elasticity for beam and column stability, E_{min}, and compression perpendicular to grain, $F_{c\perp}$, based on a deformation limit (see 4.2.6) shall be multiplied by the appropriate load duration factor, C_D, from Table 2.3.2 or Figure B1 (see Appendix B) to take into account the change in strength of wood with changes in load duration.

2.3.2.2 The load duration factor, C_D, for the shortest duration load in a combination of loads shall apply for that load combination. All applicable load combinations shall be evaluated to determine the critical load combination. Design of structural members and connections shall be based on the critical load combination (see Appendix B.2).

2.3.2.3 The load duration factors, C_D, in Table 2.3.2 and Appendix B are independent of load combination factors, and both shall be permitted to be used in design calculations (see 1.4.4 and Appendix B.4).

Table 2.3.2 Frequently Used Load Duration Factors, C_D [1]

Load Duration	C_D	Typical Design Loads
Permanent	0.9	Dead Load
Ten years	1.0	Occupancy Live Load
Two months	1.15	Snow Load
Seven days	1.25	Construction Load
Ten minutes	1.6	Wind/Earthquake Load
Impact [2]	2.0	Impact Load

1. Load duration factors shall not apply to reference modulus of elasticity, E, reference modulus of elasticity for beam and column stability, E_{min}, nor to reference compression perpendicular to grain design values, $F_{c\perp}$, based on a deformation limit.
2. Load duration factors greater than 1.6 shall not apply to structural members pressure-treated with water-borne preservatives (see Reference 30), or fire retardant chemicals. The impact load duration factor shall not apply to connections.

2.3.3 Temperature Factor, C_t

Reference design values shall be multiplied by the temperature factors, C_t, in Table 2.3.3 for structural members that will experience sustained exposure to elevated temperatures up to 150°F (see Appendix C).

2.3.4 Fire Retardant Treatment

The effects of fire retardant chemical treatment on strength shall be accounted for in the design. Adjusted design values, including adjusted connection design values, for lumber and structural glued laminated timber pressure-treated with fire retardant chemicals shall be obtained from the company providing the treatment and redrying service. Load duration factors greater than 1.6 shall not apply to structural members pressure-treated with fire retardant chemicals (see Table 2.3.2).

2.3.5 Format Conversion Factor, K_F (LRFD only)

For LRFD, reference design values shall be multiplied by the format conversion factor, K_F, specified in Appendix N.3.1. The format conversion factor, K_F, shall not apply for designs in accordance with ASD methods specified herein.

2.3.6 Resistance Factor, ϕ (LRFD only)

For LRFD, reference design values shall be multiplied by the resistance factor, ϕ, specified in Appendix N.3.2. The resistance factor, ϕ, shall not apply for designs in accordance with ASD methods specified herein.

2.3.7 Time Effect Factor, λ (LRFD only)

For LRFD, reference design values shall be multiplied by the time effect factor, λ, specified in Appendix N.3.3. The time effect factor, λ, shall not apply for designs in accordance with ASD methods specified herein.

Table 2.3.3 Temperature Factor, C_t

Reference Design Values	In-Service Moisture Conditions [1]	C_t		
		T≤100°F	100°F<T≤125°F	125°F<T≤150°F
F_t, E, E_{min}	Wet or Dry	1.0	0.9	0.9
F_b, F_v, F_c, and $F_{c\perp}$	Dry	1.0	0.8	0.7
	Wet	1.0	0.7	0.5

1. Wet and dry service conditions for sawn lumber, structural glued laminated timber, prefabricated wood I-joists, structural composite lumber, and wood structural panels are specified in 4.1.4, 5.1.5, 7.1.4, 8.1.4, and 9.3.3, respectively.

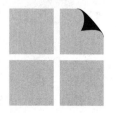

DESIGN PROVISIONS AND EQUATIONS

3

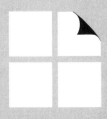

3.1 General

3.1.1 Scope

Chapter 3 establishes general design provisions that apply to all wood structural members and connections covered under this Specification. Each wood structural member or connection shall be of sufficient size and capacity to carry the applied loads without exceeding the adjusted design values specified herein. Reference design values and specific design provisions applicable to particular wood products or connections are given in other Chapters of this Specification.

3.1.2 Net Section Area

3.1.2.1 The net section area is obtained by deducting from the gross section area the projected area of all material removed by boring, grooving, dapping, notching, or other means. The net section area shall be used in calculating the load carrying capacity of a member, except as specified in 3.6.3 for columns. The effects of any eccentricity of loads applied to the member at the critical net section shall be taken into account.

3.1.2.2 For parallel to grain loading with staggered bolts, drift bolts, drift pins, or lag screws, adjacent fasteners shall be considered as occurring at the same critical section if the parallel to grain spacing between fasteners in adjacent rows is less than four fastener diameters (see Figure 3A).

Figure 3A Spacing of Staggered Fasteners

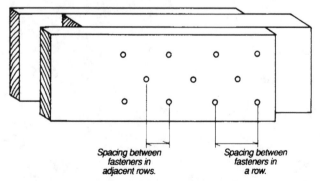

Spacing between fasteners in adjacent rows.

Spacing between fasteners in a row.

3.1.2.3 The net section area at a split ring or shear plate connection shall be determined by deducting from the gross section area the projected areas of the bolt hole and the split ring or shear plate groove within the member (see Figure 3B and Appendix K). Where split ring or shear plate connectors are staggered, adjacent connectors shall be considered as occurring at the same critical section if the parallel to grain spacing between connectors in adjacent rows is less than or equal to one connector diameter (see Figure 3A).

Figure 3B Net Cross Section at a Split Ring or Shear Plate Connection

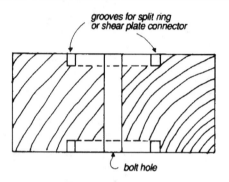

grooves for split ring or shear plate connector

bolt hole

3.1.3 Connections

Structural members and fasteners shall be arranged symmetrically at connections, unless the bending moment induced by an unsymmetrical arrangement (such as lapped joints) has been accounted for in the design. Connections shall be designed and fabricated to insure that each individual member carries its proportional stress.

3.1.4 Time Dependent Deformations

Where members of structural frames are composed of two or more layers or sections, the effect of time dependent deformations shall be accounted for in the design (see 3.5.2 and Appendix F).

3.1.5 Composite Construction

Composite constructions, such as wood-concrete, wood-steel, and wood-wood composites, shall be designed in accordance with principles of engineering mechanics using the adjusted design values for structural members and connections specified herein.

3.2 Bending Members – General

3.2.1 Span of Bending Members

For simple, continuous and cantilevered bending members, the span shall be taken as the distance from face to face of supports, plus ½ the required bearing length at each end.

3.2.2 Lateral Distribution of Concentrated Load

Lateral distribution of concentrated loads from a critically loaded bending member to adjacent parallel bending members by flooring or other cross members shall be permitted to be calculated when determining design bending moment and vertical shear force (see 15.1).

3.2.3 Notches

3.2.3.1 Bending members shall not be notched except as permitted by 4.4.3, 5.4.4, 7.4.4, and 8.4.1. A gradual taper cut from the reduced depth of the member to the full depth of the member in lieu of a square-cornered notch reduces stress concentrations.

3.2.3.2 The stiffness of a bending member, as determined from its cross section, is practically unaffected by a notch with the following dimensions:

notch depth	$\leq$	(1/6) (beam depth)
notch length	$\leq$	(1/3) (beam depth)

3.2.3.3 See 3.4.3 for effect of notches on shear strength.

3.3 Bending Members – Flexure

3.3.1 Strength in Bending

The actual bending stress or moment shall not exceed the adjusted bending design value.

3.3.2 Flexural Design Equations

3.3.2.1 The actual bending stress induced by a bending moment, M, is calculated as follows:

$$f_b = \frac{Mc}{I} = \frac{M}{S} \qquad (3.3\text{-}1)$$

For a rectangular bending member of breadth, b, and depth, d, this becomes:

$$f_b = \frac{M}{S} = \frac{6M}{bd^2} \qquad (3.3\text{-}2)$$

3.3.2.2 For solid rectangular bending members with the neutral axis perpendicular to depth at center:

$$I = \frac{bd^3}{12} = \text{moment of inertia} \qquad (3.3\text{-}3)$$

$$S = \frac{I}{c} = \frac{bd^2}{6} = \text{section modulus} \qquad (3.3\text{-}4)$$

3.3.3 Beam Stability Factor, C_L

3.3.3.1 When the depth of a bending member does not exceed its breadth, $d \leq b$, no lateral support is required and $C_L = 1.0$.

3.3.3.2 When rectangular sawn lumber bending members are laterally supported in accordance with 4.4.1, $C_L = 1.0$.

3.3.3.3 When the compression edge of a bending member is supported throughout its length to prevent lateral displacement, and the ends at points of bearing have lateral support to prevent rotation, $C_L = 1.0$.

3.3.3.4 When the depth of a bending member exceeds its breadth, $d > b$, lateral support shall be provided at points of bearing to prevent rotation and/or lateral displacement at those points. When such lateral support is provided at points of bearing, but no additional lateral support is provided throughout the length of the bending member, the unsupported length, ℓ_u, is the distance between such points of end bearing, or the length of a cantilever. When a bending member is provided with lateral support to prevent rotational and/or lateral displacement at intermediate points as well as at the ends, the unsupported length, ℓ_u, is the distance between such points of intermediate lateral support.

3.3.3.5 The effective span length, ℓ_e, for single span or cantilever bending members shall be determined in accordance with Table 3.3.3.

Table 3.3.3 Effective Length, ℓ_e, for Bending Members

Cantilever[1]	when $\ell_u/d < 7$	when $\ell_u/d \geq 7$
Uniformly distributed load	$\ell_e = 1.33\,\ell_u$	$\ell_e = 0.90\,\ell_u + 3d$
Concentrated load at unsupported end	$\ell_e = 1.87\,\ell_u$	$\ell_e = 1.44\,\ell_u + 3d$

Single Span Beam[1,2]	when $\ell_u/d < 7$	when $\ell_u/d \geq 7$
Uniformly distributed load	$\ell_e = 2.06\,\ell_u$	$\ell_e = 1.63\,\ell_u + 3d$
Concentrated load at center with no intermediate lateral support	$\ell_e = 1.80\,\ell_u$	$\ell_e = 1.37\,\ell_u + 3d$
Concentrated load at center with lateral support at center	$\ell_e = 1.11\,\ell_u$	
Two equal concentrated loads at 1/3 points with lateral support at 1/3 points	$\ell_e = 1.68\,\ell_u$	
Three equal concentrated loads at 1/4 points with lateral support at 1/4 points	$\ell_e = 1.54\,\ell_u$	
Four equal concentrated loads at 1/5 points with lateral support at 1/5 points	$\ell_e = 1.68\,\ell_u$	
Five equal concentrated loads at 1/6 points with lateral support at 1/6 points	$\ell_e = 1.73\,\ell_u$	
Six equal concentrated loads at 1/7 points with lateral support at 1/7 points	$\ell_e = 1.78\,\ell_u$	
Seven or more equal concentrated loads, evenly spaced, with lateral support at points of load application	$\ell_e = 1.84\,\ell_u$	
Equal end moments	$\ell_e = 1.84\,\ell_u$	

1. For single span or cantilever bending members with loading conditions not specified in Table 3.3.3:

   $\ell_e = 2.06\,\ell_u$ when $\ell_u/d < 7$

   $\ell_e = 1.63\,\ell_u + 3d$ when $7 \leq \ell_u/d \leq 14.3$

   $\ell_e = 1.84\,\ell_u$ when $\ell_u/d > 14.3$

2. Multiple span applications shall be based on table values or engineering analysis.

[Handwritten note:] ℓ_u = unbraced length ↳ distance between lateral supports

3.3.3.6 The slenderness ratio, R_B, for bending members shall be calculated as follows:

$$R_B = \sqrt{\frac{\ell_e d}{b^2}}$$ (3.3-5)

3.3.3.7 The slenderness ratio for bending members, R_B, shall not exceed 50.

3.3.3.8 The beam stability factor shall be calculated as follows:

$$C_L = \frac{1+\left(F_{bE}/F_b^*\right)}{1.9} - \sqrt{\left[\frac{1+\left(F_{bE}/F_b^*\right)}{1.9}\right]^2 - \frac{F_{bE}/F_b^*}{0.95}}$$ (3.3-6)

FL* IS FL' W/O CL

where:

F_b^* = reference bending design value multiplied by all applicable adjustment factors except C_{fu}, C_v, and C_L (see 2.3)

$$F_{bE} = \frac{1.20\, E_{min}'}{R_B^2}$$

3.3.3.9 See Appendix D for background information concerning beam stability calculations and Appendix F for information concerning coefficient of variation in modulus of elasticity (COV_E).

3.3.3.10 Members subjected to flexure about both principal axes (biaxial bending) shall be designed in accordance with 3.9.2.

3.4 Bending Members – Shear

3.4.1 Strength in Shear Parallel to Grain (Horizontal Shear)

3.4.1.1 The actual shear stress parallel to grain or shear force at any cross section of the bending member shall not exceed the adjusted shear design value. A check of the strength of wood bending members in shear perpendicular to grain is not required.

3.4.1.2 The shear design procedures specified herein for calculating f_v at or near points of vertical support are limited to solid flexural members such as sawn lumber, structural glued laminated timber, structural composite lumber, or mechanically laminated timber beams. Shear design at supports for built-up components containing load-bearing connections at or near points of support, such as between the web and chord of a truss, shall be based on test or other techniques.

3.4.2 Shear Design Equations

The actual shear stress parallel to grain induced in a sawn lumber, structural glued laminated timber, structural composite lumber, or timber pole or pile bending member shall be calculated as follows:

$$f_v = \frac{VQ}{Ib}$$ (3.4-1)

For a rectangular bending member of breadth, b, and depth, d, this becomes:

$$f_v = \frac{3V}{2bd}$$ (3.4-2)

3.4.3 Shear Design

3.4.3.1 When calculating the shear force, V, in bending members:

(a) For beams supported by full bearing on one surface and loads applied to the opposite surface, uniformly distributed loads within a distance from supports equal to the depth of the bending member, d, shall be permitted to be ignored. For beams supported by full bearing on one surface and loads applied to the opposite surface, concentrated loads within a distance, d, from supports shall be permitted to be multiplied by x/d where x is the distance from the beam support face to the load (see Figure 3C).

Figure 3C   Shear at Supports

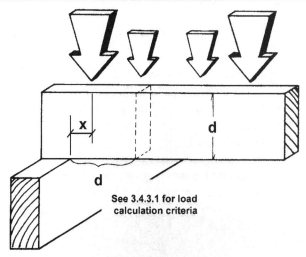

See 3.4.3.1 for load calculation criteria

(b) The largest single moving load shall be placed at a distance from the support equal to the depth of the bending member, keeping other loads in their normal relation and neglecting any load within a distance from a support equal to the depth of the bending member. This condition shall be checked at each support.

(c) With two or more moving loads of about equal weight and in proximity, loads shall be placed in the position that produces the highest shear force, V, neglecting any load within a distance from a support equal to the depth of the bending member.

3.4.3.2 For notched bending members, shear force, V, shall be determined by principles of engineering mechanics (except those given in 3.4.3.1).

(a) For bending members with rectangular cross section and notched on the tension face (see 3.2.3), the adjusted design shear, V_r', shall be calculated as follows:

$$V_r' = \left[\frac{2}{3}F_v'bd_n\right]\left[\frac{d_n}{d}\right]^2 \qquad (3.4\text{-}3)$$

where:

d = depth of unnotched bending member

d_n = depth of member remaining at a notch

F_v' = adjusted shear design value parallel to grain

(b) For bending members with circular cross section and notched on the tension face (see 3.2.3), the adjusted design shear, V_r', shall be calculated as follows:

$$V_r' = \left[\frac{2}{3}F_v'A_n\right]\left[\frac{d_n}{d}\right]^2 \qquad (3.4\text{-}4)$$

where:

A_n = cross-sectional area of notched member

(c) For bending members with other than rectangular or circular cross section and notched on the tension face (see 3.2.3), the adjusted design shear, V_r', shall be based on conventional engineering analysis of stress concentrations at notches.

(d) A gradual change in cross section compared with a square notch decreases the actual shear stress parallel to grain nearly to that computed for an unnotched bending member with a depth of d_n.

(e) When a bending member is notched on the compression face at the end as shown in Figure 3D, the adjusted design shear, V_r', shall be calculated as follows:

$$V_r' = \frac{2}{3}F_v'b\left[d - \left(\frac{d-d_n}{d_n}\right)e\right] \qquad (3.4\text{-}5)$$

where:

e = the distance the notch extends inside the inner edge of the support and must be less than or equal to the depth remaining at the notch, $e \leq d_n$. If $e > d_n$, d_n shall be used to calculate f_v using Equation 3.4-2.

d_n = depth of member remaining at a notch meeting the provisions of 3.2.3. If the end of the beam is beveled, as shown by the dashed line in Figure 3D, d_n is measured from the inner edge of the support.

Figure 3D Bending Member End-Notched on Compression Face

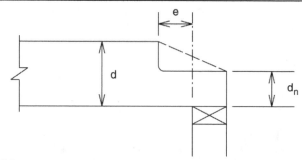

3.4.3.3 When connections in bending members are fastened with split ring connectors, shear plate connectors, bolts, or lag screws (including beams supported by such fasteners or other cases as shown in Figures 3E and 3I) the shear force, V, shall be determined by principles of engineering mechanics (except those given in 3.4.3.1).

(a) When the connection is less than five times the depth, 5d, of the member from its end, the adjusted design shear, V_r', shall be calculated as follows:

$$V_r' = \left[\frac{2}{3}F_v'bd_e\right]\left[\frac{d_e}{d}\right]^2 \qquad (3.4\text{-}6)$$

where:

for split ring or shear plate connections:

d_e = depth of member, less the distance from the unloaded edge of the member to the nearest edge of the nearest split ring or shear plate connector (see Figure 3E).

for bolt or lag screw connections:

d_e = depth of member, less the distance from the unloaded edge of the member to the center of the nearest bolt or lag screw (see Figure 3E)

(b) When the connection is at least five times the depth, 5d, of the member from its end, the adjusted design shear, V_r', shall be calculated as follows:

$$V_r' = \frac{2}{3}F_v'bd_e \qquad (3.4\text{-}7)$$

(c) When concealed hangers are used, the adjusted design shear, V_r', shall be calculated based on the provisions in 3.4.3.2 for notched bending members.

Figure 3E   Effective Depth, d_e, of Members at Connections

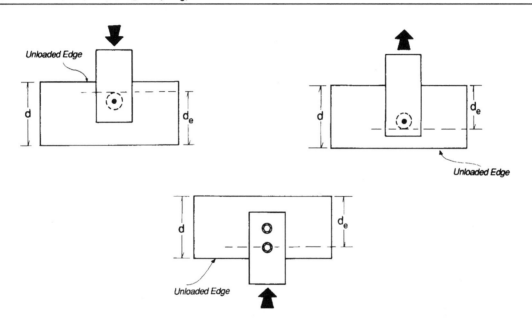

3.5 Bending Members – Deflection

3.5.1 Deflection Calculations

If deflection is a factor in design, it shall be calculated by standard methods of engineering mechanics considering bending deflections and, when applicable, shear deflections. Consideration for shear deflection is required when the reference modulus of elasticity has not been adjusted to include the effects of shear deflection (see Appendix F).

3.5.2 Long-Term Loading

Where total deflection under long-term loading must be limited, increasing member size is one way to provide extra stiffness to allow for this time dependent deformation (see Appendix F). Total deflection, Δ_T, shall be calculated as follows:

$$\Delta_T = K_{cr}\,\Delta_{LT} + \Delta_{ST}$$

where:

K_{cr} = time dependent deformation (creep) factor

= 1.5 for seasoned lumber, structural glued laminated timber, prefabricated wood I-joists, or structural composite lumber used in dry service conditions as defined in 4.1.4, 5.1.5, 7.1.4, and 8.1.4, respectively.

= 2.0 for structural glued laminated timber used in wet service conditions as defined in 5.1.5.

= 2.0 for wood structural panels used in dry service conditions as defined in 9.1.4.

= 2.0 for unseasoned lumber or for seasoned lumber used in wet service conditions as defined in 4.1.4.

Δ_{LT} = immediate deflection due to the long-term component of the design load

Δ_{ST} = deflection due to the short-term or normal component of the design load

3.6 Compression Members – General

3.6.1 Terminology

For purposes of this Specification, the term "column" refers to all types of compression members, including members forming part of trusses or other structural components.

3.6.2 Column Classifications

3.6.2.1 Simple Solid Wood Columns. Simple columns consist of a single piece or of pieces properly glued together to form a single member (see Figure 3F).

3.6.2.2 Spaced Columns, Connector Joined. Spaced columns are formed of two or more individual members with their longitudinal axes parallel, separated at the ends and middle points of their length by blocking and joined at the ends by split ring or shear plate connectors capable of developing the required shear resistance (see 15.2).

3.6.2.3 Built-Up Columns. Individual laminations of mechanically laminated built-up columns shall be designed in accordance with 3.6.3 and 3.7, except that nailed or bolted built-up columns shall be designed in accordance with 15.3.

3.6.3 Strength in Compression Parallel to Grain

The actual compression stress or force parallel to grain shall not exceed the adjusted compression design value. Calculations of f_c shall be based on the net section area (see 3.1.2) when the reduced section occurs in the critical part of the column length that is most subject to potential buckling. When the reduced section does not occur in the critical part of the column length that is most subject to potential buckling, calculations of f_c shall be based on gross section area. In addition, f_c based on net section area shall not exceed the reference compression design value parallel to grain multiplied by all applicable adjustment factors except the column stability factor, C_P.

Figure 3F   Simple Solid Column

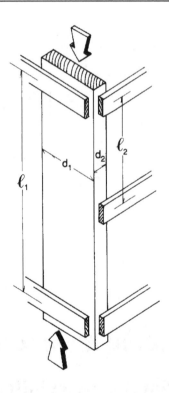

3.6.4 Compression Members Bearing End to End

For end grain bearing of wood on wood, and on metal plates or strips see 3.10.

3.6.5 Eccentric Loading or Combined Stresses

For compression members subject to eccentric loading or combined flexure and axial loading, see 3.9 and 15.4.

3.6.6 Column Bracing

Column bracing shall be installed where necessary to resist wind or other lateral forces (see Appendix A).

3.6.7 Lateral Support of Arches, Studs, and Compression Chords of Trusses

Guidelines for providing lateral support and determining ℓ_e/d in arches, studs, and compression chords of trusses are specified in Appendix A.11.

3.7 Solid Columns

3.7.1 Column Stability Factor, C$_P$

3.7.1.1 When a compression member is supported throughout its length to prevent lateral displacement in all directions, $C_P = 1.0$.

3.7.1.2 The effective column length, ℓ_e, for a solid column shall be determined in accordance with principles of engineering mechanics. One method for determining effective column length, when end-fixity conditions are known, is to multiply actual column length by the appropriate effective length factor specified in Appendix G, $\ell_e = (K_e)(\ell)$.

3.7.1.3 For solid columns with rectangular cross section, the slenderness ratio, ℓ_e/d, shall be taken as the larger of the ratios ℓ_{e1}/d_1 or ℓ_{e2}/d_2 (see Figure 3F) where each ratio has been adjusted by the appropriate buckling length coefficient, K_e, from Appendix G.

3.7.1.4 The slenderness ratio for solid columns, ℓ_e/d, shall not exceed 50, except that during construction ℓ_e/d shall not exceed 75.

3.7.1.5 The column stability factor shall be calculated as follows:

$$C_P = \frac{1 + \left(F_{cE}/F_c^*\right)}{2c} - \sqrt{\left[\frac{1 + \left(F_{cE}/F_c^*\right)}{2c}\right]^2 - \frac{F_{cE}/F_c^*}{c}} \quad (3.7\text{-}1)$$

where:

F_c^* = reference compression design value parallel to grain multiplied by all applicable adjustment factors except C_p (see 2.3)

$$F_{cE} = \frac{0.822\ E_{min}'}{\left(\ell_e/d\right)^2}$$

c = 0.8 for sawn lumber

c = 0.85 for round timber poles and piles

c = 0.9 for structural glued laminated timber or structural composite lumber

3.7.1.6 For especially severe service conditions and/or extraordinary hazard, use of lower adjusted design values may be necessary. See Appendix H for background information concerning column stability calculations and Appendix F for information concerning coefficient of variation in modulus of elasticity (COV_E).

3.7.2 Tapered Columns

For design of a column with rectangular cross section, tapered at one or both ends, the representative dimension, d, for each face of the column shall be derived as follows:

$$d = d_{min} + (d_{max} - d_{min})\left[a - 0.15\left(1 - \frac{d_{min}}{d_{max}}\right)\right] \quad (3.7\text{-}2)$$

where:

d_{min} = the minimum dimension for that face of the column

d_{max} = the maximum dimension for that face of the column

Support Conditions

Large end fixed, small end unsupported or simply supported	a = 0.70
Small end fixed, large end unsupported or simply supported	a = 0.30
Both ends simply supported:	
Tapered toward one end	a = 0.50
Tapered toward both ends	a = 0.70

For all other support conditions:

$$d = d_{min} + (d_{max} - d_{min})(1/3) \quad (3.7\text{-}3)$$

Calculations of f_c and C_P shall be based on the representative dimension, d. In addition, f_c at any cross section in the tapered column shall not exceed the reference compression design value parallel to grain multiplied by all applicable adjustment factors except the column stability factor, C_P.

3.7.3 Round Columns

The design of a column of round cross section shall be based on the design calculations for a square column of the same cross-sectional area and having the same degree of taper. Reference design values and special design provisions for round timber poles and piles are provided in Chapter 6.

3.8 Tension Members

3.8.1 Tension Parallel to Grain

The actual tension stress or force parallel to grain shall be based on the net section area (see 3.1.2) and shall not exceed the adjusted tension design value.

3.8.2 Tension Perpendicular to Grain

Designs that induce tension stress perpendicular to grain shall be avoided whenever possible (see References 16 and 19). When tension stress perpendicular to grain cannot be avoided, mechanical reinforcement sufficient to resist all such stresses shall be considered (see References 52 and 53 for additional information).

3.9 Combined Bending and Axial Loading

3.9.1 Bending and Axial Tension

Members subjected to a combination of bending and axial tension (see Figure 3G) shall be so proportioned that:

$$\frac{f_t}{F_t{}'} + \frac{f_b}{F_b^*} \leq 1.0 \tag{3.9-1}$$

and

$$\frac{f_b - f_t}{F_b^{**}} \leq 1.0 \tag{3.9-2}$$

where:

F_b^* = reference bending design value multiplied by all applicable adjustment factors except C_L

F_b^{**} = reference bending design value multiplied by all applicable adjustment factors except C_V

Figure 3G Combined Bending and Axial Tension

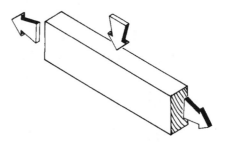

3.9.2 Bending and Axial Compression

Members subjected to a combination of bending about one or both principal axes and axial compression (see Figure 3H) shall be so proportioned that:

$$\left[\frac{f_c}{F_c{}'}\right]^2 + \frac{f_{b1}}{F_{b1}{}'\left[1 - \left(f_c/F_{cE1}\right)\right]}$$
$$+ \frac{f_{b2}}{F_{b2}{}'\left[1 - \left(f_c/F_{cE2}\right) - \left(f_{b1}/F_{bE}\right)^2\right]} \leq 1.0 \tag{3.9-3}$$

where:

$$f_c < F_{cE1} = \frac{0.822\,E_{min}'}{(\ell_{e1}/d_1)^2} \quad \text{for either uniaxial edge-wise bending or biaxial bending}$$

and

$$f_c < F_{cE2} = \frac{0.822\,E_{min}'}{(\ell_{e2}/d_2)^2} \quad \text{for uniaxial flatwise bending or biaxial bending}$$

and

$$f_{b1} < F_{bE} = \frac{1.20\,E_{min}'}{(R_B)^2} \quad \text{for biaxial bending}$$

f_{b1} = actual edgewise bending stress (bending load applied to narrow face of member)

f_{b2} = actual flatwise bending stress (bending load applied to wide face of member)

d_1 = wide face dimension (see Figure 3H)

d_2 = narrow face dimension (see Figure 3H)

Effective column lengths, ℓ_{e1} and ℓ_{e2}, shall be determined in accordance with 3.7.1.2. F_c', F_{cE1}, and F_{cE2} shall be determined in accordance with 2.3 and 3.7. F_{b1}', F_{b2}', and F_{bE} shall be determined in accordance with 2.3 and 3.3.3.

3.9.3 Eccentric Compression Loading

See 15.4 for members subjected to combined bending and axial compression due to eccentric loading, or eccentric loading in combination with other loads.

Figure 3H   Combined Bending and Axial Compression

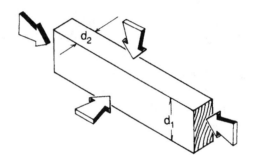

3.10 Design for Bearing

3.10.1 Bearing Parallel to Grain

3.10.1.1 The actual compressive bearing stress parallel to grain shall be based on the net bearing area and shall not exceed the reference compression design value parallel to grain multiplied by all applicable adjustment factors except the column stability factor, C_P.

3.10.1.2 F_c^*, the reference compression design values parallel to grain multiplied by all applicable adjustment factors except the column stability factor, applies to end-to-end bearing of compression members provided there is adequate lateral support and the end cuts are accurately squared and parallel.

3.10.1.3 When $f_c > (0.75)(F_c^*)$ bearing shall be on a metal plate or strap, or on other equivalently durable, rigid, homogeneous material with sufficient stiffness to distribute the applied load. When a rigid insert is required for end-to-end bearing of compression members, it shall be equivalent to 20-gage metal plate or better, inserted with a snug fit between abutting ends.

3.10.2 Bearing Perpendicular to Grain

The actual compression stress perpendicular to grain shall be based on the net bearing area and shall not exceed the adjusted compression design value perpendicular to grain, $f_{c\perp} \le F_{c\perp}'$. When calculating bearing area at the ends of bending members, no allowance shall be made for the fact that as the member bends, pressure upon the inner edge of the bearing is greater than at the member end.

3.10.3 Bearing at an Angle to Grain

The adjusted bearing design value at an angle to grain (see Figure 3I and Appendix J) shall be calculated as follows:

$$F_\theta' = \frac{F_c^* F_{c\perp}'}{F_c^* \sin^2\theta + F_{c\perp}' \cos^2\theta} \tag{3.10-1}$$

where:

θ = angle between direction of load and direction of grain (longitudinal axis of member), degrees

3.10.4 Bearing Area Factor, C_b

Reference compression design values perpendicular to grain, $F_{c\perp}$, apply to bearings of any length at the ends of a member, and to all bearings 6" or more in length at any other location. For bearings less than 6" in length and not nearer than 3" to the end of a member, the reference compression design value perpendicular to grain, $F_{c\perp}$, shall be permitted to be multiplied by the following bearing area factor, C_b:

$$C_b = \frac{\ell_b + 0.375}{\ell_b} \tag{3.10-2}$$

where:

ℓ_b = bearing length measured parallel to grain, in.

Equation 3.10-2 gives the following bearing area factors, C_b, for the indicated bearing length on such small areas as plates and washers:

Table 3.10.4 Bearing Area Factors, C_b

ℓ_b	0.5"	1"	1.5"	2"	3"	4"	6" or more
C_b	1.75	1.38	1.25	1.19	1.13	1.10	1.00

For round bearing areas such as washers, the bearing length, ℓ_b, shall be equal to the diameter.

Figure 3I Bearing at an Angle to Grain

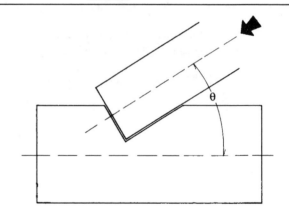

SAWN LUMBER

4

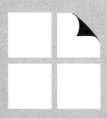

4.1 General

4.1.1 Application

Chapter 4 applies to engineering design with sawn lumber. Design procedures, reference design values and other information herein apply only to lumber complying with the requirements specified below.

4.1.2 Identification of Lumber

4.1.2.1 When the reference design values specified herein are used, the lumber, including end-jointed or edge-glued lumber, shall be identified by the grade mark of, or certificate of inspection issued by, a lumber grading or inspection bureau or agency recognized as being competent (see Reference 31). A distinct grade mark of a recognized lumber grading or inspection bureau or agency, indicating that joint integrity is subject to qualification and quality control, shall be applied to glued lumber products.

4.1.2.2 Lumber shall be specified by commercial species and grade names, or by required levels of design values as listed in Tables 4A, 4B, 4C, 4D, 4E, and 4F (published in the Supplement to this Specification).

4.1.3 Definitions

4.1.3.1 Structural sawn lumber consists of lumber classifications known as "Dimension," "Beams and Stringers," "Posts and Timbers," and "Decking," with design values assigned to each grade.

4.1.3.2 "Dimension" refers to lumber from 2" to 4" (nominal) thick, and 2" (nominal) or more in width. Dimension lumber is further classified as Structural Light Framing, Light Framing, Studs, and Joists and Planks (see References 42, 43, 44, 45, 46, 47, and 49 for additional information).

4.1.3.3 "Beams and Stringers" refers to lumber of rectangular cross section, 5" (nominal) or more thick, with width more than 2" greater than thickness, graded with respect to its strength in bending when loaded on the narrow face.

4.1.3.4 "Posts and Timbers" refers to lumber of square or approximately square cross section, 5" x 5" (nominal) and larger, with width not more than 2" greater than thickness, graded primarily for use as posts or columns carrying longitudinal load.

4.1.3.5 "Decking" refers to lumber from 2" to 4" (nominal) thick, tongued and grooved, or grooved for spline on the narrow face, and intended for use as a roof, floor, or wall membrane. Decking is graded for application in the flatwise direction, with the wide face of the decking in contact with the supporting members, as normally installed.

4.1.4 Moisture Service Condition of Lumber

The reference design values for lumber specified herein are applicable to lumber that will be used under dry service conditions such as in most covered structures, where the moisture content in use will be a maximum of 19%, regardless of the moisture content at the time of manufacture. For lumber used under conditions where the moisture content of the wood in service will exceed 19% for an extended period of time, the design values shall be multiplied by the wet service factors, C_M, specified in Tables 4A, 4B, 4C, 4D, 4E, and 4F.

4.1.5 Lumber Sizes

4.1.5.1 Lumber sizes referred to in this Specification are nominal sizes. Computations to determine the required sizes of members shall be based on the net dimensions (actual sizes) and not the nominal sizes. The dressed sizes specified in Reference 31 shall be accepted as the minimum net sizes associated with nominal dimensions (see Table 1A in the Supplement to this Specification).

4.1.5.2 For 4" (nominal) or thinner lumber, the net DRY dressed sizes shall be used in all computations of structural capacity regardless of the moisture content at the time of manufacture or use.

4.1.5.3 For 5" (nominal) and thicker lumber, the net GREEN dressed sizes shall be used in computations of structural capacity regardless of the moisture content at the time of manufacture or use.

4.1.5.4 Where a design is based on rough sizes or special sizes, the applicable moisture content and size used in design shall be clearly indicated in plans or specifications.

4.1.6 End-Jointed or Edge-Glued Lumber

Reference design values for sawn lumber are applicable to structural end-jointed or edge-glued lumber of the same species and grade. Such use shall include, but not be limited to light framing, studs, joists, planks, and decking. When finger jointed lumber is marked "STUD USE ONLY" or "VERTICAL USE ONLY" such lumber shall be limited to use where any bending or tension stresses are of short duration.

4.1.7 Resawn or Remanufactured Lumber

4.1.7.1 When structural lumber is resawn or remanufactured, it shall be regraded, and reference design values for the regraded material shall apply (see References 16, 42, 43, 44, 45, 46, 47, and 49).

4.1.7.2 When sawn lumber is cross cut to shorter lengths, the requirements of 4.1.7.1 shall not apply, except for reference bending design values for those Beam and Stringer grades where grading provisions for the middle 1/3 of the length of the piece differ from grading provisions for the outer thirds.

4.2 Reference Design Values

4.2.1 Reference Design Values

Reference design values for visually graded lumber and for mechanically graded dimension lumber are specified in Tables 4A, 4B, 4C, 4D, 4E, and 4F (published in the Supplement to this Specification). The reference design values in Tables 4A, 4B, 4C, 4D, 4E, and 4F are taken from the published grading rules of the agencies cited in References 42, 43, 44, 45, 46, 47, and 49.

4.2.2 Other Species and Grades

Reference design values for species and grades of lumber not otherwise provided herein shall be established in accordance with appropriate ASTM standards and other technically sound criteria (see References 16, 18, 19, and 31).

4.2.3 Basis for Reference Design Values

4.2.3.1 The reference design values in Tables 4A, 4B, 4C, 4D, 4E, and 4F are for the design of structures where an individual member, such as a beam, girder, post or other member, carries or is responsible for carrying its full design load. For repetitive member uses see 4.3.9.

4.2.3.2 Visually Graded Lumber. Reference design values for visually graded lumber in Tables 4A, 4B, 4C, 4D, 4E, and 4F are based on the provisions of ASTM Standards D 245 and D 1990.

4.2.3.3 Machine Stress Rated (MSR) Lumber and Machine Evaluated Lumber (MEL). Reference design values for machine stress rated lumber and machine evaluated lumber in Table 4C are determined by visual grading and nondestructive pretesting of individual pieces.

4.2.4 Modulus of Elasticity, E

4.2.4.1 Average Values. Reference design values for modulus of elasticity assigned to the visually graded species and grades of lumber listed in Tables 4A, 4B, 4C, 4D, 4E, and 4F are average values which conform to ASTM Standards D 245 and D 1990. Adjustments in modulus of elasticity have been taken to reflect increases for seasoning, increases for density where applicable, and, where required, reductions have been made to account for the effect of grade upon stiffness. Reference modulus of elasticity design values are based upon the species or species group average in accordance with ASTM Standards D 1990 and D 2555.

4.2.4.2 Special Uses. Average reference modulus of elasticity design values listed in Tables 4A, 4B, 4C, 4D, 4E, and 4F are to be used in design of repetitive member systems and in calculating the immediate deflection of single members which carry their full design load. In special applications where deflection is a critical factor, or where amount of deformation under long-term loading must be limited, the need for use of a reduced modulus of elasticity design value shall be determined. See Appendix F for provisions on design value adjustments for special end use requirements.

4.2.5 Bending, F_b

4.2.5.1 Dimension Grades. Adjusted bending design values for Dimension grades apply to members with the load applied to either the narrow or wide face.

4.2.5.2 Decking Grades. Adjusted bending design values for Decking grades apply only when the load is applied to the wide face.

4.2.5.3 Post and Timber Grades. Adjusted bending design values for Post and Timber grades apply to members with the load applied to either the narrow or wide face.

4.2.5.4 Beam and Stringer Grades. Adjusted bending design values for Beam and Stringer grades apply to members with the load applied to the narrow face. When Post and Timber sizes of lumber are graded to Beam and Stringer grade requirements, design values for the applicable Beam and Stringer grades shall be used. Such lumber shall be identified in accordance with 4.1.2.1 as conforming to Beam and Stringer grades.

4.2.5.5 Continuous or Cantilevered Beams. When Beams and Stringers are used as continuous or cantilevered beams, the design shall include a requirement that the grading provisions applicable to the middle 1/3 of the length (see References 42, 43, 44, 45, 46, 47, and 49) shall be applied to at least the middle 2/3 of the length of pieces to be used as two span continuous beams, and to the entire length of pieces to be used over three or more spans or as cantilevered beams.

4.2.6 Compression Perpendicular to Grain, $F_{c\perp}$

For sawn lumber, the reference compression design values perpendicular to grain are based on a deformation limit that has been shown by experience to provide for adequate service in typical wood frame construction. The reference compression design values perpendicular to grain specified in Tables 4A, 4B, 4C, 4D, 4E, and 4F are species group average values associated with a deformation level of 0.04" for a steel plate on wood member loading condition. One method for limiting deformation in special applications where it is critical, is use of a reduced compression design value perpendicular to grain. The following equation shall be used to calculate the compression design value perpendicular to grain for a reduced deformation level of 0.02":

$$F_{c\perp 0.02} = 0.73\, F_{c\perp} \qquad (4.2\text{-}1)$$

where:

$F_{c\perp 0.02}$ = compression perpendicular to grain design value at 0.02" deformation limit

$F_{c\perp}$ = reference compression perpendicular to grain design value at 0.04" deformation limit (as published in Tables 4A, 4B, 4C, 4D, 4E, and 4F)

4.3 Adjustment of Reference Design Values

4.3.1 General

Reference design values (F_b, F_t, F_v, $F_{c\perp}$, F_c, E, E_{min}) from Tables 4A, 4B, 4C, 4D, 4E, and 4F shall be multiplied by the adjustment factors specified in Table 4.3.1 to determine adjusted design values (F_b', F_t', F_v', $F_{c\perp}'$, F_c', E', E_{min}').

4.3.2 Load Duration Factor, C_D (ASD only)

All reference design values except modulus of elasticity, E, modulus of elasticity for beam and column stability, E_{min}, and compression perpendicular to grain, $F_{c\perp}$, shall be multiplied by load duration factors, C_D, as specified in 2.3.2.

4.3.3 Wet Service Factor, C_M

Reference design values for structural sawn lumber are based on the moisture service conditions specified in 4.1.4. When the moisture content of structural members in use differs from these moisture service conditions, reference design values shall be multiplied by the wet service factors, C_M, specified in Tables 4A, 4B, 4C, 4D, 4E, and 4F.

4.3.4 Temperature Factor, C_t

When structural members will experience sustained exposure to elevated temperatures up to 150°F (see Appendix C), reference design values shall be multiplied by the temperature factors, C_t, specified in 2.3.3.

Table 4.3.1 Applicability of Adjustment Factors for Sawn Lumber

(handwritten note: C > 1 optional / C < 1 must use)

		ASD only	ASD and LRFD										LRFD only		
		Load Duration Factor	Wet Service Factor	Temperature Factor	Beam Stability Factor	Size Factor	Flat Use Factor	Incising Factor *(southern pine)*	Repetitive Member Factor	Column Stability Factor *(buckling)*	Buckling Stiffness Factor *(ignore always >1)*	Bearing Area Factor *(always >1)*	Format Conversion Factor	Resistance Factor	Time Effect Factor
$F_b' = F_b$	x	C_D	C_M	C_t	C_L	C_F	C_{fu}	C_i	C_r	-	-	-	K_F	ϕ_b	λ
$F_t' = F_t$	x	C_D	C_M	C_t	-	C_F	-	C_i	-	-	-	-	K_F	ϕ_t	λ
$F_v' = F_v$	x	C_D	C_M	C_t	-	-	-	C_i	-	-	-	-	K_F	ϕ_v	λ
$F_{c\perp}' = F_{c\perp}$	x	-	C_M	C_t	-	-	-	C_i	-	-	-	C_b	K_F	ϕ_c	λ
$F_c' = F_c$	x	C_D	C_M	C_t	-	C_F	-	C_i	-	C_P	-	-	K_F	ϕ_c	λ
$E' = E$	x	-	C_M	C_t	-	-	-	C_i	-	-	-	-	-	-	-
$E_{min}' = E_{min}$	x	-	C_M	C_t	-	-	-	C_i	-	-	C_T	-	K_F	ϕ_s	-

4.3.5 Beam Stability Factor, C_L

Reference bending design values, F_b, shall be multiplied by the beam stability factor, C_L, specified in 3.3.3.

4.3.6 Size Factor, C_F

4.3.6.1 Reference bending, tension, and compression parallel to grain design values for visually graded dimension lumber 2" to 4" thick shall be multiplied by the size factors specified in Tables 4A and 4B.

4.3.6.2 When the depth of a rectangular sawn lumber bending member 5" or thicker exceeds 12", the reference bending design values, F_b, in Table 4D shall be multiplied by the following size factor:

$$C_F = (12 / d)^{1/9} \leq 1.0 \qquad (4.3\text{-}1)$$

4.3.6.3 For beams of circular cross section with a diameter greater than 13.5", or for 12" or larger square beams loaded in the plane of the diagonal, the size fac-tor shall be determined in accordance with 4.3.6.2 on the basis of an equivalent conventionally loaded square beam of the same cross-sectional area.

4.3.6.4 Reference bending design values for all species of 2" thick or 3" thick Decking, except Redwood, shall be multiplied by the size factors specified in Table 4E.

4.3.7 Flat Use Factor, C_{fu}

When sawn lumber 2" to 4" thick is loaded on the wide face, multiplying the reference bending design value, F_b, by the flat use factors, C_{fu}, specified in Tables 4A, 4B, 4C, and 4F, shall be permitted.

4.3.8 Incising Factor, C_i

Reference design values shall be multiplied by the following incising factor, C_i, when dimension lumber is incised parallel to grain a maximum depth of 0.4", a maximum length of 3/8", and density of incisions up to

$1100/\text{ft}^2$. Incising factors shall be determined by test or by calculation using reduced section properties for incising patterns exceeding these limits.

Table 4.3.8 Incising Factors, C_i

Design Value	C_i
E, E_{min}	0.95
F_b, F_t, F_c, F_v	0.80
$F_{c\perp}$	1.00

4.3.9 Repetitive Member Factor, C_r

Reference bending design values, F_b, in Tables 4A, 4B, 4C, and 4F for dimension lumber 2" to 4" thick shall be multiplied by the repetitive member factor, C_r = 1.15, when such members are used as joists, truss chords, rafters, studs, planks, decking, or similar members which are in contact or spaced not more than 24" on center, are not less than three in number and are joined by floor, roof or other load distributing elements adequate to support the design load. (A load distributing element is any adequate system that is designed or has been proven by experience to transmit the design load to adjacent members, spaced as described above, without displaying structural weakness or unacceptable deflection. Subflooring, flooring, sheathing, or other covering elements and nail gluing or tongue and groove joints, and through nailing generally meet these criteria.) Reference bending design values in Table 4E for visually graded Decking have already been multiplied by C_r = 1.15.

4.3.10 Column Stability Factor, C_P

Reference compression design values parallel to grain, F_c, shall be multiplied by the column stability factor, C_P, specified in 3.7.

4.3.11 Buckling Stiffness Factor, C_T

Reference modulus of elasticity for beam and column stability, E_{min}, shall be permitted to be multiplied

by the buckling stiffness factor, C_T, as specified in 4.4.2.

4.3.12 Bearing Area Factor, C_b

Reference compression design values perpendicular to grain, $F_{c\perp}$, shall be permitted to be multiplied by the bearing area factor, C_b, as specified in 3.10.4.

4.3.13 Pressure–Preservative Treatment

Reference design values apply to sawn lumber pressure-treated by an approved process and preservative (see Reference 30). Load duration factors greater than 1.6 shall not apply to structural members pressure-treated with water-borne preservatives.

4.3.14 Format Conversion Factor, K_F (LRFD only)

For LRFD, reference design values shall be multiplied by the format conversion factor, K_F, specified in Appendix N.3.1.

4.3.15 Resistance Factor, ϕ (LRFD only)

For LRFD, reference design values shall be multiplied by the resistance factor, ϕ, specified in Appendix N.3.2.

4.3.16 Time Effect Factor, λ (LRFD only)

For LRFD, reference design values shall be multiplied by the time effect factor, λ, specified in Appendix N.3.3.

4.4 Special Design Considerations

4.4.1 Stability of Bending Members

4.4.1.1 Sawn lumber bending members shall be designed in accordance with the lateral stability calculations in 3.3.3 or shall meet the lateral support requirements in 4.4.1.2 and 4.4.1.3.

4.4.1.2 As an alternative to 4.4.1.1, rectangular sawn lumber beams, rafters, joists, or other bending members, shall be designed in accordance with the following provisions to provide restraint against rotation or lateral displacement. If the depth to breadth, d/b, based on nominal dimensions is: *actual dimensions*

  (a) d/b ≤ 2; no lateral support shall be required.

  (b) 2 < d/b ≤ 4; the ends shall be held in position, as by full depth solid blocking, bridging, hangers, nailing, or bolting to other framing members, or other acceptable means.

  (c) 4 < d/b ≤ 5; the compression edge of the member shall be held in line for its entire length to prevent lateral displacement, as by adequate sheathing or subflooring, and ends at point of bearing shall be held in position to prevent rotation and/or lateral displacement.

  (d) 5 < d/b ≤ 6; bridging, full depth solid blocking or diagonal cross bracing shall be installed at intervals not exceeding 8 feet, the compression edge of the member shall be held in line as by adequate sheathing or subflooring, and the ends at points of bearing shall be held in position to prevent rotation and/or lateral displacement.

  (e) 6 < d/b ≤ 7; both edges of the member shall be held in line for their entire length and ends at points of bearing shall be held in position to prevent rotation and/or lateral displacement.

4.4.1.3 If a bending member is subjected to both flexure and axial compression, the depth to breadth ratio shall be no more than 5 to 1 if one edge is firmly held in line. If under all combinations of load, the unbraced edge of the member is in tension, the depth to breadth ratio shall be no more than 6 to 1.

4.4.2 Wood Trusses

4.4.2.1 Increased chord stiffness relative to axial loads when a 2" x 4" or smaller sawn lumber truss compression chord is subjected to combined flexure and axial compression under dry service condition and has 3/8" or thicker plywood sheathing nailed to the narrow face of the chord in accordance with code required roof sheathing fastener schedules (see References 32, 33, and 34), shall be permitted to be accounted for by multiplying the reference modulus of elasticity design value for beam and column stability, E_{min}, by the buckling stiffness factor, C_T, in column stability calculations (see 3.7 and Appendix H). When $\ell_e < 96"$, C_T shall be calculated as follows:

$$C_T = 1 + \frac{K_M \ell_e}{K_T E} \qquad (4.4\text{-}1)$$

where:

ℓ_e = effective column length of truss compression chord (see 3.7)

K_M = 2300 for wood seasoned to 19% moisture content or less at the time of plywood attachment.

   = 1200 for unseasoned or partially seasoned wood at the time of plywood attachment.

K_T = 1 − 1.645(COV$_E$)

   = 0.59 for visually graded lumber

   = 0.75 for machine evaluated lumber (MEL)

   = 0.82 for products with COV$_E$ ≤ 0.11 (see Appendix F.2)

When $\ell_e > 96"$, C_T shall be calculated based on $\ell_e = 96"$.

4.4.2.2 For additional information concerning metal plate connected wood trusses see Reference 9.

4

SAWN LUMBER

4.4.3 Notches

4.4.3.1 End notches, located at the ends of sawn lumber bending members for bearing over a support, shall be permitted, and shall not exceed 1/4 the beam depth (see Figure 4A).

4.4.3.2 Interior notches, located in the outer thirds of the span of a single span sawn lumber bending member, shall be permitted, and shall not exceed 1/6 the depth of the member. Interior notches on the tension side of 3-½" or greater thickness (4" nominal thickness) sawn lumber bending members are not permitted (see Figure 4A).

4.4.3.3 See 3.1.2 and 3.4.3 for effect of notches on strength.

Figure 4A   Notch Limitations for Sawn Lumber Beams

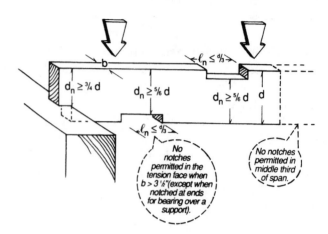

STRUCTURAL GLUED LAMINATED TIMBER

5

5.1 General

5.1.1 Application

5.1.1.1 Chapter 5 applies to engineering design with structural glued laminated timber. Basic requirements are provided in this Specification; for additional detail, see Reference 52.

5.1.1.2 Design procedures, reference design values and other information provided herein apply only to structural glued laminated timber conforming to all pertinent provisions of the specifications referenced in the footnotes to Tables 5A, 5B, 5C, and 5D and produced in accordance with ANSI/AITC A190.1.

5.1.2 Definition

The term "structural glued laminated timber" refers to an engineered, stress rated product of a timber laminating plant, comprising assemblies of specially selected and prepared wood laminations bonded together with adhesives. The grain of all laminations is approximately parallel longitudinally. The separate laminations shall not exceed 2" in net thickness and shall be of:

- one piece, or
- comprised of pieces joined to form any length, or
- pieces placed or glued edge-to-edge to make wider ones, or
- pieces bent to curved-form during gluing.

5.1.3 Standard Sizes

5.1.3.1 Normal standard finished widths of structural glued laminated members shall be as follows:

Table 5.1.3 Net Finished Widths of Structural Glued Laminated Timbers

Nominal Width (in.)	3	4	6	8	10	12	14	16
	Western Species							
Minimum Net Finished Width (in.)	2-½	3-⅛	5-⅛	6-¾	8-¾	10-¾	12-¼	14-¼
	Southern Pine							
	-	3	5	6-¾	8-½	10-½	-	-

This Specification is not intended to prohibit other finished widths when required to meet the size requirements of a design or to meet other special requirements.

5.1.3.2 The depth of straight and curved members shall be specified. The length and net dimensions of all members shall also be specified.

5.1.4 Specification

5.1.4.1 For structural glued laminated timber, the following shall be specified:
(a) Dry or wet service conditions.
(b) Laminating combinations or stress requirements.

5.1.4.2 For structural glued laminated hardwood timber, all required reference design values shall be specified for each member.

5.1.5 Service Conditions

5.1.5.1 Reference design values for dry service conditions shall apply when the moisture content in service is less than 16%, as in most covered structures.

5.1.5.2 Reference design values for glued laminated timber shall be multiplied by the wet service factors, C_M, specified in Tables 5A, 5B, 5C, and 5D when the moisture content in service is 16% or greater, as may occur in exterior and submerged construction, or humid environments.

5.2 Reference Design Values

5.2.1 Reference Design Values

Reference design values for softwood and hardwood structural glued laminated timber are specified in Tables 5A, 5B, 5C, and 5D (published in a separate Supplement to this Specification). The reference design values in Tables 5A, 5B, 5C, and 5D are a compilation of the reference design values provided in the specifications referenced in the footnotes to the tables.

5.2.2 Radial Tension, F_{rt}

For curved bending members, the following reference radial tension design values perpendicular to grain shall apply:

Southern Pine	all loading conditions	$F_{rt} = (1/3)F_v$
Douglas Fir-Larch, Douglas Fir South, Hem-Fir, Western Woods, and Canadian softwood species	wind or earthquake loading	$F_{rt} = (1/3)F_v$
	other types of loading	$F_{rt} = 15$ psi

5.2.3 Other Species and Grades

Reference design values for species and grades of structural glued laminated timber not otherwise provided herein shall be established in accordance with the principles set forth in Reference 22, or shall be based on other substantiated information from an acceptable source.

5.3 Adjustment of Reference Design Values

5.3.1 General

Reference design values (F_b, F_t, F_v, $F_{c\perp}$, F_c, F_{rt}, E, E_{min}) provided in 5.2 and Tables 5A, 5B, 5C, and 5D shall be multiplied by the adjustment factors specified in Table 5.3.1 to determine adjusted design values (F_b', F_t', F_v', $F_{c\perp}'$, F_c', F_{rt}', E', E_{min}').

5.3.2 Load Duration Factor, C_D (ASD only)

All reference design values except modulus of elasticity, E, modulus of elasticity for beam and column stability, E_{min}, and compression perpendicular to grain, $F_{c\perp}$, shall be multiplied by load duration factors, C_D, as specified in 2.3.2.

5.3.3 Wet Service Factor, C_M

Reference design values for structural glued laminated timber are based on the moisture service conditions specified in 5.1.5. When the moisture content of structural members in use differs from these moisture service conditions, reference design values shall be multiplied by the wet service factors, C_M, specified in Tables 5A, 5B, 5C, and 5D.

Table 5.3.1 Applicability of Adjustment Factors for Structural Glued Laminated Timber

		ASD only	ASD and LRFD								LRFD only		
		Load Duration Factor	Wet Service Factor	Temperature Factor	Beam Stability Factor[1]	Volume Factor[1]	Flat Use Factor	Curvature Factor	Column Stability Factor	Bearing Area Factor	Format Conversion Factor	Resistance Factor	Time Effect Factor
$F_b' = F_b$	x	C_D	C_M	C_t	C_L	C_V	C_{fu}	C_c	-	-	K_F	ϕ_b	λ
$F_t' = F_t$	x	C_D	C_M	C_t	-	-	-	-	-	-	K_F	ϕ_t	λ
$F_v' = F_v$	x	C_D	C_M	C_t	-	-	-	-	-	-	K_F	ϕ_v	λ
$F_{c\perp}' = F_{c\perp}$	x	-	C_M	C_t	-	-	-	-	-	C_b	K_F	ϕ_c	λ
$F_c' = F_c$	x	C_D	C_M	C_t	-	-	-	-	C_P	-	K_F	ϕ_c	λ
$F_{rt}' = F_{rt}$	x	C_D	C_M	C_t	-	-	-	-	-	-	K_F	ϕ_v	λ
$E' = E$	x	-	C_M	C_t	-	-	-	-	-	-	-	-	-
$E_{min}' = E_{min}$	x	-	C_M	C_t	-	-	-	-	-	-	K_F	ϕ_s	-

1. The beam stability factor, C_L, shall not apply simultaneously with the volume factor, C_v, for structural glued laminated timber bending members (see 5.3.6). Therefore, the lesser of these adjustment factors shall apply.

5.3.4 Temperature Factor, C_t

When structural members will experience sustained exposure to elevated temperatures up to 150°F (see Appendix C), reference design values shall be multiplied by the temperature factors, C_t, specified in 2.3.3.

5.3.5 Beam Stability Factor, C_L

Reference bending design values, F_b, shall be multiplied by the beam stability factor, C_L, specified in 3.3.3. The beam stability factor, C_L, shall not apply simultaneously with the volume factor, C_V, for structural glued laminated timber bending members (see 5.3.6). Therefore the lesser of these adjustment factors shall apply.

5.3.6 Volume Factor, C_v

When structural glued laminated timber is loaded perpendicular to the wide face of the laminations, reference bending design values for loading perpendicular to the wide faces of the laminations, F_{bxx}, shall be multiplied by the following volume factor:

$$C_V = \left(\frac{21}{L}\right)^{1/x} \left(\frac{12}{d}\right)^{1/x} \left(\frac{5.125}{b}\right)^{1/x} \leq 1.0 \qquad (5.3-1)$$

where:

L = length of bending member between points of zero moment, ft

d = depth of bending member, in.

b = width (breadth) of bending member. For multiple piece width layups, b = width of widest piece used in the layup. Thus, b ≤ 10.75".

x = 20 for Southern Pine

x = 10 for all other species

The volume factor, C_V, shall not apply simultaneously with the beam stability factor, C_L (see 3.3.3). Therefore, the lesser of these adjustment factors shall apply.

5.3.7 Flat Use Factor, C_{fu}

When structural glued laminated timber is loaded parallel to the wide face of the laminations and the member dimension parallel to the wide face of the laminations is less than 12", multiplying the reference bending design value for loading parallel to the wide faces of the laminations, F_{byy}, by the flat use factors, C_{fu}, specified in Tables 5A, 5B, 5C, and 5D, shall be permitted.

5.3.8 Curvature Factor, C_c

For curved portions of bending members, the reference bending design value shall be multiplied by the following curvature factor:

$$C_c = 1 - (2000)(t / R)^2 \qquad (5.3\text{-}2)$$

where:

t = thickness of lamination, in.

R = radius of curvature of inside face of lamination, in.

$t/R \leq 1/100$ for hardwoods and Southern Pine

$t/R \leq 1/125$ for other softwoods

The curvature factor shall not apply to reference design values in the straight portion of a member, regardless of curvature elsewhere.

5.3.9 Column Stability Factor, C_P

Reference compression design values parallel to grain, F_c, shall be multiplied by the column stability factor, C_P, specified in 3.7.

5.3.10 Bearing Area Factor, C_b

Reference compression design values perpendicular to grain, $F_{c\perp}$, shall be permitted to be multiplied by the bearing area factor, C_b, as specified in 3.10.4.

5.3.11 Pressure-Preservative Treatment

Reference design values apply to structural glued laminated timber treated by an approved process and preservative (see Reference 30). Load duration factors greater than 1.6 shall not apply to structural members pressure-treated with water-borne preservatives.

5.3.12 Format Conversion Factor, K_F (LRFD only)

For LRFD, reference design values shall be multiplied by the format conversion factor, K_F, specified in Appendix N.3.1.

5.3.13 Resistance Factor, ϕ (LRFD only)

For LRFD, reference design values shall be multiplied by the resistance factor, ϕ, specified in Appendix N.3.2.

5.3.14 Time Effect Factor, λ (LRFD only)

For LRFD, reference design values shall be multiplied by the time effect factor, λ, specified in Appendix N.3.3.

5.4 Special Design Considerations

5.4.1 Radial Stress

5.4.1.1 The actual radial stress induced by a bending moment in a curved member of constant rectangular cross section is:

$$f_r = \frac{3M}{2Rbd} \qquad (5.4\text{-}1)$$

where:

 M = bending moment, in.-lbs

 R = radius of curvature at center line of member, in.

Curved bending members having a varying rectangular cross section (see Figure 5A) and taper cut structural glued laminated bending members shall be designed in accordance with Reference 52.

Figure 5A   Curved Bending Member

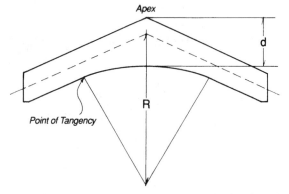

Apex

d

R

Point of Tangency

5.4.1.2 When the bending moment is in the direction tending to decrease curvature (increase the radius), the actual radial stress shall not exceed the adjusted radial tension design value perpendicular to grain, $f_r \le F_{rt}'$, unless mechanical reinforcing sufficient to resist all radial stresses is used (see Reference 52). In no case shall $f_r > (1/3)F_v'$.

5.4.1.3 When the bending moment is in the direction tending to increase curvature (decrease the radius), the actual radial stress shall not exceed the adjusted compression design value perpendicular to grain, $f_r \le F_{c\perp}'$.

5.4.2 Lateral Stability for Structural Glued Laminated Timber

5.4.2.1 Bending members shall be laterally supported in accordance with 3.3.3, taking into account the provisions of Appendix A.11. The modulus of elasticity of beams loaded parallel to the wide face of the laminations, $E_{y\min}$, shall be used in beam stability factor calculations.

5.4.2.2 The ratio of tangent point depth to breadth of arches (d/b) shall not exceed 6, based on actual dimensions, when one edge of the arch is braced by decking fastened directly to the arch, or braced at frequent intervals as by girts or roof purlins. When such lateral bracing is not present, d/b shall not exceed 5. Arches shall be designed for lateral stability in accordance with the provisions of 3.7 and 3.9.2.

5.4.3 Deflection

Reference design values for modulus of elasticity in Tables 5A, 5B, 5C, and 5D are average values which include the effects of the grade and placement of laminations used. In special applications where deflection is a critical factor, or where deformation under long-term loading must be limited, the need for use of a reduced reference modulus of elasticity shall be determined. See Appendix F for provisions on design value adjustments for special end use requirements.

5.4.4 Notches

5.4.4.1 The tension side of structural glued laminated timber bending members shall not be notched, except at ends of members for bearing over a support, and notch depth shall not exceed the lesser of 1/10 the depth of the member or 3". The compression side of structural glued laminated timber bending members shall not be notched, except at ends of members, and the notch depth on the compression side shall not exceed 2/5 the depth of the member. Compression side end-notches shall not extend into the middle 1/3 of the span.

> **Exception:** A taper cut on the compression edge at the end of a structural glued laminated timber bending member shall not exceed 2/3 the depth of the member and the length shall not exceed three times the depth of the member, 3d. For tapered beams where the taper extends into the middle 1/3 of the span, special design provisions shall be required.

5.4.4.2 See 3.1.2 and 3.4.3 for effect of notches on strength.

ROUND TIMBER POLES AND PILES

6

6.1 General

6.1.1 Application

6.1.1.1 Chapter 6 applies to engineering design with round timber poles and piles. Design procedures and reference design values herein pertain to the load carrying capacity of poles and piles as structural wood members.

6.1.1.2 This Specification does not apply to the load supporting capacity of the soil.

6.1.2 Specifications

6.1.2.1 The procedures and reference design values herein apply only to timber piles conforming to applicable provisions of ASTM Standard D 25 and only to poles conforming to applicable provisions of ASTM Standard D 3200.

6.1.2.2 Specifications for round timber poles and piles shall include the standard for preservative treatment, pile length, and nominal tip circumference or nominal circumference 3 feet from the butt. Specifications for piles shall state whether piles are to be used as foundation piles, land and fresh water piles, or marine piles.

6.1.3 Standard Sizes

6.1.3.1 Standard sizes for round timber piles are given in ASTM Standard D 25.

6.1.3.2 Standard sizes for round timber poles are given in ASTM Standard D 3200.

6.1.4 Preservative Treatment

6.1.4.1 Reference design values apply to timber poles or piles treated by an approved process and preservative (see Reference 30). Load duration factors greater than 1.6 shall not apply to structural members pressure-treated with water-borne preservatives.

6.1.4.2 Untreated timber poles and piles shall not be used unless the cutoff is below the lowest ground water level expected during the life of the structure, but in no case less than 3 feet below the existing ground water level unless approved by the authority having jurisdiction.

6.2 Reference Design Values

6.2.1 Reference Design Values

6.2.1.1 Reference design values for round timber piles are specified in Table 6A. Reference design values in Table 6A are based on the provisions of ASTM Standard D 2899.

6.2.1.2 Reference design values for round timber poles are specified in Table 6B. Reference design values in Table 6B are based on provisions of ASTM Standard D 3200.

6.2.2 Other Species or Grades

Reference design values for piles of other species or grades shall be determined in accordance with ASTM Standard D 2899.

Table 6A   Reference Design Values for Treated Round Timber Piles

Species	Reference design values for normal load duration and wet service conditions, psi					
	F_c	F_b	F_v	$F_{c\perp}$	E	E_{min}
Pacific Coast Douglas Fir[1]	1250	2450	115	230	1,500,000	790,000
Red Oak[2]	1100	2450	135	350	1,250,000	660,000
Red Pine[3]	900	1900	85	155	1,280,000	680,000
Southern Pine[4]	1200	2400	110	250	1,500,000	790,000

1. Pacific Coast Douglas Fir reference design values apply to this species as defined in ASTM Standard D 1760. For connection design use Douglas Fir-Larch reference design values.
2. Red Oak reference design values apply to Northern and Southern Red Oak.
3. Red Pine reference design values apply to Red Pine grown in the United States. For connection design use Northern Pine reference design values.
4. Southern Pine reference design values apply to Loblolly, Longleaf, Shortleaf, and Slash Pines.

Table 6B   Reference Design Values for Poles Graded in Accordance with ASTM D 3200

Species	Reference design values for normal load duration and wet service conditions, psi					
	F_b	F_v	$F_{c\perp}$	F_c	E	E_{min}
Pacific Coast Douglas Fir	1850	115	375	1000	1,500,000	790,000
Jack Pine	1500	95	280	800	1,070,000	570,000
Lodgepole Pine	1350	85	240	700	1,080,000	570,000
Northern White Cedar	1050	80	225	525	640,000	340,000
Ponderosa Pine	1300	90	320	650	1,000,000	530,000
Red Pine	1450	85	265	725	1,280,000	680,000
Southern Pine	1700	105	320	900	1,400,000	740,000
Western Hemlock	1650	115	245	900	1,310,000	690,000
Western Larch	2050	120	375	1075	1,460,000	770,000
Western Red Cedar	1350	95	255	750	940,000	500,000

6.3 Adjustment of Reference Design Values

6.3.1 Applicability of Adjustment Factors

Reference design values (F_c, F_b, F_v, $F_{c\perp}$, E, E_{min}) shall be multiplied by all applicable adjustment factors to determine adjusted design values (F_c', F_b', F_v', $F_{c\perp}'$, E', E_{min}'). Table 6.3.1 specifies the adjustment factors which apply to each reference design value for round timber poles and piles.

6.3.2 Load Duration Factor, C_D (ASD only)

All reference design values except modulus of elasticity, E, and modulus of elasticity for beam and column stability, E_{min}, for poles and piles and compression perpendicular to grain $F_{c\perp}$, for poles shall be multiplied

by load duration factors, C_D, as specified in 2.3.2. Load duration factors greater than 1.6 shall not apply to timber poles or piles pressure-treated with water-borne preservatives, (see Reference 30), nor to structural members pressure-treated with fire retardant chemicals (see Table 2.3.2).

6.3.3 Wet Service Factor, C_M

Reference design values apply to wet or dry service conditions.

6.3.4 Temperature Factor, C_t

Reference design values shall be multiplied by temperature factors, C_t, as specified in 2.3.3.

Table 6.3.1 Applicability of Adjustment Factors for Round Timber Poles and Piles

		ASD only	ASD and LRFD							LRFD only		
		Load Duration Factor	Temperature Factor	Untreated Factor	Size Factor	Column Stability Factor	Critical Section Factor	Bearing Area Factor	Single Pile Factor	Format Conversion Factor	Resistance Factor	Time Effect Factor
$F_c' = F_c$	x	C_D	C_t	C_u	-	C_P	C_{cs}	-	C_{sp}	K_F	ϕ_c	λ
$F_b' = F_b$	x	C_D	C_t	C_u	C_F	-	-	-	C_{sp}	K_F	ϕ_b	λ
$F_v' = F_v$	x	C_D	C_t	C_u	-	-	-	-	-	K_F	ϕ_v	λ
$F_{c\perp}' = F_{c\perp}$	x	C_D^1	C_t	C_u	-	-	-	C_b	-	K_F	ϕ_c	λ
$E' = E$	x	-	C_t	-	-	-	-	-	-	-	-	-
$E_{min}' = E_{min}$	x	-	C_t	-	-	-	-	-	-	K_F	ϕ_s	-

1. The C_D factor shall not apply to compression perpendicular to grain values for poles.

6.3.5 Untreated Factor, C_u

Reference design values include an adjustment to compensate for strength reduction due to steam conditioning or boultonizing prior to treatment (see Reference 20). Where poles or piles are air dried or kiln dried prior to pressure treatment, or where untreated poles or piles are used, all reference design values except modulus of elasticity, E, and modulus of elasticity for beam and column stability, E_{min}, shall be permitted to be multiplied by the untreated factors, C_u, in Table 6.3.5.

Table 6.3.5 Untreated Factors, C_u, for Timber Poles and Piles

Species	C_u
Pacific Coast Douglas Fir, Red Oak, Red Pine	1.11
Southern Pine	1.18

6.3.6 Beam Stability Factor, C_L

Reference bending design values, F_b, for round timber poles or piles shall not be adjusted for beam stability.

6.3.7 Size Factor, C_F

When pole or pile circumference exceeds 43" (diameter exceeds 13.5") at the critical section in bending, the reference bending design value, F_b, shall be multiplied by the size factor, C_F, specified in 4.3.6.2 and 4.3.6.3.

6.3.8 Column Stability Factor, C_P

Reference compression design values parallel to grain, F_c, for the portion of a timber pole or pile standing unbraced in air, water, or material not capable of lateral support shall be multiplied by the column stability factor, C_P, specified in 3.7.

6.3.9 Critical Section Factor, C_{cs}

Reference compression design values parallel to grain, F_c, for round timber piles are based on the strength at the tip of the pile. Reference compression design values parallel to grain, F_c, for Pacific Coast Douglas Fir and Southern Pine in Table 6A shall be permitted to be increased 0.2% for each foot of length from the tip of the pile to the critical section. The critical section factor, C_{cs}, shall be determined as follows:

$$C_{cs} = 1.0 + (L_c)(0.002) \qquad (6.3-1)$$

where:

L_c = length from tip of pile to critical section, ft

The increase for location of critical section shall not exceed 10% for any pile ($C_{cs} \leq 1.10$). The critical section factors, C_{cs}, are independent of tapered column provisions in 3.7.2 and both shall be permitted to be used in design calculations.

6.3.10 Bearing Area Factor, C_b

Reference compression design values perpendicular to grain, $F_{c\perp}$, for timber poles or piles shall be permitted to be multiplied by the bearing area factor, C_b, specified in 3.10.4.

6.3.11 Single Pile Factor, C_{sp}

Reference bending design values, F_b, and reference compression design values parallel to grain, F_c, are intended for use when the design encompasses load sharing principles such as occur in a pile cluster. When piles are used in such a manner that each pile supports its own specific load, reference bending design values and reference compression design values parallel to grain shall be multiplied by the single pile factors, C_{sp}, in Table 6.3.11.

Table 6.3.11 Single Pile Factors, C_{sp}, for Round Timber Piles

Reference Design Value	C_{sp}
F_c	0.80
F_b	0.77

6.3.12 Format Conversion Factor, K_F (LRFD only)

For LRFD, reference design values shall be multiplied by the format conversion factor, K_F, specified in Appendix N.3.1.

6.3.13 Resistance Factor, ϕ (LRFD only)

For LRFD, reference design values shall be multiplied by the resistance factor, ϕ, specified in Appendix N.3.2.

6.3.14 Time Effect Factor, λ (LRFD only)

For LRFD, reference design values shall be multiplied by the time effect factor, λ, specified in Appendix N.3.3.

PREFABRICATED WOOD I-JOISTS

7

7.1 General

7.1.1 Application

Chapter 7 applies to engineering design with prefabricated wood I-joists. Basic requirements are provided in this Specification. Design procedures and other information provided herein apply only to prefabricated wood I-joists conforming to all pertinent provisions of ASTM D 5055.

7.1.2 Definition

The term "prefabricated wood I-joist" refers to a structural member manufactured using sawn or structural composite lumber flanges and wood structural panel webs bonded together with exterior exposure adhesives, forming an "I" cross-sectional shape.

7.1.3 Identification

When the design procedures and other information provided herein are used, the prefabricated wood I-joists shall be identified with the manufacturer's name and the quality assurance agency's name.

7.1.4 Service Conditions

Reference design values reflect dry service conditions, where the moisture content in service is less than 16%, as in most covered structures. I-joists shall not be used in higher moisture service conditions unless specifically permitted by the I-joist manufacturer.

7.2 Reference Design Values

Reference design values for prefabricated wood I-joists shall be obtained from the prefabricated wood I-joist manufacturer's literature or code evaluation reports.

7.3 Adjustment of Reference Design Values

7.3.1 General

Reference design values (M_r, V_r, R_r, EI, $(EI)_{min}$, K) shall be multiplied by the adjustment factors specified in Table 7.3.1 to determine adjusted design values (M_r', V_r', R_r', EI', $(EI)_{min}'$, K').

7.3.2 Load Duration Factor, C_D (ASD only)

All reference design values except stiffness, EI, $(EI)_{min}$, and K, shall be multiplied by load duration factors, C_D, as specified in 2.3.2.

7.3.3 Wet Service Factor, C_M

Reference design values for prefabricated wood I-joists are applicable to dry service conditions as specified in 7.1.4 where $C_M = 1.0$. When the service conditions differ from the specified conditions, adjustments for high moisture shall be in accordance with information provided by the prefabricated wood I-joist manufacturer.

7.3.4 Temperature Factor, C_t

When structural members will experience sustained exposure to elevated temperatures up to 150°F (see Appendix C), reference design values shall be multiplied by the temperature factors, C_t, specified in 2.3.3. For M_r, V_r, R_r, EI, $(EI)_{min}$, and K use C_t for F_b, F_v, F_v, E, E_{min}, and F_v, respectively.

Table 7.3.1 Applicability of Adjustment Factors for Prefabricated Wood I-Joists

		ASD only	ASD and LRFD				LRFD only		
		Load Duration Factor	Wet Service Factor	Temperature Factor	Beam Stability Factor	Repetitive Member Factor	Format Conversion Factor	Resistance Factor	Time Effect Factor
$M_r' = M_r$	x	C_D	C_M	C_t	C_L	C_r	K_F	ϕ_b	λ
$V_r' = V_r$	x	C_D	C_M	C_t	-	-	K_F	ϕ_v	λ
$R_r' = R_r$	x	C_D	C_M	C_t	-	-	K_F	ϕ_v	λ
$EI' = EI$	x	-	C_M	C_t	-	-	-	-	-
$(EI)_{min}' = (EI)_{min}$	x	-	C_M	C_t	-	-	K_F	ϕ_s	-
$K' = K$	x	-	C_M	C_t	-	-	-	-	-

7.3.5 Beam Stability Factor, C_L

Lateral stability of prefabricated wood I-joists shall be considered. One acceptable method is the procedure of 3.7.1 using the section properties of the compression flange only. The compression flange shall be evaluated as a column continuously restrained in the direction of the web. C_P of the compression flange shall be used as C_L of the joist. Prefabricated wood I-joists shall be restrained against lateral movement and rotation at supports.

7.3.6 Repetitive Member Factor, C_r

For prefabricated wood I-joists with structural composite lumber flanges or sawn lumber flanges, reference moment design resistances shall be multiplied by the repetitive member factor, $C_r = 1.0$.

7.3.7 Pressure-Preservative Treatment

Adjustments to reference design values to account for the effects of pressure-preservative treatment shall be in accordance with information provided by the prefabricated wood I-joist manufacturer.

7.3.8 Format Conversion Factor, K_F (LRFD only)

For LRFD, reference design values shall be multiplied by the format conversion factor, K_F, provided by the wood I-joist manufacturer.

7

PREFABRICATED WOOD I-JOISTS

7.3.9 Resistance Factor, ϕ (LRFD only)

For LRFD, reference design values shall be multiplied by the resistance factor, ϕ, specified in Appendix N.3.2.

7.3.10 Time Effect Factor, λ (LRFD only)

For LRFD, reference design values shall be multiplied by the time effect factor, λ, specified in Appendix N.3.3.

7.4 Special Design Considerations

7.4.1 Bearing

Reference bearing design values, as a function of bearing length, for prefabricated wood I-joists with and without web stiffeners shall be obtained from the prefabricated wood I-joist manufacturer's literature or code evaluation reports.

7.4.2 Load Application

Prefabricated wood I-joists act primarily to resist loads applied to the top flange. Web stiffener requirements, if any, at concentrated loads applied to the top flange and design values to resist concentrated loads applied to the web or bottom flange shall be obtained from the prefabricated wood I-joist manufacturer's literature or code evaluation reports.

7.4.3 Web Holes

The effects of web holes on strength shall be accounted for in the design. Determination of critical shear at a web hole shall consider load combinations of 1.4.4 and partial span loadings defined as live or snow loads applied from each adjacent bearing to the opposite edge of a rectangular hole (centerline of a circular hole). The effects of web holes on deflection are negligible when the number of holes is limited to 3 or less per span. Reference design values for prefabricated wood I-joists with round or rectangular holes shall be obtained from the prefabricated wood I-joist manufacturer's literature or code evaluation reports.

7.4.4 Notches

Notched flanges at or between bearings significantly reduces prefabricated wood I-joist capacity and is beyond the scope of this document. See the manufacturer for more information.

7.4.5 Deflection

Both bending and shear deformations shall be considered in deflection calculations, in accordance with the prefabricated wood I-joist manufacturer's literature or code evaluation reports.

7.4.6 Vertical Load Transfer

I-joists supporting bearing walls located directly above the I-joist support require rim joists, blocking panels, or other means to directly transfer vertical loads from the bearing wall to the supporting structure below.

7.4.7 Shear

Provisions of 3.4.3.1 for calculating shear force, V, shall not be used for design of prefabricated wood I-joist bending members.

STRUCTURAL COMPOSITE LUMBER

8

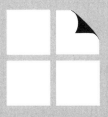

8.1 General

8.1.1 Application

Chapter 8 applies to engineering design with structural composite lumber. Basic requirements are provided in this Specification. Design procedures and other information provided herein apply only to structural composite lumber conforming to all pertinent provisions of ASTM D5456.

8.1.2 Definitions

8.1.2.1 The term "laminated veneer lumber" refers to a composite of wood veneer sheet elements with wood fiber primarily oriented along the length of the member. Veneer thickness shall not exceed 0.25".

8.1.2.2 The term "parallel strand lumber" refers to a composite of wood strand elements with wood fibers primarily oriented along the length of the member. The least dimension of the strands shall not exceed 0.25" and the average length shall be a minimum of 150 times the least dimension.

8.1.2.3 The term "structural composite lumber" refers to either laminated veneer lumber or parallel strand lumber. These materials are structural members bonded with an exterior adhesive.

8.1.3 Identification

When the design procedures and other information provided herein are used, the structural composite lumber shall be identified with the manufacturer's name and the quality assurance agency's name.

8.1.4 Service Conditions

Reference design values reflect dry service conditions, where the moisture content in service is less than 16%, as in most covered structures. Structural composite lumber shall not be used in higher moisture service conditions unless specifically permitted by the structural composite lumber manufacturer.

8.2 Reference Design Values

Reference design values for structural composite lumber shall be obtained from the structural composite lumber manufacturer's literature or code evaluation report. In special applications where deflection is a critical factor, or where deformation under long-term loading must be limited, the need for use of a reduced modulus of elasticity shall be determined. See Appendix F for provisions on adjusted values for special end use requirements.

8.3 Adjustment of Reference Design Values

8.3.1 General

Reference design values (F_b, F_t, F_v, $F_{c\perp}$, F_c, E, E_{min}) shall be multiplied by the adjustment factors specified in Table 8.3.1 to determine adjusted design values (F_b', F_t', F_v', $F_{c\perp}'$, F_c', E', E_{min}').

Table 8.3.1 Applicability of Adjustment Factors for Structural Composite Lumber

	ASD only	ASD and LRFD							LRFD only		
	Load Duration Factor	Wet Service Factor	Temperature Factor	Beam Stability Factor [1]	Volume Factor [1]	Repetitive Member Factor	Column Stability Factor	Bearing Area Factor	Format Conversion Factor	Resistance Factor	Time Effect Factor
$F_b' = F_b \quad x$	C_D	C_M	C_t	C_L	C_V	C_r	–	–	K_F	ϕ_b	λ
$F_t' = F_t \quad x$	C_D	C_M	C_t	–	–	–	–	–	K_F	ϕ_t	λ
$F_v' = F_v \quad x$	C_D	C_M	C_t	–	–	–	–	–	K_F	ϕ_v	λ
$F_{c\perp}' = F_{c\perp} \quad x$	–	C_M	C_t	–	–	–	–	C_b	K_F	ϕ_c	λ
$F_c' = F_c \quad x$	C_D	C_M	C_t	–	–	–	C_P	–	K_F	ϕ_c	λ
$E' = E \quad x$	–	C_M	C_t	–	–	–	–	–	–	–	–
$E_{min}' = E_{min} \quad x$	–	C_M	C_t	–	–	–	–	–	K_F	ϕ_s	–

1. See 8.3.6 for information on simultaneous application of the volume factor, C_V, and the beam stability factor, C_L.

8.3.2 Load Duration Factor, C_D (ASD only)

All reference design values except modulus of elasticity, E, modulus of elasticity for beam and column stability, E_{min}, and compression perpendicular to grain, $F_{c\perp}$, shall be multiplied by load duration factors, C_D, as specified in 2.3.2.

8.3.3 Wet Service Factor, C_M

Reference design values for structural composite lumber are applicable to dry service conditions as specified in 8.1.4 where $C_M = 1.0$. When the service conditions differ from the specified conditions, adjustments for high moisture shall be in accordance with information provided by the structural composite lumber manufacturer.

8.3.4 Temperature Factor, C_t

When structural members will experience sustained exposure to elevated temperatures up to 150°F (see Appendix C), reference design values shall be multiplied by the temperature factors, C_t, specified in 2.3.3.

8.3.5 Beam Stability Factor, C_L

Structural composite lumber bending members shall be laterally supported in accordance with 3.3.3.

8.3.6 Volume Factor, C_V

Reference bending design values, F_b, for structural composite lumber shall be multiplied by the volume factor, C_V, and shall be obtained from the structural composite lumber manufacturer's literature or code evaluation reports. When $C_V \leq 1.0$, the volume factor, C_V, shall not apply simultaneously with the beam stability factor, C_L (see 3.3.3) and therefore, the lesser of these adjustment factors shall apply. When $C_V > 1.0$, the volume factor, C_V, shall apply simultaneously with the beam stability factor, C_L (see 3.3.3).

8.3.7 Repetitive Member Factor, C_r

Reference bending design values, F_b, shall be multiplied by the repetitive member factor, $C_r = 1.04$, when such members are used as joists, studs, or similar members which are in contact or spaced not more than 24" on center, are not less than 3 in number and are joined by floor, roof, or other load distributing elements adequate to support the design load. (A load distributing element is any adequate system that is designed or has been proven by experience to transmit the design load to adjacent members, spaced as described above, without displaying structural weakness or unacceptable deflection. Subflooring, flooring, sheathing, or other covering elements and nail gluing or tongue and groove joints, and through nailing generally meet these criteria.)

8.3.8 Column Stability Factor, C_P

Reference compression design values parallel to grain, F_c, shall be multiplied by the column stability factor, C_P, specified in 3.7.

8.3.9 Bearing Area Factor, C_b

Reference compression design values perpendicular to grain, $F_{c\perp}$, shall be permitted to be multiplied by the bearing area factor, C_b, as specified in 3.10.4.

8.3.10 Pressure-Preservative Treatment

Adjustments to reference design values to account for the effects of pressure-preservative treatment shall be in accordance with information provided by the structural composite lumber manufacturer.

8.3.11 Format Conversion Factor, K_F (LRFD only)

For LRFD, reference design values shall be multiplied by the format conversion factor, K_F, specified in Appendix N.3.1.

8.3.12 Resistance Factor, ϕ (LRFD only)

For LRFD, reference design values shall be multiplied by the resistance factor, ϕ, specified in Appendix N.3.2.

8.3.13 Time Effect Factor, λ (LRFD only)

For LRFD, reference design values shall be multiplied by the time effect factor, λ, specified in Appendix N.3.3.

8.4 Special Design Considerations

8.4.1 Notches

8.4.1.1 The tension side of structural composite bending members shall not be notched, except at ends of members for bearing over a support, and notch depth shall not exceed 1/10 the depth of the member. The compression side of structural composite bending members shall not be notched, except at ends of members, and the notch depth on the compression side shall not exceed 2/5 the depth of the member. Compression side end-notches shall not extend into the middle third of the span.

8.4.1.2 See 3.1.2 and 3.4.3 for effect of notches on strength.

WOOD STRUCTURAL PANELS

9

9.1 General

9.1.1 Application

Chapter 9 applies to engineering design with the following wood structural panels: plywood, oriented strand board, and composite panels. Basic requirements are provided in this Specification. Design procedures and other information provided herein apply only to wood structural panels complying with the requirements specified in this Chapter.

9.1.2 Identification

9.1.2.1 When design procedures and other information herein are used, the wood structural panel shall be identified for grade and glue type by the trademarks of an approved testing and grading agency.

9.1.2.2 Wood structural panels shall be specified by span rating, nominal thickness, exposure rating, and grade.

9.1.3 Definitions

9.1.3.1 The term "wood structural panel" refers to a wood-based panel product bonded with a waterproof adhesive. Included under this designation are plywood, oriented strand board (OSB) and composite panels. These panel products meet the requirements of USDOC PS 1 or PS 2 and are intended for structural use in residential, commercial, and industrial applications.

9.1.3.2 The term "composite panel" refers to a wood structural panel comprised of wood veneer and reconstituted wood-based material and bonded with waterproof adhesive.

9.1.3.3 The term "oriented strand board" refers to a mat-formed wood structural panel comprised of thin rectangular wood strands arranged in cross-aligned layers with surface layers normally arranged in the long panel direction and bonded with waterproof adhesive.

9.1.3.4 The term "plywood" refers to a wood structural panel comprised of plies of wood veneer arranged in cross-aligned layers. The plies are bonded with an adhesive that cures on application of heat and pressure.

9.1.4 Service Conditions

9.1.4.1 Reference design values reflect dry service conditions, where the moisture content in service is less than 16%, as in most covered structures.

9.2 Reference Design Values

9.2.1 Panel Stiffness and Strength

9.2.1.1 Reference panel stiffness and strength design values (the product of material and section properties) shall be obtained from an approved source.

9.2.1.2 Due to the orthotropic nature of panels, reference design values shall be provided for the primary and secondary strength axes. The appropriate reference design values shall be applied when designing for each panel orientation. When forces act at an angle to the principal axes of the panel, the capacity of the panel at the angle shall be calculated by adjusting the reference design values for the principal axes using principles of engineering mechanics.

9.2.2 Strength and Elastic Properties

Where required, strength and elastic parameters shall be calculated from reference strength and stiffness design values, respectively, on the basis of tabulated design section properties.

9.2.3 Design Thickness

Nominal thickness shall be used in design calculations. The relationships between span ratings and nominal thicknesses are provided with associated reference design values.

9.2.4 Design Section Properties

Design section properties shall be assigned on the basis of span rating or design thickness and are provided on a per-foot-of-panel-width basis.

9.3 Adjustment of Reference Design Values

9.3.1 General

Reference design values shall be multiplied by the adjustment factors specified in Table 9.3.1 to determine adjusted design values.

9.3.2 Load Duration Factor, C_D (ASD only)

All reference strength design values (F_bS, F_tA, F_vt_v, $F_s(Ib/Q)$, F_cA) shall be multiplied by load duration factors, C_D, as specified in 2.3.2.

9.3.3 Wet Service Factor, C_M, and Temperature Factor, C_t

Reference design values for wood structural panels are applicable to dry service conditions as specified in 9.1.4 where $C_M = 1.0$ and $C_t = 1.0$. When the service conditions differ from the specified conditions, adjustments for high moisture and/or high temperature shall be based on information from an approved source.

Table 9.3.1 Applicability of Adjustment Factors for Wood Structural Panels

		ASD only	ASD and LRFD				LRFD only		
		Load Duration Factor	Wet Service Factor	Temperature Factor	Grade & Construction Factor	Panel Size Factor	Format Conversion Factor	Resistance Factor	Time Effect Factor
$F_bS' = F_bS$	x	C_D	C_M	C_t	C_G	C_s	K_F	ϕ_b	λ
$F_tA' = F_tA$	x	C_D	C_M	C_t	C_G	C_s	K_F	ϕ_t	λ
$F_vt_v' = F_vt_v$	x	C_D	C_M	C_t	C_G	-	K_F	ϕ_v	λ
$F_s(Ib/Q)' = F_s(Ib/Q)$	x	C_D	C_M	C_t	C_G	-	K_F	ϕ_v	λ
$F_cA' = F_cA$	x	C_D	C_M	C_t	C_G	-	K_F	ϕ_c	λ
$EI' = EI$	x	-	C_M	C_t	C_G	-	-	-	-
$EA' = EA$	x	-	C_M	C_t	C_G	-	-	-	-
$G_vt_v' = G_vt_v$	x	-	C_M	C_t	C_G	-	-	-	-
$F_{c\perp}' = F_{c\perp}$	x	-	C_M	C_t	C_G	-	K_F	ϕ_c	λ

9

WOOD STRUCTURAL PANELS

9.3.4 Grade and Construction Factor, C_G, and Panel Size Factor, C_s

Other adjustments to reference panel design values for grade and construction and panel size shall be based on information from an approved source.

9.3.5 Format Conversion Factor, K_F (LRFD only)

For LRFD, reference design values shall be multiplied by the format conversion factor, K_F, specified in Appendix N.3.1.

9.3.6 Resistance Factor, ϕ (LRFD only)

For LRFD, reference design values shall be multiplied by the resistance factor, ϕ, specified in Appendix N.3.2.

9.3.7 Time Effect Factor, λ (LRFD only)

For LRFD, reference design values shall be multiplied by the time effect factor, λ, specified in Appendix N.3.3.

9.4 Design Considerations

9.4.1 Flatwise Bending

Wood structural panels shall be designed for flexure by checking bending moment, shear, and deflection. Adjusted planar shear shall be used as the shear resistance in checking the shear for panels in flatwise bending. Appropriate beam equations shall be used with the design spans as defined below.
 (a) Bending moment-distance between center-line of supports.
 (b) Shear-clear span.
 (c) Deflection-clear span plus the support width factor. For 2" nominal and 4" nominal framing, the support width factor is equal to 0.25" and 0.625", respectively.

9.4.2 Tension in the Plane of the Panel

When wood structural panels are loaded in axial tension, the orientation of the primary strength axis of the panel with respect to the direction of loading, shall be considered in determining adjusted tensile capacity.

9.4.3 Compression in the Plane of the Panel

When wood structural panels are loaded in axial compression, the orientation of the primary strength axis of the panel with respect to the direction of loading, shall be considered in determining the adjusted compressive capacity. In addition, panels shall be designed to prevent buckling.

9.4.4 Planar (Rolling) Shear

The adjusted planar (rolling) shear shall be used in design when the shear force is applied in the plane of wood structural panels.

9.4.5 Through-the-Thickness Shear

The adjusted through-the-thickness shear shall be used in design when the shear force is applied through-the-thickness of wood structural panels.

9.4.6 Bearing

The adjusted bearing design value of wood structural panels shall be used in design when the load is applied perpendicular to the panel face.

MECHANICAL CONNECTIONS

10

10.1 General

10.1.1 Scope

10.1.1.1 Chapter 10 applies to the engineering design of connections using bolts, lag screws, split ring or shear plate connectors, drift bolts, drift pins, wood screws, nails, spikes, timber rivets, metal connector plates or spike grids in sawn lumber, structural glued laminated timber, timber poles, timber piles, structural composite lumber, prefabricated wood I-joists, and wood structural panels. Except where specifically limited elsewhere herein, the provisions of Chapter 10 shall apply to all fastener types covered in Chapters 11, 12, and 13.

10.1.1.2 The requirements of 3.1.3, 3.1.4, and 3.1.5 shall be accounted for in the design of connections.

10.1.1.3 Connection design provisions in Chapters 10, 11, 12, and 13 shall not preclude the use of connections where it is demonstrated by analysis based on generally recognized theory, full-scale, or prototype loading tests, studies of model analogues or extensive experience in use that the connections will perform satisfactorily in their intended end uses (see 1.1.1.3).

10.1.2 Stresses in Members at Connections

Structural members shall be checked for load carrying capacity at connections in accordance with all applicable provisions of this standard including 3.1.2, 3.1.3, and 3.4.3.3. Local stresses in connections using multiple fasteners shall be checked in accordance with principles of engineering mechanics. One method for determining these stresses is provided in Appendix E.

10.1.3 Eccentric Connections

Eccentric connections that induce tension stress perpendicular to grain in the wood shall not be used unless appropriate engineering procedures or tests are employed in the design of such connections to insure that all applied loads will be safely carried by the members and connections. Connections similar to those in Figure 10A are examples of connections requiring appropriate engineering procedures or tests.

10.1.4 Mixed Fastener Connections

Methods of analysis and test data for establishing reference design values for connections made with more than one type of fastener have not been developed. Reference design values and design value adjustments for mixed fastener connections shall be based on tests or other analysis (see 1.1.1.3).

10.1.5 Connection Fabrication

Reference lateral design values for connections in Chapters 11, 12, and 13 are based on:

(a) the assumption that the faces of the members are brought into contact when the fasteners are installed, and

(b) allowance for member shrinkage due to seasonal variations in moisture content (see 10.3.3).

Figure 10A Eccentric Connections

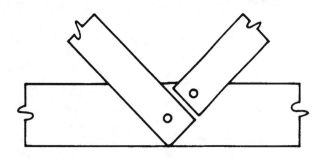

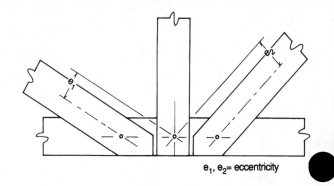

e_1, e_2= eccentricity

10.2 Reference Design Values

10.2.1 Single Fastener Connections

10.2.1.1 Chapters 11, 12, and 13 contain tabulated reference design values and design provisions for calculating reference design values for various types of single fastener connections. Reference design values for connections in a given species apply to all grades of that species unless otherwise indicated. Dowel-type fastener connection reference design values for one species of wood are also applicable to other species having the same or higher dowel bearing strength, F_e.

10.2.1.2 Design provisions and reference design values for dowel-type fastener connections such as bolts, lag screws, wood screws, nails and spikes, drift bolts, and drift pins are provided in Chapter 11.

10.2.1.3 Design provisions and reference design values for split ring and shear plate connections are provided in Chapter 12.

10.2.1.4 Design provisions and reference design values for timber rivet connections are provided in Chapter 13.

10.2.1.5 Wood to wood connections involving spike grids for load transfer shall be designed in accordance with principles of engineering mechanics (see Reference 50 for additional information).

10.2.1.6 Metal plate connected wood truss construction shall be designed in accordance with ANSI/TPI 1.

10.2.2 Multiple Fastener Connections

When a connection contains two or more fasteners of the same type and similar size, each of which exhibits the same yield mode (see Appendix I), the total ad-justed design value for the connection shall be the sum of the adjusted design values for each individual fastener. Local stresses in connections using multiple fasteners shall be evaluated in accordance with principles of engineering mechanics (see 10.1.2).

10.2.3 Design of Metal Parts

Metal plates, hangers, fasteners, and other metal parts shall be designed in accordance with applicable metal design procedures to resist failure in tension, shear, bearing (metal on metal), bending, and buckling (see References 39, 40, and 41). When the capacity of a connection is controlled by metal strength rather than wood strength, metal strength shall not be multiplied by the adjustment factors in this Specification. In addition, metal strength shall not be increased by wind and earthquake factors if design loads have already been reduced by load combination factors (see Reference 5 for additional information).

10.2.4 Design of Concrete or Masonry Parts

Concrete footers, walls, and other concrete or masonry parts shall be designed in accordance with accepted practices (see References 1 and 2). When the capacity of a connection is controlled by concrete or masonry strength rather than wood strength, concrete or masonry strength shall not be multiplied by the adjustment factors in this Specification. In addition, concrete or masonry strength shall not be increased by wind and earthquake factors if design loads have already been reduced by load combination factors (see Reference 5 for additional information).

10.3 Adjustment of Reference Design Values

10.3.1 Applicability of Adjustment Factors

Reference design values (Z, W) shall be multiplied by all applicable adjustment factors to determine adjusted design values (Z', W'). Table 10.3.1 specifies the adjustment factors which apply to reference lateral design values (Z) and reference withdrawal design values (W) for each fastener type. The actual load applied to a connection shall not exceed the adjusted design value (Z', W') for the connection.

10

MECHANICAL CONNECTIONS

Table 10.3.1   Applicability of Adjustment Factors for Connections

		ASD Only	ASD and LRFD										LRFD Only		
		Load Duration Factor [1]	Wet Service Factor [2]	Temperature Factor	Group Action Factor	Geometry Factor [3]	Penetration Depth Factor [3]	End Grain Factor [3]	Metal Side Plate Factor [3]	Diaphragm Factor [3]	Toe-Nail Factor [3]	Format Conversion Factor	Resistance Factor	Time Effect Factor
Lateral Loads															
Dowel-type Fasteners	$Z' = Z$ x	C_D	C_M	C_t	C_g	C_Δ	-	C_{eg}	-	C_{di}	C_{tn}	K_F	ϕ_z	λ
Split Ring and Shear Plate Connectors	$P' = P$ x	C_D	C_M	C_t	C_g	C_Δ	C_d	-	C_{st}	-	-	K_F	ϕ_z	λ
	$Q' = Q$ x	C_D	C_M	C_t	C_g	C_Δ	C_d	-	-	-	-	K_F	ϕ_z	λ
Timber Rivets	$P' = P$ x	C_D^4	C_M	C_t	-	-	-	-	C_{st}^5	-	-	K_F	ϕ_z	λ
	$Q' = Q$ x	C_D^4	C_M	C_t	-	C_Δ^6	-	-	C_{st}^5	-	-	K_F	ϕ_z	λ
Metal Plate Connectors	$Z' = Z$ x	C_D	C_M	C_t	-	-	-	-	-	-	-	K_F	ϕ_z	λ
Spike Grids	$Z' = Z$ x	C_D	C_M	C_t	-	C_Δ	-	-	-	-	-	K_F	ϕ_z	λ
Withdrawal Loads															
Nails, spikes, lag screws, wood screws, and drift pins	$W' = W$ x	C_D	C_M	C_t	-	-	-	C_{eg}	-	-	C_{tn}	K_F	ϕ_z	λ

1. The load duration factor, C_D, shall not exceed 1.6 for connections (see 10.3.2).
2. The wet service factor, C_M, shall not apply to toe-nails loaded in withdrawal (see 11.5.4.1).
3. Specific information concerning geometry factors C_Δ, penetration depth factors C_d, end grain factors, C_{eg}, metal side plate factors, C_{st}, diaphragm factors, C_{di}, and toe-nail factors, C_{tn}, is provided in Chapters 11, 12, and 13.
4. The load duration factor, C_D, is only applied when wood capacity (P_w, Q_w) controls (see Chapter 13).
5. The metal side plate factor, C_{st}, is only applied when rivet capacity (P_r, Q_r) controls (see Chapter 13).
6. The geometry factor, C_Δ, is only applied when wood capacity, Q_w, controls (see Chapter 13).

10.3.2 Load Duration Factor, C_D (ASD only)

Reference design values shall be multiplied by the load duration factors, $C_D \leq 1.6$, specified in 2.3.2 and Appendix B, except when the capacity of the connection is controlled by metal strength or strength of concrete/masonry (see 10.2.3, 10.2.4, and Appendix B.3). The impact load duration factor shall not apply to connections.

10.3.3 Wet Service Factor, C_M

Reference design values are for connections in wood seasoned to a moisture content of 19% or less and used under continuously dry conditions, as in most covered structures. For connections in wood that is unsea-

soned or partially seasoned, or when connections are exposed to wet service conditions in use, reference design values shall be multiplied by the wet service factors, C_M, specified in Table 10.3.3.

10.3.4 Temperature Factor, C_t

Reference design values shall be multiplied by the temperature factors, C_t, in Table 10.3.4 for connections that will experience sustained exposure to elevated temperatures up to 150°F (see Appendix C).

Table 10.3.3 Wet Service Factors, C$_M$, for Connections

| Fastener Type | Moisture Content | | C$_M$ |
	At Time of Fabrication	In-Service	
Lateral Loads			
Shear Plates & Split Rings[1]	≤ 19%	≤ 19%	1.0
	> 19%	≤ 19%	0.8
	any	> 19%	0.7
Metal Connector Plates[2]	≤ 19%	≤ 19%	1.0
	> 19%	≤ 19%	0.8
	any	> 19%	0.8
Dowel-type Fasteners	≤ 19%	≤ 19%	1.0
	> 19%	≤ 19%	0.4[3]
	any	> 19%	0.7
Timber Rivets	≤ 19%	≤ 19%	1.0
	≤ 19%	> 19%	0.8
Withdrawal Loads			
Lag Screws & Wood Screws	any	≤ 19%	1.0
	any	> 19%	0.7
Nails & Spikes	≤ 19%	≤ 19%	1.0
	> 19%	≤ 19%	0.25
	≤ 19%	> 19%	0.25
	> 19%	> 19%	1.0
Threaded Hardened Nails	any	any	1.0

1. For split ring or shear plate connectors, moisture content limitations apply to a depth of 3/4" below the surface of the wood.
2. For more information on metal connector plates see Reference 9.
3. C$_M$ = 0.7 for dowel-type fasteners with diameter, D, less than 1/4".
   C$_M$ = 1.0 for dowel-type fastener connections with:
   1) one fastener only, or
   2) two or more fasteners placed in a single row parallel to grain, or
   3) fasteners placed in two or more rows parallel to grain with separate splice plates for each row.

Table 10.3.4 Temperature Factors, C$_t$, for Connections

| In-Service Moisture Conditions[1] | C$_t$ | | |
	T≤100°F	100°F<T≤125°F	125°F<T≤150°F
Dry	1.0	0.8	0.7
Wet	1.0	0.7	0.5

1. Wet and dry service conditions for connections are specified in 10.3.3.

10.3.5 Fire Retardant Treatment

Adjusted design values for connections in lumber and structural glued laminated timber pressure-treated with fire retardant chemicals shall be obtained from the company providing the treatment and redrying service (see 2.3.4). The impact load duration factor shall not apply to connections in wood pressure-treated with fire retardant chemicals (see Table 2.3.2).

10.3.6 Group Action Factors, C_g

10.3.6.1 Reference lateral design values for split ring connectors, shear plate connectors, or dowel-type fasteners with $D \le 1"$ in a row shall be multiplied by the following group action factor, C_g:

$$C_g = \left[\frac{m(1-m^{2n})}{n\left[(1+R_{EA}m^n)(1+m)-1+m^{2n}\right]}\right]\left[\frac{1+R_{EA}}{1-m}\right] \quad (10.3\text{-}1)$$

where:

C_g = 1.0 for dowel type fasteners with $D < 1/4"$. Reference design values for timber rivet connections account for group action effects and do not require further modification by the group action factor.

n = number of fasteners in a row

R_{EA} = the lesser of $\dfrac{E_s A_s}{E_m A_m}$ or $\dfrac{E_m A_m}{E_s A_s}$

E_m = modulus of elasticity of main member, psi

E_s = modulus of elasticity of side members, psi

A_m = gross cross-sectional area of main member, in.^{2}

A_s = sum of gross cross-sectional areas of side members, in.^{2}

$m = u - \sqrt{u^2 - 1}$

$u = 1 + \gamma\dfrac{s}{2}\left[\dfrac{1}{E_m A_m} + \dfrac{1}{E_s A_s}\right]$

s = center to center spacing between adjacent fasteners in a row, in.

γ = load/slip modulus for a connection, lbs./in.

= 500,000 lbs./in. for 4" split ring or shear plate connectors

= 400,000 lbs./in. for 2-1/2" split ring or 2-5/8" shear plate connectors

= $(180,000)(D^{1.5})$ for dowel-type fasteners in wood-to-wood connections

= $(270,000)(D^{1.5})$ for dowel-type fasteners in wood-to-metal connections

D = diameter of bolt or lag screw, in.

Group action factors for various connection geometries are provided in Tables 10.3.6A, 10.3.6B, 10.3.6C, and 10.3.6D.

10.3.6.2 For determining group action factors, a row of fasteners is defined as any of the following:
(a) Two or more split rings or shear plate connector units, as defined in 12.1.1, aligned with the direction of load.
(b) Two or more dowel-type fasteners of the same diameter loaded in single or multiple shear and aligned with the direction of load.

When fasteners in adjacent rows are staggered and the distance between adjacent rows is less than 1/4 the distance between the closest fasteners in adjacent rows measured parallel to the rows, the adjacent rows shall be considered as one row for purposes of determining group action factors. For groups of fasteners having an even number of rows, this principle shall apply to each pair of rows. For groups of fasteners having an odd number of rows, the most conservative interpretation shall apply (see Figure 10B).

10.3.6.3 Gross section areas shall be used, with no reductions for net section, when calculating A_m and A_s for determining group action factors. When a member is loaded perpendicular to grain its equivalent cross-sectional area shall be the product of the thickness of the member and the overall width of the fastener group (see Figure 10B). When only one row of fasteners is used, the width of the fastener group shall be the minimum parallel to grain spacing of the fasteners.

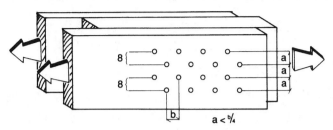

Consider as 2 rows of 8 fasteners

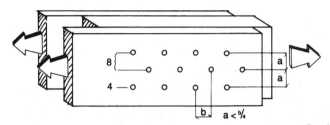

Consider as 1 row of 8 fasteners and 1 row of 4 fasteners

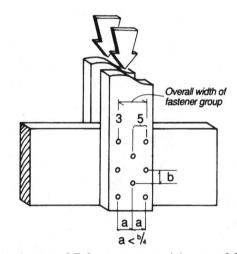

Consider as 1 row of 5 fasteners and 1 row of 3 fasteners

10.3.7 Format Conversion Factor, K$_F$ (LRFD only)

For LRFD, reference design values shall be multiplied by the format conversion factor, K$_F$, specified in Appendix N.3.1.

10.3.8 Resistance Factor, ϕ (LRFD only)

For LRFD, reference design values shall be multiplied by the resistance factor, ϕ, specified in Appendix N.3.2.

10.3.9 Time Effect Factor, λ (LRFD only)

For LRFD, reference design values shall be multiplied by the time effect factor, λ, specified in Appendix N.3.3.

10

MECHANICAL CONNECTIONS

Table 10.3.6A Group Action Factors, C_g, for Bolt or Lag Screw Connections with Wood Side Members[2]

A_s/A_m[1]	A_s[1] in.[2]	Number of fasteners in a row										
		2	3	4	5	6	7	8	9	10	11	12
0.5	5	0.98	0.92	0.84	0.75	0.68	0.61	0.55	0.50	0.45	0.41	0.38
	12	0.99	0.96	0.92	0.87	0.81	0.76	0.70	0.65	0.61	0.57	0.53
	20	0.99	0.98	0.95	0.91	0.87	0.83	0.78	0.74	0.70	0.66	0.62
	28	1.00	0.98	0.96	0.93	0.90	0.87	0.83	0.79	0.76	0.72	0.69
	40	1.00	0.99	0.97	0.95	0.93	0.90	0.87	0.84	0.81	0.78	0.75
	64	1.00	0.99	0.98	0.97	0.95	0.93	0.91	0.89	0.87	0.84	0.82
1	5	1.00	0.97	0.91	0.85	0.78	0.71	0.64	0.59	0.54	0.49	0.45
	12	1.00	0.99	0.96	0.93	0.88	0.84	0.79	0.74	0.70	0.65	0.61
	20	1.00	0.99	0.98	0.95	0.92	0.89	0.86	0.82	0.78	0.75	0.71
	28	1.00	0.99	0.98	0.97	0.94	0.92	0.89	0.86	0.83	0.80	0.77
	40	1.00	1.00	0.99	0.98	0.96	0.94	0.92	0.90	0.87	0.85	0.82
	64	1.00	1.00	0.99	0.98	0.97	0.96	0.95	0.93	0.91	0.90	0.88

For $D = 1''$, $s = 4''$, $E = 1,400,000$ psi

1. When $A_s/A_m > 1.0$, use A_m/A_s and use A_m instead of A_s.
2. Tabulated group action factors (C_g) are conservative for $D < 1''$, $s < 4''$, or $E > 1,400,000$ psi.

Table 10.3.6B Group Action Factors, C_g, for 4" Split Ring or Shear Plate Connectors with Wood Side Members[2]

A_s/A_m[1]	A_s[1] in.[2]	Number of fasteners in a row										
		2	3	4	5	6	7	8	9	10	11	12
0.5	5	0.90	0.73	0.59	0.48	0.41	0.35	0.31	0.27	0.25	0.22	0.20
	12	0.95	0.83	0.71	0.60	0.52	0.45	0.40	0.36	0.32	0.29	0.27
	20	0.97	0.88	0.78	0.69	0.60	0.53	0.47	0.43	0.39	0.35	0.32
	28	0.97	0.91	0.82	0.74	0.66	0.59	0.53	0.48	0.44	0.40	0.37
	40	0.98	0.93	0.86	0.79	0.72	0.65	0.59	0.54	0.49	0.45	0.42
	64	0.99	0.95	0.91	0.85	0.79	0.73	0.67	0.62	0.58	0.54	0.50
1	5	1.00	0.87	0.72	0.59	0.50	0.43	0.38	0.34	0.30	0.28	0.25
	12	1.00	0.93	0.83	0.72	0.63	0.55	0.48	0.43	0.39	0.36	0.33
	20	1.00	0.95	0.88	0.79	0.71	0.63	0.57	0.51	0.46	0.42	0.39
	28	1.00	0.97	0.91	0.83	0.76	0.69	0.62	0.57	0.52	0.47	0.44
	40	1.00	0.98	0.93	0.87	0.81	0.75	0.69	0.63	0.58	0.54	0.50
	64	1.00	0.98	0.95	0.91	0.87	0.82	0.77	0.72	0.67	0.62	0.58

$s = 9''$, $E = 1,400,000$ psi

1. When $A_s/A_m > 1.0$, use A_m/A_s and use A_m instead of A_s.
2. Tabulated group action factors (C_g) are conservative for 2-1/2" split ring connectors, 2-5/8" shear plate connectors, $s < 9''$, or $E > 1,400,000$ psi.

Table 10.3.6C Group Action Factors, C_g, for Bolt or Lag Screw Connections with Steel Side Plates[1]

A_m/A_s	A_m in.^{2}	Number of fasteners in a row										
		2	3	4	5	6	7	8	9	10	11	12
12	5	0.97	0.89	0.80	0.70	0.62	0.55	0.49	0.44	0.40	0.37	0.34
	8	0.98	0.93	0.85	0.77	0.70	0.63	0.57	0.52	0.47	0.43	0.40
	16	0.99	0.96	0.92	0.86	0.80	0.75	0.69	0.64	0.60	0.55	0.52
	24	0.99	0.97	0.94	0.90	0.85	0.81	0.76	0.71	0.67	0.63	0.59
	40	1.00	0.98	0.96	0.94	0.90	0.87	0.83	0.79	0.76	0.72	0.69
	64	1.00	0.99	0.98	0.96	0.94	0.91	0.88	0.86	0.83	0.80	0.77
	120	1.00	0.99	0.99	0.98	0.96	0.95	0.93	0.91	0.90	0.87	0.85
	200	1.00	1.00	0.99	0.99	0.98	0.97	0.96	0.95	0.93	0.92	0.90
18	5	0.99	0.93	0.85	0.76	0.68	0.61	0.54	0.49	0.44	0.41	0.37
	8	0.99	0.95	0.90	0.83	0.75	0.69	0.62	0.57	0.52	0.48	0.44
	16	1.00	0.98	0.94	0.90	0.85	0.79	0.74	0.69	0.65	0.60	0.56
	24	1.00	0.98	0.96	0.93	0.89	0.85	0.80	0.76	0.72	0.68	0.64
	40	1.00	0.99	0.97	0.95	0.93	0.90	0.87	0.83	0.80	0.77	0.73
	64	1.00	0.99	0.98	0.97	0.95	0.93	0.91	0.89	0.86	0.83	0.81
	120	1.00	1.00	0.99	0.98	0.97	0.96	0.95	0.93	0.92	0.90	0.88
	200	1.00	1.00	0.99	0.99	0.98	0.98	0.97	0.96	0.95	0.94	0.92
24	40	1.00	0.99	0.97	0.95	0.93	0.89	0.86	0.83	0.79	0.76	0.72
	64	1.00	0.99	0.98	0.97	0.95	0.93	0.91	0.88	0.85	0.83	0.80
	120	1.00	1.00	0.99	0.98	0.97	0.96	0.95	0.93	0.91	0.90	0.88
	200	1.00	1.00	0.99	0.99	0.98	0.98	0.97	0.96	0.95	0.93	0.92
30	40	1.00	0.98	0.96	0.93	0.89	0.85	0.81	0.77	0.73	0.69	0.65
	64	1.00	0.99	0.97	0.95	0.93	0.90	0.87	0.83	0.80	0.77	0.73
	120	1.00	0.99	0.99	0.97	0.96	0.94	0.92	0.90	0.88	0.85	0.83
	200	1.00	1.00	0.99	0.98	0.97	0.96	0.95	0.94	0.92	0.90	0.89
35	40	0.99	0.97	0.94	0.91	0.86	0.82	0.77	0.73	0.68	0.64	0.60
	64	1.00	0.98	0.96	0.94	0.91	0.87	0.84	0.80	0.76	0.73	0.69
	120	1.00	0.99	0.98	0.97	0.95	0.92	0.90	0.88	0.85	0.82	0.79
	200	1.00	0.99	0.99	0.98	0.97	0.95	0.94	0.92	0.90	0.88	0.86
42	40	0.99	0.97	0.93	0.88	0.83	0.78	0.73	0.68	0.63	0.59	0.55
	64	0.99	0.98	0.95	0.92	0.88	0.84	0.80	0.76	0.72	0.68	0.64
	120	1.00	0.99	0.97	0.95	0.93	0.90	0.88	0.85	0.81	0.78	0.75
	200	1.00	0.99	0.98	0.97	0.96	0.94	0.92	0.90	0.88	0.85	0.83
50	40	0.99	0.96	0.91	0.85	0.79	0.74	0.68	0.63	0.58	0.54	0.51
	64	0.99	0.97	0.94	0.90	0.85	0.81	0.76	0.72	0.67	0.63	0.59
	120	1.00	0.98	0.97	0.94	0.91	0.88	0.85	0.81	0.78	0.74	0.71
	200	1.00	0.99	0.98	0.96	0.95	0.92	0.90	0.87	0.85	0.82	0.79

For D = 1", s = 4", E_{wood} = 1,400,000 psi, E_{steel} = 30,000,000 psi

1. Tabulated group action factors (C_g) are conservative for D < 1" or s < 4".

10

MECHANICAL CONNECTIONS

Table 10.3.6D Group Action Factors, C_g, for 4" Shear Plate Connectors with Steel Side Plates[1]

$s = 9"$, $E_{wood} = 1,400,000$ psi, $E_{steel} = 30,000,000$ psi

A_m/A_s	A_m in.^{2}	Number of fasteners in a row										
		2	3	4	5	6	7	8	9	10	11	12
12	5	0.91	0.75	0.60	0.50	0.42	0.36	0.31	0.28	0.25	0.23	0.21
	8	0.94	0.80	0.67	0.56	0.47	0.41	0.36	0.32	0.29	0.26	0.24
	16	0.96	0.87	0.76	0.66	0.58	0.51	0.45	0.40	0.37	0.33	0.31
	24	0.97	0.90	0.82	0.73	0.64	0.57	0.51	0.46	0.42	0.39	0.35
	40	0.98	0.94	0.87	0.80	0.73	0.66	0.60	0.55	0.50	0.46	0.43
	64	0.99	0.96	0.91	0.86	0.80	0.74	0.69	0.63	0.59	0.55	0.51
	120	0.99	0.98	0.95	0.91	0.87	0.83	0.79	0.74	0.70	0.66	0.63
	200	1.00	0.99	0.97	0.95	0.92	0.89	0.85	0.82	0.79	0.75	0.72
18	5	0.97	0.83	0.68	0.56	0.47	0.41	0.36	0.32	0.28	0.26	0.24
	8	0.98	0.87	0.74	0.62	0.53	0.46	0.40	0.36	0.32	0.30	0.27
	16	0.99	0.92	0.82	0.73	0.64	0.56	0.50	0.45	0.41	0.37	0.34
	24	0.99	0.94	0.87	0.78	0.70	0.63	0.57	0.51	0.47	0.43	0.39
	40	0.99	0.96	0.91	0.85	0.78	0.72	0.66	0.60	0.55	0.51	0.47
	64	1.00	0.97	0.94	0.89	0.84	0.79	0.74	0.69	0.64	0.60	0.56
	120	1.00	0.99	0.97	0.94	0.90	0.87	0.83	0.79	0.75	0.71	0.67
	200	1.00	0.99	0.98	0.96	0.94	0.91	0.89	0.86	0.82	0.79	0.76
24	40	1.00	0.96	0.91	0.84	0.77	0.71	0.65	0.59	0.54	0.50	0.46
	64	1.00	0.98	0.94	0.89	0.84	0.78	0.73	0.68	0.63	0.58	0.54
	120	1.00	0.99	0.96	0.94	0.90	0.86	0.82	0.78	0.74	0.70	0.66
	200	1.00	0.99	0.98	0.96	0.94	0.91	0.88	0.85	0.82	0.78	0.75
30	40	0.99	0.93	0.86	0.78	0.70	0.63	0.57	0.52	0.47	0.43	0.40
	64	0.99	0.96	0.90	0.84	0.78	0.71	0.66	0.60	0.56	0.51	0.48
	120	0.99	0.98	0.94	0.90	0.86	0.81	0.76	0.71	0.67	0.63	0.59
	200	1.00	0.98	0.96	0.94	0.91	0.87	0.83	0.79	0.76	0.72	0.68
35	40	0.98	0.91	0.83	0.74	0.66	0.59	0.53	0.48	0.43	0.40	0.36
	64	0.99	0.94	0.88	0.81	0.73	0.67	0.61	0.56	0.51	0.47	0.43
	120	0.99	0.97	0.93	0.88	0.82	0.77	0.72	0.67	0.62	0.58	0.54
	200	1.00	0.98	0.95	0.92	0.88	0.84	0.80	0.76	0.71	0.68	0.64
42	40	0.97	0.88	0.79	0.69	0.61	0.54	0.48	0.43	0.39	0.36	0.33
	64	0.98	0.92	0.84	0.76	0.69	0.62	0.56	0.51	0.46	0.42	0.39
	120	0.99	0.95	0.90	0.85	0.78	0.72	0.67	0.62	0.57	0.53	0.49
	200	0.99	0.97	0.94	0.90	0.85	0.80	0.76	0.71	0.67	0.62	0.59
50	40	0.95	0.86	0.75	0.65	0.56	0.49	0.44	0.39	0.35	0.32	0.30
	64	0.97	0.90	0.81	0.72	0.64	0.57	0.51	0.46	0.42	0.38	0.35
	120	0.98	0.94	0.88	0.81	0.74	0.68	0.62	0.57	0.52	0.48	0.45
	200	0.99	0.96	0.92	0.87	0.82	0.77	0.71	0.66	0.62	0.58	0.54

1. Tabulated group action factors (C_g) are conservative for 2-5/8" shear plate connectors or $s < 9"$.

DOWEL-TYPE FASTENERS

(BOLTS, LAG SCREWS, WOOD SCREWS, NAILS/SPIKES, DRIFT BOLTS, AND DRIFT PINS)

11

11.1 General

11.1.1 Terminology

11.1.1.1 "Edge distance" is the distance from the edge of a member to the center of the nearest fastener, measured perpendicular to grain. When a member is loaded perpendicular to grain, the loaded edge shall be defined as the edge in the direction toward which the fastener is acting. The unloaded edge shall be defined as the edge opposite the loaded edge (see Figure 11G).

11.1.1.2 "End distance" is the distance measured parallel to grain from the square-cut end of a member to the center of the nearest bolt (see Figure 11G).

11.1.1.3 "Spacing" is the distance between centers of fasteners measured along a line joining their centers (see Figure 11G).

11.1.1.4 A "row of fasteners" is defined as two or more fasteners aligned with the direction of load (see Figure 11G).

11.1.1.5 End distance, edge distance, and spacing requirements herein are based on wood properties. Wood-to-metal and wood-to-concrete connections are subject to placement provisions as shown in 11.5.1, however, applicable end and edge distance and spacing requirements for metal and concrete, also apply (see 10.2.3 and 10.2.4).

11.1.2 Bolts

11.1.2.1 Installation requirements apply to bolts meeting requirements of ANSI/ASME Standard B18.2.1.

11.1.2.2 Holes shall be a minimum of 1/32" to a maximum of 1/16" larger than the bolt diameter. Holes shall be accurately aligned in main members and side plates. Bolts shall not be forcibly driven.

11.1.2.3 A metal plate, metal strap, or washer not less than a standard cut washer shall be between the wood and the bolt head and between the wood and the nut.

11.1.2.4 Edge distance, end distance, and fastener spacing shall not be less than the requirements in Tables 11.5.1A through D.

11.1.3 Lag Screws

11.1.3.1 Installation requirements apply to lag screws meeting requirements of ANSI/ASME Standard B18.2.1. See Appendix L for lag screw dimensions.

11.1.3.2 Lead holes for lag screws loaded laterally and in withdrawal shall be bored as follows to avoid splitting of the wood member during connection fabrication:

(a) The clearance hole for the shank shall have the same diameter as the shank, and the same depth of penetration as the length of unthreaded shank.

(b) The lead hole for the threaded portion shall have a diameter equal to 65% to 85% of the shank diameter in wood with $G > 0.6$, 60% to 75% in wood with $0.5 < G \leq 0.6$, and 40% to 70% in wood with $G \leq 0.5$ (see Table 11.3.2A) and a length equal to at least the length of the threaded portion. The larger percentile in each range shall apply to lag screws of greater diameters.

11.1.3.3 Lead holes or clearance holes shall not be required for 3/8" and smaller diameter lag screws loaded primarily in withdrawal in wood with $G \leq 0.5$ (see Table 11.3.2A), provided that edge distances, end distances, and spacing are sufficient to prevent unusual splitting.

11.1.3.4 The threaded portion of the lag screw shall be inserted in its lead hole by turning with a wrench, not by driving with a hammer.

11.1.3.5 No reduction to reference design values is anticipated if soap or other lubricant is used on the lag screw or in the lead holes to facilitate insertion and to prevent damage to the lag screw.

11.1.3.6 Minimum penetration (not including the length of the tapered tip) of the lag screw into the main member for single shear connections or the side member for double shear connections shall be four times the diameter, $p_{min} = 4D$.

11.1.3.7 Edge distance, end distance, and fastener spacing shall not be less than the requirements in Tables 11.5.1A through E.

11.1.4 Wood Screws

11.1.4.1 Installation requirements apply to wood screws meeting requirements of ANSI/ASME Standard B18.6.1.

11.1.4.2 Lead holes for wood screws loaded in withdrawal shall have a diameter equal to approximately 90% of the wood screw root diameter in wood with $G > 0.6$, and approximately 70% of the wood screw root diameter in wood with $0.5 < G \leq 0.6$. Wood with $G \leq 0.5$ (see Table 11.3.2A) is not required to have a lead hole for insertion of wood screws.

11.1.4.3 Lead holes for wood screws loaded laterally shall be bored as follows:

(a) For wood with G > 0.6 (see Table 11.3.2A), the part of the lead hole receiving the shank shall have about the same diameter as the shank, and that receiving the threaded portion shall have about the same diameter as the screw at the root of the thread (see Reference 8).

(b) For G ≤ 0.6 (see Table 11.3.2A), the part of the lead hole receiving the shank shall be about 7/8 the diameter of the shank and that receiving the threaded portion shall be about 7/8 the diameter of the screw at the root of the thread (see Reference 8).

11.1.4.4 The wood screw shall be inserted in its lead hole by turning with a screw driver or other tool, not by driving with a hammer.

11.1.4.5 No reduction to reference design values is anticipated if soap or other lubricant is used on the wood screw or in the lead holes to facilitate insertion and to prevent damage to the wood screw.

11.1.4.6 Minimum penetration of the wood screw into the main member for single shear connections or the side member for double shear connections shall be six times the diameter, $p_{min} = 6D$.

11.1.4.7 Edge distances, end distances, and spacings shall be sufficient to prevent splitting of the wood.

11.1.5 Nails and Spikes

11.1.5.1 Installation requirements apply to common steel wire nails and spikes, box nails, and threaded hardened-steel nails meeting requirements in ASTM F1667. Nail specifications for engineered construction shall include the minimum lengths and diameters for the nails and spikes to be used.

11.1.5.2 Threaded, hardened-steel nails, and spikes shall be made of high carbon steel wire, headed, pointed, annularly or helically threaded, and heat-treated and tempered to provide greater yield strength than for common wire nails of corresponding size.

11.1.5.3 Reference design values herein apply to nailed and spiked connections either with or without bored holes. When a bored hole is desired to prevent splitting of wood, the diameter of the bored hole shall not exceed 90% of the nail or spike diameter for wood with G > 0.6, nor 75% of the nail or spike diameter for wood with G ≤ 0.6 (see Table 11.3.2A).

11.1.5.4 Toe-nails shall be driven at an angle of approximately 30° with the member and started approximately 1/3 the length of the nail from the member end (see Figure 11A).

Figure 11A   Toe-Nail Connection

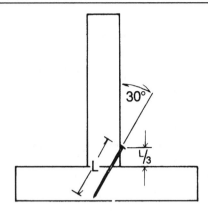

11.1.5.5 Minimum penetration of the nail or spike into the main member for single shear connections or the side member for double shear connections shall be six times the diameter, $p_{min} = 6D$.

Exception: Symmetric double shear connections when 12d or smaller nails extend at least three diameters beyond the side member and are clinched, and side members are at least 3/8" thick.

11.1.5.6 Edge distances, end distances, and spacings shall be sufficient to prevent splitting of the wood.

11.1.6 Drift Bolts and Drift Pins

11.1.6.1 Lead holes shall be drilled 0" to 1/32" smaller than the actual pin diameter.

11.1.6.2 Additional penetration of pin into members shall be provided in lieu of the washer, head, and nut on a common bolt (see Reference 53 for additional information).

11.1.6.3 Edge distance, end distance, and fastener spacing shall not be less than the requirements in Tables 11.5.1A through D.

11.1.7 Other Dowel-Type Fasteners

When fastener type or connection fabrication and assembly requirements vary from those specified in 11.1.2, 11.1.3, 11.1.4, 11.1.5, and 11.1.6, provisions of 11.3 shall be permitted to be used in calculation of reference lateral design values provided allowance is made to account for such variation. Edge distances, end distances, and spacings shall be sufficient to prevent splitting of the wood.

11.2 Reference Withdrawal Design Values

11.2.1 Lag Screws

11.2.1.1 The reference withdrawal design values, in lb/in. of penetration, for a single lag screw inserted in side grain, with the lag screw axis perpendicular to the wood fibers, shall be determined from Table 11.2A or Equation 11.2-1, within the range of specific gravities and screw diameters given in Table 11.2A. Reference withdrawal design values, W, shall be multiplied by all applicable adjustment factors (see Table 10.3.1) to obtain adjusted withdrawal design values, W'.

$$W = 1800\ G^{3/2}D^{3/4} \qquad\qquad (11.2\text{-}1)$$

11.2.1.2 When lag screws are loaded in withdrawal from end grain, reference withdrawal design values, W, shall be multiplied by the end grain factor, $C_{eg} = 0.75$.

11.2.1.3 When lag screws are loaded in withdrawal, the tensile strength of the lag screw at the net (root) section shall not be exceeded (see 10.2.3).

Table 11.2A Lag Screw Reference Withdrawal Design Values (W)[1]

Tabulated withdrawal design values (W) are in pounds per inch of thread penetration into side grain of main member. Length of thread penetration in main member shall not include the length of the tapered tip (see Appendix L).

Specific Gravity, G	Lag Screw Unthreaded Shank Diameter, D										
	1/4"	5/16"	3/8"	7/16"	1/2"	5/8"	3/4"	7/8"	1"	1-1/8"	1-1/4"
0.73	397	469	538	604	668	789	905	1016	1123	1226	1327
0.71	381	450	516	579	640	757	868	974	1077	1176	1273
0.68	357	422	484	543	600	709	813	913	1009	1103	1193
0.67	349	413	473	531	587	694	796	893	987	1078	1167
0.58	281	332	381	428	473	559	641	719	795	869	940
0.55	260	307	352	395	437	516	592	664	734	802	868
0.51	232	274	314	353	390	461	528	593	656	716	775
0.50	225	266	305	342	378	447	513	576	636	695	752
0.49	218	258	296	332	367	434	498	559	617	674	730
0.47	205	242	278	312	345	408	467	525	580	634	686
0.46	199	235	269	302	334	395	453	508	562	613	664
0.44	186	220	252	283	312	369	423	475	525	574	621
0.43	179	212	243	273	302	357	409	459	508	554	600
0.42	173	205	235	264	291	344	395	443	490	535	579
0.41	167	198	226	254	281	332	381	428	473	516	559
0.40	161	190	218	245	271	320	367	412	455	497	538
0.39	155	183	210	236	261	308	353	397	438	479	518
0.38	149	176	202	227	251	296	340	381	422	461	498
0.37	143	169	194	218	241	285	326	367	405	443	479
0.36	137	163	186	209	231	273	313	352	389	425	460
0.35	132	156	179	200	222	262	300	337	373	407	441
0.31	110	130	149	167	185	218	250	281	311	339	367

1. Tabulated withdrawal design values (W) for lag screw connections shall be multiplied by all applicable adjustment factors (see Table 10.3.1).

11.2.2 Wood Screws

11.2.2.1 The reference withdrawal design value, in lb/in. of penetration, for a single wood screw (cut thread or rolled thread) inserted in side grain, with the wood screw axis perpendicular to the wood fibers, shall be determined from Table 11.2B or Equation 11.2-2, within the range of specific gravities and screw diameters given in Table 11.2B. Reference withdrawal design values, W, shall be multiplied by all applicable adjustment factors (see Table 10.3.1) to obtain adjusted withdrawal design values, W'.

$$W = 2850\, G^2 D \qquad (11.2\text{-}2)$$

11.2.2.2 Wood screws shall not be loaded in withdrawal from end grain of wood.

11.2.2.3 When wood screws are loaded in withdrawal, the adjusted tensile strength of the wood screw at net (root) section shall not be exceeded (see 10.2.3).

11.2.3 Nails and Spikes

11.2.3.1 The reference withdrawal design value, in lb/in. of penetration, for a single nail or spike driven in the side grain of the main member, with the nail or spike axis perpendicular to the wood fibers, shall be determined from Table 11.2C or Equation 11.2-3, within the range of specific gravities and nail or spike diameters given in Table 11.2C. Reference withdrawal design values, W, shall be multiplied by all applicable adjustment factors (see Table 10.3.1) to obtain adjusted withdrawal design values, W'.

$$W = 1380\, G^{5/2} D \qquad (11.2\text{-}3)$$

11.2.3.2 Nails and spikes shall not be loaded in withdrawal from end grain of wood.

11.2.4 Drift Bolts and Drift Pins

Drift bolt and drift pin connections loaded in withdrawal shall be designed in accordance with principles of engineering mechanics.

Table 11.2B   Cut Thread or Rolled Thread Wood Screw Reference Withdrawal Design Values (W)[1]

Tabulated withdrawal design values (W) are in pounds per inch of thread penetration into side grain of main member. Thread length is approximately 2/3 the total wood screw length (see Appendix L).

Specific Gravity, G	Wood Screw Number											
	6	7	8	9	10	12	14	16	18	20	24
0.73	209	229	249	268	288	327	367	406	446	485	564
0.71	198	216	235	254	272	310	347	384	421	459	533
0.68	181	199	216	233	250	284	318	352	387	421	489
0.67	176	193	209	226	243	276	309	342	375	409	475
0.58	132	144	157	169	182	207	232	256	281	306	356
0.55	119	130	141	152	163	186	208	231	253	275	320
0.51	102	112	121	131	141	160	179	198	217	237	275
0.50	98	107	117	126	135	154	172	191	209	228	264
0.49	94	103	112	121	130	147	165	183	201	219	254
0.47	87	95	103	111	119	136	152	168	185	201	234
0.46	83	91	99	107	114	130	146	161	177	193	224
0.44	76	83	90	97	105	119	133	148	162	176	205
0.43	73	79	86	93	100	114	127	141	155	168	196
0.42	69	76	82	89	95	108	121	134	147	161	187
0.41	66	72	78	85	91	103	116	128	141	153	178
0.40	63	69	75	81	86	98	110	122	134	146	169
0.39	60	65	71	77	82	93	105	116	127	138	161
0.38	57	62	67	73	78	89	99	110	121	131	153
0.37	54	59	64	69	74	84	94	104	114	125	145
0.36	51	56	60	65	70	80	89	99	108	118	137
0.35	48	53	57	62	66	75	84	93	102	111	130
0.31	38	41	45	48	52	59	66	73	80	87	102

1. Tabulated withdrawal design values (W) for wood screw connections shall be multiplied by all applicable adjustment factors (see Table 10.3.1).

Table 11.2C   Nail and Spike Reference Withdrawal Design Values (W)[1]

Tabulated withdrawal design values (W) are in pounds per inch of penetration into side grain of main member (see Appendix L).

Specific Gravity, G	Common Wire Nails, Box Nails, and Common Wire Spikes Diameter, D															Threaded Nails Wire Diameter, D				
	0.099"	0.113"	0.128"	0.131"	0.135"	0.148"	0.162"	0.192"	0.207"	0.225"	0.244"	0.263"	0.283"	0.312"	0.375"	0.120"	0.135"	0.148"	0.177"	0.207"
0.73	62	71	80	82	85	93	102	121	130	141	153	165	178	196	236	82	93	102	121	141
0.71	58	66	75	77	79	87	95	113	121	132	143	154	166	183	220	77	87	95	113	132
0.68	52	59	67	69	71	78	85	101	109	118	128	138	149	164	197	69	78	85	101	118
0.67	50	57	65	66	68	75	82	97	105	114	124	133	144	158	190	66	75	82	97	114
0.58	35	40	45	46	48	52	57	68	73	80	86	93	100	110	133	46	52	57	68	80
0.55	31	35	40	41	42	46	50	59	64	70	76	81	88	97	116	41	46	50	59	70
0.51	25	29	33	34	35	38	42	49	53	58	63	67	73	80	96	34	38	42	49	58
0.50	24	28	31	32	33	36	40	47	50	55	60	64	69	76	91	32	36	40	47	55
0.49	23	26	30	30	31	34	38	45	48	52	57	61	66	72	87	30	34	38	45	52
0.47	21	24	27	27	28	31	34	40	43	47	51	55	59	65	78	27	31	34	40	47
0.46	20	22	25	26	27	29	32	38	41	45	48	52	56	62	74	26	29	32	38	45
0.44	18	20	23	23	24	26	29	34	37	40	43	47	50	55	66	23	26	29	34	40
0.43	17	19	21	22	23	25	27	32	35	38	41	44	47	52	63	22	25	27	32	38
0.42	16	18	20	21	21	23	26	30	33	35	38	41	45	49	59	21	23	26	30	35
0.41	15	17	19	19	20	22	24	29	31	33	36	39	42	46	56	19	22	24	29	33
0.40	14	16	18	18	19	21	23	27	29	31	34	37	40	44	52	18	21	23	27	31
0.39	13	15	17	17	18	19	21	25	27	29	32	34	37	41	49	17	19	21	25	29
0.38	12	14	16	16	17	18	20	24	25	28	30	32	35	38	46	16	18	20	24	28
0.37	11	13	15	15	16	17	19	22	24	26	28	30	33	36	43	15	17	19	22	26
0.36	11	12	14	14	14	16	17	21	22	24	26	28	30	33	40	14	16	17	21	24
0.35	10	11	13	13	14	15	16	19	21	23	24	26	28	31	38	13	15	16	19	23
0.31	7	8	9	10	10	11	12	14	15	17	18	19	21	23	28	10	11	12	14	17

1. Tabulated withdrawal design values (W) for nail or spike connections shall be multiplied by all applicable adjustment factors (see Table 10.3.1).

11.3 Reference Lateral Design Values

11.3.1 Yield Limit Equations

For single shear and symmetric double shear connections using dowel-type fasteners (see Appendix I, Figures 11B and 11C) where:

(a) the faces of the connected members are in contact

(b) the load acts perpendicular to the axis of the dowel

(c) edge distances, end distances, and spacing are not less than the requirements in 11.5, and

(d) the depth of fastener penetration in the main member for single shear connections or the side member holding the point for double shear connections is greater than or equal to the minimum penetration required (see 11.1).

The reference design value, Z, shall be the minimum computed yield mode value using equations in Tables 11.3.1A and B. Reference design values for connections with bolts (see Tables 11A through I), lag screws (see Tables 11J and K), wood screws (see Tables 11L and M), and nails and spikes (see Tables 11N through R) are calculated for common connection conditions in accordance with yield mode equations in Tables 11.3.1A and B.

Table 11.3.1A   Yield Limit Equations

Yield Mode	Single Shear		Double Shear	
I_m	$Z = \dfrac{D\,\ell_m\,F_{em}}{R_d}$	(11.3-1)	$Z = \dfrac{D\,\ell_m\,F_{em}}{R_d}$	(11.3-7)
I_s	$Z = \dfrac{D\,\ell_s\,F_{es}}{R_d}$	(11.3-2)	$Z = \dfrac{2D\,\ell_s\,F_{es}}{R_d}$	(11.3-8)
II	$Z = \dfrac{k_1\,D\,\ell_s\,F_{es}}{R_d}$	(11.3-3)		
III_m	$Z = \dfrac{k_2\,D\,\ell_m\,F_{em}}{(1+2R_e)\,R_d}$	(11.3-4)		
III_s	$Z = \dfrac{k_3\,D\,\ell_s\,F_{em}}{(2+R_e)\,R_d}$	(11.3-5)	$Z = \dfrac{2k_3\,D\,\ell_s\,F_{em}}{(2+R_e)\,R_d}$	(11.3-9)
IV	$Z = \dfrac{D^2}{R_d}\sqrt{\dfrac{2F_{em}\,F_{yb}}{3(1+R_e)}}$	(11.3-6)	$Z = \dfrac{2D^2}{R_d}\sqrt{\dfrac{2F_{em}\,F_{yb}}{3(1+R_e)}}$	(11.3-10)

Notes:

$$k_1 = \frac{\sqrt{R_e + 2R_e^2(1+R_t+R_t^2)+R_t^2 R_e^3} - R_e(1+R_t)}{(1+R_e)}$$

$$k_2 = -1 + \sqrt{2(1+R_e) + \frac{2F_{yb}(1+2R_e)D^2}{3F_{em}\ell_m^2}}$$

$$k_3 = -1 + \sqrt{\frac{2(1+R_e)}{R_e} + \frac{2F_{yb}(2+R_e)D^2}{3F_{em}\ell_s^2}}$$

D = diameter, in. (see 11.3.6)
F_{yb} = dowel bending yield strength, psi
R_d = reduction term (see Table 11.3.1B)
R_e = F_{em}/F_{es}
R_t = ℓ_m/ℓ_s
ℓ_m = main member dowel bearing length, in.
ℓ_s = side member dowel bearing length, in.
F_{em} = main member dowel bearing strength, psi (see Table 11.3.2)
F_{es} = side member dowel bearing strength, psi (see Table 11.3.2)

DOWEL-TYPE FASTENERS

11

Table 11.3.1B Reduction Term, R_d

Fastener Size	Yield Mode	Reduction Term, R_d
$0.25" \leq D \leq 1"$	I_m, I_s	$4 K_\theta$
	II	$3.6 K_\theta$
	III_m, III_s, IV	$3.2 K_\theta$
$D < 0.25"$	$I_m, I_s, II, III_m, III_s, IV$	$K_D{}^1$

Notes:
$K_\theta = 1 + 0.25(\theta/90)$
θ = maximum angle of load to grain $(0° \leq \theta \leq 90°)$ for any member in a connection
D = diameter, in. (see 11.3.6)
$K_D = 2.2$ for $D \leq 0.17"$
$K_D = 10D + 0.5$ for $0.17" < D < 0.25"$

1. For threaded fasteners where nominal diameter (see Appendix L) is greater than or equal to 0.25" and root diameter is less than 0.25", $R_d = K_D K_\theta$.

11.3.2 Dowel Bearing Strength

11.3.2.1 Dowel bearing strengths, F_e, for parallel or perpendicular to grain loading are provided for dowel-type fasteners with $1/4" \leq D \leq 1"$ in Table 11.3.2. When fastener diameter, $D < 1/4"$, a single dowel bearing strength, F_e, is used for both parallel and perpendicular to grain loading.

11.3.2.2 Dowel bearing strengths, F_e, for wood structural panels are provided in Table 11.3.2B.

11.3.2.3 Dowel bearing strengths, F_e, for structural composite lumber shall be obtained from the manufacturer's literature or code evaluation report.

11.3.2.4 When dowel-type fasteners with $D \geq 1/4"$ are inserted into the end grain of the main member, with the fastener axis parallel to the wood fibers, $F_{e\perp}$ shall be used in determination of the dowel bearing strength of the main member, F_{em}.

11.3.3 Dowel Bearing Strength at an Angle to Grain

When a member in a connection is loaded at an angle to grain, the dowel bearing strength, $F_{e\theta}$, for the member shall be determined as follows (see Appendix J):

$$F_{e\theta} = \frac{F_{e\parallel} F_{e\perp}}{F_{e\parallel} \sin^2 \theta + F_{e\perp} \cos^2 \theta} \qquad (11.3\text{-}11)$$

where:

θ = angle between direction of load and direction of grain (longitudinal axis of member).

Figure 11B   Single Shear Bolted Connections

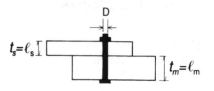

Figure 11C   Double Shear Bolted Connections

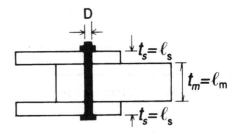

11.3.4 Dowel Bearing Length

11.3.4.1 Dowel bearing length in the side member(s) and main member, ℓ_s and ℓ_m, represent the length of dowel bearing perpendicular to the application of load. The length of dowel bearing shall not include the tapered tip of a fastener for fastener penetration lengths less than 10D.

11.3.5 Dowel Bending Yield Strength

11.3.5.1 Reference design values for bolts, lag screws, wood screws, nails, and spikes are based on bending yield strengths provided in Tables 11A through 11R.

11.3.5.2 Dowel bending yield strengths, F_{yb}, used in calculation of reference design values shall be based on yield strength derived using methods provided in ASTM F 1575 or the tensile yield strength derived using procedures of ASTM F 606.

11.3.6 Dowel Diameter

11.3.6.1 When used in Tables 11.3-1A and 11.3-1B, the fastener diameter shall be taken as D for unthreaded full-body diameter fasteners and D_r for reduced body diameter fasteners or threaded fasteners except as provided in 11.3.6.2. For bolts meeting the requirements of ANSI/ASME Standard B18.2.1 for full-body diameter bolts, the fastener diameter shall be taken as D (see Appendix L).

Table 11.3.2 Dowel Bearing Strengths

Specific[1] Gravity, G	F_e D<1/4"	$F_{e\parallel}$ D≥1/4"	Dowel bearing strength in pounds per square inch (psi)[2] $F_{e\perp}$								
			D=1/4"	D=5/16"	D=3/8"	D=7/16"	D=1/2"	D=5/8"	D=3/4"	D=7/8"	D=1"
0.73	9300	8200	7750	6900	6300	5850	5450	4900	4450	4150	3850
0.72	9050	8050	7600	6800	6200	5750	5350	4800	4350	4050	3800
0.71	8850	7950	7400	6650	6050	5600	5250	4700	4300	3950	3700
0.70	8600	7850	7250	6500	5950	5500	5150	4600	4200	3900	3650
0.69	8400	7750	7100	6350	5800	5400	5050	4500	4100	3800	3550
0.68	8150	7600	6950	6250	5700	5250	4950	4400	4050	3750	3500
0.67	7950	7500	6850	6100	5550	5150	4850	4300	3950	3650	3400
0.66	7750	7400	6700	5950	5450	5050	4700	4200	3850	3550	3350
0.65	7500	7300	6550	5850	5350	4950	4600	4150	3750	3500	3250
0.64	7300	7150	6400	5700	5200	4850	4500	4050	3700	3400	3200
0.63	7100	7050	6250	5600	5100	4700	4400	3950	3600	3350	3100
0.62	6900	6950	6100	5450	5000	4600	4300	3850	3500	3250	3050
0.61	6700	6850	5950	5350	4850	4500	4200	3750	3450	3200	3000
0.60	6500	6700	5800	5200	4750	4400	4100	3700	3350	3100	2900
0.59	6300	6600	5700	5100	4650	4300	4000	3600	3300	3050	2850
0.58	6100	6500	5550	4950	4500	4200	3900	3500	3200	2950	2750
0.57	5900	6400	5400	4850	4400	4100	3800	3400	3100	2900	2700
0.56	5700	6250	5250	4700	4300	4000	3700	3350	3050	2800	2650
0.55	5550	6150	5150	4600	4200	3900	3650	3250	2950	2750	2550
0.54	5350	6050	5000	4450	4100	3750	3550	3150	2900	2650	2500
0.53	5150	5950	4850	4350	3950	3650	3450	3050	2800	2600	2450
0.52	5000	5800	4750	4250	3850	3550	3350	3000	2750	2550	2350
0.51	4800	5700	4600	4100	3750	3450	3250	2900	2650	2450	2300
0.50	4650	5600	4450	4000	3650	3400	3150	2800	2600	2400	2250
0.49	4450	5500	4350	3900	3550	3300	3050	2750	2500	2300	2150
0.48	4300	5400	4200	3750	3450	3200	3000	2650	2450	2250	2100
0.47	4150	5250	4100	3650	3350	3100	2900	2600	2350	2200	2050
0.46	4000	5150	3950	3550	3250	3000	2800	2500	2300	2100	2000
0.45	3800	5050	3850	3450	3150	2900	2700	2400	2200	2050	1900
0.44	3650	4950	3700	3300	3050	2800	2600	2350	2150	2000	1850
0.43	3500	4800	3600	3200	2950	2700	2550	2250	2050	1900	1800
0.42	3350	4700	3450	3100	2850	2600	2450	2200	2000	1850	1750
0.41	3200	4600	3350	3000	2750	2550	2350	2100	1950	1800	1650
0.40	3100	4500	3250	2900	2650	2450	2300	2050	1850	1750	1600
0.39	2950	4350	3100	2800	2550	2350	2200	1950	1800	1650	1550
0.38	2800	4250	3000	2700	2450	2250	2100	1900	1750	1600	1500
0.37	2650	4150	2900	2600	2350	2200	2050	1850	1650	1550	1450
0.36	2550	4050	2750	2500	2250	2100	1950	1750	1600	1500	1400
0.35	2400	3900	2650	2400	2150	2000	1900	1700	1550	1400	1350
0.34	2300	3800	2550	2300	2100	1950	1800	1600	1450	1350	1300
0.33	2150	3700	2450	2200	2000	1850	1750	1550	1400	1300	1200
0.32	2050	3600	2350	2100	1900	1750	1650	1500	1350	1250	1150
0.31	1900	3450	2250	2000	1800	1700	1600	1400	1300	1200	1100

1. Specific gravity based on weight and volume when oven-dry (see Table 11.3.2A). Different specific gravities (G) are possible for different grades of MSR and MEL lumber (see Table 4C, Footnote 2).

2. $F_{e\parallel} = 11200G$; $F_{e\perp} = 6100G^{1.45}/\sqrt{D}$; F_e for D < 1/4" = $16600 G^{1.84}$; Tabulated values are rounded to the nearest 50 psi.

Table 11.3.2A   Assigned Specific Gravities

Species Combination	Specific[1] Gravity, G	Species Combinations of MSR and MEL Lumber	Specific[1] Gravity, G
Aspen	0.39	Douglas Fir-Larch	
Alaska Cedar	0.47	E=1,900,000 psi and lower grades of MSR	0.50
Alaska Hemlock	0.46	E=2,000,000 psi grades of MSR	0.51
Alaska Spruce	0.41	E=2,100,000 psi grades of MSR	0.52
Alaska Yellow Cedar	0.46	E=2,200,000 psi grades of MSR	0.53
Balsam Fir	0.36	E=2,300,000 psi grades of MSR	0.54
Beech-Birch-Hickory	0.71	E=2,400,000 psi grades of MSR	0.55
Coast Sitka Spruce	0.39	Douglas Fir-Larch (North)	
Cottonwood	0.41	E=1,900,000 psi and lower grades of MSR and MEL	0.49
Douglas Fir-Larch	0.50	E=2,000,000 psi to 2,200,000 psi grades of MSR and MEL	0.53
Douglas Fir-Larch (North)	0.49	E=2,300,000 psi and higher grades of MSR and MEL	0.57
Douglas Fir-South	0.46	Douglas Fir-Larch (South)	
Eastern Hemlock	0.41	E=1,000,000 psi and higher grades of MSR	0.46
Eastern Hemlock-Balsam Fir	0.36	Engelmann Spruce-Lodgepole Pine	
Eastern Hemlock-Tamarack	0.41	E=1,400,000 psi and lower grades of MSR	0.38
Eastern Hemlock-Tamarack (North)	0.47	E=1,500,000 psi and higher grades of MSR	0.46
Eastern Softwoods	0.36	Hem-Fir	
Eastern Spruce	0.41	E=1,500,000 psi and lower grades of MSR	0.43
Eastern White Pine	0.36	E=1,600,000 psi grades of MSR	0.44
Engelmann Spruce-Lodgepole Pine	0.38	E=1,700,000 psi grades of MSR	0.45
Hem-Fir	0.43	E=1,800,000 psi grades of MSR	0.46
Hem-Fir (North)	0.46	E=1,900,000 psi grades of MSR	0.47
Mixed Maple	0.55	E=2,000,000 psi grades of MSR	0.48
Mixed Oak	0.68	E=2,100,000 psi grades of MSR	0.49
Mixed Southern Pine	0.51	E=2,200,000 psi grades of MSR	0.50
Mountain Hemlock	0.47	E=2,300,000 psi grades of MSR	0.51
Northern Pine	0.42	E=2,400,000 psi grades of MSR	0.52
Northern Red Oak	0.68	Hem-Fir (North)	
Northern Species	0.35	E=1,000,000 psi and higher grades of MSR and MEL	0.46
Northern White Cedar	0.31	Southern Pine	
Ponderosa Pine	0.43	E=1,700,000 psi and lower grades of MSR and MEL	0.55
Red Maple	0.58	E=1,800,000 psi and higher grades of MSR and MEL	0.57
Red Oak	0.67	Spruce-Pine-Fir	
Red Pine	0.44	E=1,700,000 psi and lower grades of MSR and MEL	0.42
Redwood, close grain	0.44	E=1,800,000 psi and 1,900,000 grades of MSR and MEL	0.46
Redwood, open grain	0.37	E=2,000,000 psi and higher grades of MSR and MEL	0.50
Sitka Spruce	0.43	Spruce-Pine-Fir (South)	
Southern Pine	0.55	E=1,100,000 psi and lower grades of MSR	0.36
Spruce-Pine-Fir	0.42	E=1,200,000 psi to 1,900,000 psi grades of MSR	0.42
Spruce-Pine-Fir (South)	0.36	E=2,000,000 psi and higher grades of MSR	0.50
Western Cedars	0.36	Western Cedars	
Western Cedars (North)	0.35	E=1,000,000 psi and higher grades of MSR	0.36
Western Hemlock	0.47	Western Woods	
Western Hemlock (North)	0.46	E=1,000,000 psi and higher grades of MSR	0.36
Western White Pine	0.40		
Western Woods	0.36		
White Oak	0.73		
Yellow Poplar	0.43		

1. Specific gravity based on weight and volume when oven-dry. Different specific gravities (G) are possible for different grades of MSR and MEL lumber (see Table 4C, Footnote 2).

Table 11.3.2B Dowel Bearing Strengths for Wood Structural Panels

Wood Structural Panel	Specific[1] Gravity, G	Dowel Bearing Strength, F_e, in pounds per square inch (psi)
Plywood		
Structural 1, Marine	0.50	4650
Other Grades[1]	0.42	3350
Oriented Strand Board		
All Grades	0.50	4650

1. Use G = 0.42 when species of the plies is not known. When species of the plies is known, specific gravity listed for the actual species and the corresponding dowel bearing strength may be used, or the weighted average may be used for mixed species.

11.3.6.2 For threaded full-body fasteners (see Appendix L), D shall be permitted to be used in lieu of D_r when the bearing length of the threads does not exceed ¼ of the full bearing length in the member holding the threads. Alternatively, a more detailed analysis accounting for the moment and bearing resistance of the threaded portion of the fastener shall be permitted (see Appendix I).

11.3.7 Asymmetric Three Member Connections, Double Shear

Reference design values, Z, for asymmetric three member connections shall be the minimum computed yield mode value for symmetric double shear connections using the smaller dowel bearing length in the side member as ℓ_s and the minimum dowel diameter, D, occurring in either of the connection shear planes.

Figure 11D Multiple Shear Bolted Connections

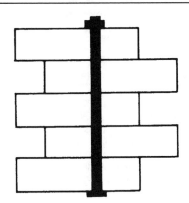

11.3.8 Multiple Shear Connections

For a connection with four or more members (see Figure 11D), each shear plane shall be evaluated as a single shear connection. The reference design value for the connection shall be the lowest reference design value for any single shear plane, multiplied by the number of shear planes.

11.3.9 Load at an Angle to Fastener Axis

11.3.9.1 When the applied load in a single shear (two member) connection is at an angle (other than 90º) with the fastener axis, the fastener lengths in the two members shall be designated ℓ_s and ℓ_m (see Figure 11E). The component of the load acting at 90° with the fastener axis shall not exceed the adjusted design value, Z', for a connection in which two members at 90° with the fastener axis have thicknesses $t_s = \ell_s$ and $t_m = \ell_m$. Ample bearing area shall be provided to resist the load component acting parallel to the fastener axis.

11.3.9.2 For toe-nailed connections, use the minimum of t_s or L/3 for ℓ_s (see Figure 11A).

11.3.10 Drift Bolts and Drift Pins

Adjusted lateral design values for drift bolts and drift pins driven in the side grain of wood shall not exceed 75% of the adjusted lateral design values for common bolts of the same diameter and length in main member.

Figure 11E Shear Area for Bolted Connections

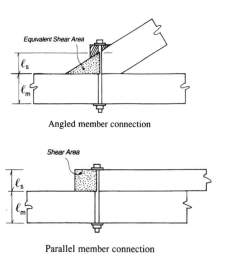

Angled member connection

Parallel member connection

11.4 Combined Lateral and Withdrawal Loads

11.4.1 Lag Screws and Wood Screws

When a lag screw or wood screw is subjected to combined lateral and withdrawal loading, as when the fastener is inserted perpendicular to the fiber and the load acts at an angle, α, to the wood surface (see Figure 11F), the adjusted design value shall be determined as follows (see Appendix J):

$$Z_\alpha' = \frac{(W'p)Z'}{(W'p)\cos^2\alpha + Z'\sin^2\alpha} \qquad (11.4\text{-}1)$$

where:

α = angle between wood surface and direction of applied load

p = length of thread penetration in main member, in.

11.4.2 Nails and Spikes

When a nail or spike is subjected to combined lateral and withdrawal loading, as when the nail or spike is inserted perpendicular to the fiber and the load acts at an angle, α, to the wood surface, the adjusted design value shall be determined as follows:

$$Z_\alpha' = \frac{(W'p)Z'}{(W'p)\cos\alpha + Z'\sin\alpha} \qquad (11.4\text{-}2)$$

where:

α = angle between wood surface and direction of applied load

p = length of penetration in main member, in.

Figure 11F Combined Lateral and Withdrawal Loading

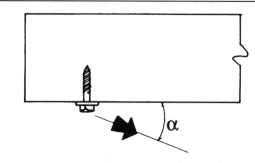

11.5 Adjustment of Reference Design Values

11.5.1 Geometry Factor, C_Δ

11.5.1.1 When $D < 1/4"$, $C_\Delta = 1.0$.

11.5.1.2 When $D \geq 1/4"$ and the end distance or spacing provided for dowel-type fasteners is less than the minimum required for $C_\Delta = 1.0$ for any condition in (a), (b), or (c), reference design values shall be multiplied by the smallest applicable geometry factor, C_Δ, determined in (a), (b), or (c). The smallest geometry factor for any fastener in a group shall apply to all fasteners in the group. For multiple shear connections or for asymmetric three member connections, the smallest geometry factor, C_Δ, for any shear plane shall apply to all fasteners in the connection. Provisions for C_Δ are based on an assumption that edge distance and spacing between rows of fasteners is in accordance with Table 11.5.1A and Table 11.5.1D and applicable requirements of 11.1.

Table 11.5.1A Edge Distance Requirements [1,2]

Direction of Loading	Minimum Edge Distance
Parallel to Grain:	
when $\ell/D \leq 6$	1.5D
when $\ell/D > 6$	1.5D or ½ the spacing between rows, whichever is greater
Perpendicular to Grain:[2]	
loaded edge	4D
unloaded edge	1.5D

1. The ℓ/D ratio used to determine the minimum edge distance shall be the lesser of:
   (a) length of fastener in wood main member/D = ℓ_m/D
   (b) total length of fastener in wood side member(s)/D = ℓ_s/D
2. Heavy or medium concentrated loads shall not be suspended below the neutral axis of a single sawn lumber or structural glued laminated timber beam except where mechanical or equivalent reinforcement is provided to resist tension stresses perpendicular to grain (see 3.8.2 and 10.1.3).

Figure 11G   Bolted Connection Geometry

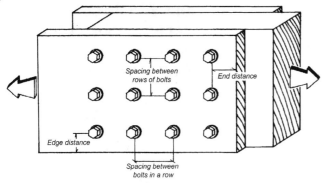

Parallel to grain loading in all wood members ($Z_\parallel$)

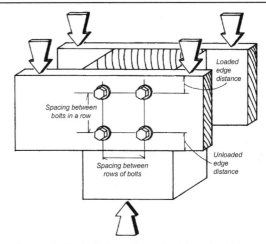

Perpendicular to grain loading in the side member
and parallel to grain loading in the main member ($Z_{s\perp}$)

(a) When dowel-type fasteners are used and the actual end distance for parallel or perpendicular to grain loading is greater than or equal to the minimum end distance (see Table 11.5.1B) for $C_\Delta = 0.5$, but less than the minimum end distance for $C_\Delta = 1.0$, the geometry factor, C_Δ, shall be determined as follows:

$$C_\Delta = \frac{\text{actual end distance}}{\text{minimum end distance for } C_\Delta = 1.0}$$

(b) For loading at an angle to the fastener, when dowel-type fasteners are used, the minimum shear area for $C_\Delta = 1.0$ shall be equivalent to the shear area for a parallel member connection with minimum end distance for $C_\Delta = 1.0$ (see Table 11.5.1B and Figure 11E). The minimum shear area for $C_\Delta = 0.5$ shall be equivalent to ½ the minimum shear area for $C_\Delta = 1.0$. When the actual shear area is greater than or equal to the minimum shear area for $C_\Delta = 0.5$, but less than the minimum shear area for $C_\Delta = 1.0$, the geometry factor, C_Δ, shall be determined as follows:

$$C_\Delta = \frac{\text{actual shear area}}{\text{minimum shear area for } C_\Delta = 1.0}$$

(c) When the actual spacing between dowel-type fasteners in a row for parallel or perpendicular to grain loading is greater than or equal to the minimum spacing (see Table 11.5.1C), but less than the minimum spacing for $C_\Delta = 1.0$, the geometry factor, C_Δ, shall be determined as follows:

$$C_\Delta = \frac{\text{actual spacing}}{\text{minimum spacing for } C_\Delta = 1.0}$$

Table 11.5.1B   End Distance Requirements

| | End Distances | |
| | Minimum end distance for $C_\Delta = 0.5$ | Minimum end distance for $C_\Delta = 1.0$ |
Direction of Loading		
Perpendicular to Grain	2D	4D
Parallel to Grain, Compression: (fastener bearing away from member end)	2D	4D
Parallel to Grain, Tension: (fastener bearing toward member end)		
for softwoods	3.5D	7D
for hardwoods	2.5D	5D

Table 11.5.1C Spacing Requirements for Fasteners in a Row

| | Spacing | |
Direction of Loading	Minimum spacing	Minimum spacing for $C_\Delta = 1.0$
Parallel to Grain	3D	4D
Perpendicular to Grain	3D	Required spacing for attached members

Table 11.5.1D Spacing Requirements Between Rows [1,2]

Direction of Loading	Minimum Spacing
Parallel to Grain	1.5D
Perpendicular to Grain:	
when $\ell/D \leq 2$	2.5D
when $2 < \ell/D < 6$	$(5\ell + 10D)\,/\,8$
when $\ell/D \geq 6$	5D

1. The ℓ/D ratio used to determine the minimum edge distance shall be the lesser of:
   (a) length of fastener in wood main member/D = ℓ_m/D
   (b) total length of fastener in wood side member(s)/D = ℓ_s/D
2. The spacing between outer rows of fasteners paralleling the member on a single splice plate shall not exceed 5" (see Figure 11H).

11.5.2 End Grain Factor, C_{eg}

11.5.2.1 When lag screws are loaded in withdrawal from end grain, the reference withdrawal design values, W, shall be multiplied by the end grain factor, $C_{eg} = 0.75$.

11.5.2.2 When dowel-type fasteners are inserted in the end grain of the main member, with the fastener axis parallel to the wood fibers, reference lateral design values, Z, shall be multiplied by the end grain factor, $C_{eg} = 0.67$.

11.5.3 Diaphragm Factor, C_{di}

When nails or spikes are used in diaphragm construction, reference lateral design values, Z, shall be multiplied by the diaphragm factor, $C_{di} = 1.1$.

11.5.4 Toe-Nail Factor, C_{tn}

11.5.4.1 When toe-nailed connections are used, reference withdrawal design values, W, for the nails or spikes shall be multiplied by the toe-nail factor, $C_{tn} = 0.67$. The wet service factor, C_M, shall not apply for toe-nailed connections loaded in withdrawal.

11.5.4.2 When toe-nailed connections are used, reference lateral design values, Z, shall be multiplied by the toe-nail factor, $C_{tn} = 0.83$.

Table 11.5.1E Edge and End Distance and Spacing Requirements for Lag Screws Loaded in Withdrawal and Not Loaded Laterally

Orientation	Minimum Distance/Spacing
Edge Distance	1.5D
End Distance	4D
Spacing	4D

Figure 11H Spacing Between Outer Rows of Bolts

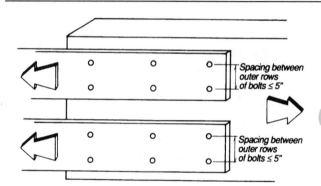

11.6 Multiple Fasteners

11.6.1 Symmetrically Staggered Fasteners

When a connection contains multiple fasteners, fasteners shall be staggered symmetrically in members loaded perpendicular to grain whenever possible (see 3.1.2.2 and 10.3.6.2 for special design provisions when bolts, lag screws, or drift pins are staggered).

11.6.2 Fasteners Loaded at an Angle to Grain

When a multiple fastener connection is loaded at an angle to grain, the gravity axis of each member shall pass through the center of resistance of the group of fasteners to insure uniform stress in the main member and a uniform distribution of load to all fasteners.

11.6.3 Local Stresses in Connections

Local stresses in connections using multiple fasteners shall be evaluated in accordance with principles of engineering mechanics (see 10.1.2).

DOWEL-TYPE FASTENERS

11

Table 11A   BOLTS: Reference Lateral Design Values (Z) for Single Shear (two member) Connections[1,2]

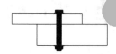

for sawn lumber or SCL with both members of identical specific gravity

Main Member t_m in.	Side Member t_s in.	Bolt Diameter D in.	G=0.67 Red Oak $Z_\parallel$ lbs.	$Z_{s\perp}$ lbs.	$Z_{m\perp}$ lbs.	$Z_\perp$ lbs.	G=0.55 Mixed Maple Southern Pine $Z_\parallel$ lbs.	$Z_{s\perp}$ lbs.	$Z_{m\perp}$ lbs.	$Z_\perp$ lbs.	G=0.50 Douglas Fir-Larch $Z_\parallel$ lbs.	$Z_{s\perp}$ lbs.	$Z_{m\perp}$ lbs.	$Z_\perp$ lbs.	G=0.49 Douglas Fir-Larch(N) $Z_\parallel$ lbs.	$Z_{s\perp}$ lbs.	$Z_{m\perp}$ lbs.	$Z_\perp$ lbs.	G=0.46 Douglas Fir(S) Hem-Fir(N) $Z_\parallel$ lbs.	$Z_{s\perp}$ lbs.	$Z_{m\perp}$ lbs.	$Z_\perp$ lbs.
1-1/2	1-1/2	1/2	650	420	420	330	530	330	330	250	480	300	300	220	470	290	290	210	440	270	270	190
		5/8	810	500	500	370	660	400	400	280	600	360	360	240	590	350	350	240	560	320	320	220
		3/4	970	580	580	410	800	460	460	310	720	420	420	270	710	400	400	260	670	380	380	240
		7/8	1130	660	660	440	930	520	520	330	850	470	470	290	830	460	460	280	780	420	420	250
		1	1290	740	740	470	1060	580	580	350	970	530	530	310	950	510	510	300	890	480	480	280
1-3/4	1-3/4	1/2	760	490	490	390	620	390	390	290	560	350	350	250	550	340	340	250	520	320	320	230
		5/8	940	590	590	430	770	470	470	330	700	420	420	280	690	410	410	280	650	380	380	250
		3/4	1130	680	680	480	930	540	540	360	850	480	480	310	830	470	470	300	780	440	440	280
		7/8	1320	770	770	510	1080	610	610	390	990	550	550	340	970	530	530	320	910	500	500	300
		1	1510	860	860	550	1240	680	680	410	1130	610	610	360	1110	600	600	350	1040	560	560	320
2-1/2	1-1/2	1/2	770	480	540	440	660	400	420	350	610	370	370	310	610	360	360	300	580	340	330	270
		5/8	1070	660	630	520	930	560	490	390	850	520	430	340	830	520	420	330	780	470	390	300
		3/4	1360	890	720	570	1120	660	560	430	1020	590	500	380	1000	560	480	360	940	520	450	330
		7/8	1590	960	800	620	1300	720	620	470	1190	630	550	410	1170	600	540	390	1090	550	500	360
		1	1820	1020	870	660	1490	770	680	490	1360	680	610	440	1330	650	590	420	1250	600	550	390
3-1/2	1-1/2	1/2	770	480	560	440	660	400	460	360	610	370	430	330	610	360	420	320	580	340	400	310
		5/8	1070	760	760	590	940	560	620	500	880	520	540	460	870	520	530	450	830	470	490	410
		3/4	1450	890	900	770	1270	660	690	580	1200	590	610	510	1190	560	590	490	1140	520	550	450
		7/8	1890	960	990	830	1680	720	770	630	1590	630	680	550	1570	600	650	530	1470	550	600	480
		1	2410	1020	1080	890	2010	770	830	670	1830	680	740	590	1790	650	710	560	1680	600	660	520
3-1/2	1-3/4	1/2	830	510	590	480	720	420	510	390	670	380	470	350	660	380	460	340	620	360	440	320
		5/8	1160	680	820	620	1000	580	640	520	930	530	560	460	920	530	550	450	880	500	510	410
		3/4	1530	900	940	780	1330	770	720	580	1250	680	640	520	1240	660	620	500	1190	600	580	460
		7/8	1970	1120	1040	840	1730	840	810	640	1620	740	710	550	1590	700	690	530	1490	640	640	490
		1	2480	1190	1130	900	2030	890	880	670	1850	790	780	590	1820	750	760	570	1700	700	700	530
3-1/2	3-1/2	1/2	830	590	590	530	750	520	520	460	720	490	490	430	710	480	480	420	690	460	460	410
		5/8	1290	880	880	780	1170	780	780	650	1120	700	700	560	1110	690	690	550	1070	650	650	500
		3/4	1860	1190	1190	950	1690	960	960	710	1610	870	870	630	1600	850	850	600	1540	800	800	560
		7/8	2540	1410	1410	1030	2170	1160	1160	800	1970	1060	1060	700	1940	1040	1040	650	1810	980	980	590
		1	3020	1670	1670	1100	2480	1360	1360	820	2260	1230	1230	720	2210	1190	1190	690	2070	1110	1110	640
5-1/4	1-1/2	5/8	1070	660	760	590	940	560	640	500	880	520	590	460	870	520	590	450	830	470	560	430
		3/4	1450	890	990	780	1270	660	850	660	1200	590	790	590	1190	560	780	560	1140	520	740	520
		7/8	1890	960	1260	960	1680	720	1060	720	1590	630	940	630	1570	600	900	600	1520	550	830	550
		1	2410	1020	1500	1020	2150	770	1140	770	2050	680	1010	680	2030	650	970	650	1930	600	910	600
5-1/4	1-3/4	5/8	1160	680	820	620	1000	580	690	520	930	530	630	470	920	530	630	470	880	500	590	440
		3/4	1530	900	1050	800	1330	770	850	660	1250	680	830	620	1240	660	810	620	1190	600	780	590
		7/8	1970	1120	1320	1000	1730	840	1090	840	1640	740	960	740	1620	700	920	700	1550	640	850	640
		1	2480	1190	1530	1190	2200	890	1170	890	2080	790	1040	790	2060	750	1000	750	1990	700	930	700
5-1/4	3-1/2	5/8	1290	880	880	780	1170	780	780	680	1120	700	730	630	1110	690	720	620	1070	650	690	580
		3/4	1860	1190	1240	1080	1690	960	1090	850	1610	870	1030	780	1600	850	1010	750	1540	800	970	710
		7/8	2540	1410	1640	1260	2300	1160	1380	1000	2190	1060	1230	870	2170	1040	1190	840	2060	980	1100	770
		1	3310	1670	1940	1420	2870	1390	1520	1060	2660	1290	1360	940	2630	1260	1320	900	2500	1210	1230	830
5-1/2	1-1/2	5/8	1070	660	760	590	940	560	640	500	880	520	590	460	870	520	590	450	830	470	560	430
		3/4	1450	890	990	780	1270	660	850	660	1200	590	790	590	1190	560	780	560	1140	520	740	520
		7/8	1890	960	1260	960	1680	720	1090	720	1590	630	980	630	1570	600	940	600	1520	550	860	550
		1	2410	1020	1560	1020	2150	770	1190	770	2050	680	1060	680	2030	650	1010	650	1930	600	940	600
5-1/2	3-1/2	5/8	1290	880	880	780	1170	780	780	680	1120	700	730	630	1110	690	720	620	1070	650	690	580
		3/4	1860	1190	1240	1080	1690	960	1090	850	1610	870	1030	780	1600	850	1010	750	1540	800	970	710
		7/8	2540	1410	1640	1260	2300	1160	1410	1020	2190	1060	1260	910	2170	1040	1220	870	2060	980	1130	790
		1	3310	1670	1980	1470	2870	1390	1550	1090	2660	1290	1390	970	2630	1260	1340	930	2500	1210	1250	860
7-1/2	1-1/2	5/8	1070	660	760	590	940	560	640	500	880	520	590	460	870	520	590	450	830	470	560	430
		3/4	1450	890	990	780	1270	660	850	660	1200	590	790	590	1190	560	780	560	1140	520	740	520
		7/8	1890	960	1260	960	1680	720	1090	720	1590	630	1010	630	1570	600	990	600	1520	550	950	550
		1	2410	1020	1560	1020	2150	770	1350	770	2050	680	1270	680	2030	650	1240	650	1930	600	1190	600
7-1/2	3-1/2	5/8	1290	880	880	780	1170	780	780	680	1120	700	730	630	1110	690	720	620	1070	650	690	580
		3/4	1860	1190	1240	1080	1690	960	1090	850	1610	870	1030	780	1600	850	1010	750	1540	800	970	710
		7/8	2540	1410	1640	1260	2300	1160	1450	1020	2190	1060	1360	910	2170	1040	1340	870	2060	980	1280	850
		1	3310	1670	2090	1470	2870	1390	1830	1210	2660	1290	1630	1110	2630	1260	1570	1080	2500	1210	1470	1030

1. Tabulated lateral design values (Z) for bolted connections shall be multiplied by all applicable adjustment factors (see Table 10.3.1).
2. Tabulated lateral design values (Z) are for "full diameter" bolts (see Appendix L) with bending yield strength (F_{yb}) of 45,000 psi.

Table 11A (Cont.) BOLTS: Reference Lateral Design Values (Z) for Single Shear (two member) Connections[1,2]

for sawn lumber or SCL with both members of identical specific gravity

Thickness Main Member t_m (in.)	Side Member t_s (in.)	Bolt Diameter D (in.)	G=0.43 Hem-Fir $Z_\parallel$ lbs.	$Z_{s\perp}$ lbs.	$Z_{m\perp}$ lbs.	$Z_\perp$ lbs.	G=0.42 SPF $Z_\parallel$ lbs.	$Z_{s\perp}$ lbs.	$Z_{m\perp}$ lbs.	$Z_\perp$ lbs.	G=0.37 Redwood $Z_\parallel$ lbs.	$Z_{s\perp}$ lbs.	$Z_{m\perp}$ lbs.	$Z_\perp$ lbs.	G=0.36 E.Softwds $Z_\parallel$ lbs.	$Z_{s\perp}$ lbs.	$Z_{m\perp}$ lbs.	$Z_\perp$ lbs.	G=0.35 Northern $Z_\parallel$ lbs.	$Z_{s\perp}$ lbs.	$Z_{m\perp}$ lbs.	$Z_\perp$ lbs.
1-1/2	1-1/2	1/2	410	250	250	180	410	240	240	170	360	210	210	140	350	200	200	130	340	200	200	130
		5/8	520	300	300	190	510	290	290	190	450	250	250	160	440	240	240	150	420	240	240	150
		3/4	620	350	350	210	610	340	340	210	540	290	290	170	520	280	280	170	500	270	270	160
		7/8	720	390	390	230	710	380	380	220	630	330	330	190	610	320	320	180	590	310	310	170
		1	830	440	440	250	810	430	430	240	720	370	370	200	700	360	360	190	670	350	350	190
1-3/4	1-3/4	1/2	480	290	290	210	470	280	280	200	420	250	250	170	410	240	240	160	390	230	230	150
		5/8	600	350	350	230	590	340	340	220	520	290	290	190	510	280	280	180	490	270	270	170
		3/4	720	400	400	240	710	390	390	240	630	340	340	200	610	330	330	190	590	320	320	190
		7/8	850	460	460	270	830	450	450	260	730	390	390	220	710	380	380	210	690	360	360	200
		1	970	510	510	290	950	500	500	280	840	430	430	230	820	420	420	230	790	410	410	220
2-1/2	1-1/2	1/2	550	320	310	250	540	320	300	240	500	290	250	200	490	280	240	190	470	280	240	180
		5/8	730	420	360	270	710	410	350	270	630	350	300	220	610	330	290	210	590	320	280	210
		3/4	870	460	410	300	850	450	400	290	750	370	340	240	740	360	330	230	710	350	320	230
		7/8	1020	500	450	320	1000	490	440	310	880	410	380	260	860	390	370	250	830	370	350	240
		1	1160	540	500	350	1140	530	490	340	1010	440	440	280	980	420	410	270	940	410	390	260
3-1/2	1-1/2	1/2	550	320	380	290	540	320	370	280	500	290	320	250	490	280	300	250	480	280	290	240
		5/8	790	420	440	370	780	410	430	360	720	350	370	300	710	330	350	290	700	320	340	280
		3/4	1100	460	500	400	1080	450	480	390	1010	370	410	320	990	360	400	310	950	350	380	300
		7/8	1370	500	550	430	1340	490	540	420	1180	410	460	350	1160	390	440	340	1110	370	420	320
		1	1570	540	600	470	1530	530	590	460	1350	440	500	380	1320	420	480	370	1270	410	470	350
3-1/2	1-3/4	1/2	590	340	400	300	580	330	390	290	530	300	330	260	520	290	320	250	510	280	310	250
		5/8	840	480	460	370	820	470	450	360	760	400	390	310	740	380	370	290	730	370	360	280
		3/4	1130	540	520	410	1120	530	510	400	1030	430	430	330	1000	420	420	320	970	410	410	310
		7/8	1390	580	580	440	1360	570	570	430	1200	470	480	360	1170	460	470	350	1130	430	440	320
		1	1590	630	640	480	1550	610	630	460	1370	510	530	380	1340	490	520	370	1290	470	500	360
3-1/2	3-1/2	1/2	660	440	440	390	660	430	430	380	620	400	400	330	610	390	390	310	600	380	380	310
		5/8	1040	600	600	450	1020	590	590	440	960	520	520	370	950	500	500	350	930	490	490	340
		3/4	1450	740	740	500	1420	730	730	480	1250	650	650	400	1220	630	630	390	1180	620	620	370
		7/8	1690	910	910	540	1660	890	890	520	1460	770	770	470	1430	750	750	450	1370	720	720	390
		1	1930	1030	1030	580	1890	1000	1000	560	1670	870	870	470	1630	840	840	450	1570	810	810	430
5-1/4	1-1/2	5/8	790	420	530	410	780	410	520	400	720	350	470	350	710	330	460	330	700	320	450	320
		3/4	1100	460	690	460	1080	450	670	450	1010	370	560	370	990	360	540	360	970	350	530	350
		7/8	1460	500	750	500	1440	490	730	490	1350	410	620	410	1330	390	600	390	1280	370	560	370
		1	1800	540	820	540	1760	530	800	530	1560	440	670	440	1520	420	650	420	1460	410	630	410
5-1/4	1-3/4	5/8	840	480	560	410	820	470	550	400	760	400	500	370	740	380	480	360	730	370	470	350
		3/4	1130	540	700	540	1120	530	680	530	1040	430	570	430	1020	420	560	420	1000	410	540	410
		7/8	1490	580	770	580	1470	570	750	570	1370	470	640	470	1350	460	620	460	1320	430	580	430
		1	1910	630	850	630	1890	610	820	610	1760	510	690	510	1740	490	670	490	1700	470	650	470
5-1/4	3-1/2	5/8	1040	600	660	530	1020	590	650	520	960	520	610	460	950	500	590	440	930	490	580	430
		3/4	1490	740	900	640	1480	730	880	620	1390	650	750	520	1370	630	730	500	1330	620	710	480
		7/8	1950	920	1010	690	1920	910	990	670	1740	820	850	560	1710	800	830	550	1660	770	780	510
		1	2370	1140	1130	750	2330	1120	1100	730	2120	1020	940	600	2080	980	940	600	2030	950	880	560
5-1/2	1-1/2	5/8	790	420	530	410	780	410	520	400	720	350	470	350	710	330	460	330	700	320	450	320
		3/4	1100	460	700	460	1080	450	690	450	1010	370	580	370	990	360	570	360	970	350	550	350
		7/8	1460	500	780	500	1440	490	760	490	1350	410	650	410	1330	390	630	390	1280	370	590	370
		1	1800	540	860	540	1760	530	830	530	1560	440	700	440	1520	420	680	420	1460	410	650	410
5-1/2	3-1/2	5/8	1040	600	660	530	1020	590	650	520	960	520	610	460	950	500	590	440	930	490	580	430
		3/4	1490	740	920	650	1480	730	900	640	1390	650	770	530	1370	630	750	520	1330	620	720	500
		7/8	1950	920	1030	720	1920	910	1010	700	1740	820	870	590	1710	800	840	570	1660	770	800	530
		1	2370	1140	1150	780	2330	1120	1120	760	2120	1020	960	650	2080	980	930	600	2030	950	890	580
7-1/2	1-1/2	5/8	790	420	530	410	780	410	520	400	720	350	470	350	710	330	460	330	700	320	450	320
		3/4	1100	460	700	460	1080	450	690	450	1010	370	630	370	990	360	620	360	970	350	600	350
		7/8	1460	500	900	500	1440	490	890	490	1350	410	810	410	1330	390	800	390	1280	370	770	370
		1	1800	540	1130	540	1760	530	1110	530	1560	440	920	440	1520	420	890	420	1460	410	860	410
7-1/2	3-1/2	5/8	1040	600	660	530	1020	590	650	520	960	520	610	460	950	500	590	440	930	490	580	430
		3/4	1490	740	920	650	1480	730	910	640	1390	650	840	560	1370	630	820	550	1330	620	810	540
		7/8	1950	920	1210	790	1920	910	1180	780	1740	820	1010	700	1710	800	980	680	1660	770	920	650
		1	2370	1140	1340	970	2330	1120	1300	950	2120	1020	1100	820	2080	980	1070	790	2030	950	1030	760

1. Tabulated lateral design values (Z) for bolted connections shall be multiplied by all applicable adjustment factors (see Table 10.3.1).
2. Tabulated lateral design values (Z) are for "full diameter" bolts (see Appendix L) with bending yield strength (F_{yb}) of 45,000 psi.

Table 11B BOLTS: Reference Lateral Design Values (Z) for Single Shear (two member) Connections[1,2]

for sawn lumber or SCL with 1/4" ASTM A 36 steel side plate

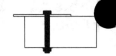

Thickness			G=0.67 Red Oak		G=0.55 Mixed Maple Southern Pine		G=0.50 Douglas Fir-Larch		G=0.49 Douglas Fir-Larch(N)		G=0.46 Douglas Fir(S) Hem-Fir(N)		G=0.43 Hem-Fir		G=0.42 Spruce-Pine-Fir		G=0.37 Redwood (open grain)		G=0.36 Eastern Softwoods Spruce-Pine-Fir(S) Western Cedars Western Woods		G=0.35 Northern Species	
Main Member t_m in.	Side Member t_s in.	Bolt Diameter D in.	$Z_{\|\|}$ lbs.	$Z_\perp$ lbs.	$Z_{\|\|}$ lbs.	$Z_\perp$ lbs.	$Z_{\|\|}$ lbs.	$Z_\perp$ lbs.	$Z_{\|\|}$ lbs.	$Z_\perp$ lbs.	$Z_{\|\|}$ lbs.	$Z_\perp$ lbs.	$Z_{\|\|}$ lbs.	$Z_\perp$ lbs.	$Z_{\|\|}$ lbs.	$Z_\perp$ lbs.	$Z_{\|\|}$ lbs.	$Z_\perp$ lbs.	$Z_{\|\|}$ lbs.	$Z_\perp$ lbs.	$Z_{\|\|}$ lbs.	$Z_\perp$ lbs.
1-1/2	1/4	1/2	730	420	620	350	580	310	580	310	550	290	520	280	510	270	470	240	460	240	450	230
		5/8	910	480	780	400	730	360	720	360	690	340	650	320	640	320	590	290	580	280	560	270
		3/4	1090	550	940	450	870	420	860	410	820	390	780	360	770	360	710	320	690	320	680	310
		7/8	1270	600	1090	510	1020	470	1010	450	960	430	910	410	900	400	820	370	810	360	790	350
		1	1460	660	1250	550	1170	510	1150	500	1100	480	1040	450	1030	450	940	400	930	400	900	390
1-3/4	1/4	1/2	810	460	690	370	640	340	630	330	600	310	570	290	560	280	510	250	500	250	490	240
		5/8	1020	520	870	430	800	390	790	380	750	360	710	340	700	330	640	300	630	290	610	280
		3/4	1220	590	1040	480	960	440	950	430	900	410	860	380	840	370	770	330	750	330	730	320
		7/8	1420	650	1210	540	1130	490	1110	480	1050	450	1000	420	980	420	890	380	880	370	850	360
		1	1630	710	1380	580	1290	540	1270	520	1200	500	1140	470	1120	460	1020	410	1000	410	980	400
2-1/2	1/4	1/2	930	600	860	470	830	410	820	400	780	380	740	350	720	340	650	300	640	290	620	280
		5/8	1370	670	1150	530	1050	470	1040	470	980	430	920	400	910	390	810	340	800	330	770	320
		3/4	1640	750	1370	590	1270	530	1250	520	1180	490	1110	450	1090	440	980	380	960	370	930	360
		7/8	1910	820	1600	650	1480	590	1450	570	1370	530	1290	490	1270	480	1140	420	1120	410	1080	400
		1	2190	880	1830	700	1690	640	1660	620	1570	580	1480	540	1450	530	1300	460	1280	450	1240	440
3-1/2	1/4	1/2	930	620	860	550	830	510	820	510	800	480	770	450	770	430	720	370	720	360	710	350
		5/8	1370	860	1260	690	1210	610	1200	600	1160	550	1130	500	1120	490	1060	420	1050	410	1020	400
		3/4	1900	990	1740	760	1670	680	1660	660	1580	610	1480	560	1450	540	1290	460	1260	450	1220	440
		7/8	2530	1070	2170	840	1990	740	1950	710	1840	660	1720	610	1690	590	1510	510	1480	500	1430	470
		1	2980	1150	2480	890	2270	800	2230	770	2100	730	1970	660	1930	650	1720	560	1690	540	1630	530
5-1/4	1/4	5/8	1370	860	1260	760	1210	710	1200	700	1160	670	1130	640	1120	630	1060	580	1050	560	1030	540
		3/4	1900	1140	1740	1000	1670	940	1660	930	1610	860	1560	770	1550	760	1460	640	1450	620	1420	600
		7/8	2530	1460	2320	1190	2220	1050	2200	1010	2140	920	2070	840	2050	820	1940	700	1920	680	1890	640
		1	3260	1660	2980	1270	2860	1130	2840	1080	2750	1010	2670	920	2640	890	2490	750	2450	730	2360	710
5-1/2	1/4	5/8	1370	860	1260	760	1210	710	1200	700	1160	670	1130	640	1120	630	1060	580	1050	570	1030	560
		3/4	1900	1140	1740	1000	1670	940	1660	930	1610	890	1560	810	1550	790	1460	660	1450	640	1420	620
		7/8	2530	1460	2320	1240	2220	1090	2200	1050	2140	960	2070	880	2050	860	1940	730	1920	710	1890	660
		1	3260	1730	2980	1320	2860	1170	2840	1130	2750	1050	2670	950	2640	930	2490	780	2470	760	2420	740
7-1/2	1/4	5/8	1370	860	1260	760	1210	710	1200	700	1160	670	1130	640	1120	630	1060	580	1050	570	1030	560
		3/4	1900	1140	1740	1000	1670	940	1660	930	1610	890	1560	850	1550	840	1460	760	1450	750	1420	740
		7/8	2530	1460	2320	1280	2220	1210	2200	1180	2140	1130	2070	1080	2050	1070	1940	960	1920	930	1890	870
		1	3260	1820	2980	1590	2860	1500	2840	1470	2750	1400	2670	1270	2640	1230	2490	1030	2470	1000	2420	960
9-1/2	1/4	3/4	1900	1140	1740	1000	1670	940	1660	930	1610	890	1560	850	1550	840	1460	760	1450	750	1420	740
		7/8	2530	1460	2320	1280	2220	1210	2200	1180	2140	1130	2070	1080	2050	1070	1940	980	1920	970	1890	930
		1	3260	1820	2980	1590	2860	1500	2840	1470	2750	1420	2670	1350	2640	1330	2490	1220	2470	1200	2420	1180
11-1/2	1/4	7/8	2530	1460	2320	1280	2220	1210	2200	1180	2140	1130	2070	1080	2050	1070	1940	980	1920	970	1890	930
		1	3260	1820	2980	1590	2860	1500	2840	1470	2750	1420	2670	1350	2640	1330	2490	1220	2470	1200	2420	1180
13-1/2	1/4	1	3260	1820	2980	1590	2860	1500	2840	1470	2750	1420	2670	1350	2640	1330	2490	1220	2470	1200	2420	1180

1. Tabulated lateral design values (Z) for bolted connections shall be multiplied by all applicable adjustment factors (see Table 10.3.1).
2. Tabulated lateral design values (Z) are for "full diameter" bolts (see Appendix L) with bending yield strength (F_{yb}) of 45,000 psi and dowel bearing strength (F_e) of 87,000 psi for ASTM A 36 steel.

Table 11C BOLTS: Reference Lateral Design Values (Z) for Single Shear (two member) Connections[1,2]

for structural glued laminated timber main member with sawn lumber side member of identical specific gravity

Thickness Main Member t_m (in.)	Side Member t_s (in.)	Bolt Diameter D (in.)	G=0.55 Southern Pine $Z_{\parallel}$	$Z_{s\perp}$	$Z_{m\perp}$	$Z_\perp$	G=0.50 Douglas Fir-Larch $Z_{\parallel}$	$Z_{s\perp}$	$Z_{m\perp}$	$Z_\perp$	G=0.46 Douglas Fir(S) $Z_{\parallel}$	$Z_{s\perp}$	$Z_{m\perp}$	$Z_\perp$	G=0.43 Hem-Fir $Z_{\parallel}$	$Z_{s\perp}$	$Z_{m\perp}$	$Z_\perp$	G=0.42 Spruce-Pine-Fir $Z_{\parallel}$	$Z_{s\perp}$	$Z_{m\perp}$	$Z_\perp$	G=0.36 Spruce-Pine-Fir(S) Western Woods $Z_{\parallel}$	$Z_{s\perp}$	$Z_{m\perp}$	$Z_\perp$
2-1/2	1-1/2	1/2	–	–	470	360	610	370	370	310	580	340	330	270	550	320	310	250	540	320	300	240	490	280	240	190
		5/8	–	–	550	460	850	520	430	340	780	470	390	300	730	420	360	270	710	410	350	270	610	330	290	210
		3/4	–	–	620	500	1020	590	500	380	940	520	450	330	870	460	410	300	850	450	400	290	740	360	330	230
		7/8	–	–	690	540	1190	630	550	410	1090	550	500	360	1020	500	450	320	1000	490	440	310	860	390	370	250
		1	–	–	750	580	1360	680	610	440	1250	600	550	390	1160	540	500	350	1140	530	490	340	980	420	410	270
3	1-1/2	1/2	660	400	470	360	–	–	–	–	–	–	–	–	–	–	–	–	–	–	–	–	–	–	–	–
		5/8	940	560	550	460	–	–	–	–	–	–	–	–	–	–	–	–	–	–	–	–	–	–	–	–
		3/4	1270	660	620	500	–	–	–	–	–	–	–	–	–	–	–	–	–	–	–	–	–	–	–	–
		7/8	1520	720	690	540	–	–	–	–	–	–	–	–	–	–	–	–	–	–	–	–	–	–	–	–
		1	1740	770	750	580	–	–	–	–	–	–	–	–	–	–	–	–	–	–	–	–	–	–	–	–
3-1/8	1-1/2	1/2	–	–	–	–	610	370	430	330	580	340	390	310	550	320	360	290	540	320	340	280	490	280	280	230
		5/8	–	–	–	–	880	520	500	410	830	470	450	370	790	420	410	330	780	410	400	320	710	330	330	260
		3/4	–	–	–	–	1200	590	570	460	1130	520	510	410	1060	460	460	360	1040	450	450	350	890	360	370	280
		7/8	–	–	–	–	1440	630	630	490	1320	550	560	430	1230	500	510	390	1210	490	500	380	1040	390	410	310
		1	–	–	–	–	1640	680	690	530	1510	600	620	470	1410	540	560	420	1380	530	550	410	1190	420	450	330
5	1-1/2	5/8	940	560	640	500	–	–	–	–	–	–	–	–	–	–	–	–	–	–	–	–	–	–	–	–
		3/4	1270	660	850	660	–	–	–	–	–	–	–	–	–	–	–	–	–	–	–	–	–	–	–	–
		7/8	1680	720	1020	720	–	–	–	–	–	–	–	–	–	–	–	–	–	–	–	–	–	–	–	–
		1	2150	770	1100	770	–	–	–	–	–	–	–	–	–	–	–	–	–	–	–	–	–	–	–	–
5-1/8	1-1/2	5/8	–	–	–	–	880	520	590	460	830	470	560	430	790	420	530	410	780	410	520	400	710	330	460	330
		3/4	–	–	–	–	1200	590	790	590	1140	520	740	520	1100	460	670	460	1080	450	660	450	990	360	530	360
		7/8	–	–	–	–	1590	630	920	630	1520	550	810	550	1460	500	740	500	1440	490	720	490	1330	390	590	390
		1	–	–	–	–	2050	680	990	680	1930	600	890	600	1800	540	810	540	1760	530	780	530	1520	420	640	420
6-3/4	1-1/2	5/8	940	560	640	500	880	520	590	460	830	470	560	430	790	420	530	410	780	410	520	400	710	330	460	330
		3/4	1270	660	850	660	1200	590	790	590	1140	520	740	520	1100	460	700	460	1080	450	690	450	990	360	620	360
		7/8	1680	720	1090	720	1590	630	1010	630	1520	550	950	550	1460	500	900	500	1440	490	890	490	1330	390	750	390
		1	2150	770	1350	770	2050	680	1270	680	1930	600	1140	600	1800	540	1030	540	1760	530	1000	530	1520	420	810	420

(All Z values in lbs.)

1. Tabulated lateral design values (Z) for bolted connections shall be multiplied by all applicable adjustment factors (see Table 10.3.1).
2. Tabulated lateral design values (Z) are for "full diameter" (see Appendix L) bolts with bending yield strength (F_{yb}) of 45,000 psi.

Table 11D BOLTS: Reference Lateral Design Values (Z) for Single Shear (two member) Connections[1,2]

for structural glued laminated timber with 1/4" ASTM A 36 steel side plate

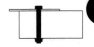

| Thickness | | | G=0.55 Southern Pine | | G=0.50 Douglas Fir-Larch | | G=0.46 Douglas Fir(S) Hem-Fir(N) | | G=0.43 Hem-Fir | | G=0.42 Spruce-Pine-Fir | | G=0.36 Spruce-Pine-Fir(S) Western Woods | |
Main Member t_m in.	Side Member t_s in.	Bolt Diameter D in.	$Z_\parallel$ lbs.	$Z_\perp$ lbs.	$Z_\parallel$ lbs.	$Z_\perp$ lbs.	$Z_\parallel$ lbs.	$Z_\perp$ lbs.	$Z_\parallel$ lbs.	$Z_\perp$ lbs.	$Z_\parallel$ lbs.	$Z_\perp$ lbs.	$Z_\parallel$ lbs.	$Z_\perp$ lbs.
2-1/2	1/4	1/2	-	-	830	410	780	380	740	350	720	340	640	290
		5/8	-	-	1050	470	980	430	920	400	910	390	800	330
		3/4	-	-	1270	530	1180	490	1110	450	1090	440	960	370
		7/8	-	-	1480	590	1370	530	1290	490	1270	480	1120	410
		1	-	-	1690	640	1570	580	1480	540	1450	530	1280	450
3	1/4	1/2	860	540	-	-	-	-	-	-	-	-	-	-
		5/8	1260	610	-	-	-	-	-	-	-	-	-	-
		3/4	1610	670	-	-	-	-	-	-	-	-	-	-
		7/8	1880	740	-	-	-	-	-	-	-	-	-	-
		1	2150	790	-	-	-	-	-	-	-	-	-	-
3-1/8	1/4	1/2	-	-	830	490	800	440	770	410	770	400	720	330
		5/8	-	-	1210	550	1160	500	1110	460	1090	450	960	380
		3/4	-	-	1540	620	1420	560	1340	510	1310	500	1150	420
		7/8	-	-	1790	680	1660	610	1560	560	1530	550	1340	470
		1	-	-	2050	740	1900	670	1780	610	1750	600	1530	510
5	1/4	5/8	1260	760	-	-	-	-	-	-	-	-	-	-
		3/4	1740	1000	-	-	-	-	-	-	-	-	-	-
		7/8	2320	1140	-	-	-	-	-	-	-	-	-	-
		1	2980	1210	-	-	-	-	-	-	-	-	-	-
5-1/8	1/4	5/8	-	-	1210	710	1160	670	1130	640	1120	630	1050	550
		3/4	-	-	1670	940	1610	840	1560	760	1550	740	1450	610
		7/8	-	-	2220	1020	2140	900	2070	830	2050	810	1920	670
		1	-	-	2860	1100	2750	990	2670	900	2640	880	2390	720
6-3/4	1/4	5/8	1260	760	1210	710	1160	670	1130	640	1120	630	1050	570
		3/4	1740	1000	1670	940	1610	890	1560	850	1550	840	1450	750
		7/8	2320	1280	2220	1210	2140	1130	2070	1060	2050	1030	1920	850
		1	2980	1590	2860	1420	2750	1270	2670	1150	2640	1120	2470	910
8-1/2	1/4	3/4	1740	1000	-	-	-	-	-	-	-	-	-	-
		7/8	2320	1280	-	-	-	-	-	-	-	-	-	-
		1	2980	1590	-	-	-	-	-	-	-	-	-	-
8-3/4	1/4	3/4	-	-	1670	940	1610	890	1560	850	1550	840	1450	750
		7/8	-	-	2220	1210	2140	1130	2070	1080	2050	1070	1920	970
		1	-	-	2860	1500	2750	1420	2670	1350	2640	1330	2470	1150
10-1/2	1/4	7/8	2320	1280	-	-	-	-	-	-	-	-	-	-
		1	2980	1590	-	-	-	-	-	-	-	-	-	-
10-3/4	1/4	7/8	-	-	2220	1210	2140	1130	2070	1080	2050	1070	1920	970
		1	-	-	2860	1500	2750	1420	2670	1350	2640	1330	2470	1200
12-1/4	1/4	7/8	-	-	2220	1210	2140	1130	2070	1080	2050	1070	1920	970
		1	-	-	2860	1500	2750	1420	2670	1350	2640	1330	2470	1200
14-1/4	1/4	1	-	-	2860	1500	2750	1420	2670	1350	2640	1330	2470	1200

1. Tabulated lateral design values (Z) for bolted connections shall be multiplied by all applicable adjustment factors (see Table 10.3.1).
2. Tabulated lateral design values (Z) are for "full diameter" bolts (see Appendix L) with bending yield strength (F_{yb}) of 45,000 psi and dowel bearing strength (F_e) of 87,000 psi for ASTM A 36 steel.

BOLTS

Table 11E BOLTS: Reference Lateral Design Values (Z) for Single Shear (two member) Connections[1,2,3,4]

for sawn lumber or SCL to concrete

Embedment Depth in Concrete t_m in.	Side Member t_s in.	Bolt Diameter D in.	G=0.67 Red Oak $Z_\parallel$ lbs.	$Z_\perp$ lbs.	G=0.55 Mixed Maple Southern Pine $Z_\parallel$ lbs.	$Z_\perp$ lbs.	G=0.50 Douglas Fir-Larch $Z_\parallel$ lbs.	$Z_\perp$ lbs.	G=0.49 Douglas Fir-Larch(N) $Z_\parallel$ lbs.	$Z_\perp$ lbs.	G=0.46 Douglas Fir(S) Hem-Fir(N) $Z_\parallel$ lbs.	$Z_\perp$ lbs.
6.0 and greater	1-1/2	1/2	770	480	680	410	650	380	640	380	620	360
		5/8	1070	660	970	580	930	530	920	520	890	470
		3/4	1450	890	1330	660	1270	590	1260	560	1230	520
		7/8	1890	960	1750	720	1690	630	1680	600	1640	550
		1	2410	1020	2250	770	2100	680	2060	650	1930	600
	1-3/4	1/2	830	510	740	430	700	400	690	390	670	370
		5/8	1160	680	1030	600	980	550	970	550	940	530
		3/4	1530	900	1390	770	1330	680	1310	660	1270	600
		7/8	1970	1120	1800	840	1730	740	1720	700	1680	640
		1	2480	1190	2290	890	2210	790	2200	750	2150	700
	2-1/2	1/2	830	590	790	520	770	470	760	460	750	440
		5/8	1290	800	1230	670	1180	610	1170	610	1120	570
		3/4	1840	1000	1630	850	1540	800	1520	780	1460	750
		7/8	2290	1240	2050	1080	1940	1020	1920	1000	1860	920
		1	2800	1520	2530	1280	2410	1130	2390	1080	2310	1000
	3-1/2	1/2	830	590	790	540	770	510	760	500	750	490
		5/8	1290	880	1230	810	1200	730	1190	720	1170	670
		3/4	1860	1190	1770	980	1720	900	1720	880	1680	830
		7/8	2540	1410	2410	1190	2320	1100	2290	1070	2200	1020
		1	3310	1670	2970	1420	2800	1330	2770	1300	2660	1260

Embedment Depth in Concrete t_m in.	Side Member t_s in.	Bolt Diameter D in.	G=0.43 Hem-Fir $Z_\parallel$ lbs.	$Z_\perp$ lbs.	G=0.42 Spruce-Pine-Fir $Z_\parallel$ lbs.	$Z_\perp$ lbs.	G=0.37 Redwood (open grain) $Z_\parallel$ lbs.	$Z_\perp$ lbs.	G=0.36 Eastern Softwoods Spruce-Pine-Fir(S) Western Cedars Western Woods $Z_\parallel$ lbs.	$Z_\perp$ lbs.	G=0.35 Northern Species $Z_\parallel$ lbs.	$Z_\perp$ lbs.
6.0 and greater	1-1/2	1/2	590	340	590	340	550	310	540	290	530	290
		5/8	860	420	850	410	810	350	800	330	780	320
		3/4	1200	460	1190	450	1130	370	1120	360	1100	350
		7/8	1580	500	1540	490	1360	410	1330	390	1280	370
		1	1800	540	1760	530	1560	440	1520	420	1460	410
	1-3/4	1/2	640	360	630	350	580	320	580	310	560	310
		5/8	910	490	900	480	840	400	830	380	810	370
		3/4	1230	540	1220	530	1160	430	1140	420	1120	410
		7/8	1630	580	1610	570	1540	470	1520	460	1490	430
		1	2090	630	2060	610	1820	510	1770	490	1710	470
	2-1/2	1/2	730	410	730	400	700	360	690	340	680	340
		5/8	1070	540	1060	530	980	480	960	470	940	460
		3/4	1400	710	1380	700	1290	620	1270	600	1240	580
		7/8	1790	830	1770	810	1660	680	1640	660	1600	610
		1	2230	900	2210	880	2080	730	2060	700	2030	680
	3-1/2	1/2	730	470	730	470	700	430	690	410	690	400
		5/8	1140	620	1140	610	1090	550	1080	530	1070	520
		3/4	1650	780	1640	770	1540	680	1510	670	1470	660
		7/8	2100	960	2070	950	1910	870	1880	850	1840	820
		1	2550	1190	2520	1180	2340	1020	2310	980	2260	950

1. Tabulated lateral design values (Z) for bolted connections shall be multiplied by all applicable adjustment factors (see Table 10.3.1).
2. Tabulated lateral design values (Z) are for "full diameter" bolts (see Appendix L) with bending yield strength (F_{yb}) of 45,000 psi.
3. Tabulated lateral design values (Z) are based on dowel bearing strength (F_e) of 7,500 psi for concrete with minimum $f_c' = 2,500$ psi.
4. Six inch anchor embedment assumed.

DOWEL-TYPE FASTENERS

11

BOLTS

Table 11F BOLTS: Reference Lateral Design Values (Z) for Double Shear (three member) Connections[1,2]

for sawn lumber or SCL with all members of identical specific gravity

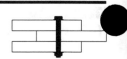

t_m (in.)	t_s (in.)	D (in.)	G=0.67 Red Oak $Z_{\parallel}$ lbs.	$Z_{s\perp}$ lbs.	$Z_{m\perp}$ lbs.	G=0.55 Mixed Maple Southern Pine $Z_{\parallel}$ lbs.	$Z_{s\perp}$ lbs.	$Z_{m\perp}$ lbs.	G=0.50 Douglas Fir-Larch $Z_{\parallel}$ lbs.	$Z_{s\perp}$ lbs.	$Z_{m\perp}$ lbs.	G=0.49 Douglas Fir-Larch(N) $Z_{\parallel}$ lbs.	$Z_{s\perp}$ lbs.	$Z_{m\perp}$ lbs.	G=0.46 Douglas Fir(S) Hem-Fir(N) $Z_{\parallel}$ lbs.	$Z_{s\perp}$ lbs.	$Z_{m\perp}$ lbs.
1-1/2	1-1/2	1/2	1410	960	730	1150	800	550	1050	730	470	1030	720	460	970	680	420
		5/8	1760	1310	810	1440	1130	610	1310	1040	530	1290	1030	520	1210	940	470
		3/4	2110	1690	890	1730	1330	660	1580	1170	590	1550	1130	560	1450	1040	520
		7/8	2460	1920	960	2020	1440	720	1840	1260	630	1800	1210	600	1690	1100	550
		1	2810	2040	1020	2310	1530	770	2100	1350	680	2060	1290	650	1930	1200	600
1-3/4	1-3/4	1/2	1640	1030	850	1350	850	640	1230	770	550	1200	750	530	1130	710	490
		5/8	2050	1370	940	1680	1160	710	1530	1070	610	1500	1060	600	1410	1000	550
		3/4	2460	1810	1040	2020	1550	770	1840	1370	680	1800	1310	660	1690	1210	600
		7/8	2870	2240	1120	2350	1680	840	2140	1470	740	2110	1410	700	1970	1290	640
		1	3280	2380	1190	2690	1790	890	2450	1580	790	2410	1510	750	2250	1400	700
2-1/2	1-1/2	1/2	1530	960	1120	1320	800	910	1230	730	790	1210	720	760	1160	680	700
		5/8	2150	1310	1340	1870	1130	1020	1760	1040	880	1740	1030	860	1660	940	780
		3/4	2890	1770	1480	2550	1330	1110	2400	1170	980	2380	1130	940	2280	1040	860
		7/8	3780	1920	1600	3360	1440	1200	3060	1260	1050	3010	1210	1010	2820	1100	920
		1	4690	2040	1700	3840	1530	1280	3500	1350	1130	3440	1290	1080	3220	1200	1000
3-1/2	1-1/2	1/2	1530	960	1120	1320	800	940	1230	730	860	1210	720	850	1160	680	810
		5/8	2150	1310	1510	1870	1130	1290	1760	1040	1190	1740	1030	1170	1660	940	1090
		3/4	2890	1770	1980	2550	1330	1550	2400	1170	1370	2380	1130	1310	2280	1040	1210
		7/8	3780	1920	2240	3360	1440	1680	3180	1260	1470	3150	1210	1410	3030	1100	1290
		1	4820	2040	2380	4310	1530	1790	4090	1350	1580	4050	1290	1510	3860	1200	1400
	1-3/4	1/2	1660	1030	1180	1430	850	1030	1330	770	940	1310	750	920	1250	710	870
		5/8	2310	1370	1630	1990	1160	1380	1860	1070	1230	1840	1060	1200	1760	1000	1090
		3/4	3060	1810	2070	2670	1550	1550	2510	1370	1370	2480	1310	1310	2370	1210	1210
		7/8	3940	2240	2240	3470	1680	1680	3270	1470	1470	3240	1410	1410	3110	1290	1290
		1	4960	2380	2380	4400	1790	1790	4170	1580	1580	4120	1510	1510	3970	1400	1400
	3-1/2	1/2	1660	1180	1180	1500	1040	1040	1430	970	970	1420	960	960	1370	920	920
		5/8	2590	1770	1770	2340	1560	1420	2240	1410	1230	2220	1390	1200	2150	1290	1090
		3/4	3730	2380	2070	3380	1910	1550	3220	1750	1370	3190	1700	1310	3090	1610	1210
		7/8	5080	2820	2240	4600	2330	1680	4290	2130	1470	4210	2070	1410	3940	1960	1290
		1	6560	3340	2380	5380	2780	1790	4900	2580	1580	4810	2520	1510	4510	2410	1400
5-1/4	1-1/2	5/8	2150	1310	1510	1870	1130	1290	1760	1040	1190	1740	1030	1170	1660	940	1110
		3/4	2890	1770	1980	2550	1330	1690	2400	1170	1580	2380	1130	1550	2280	1040	1480
		7/8	3780	1920	2520	3360	1440	2170	3180	1260	2030	3150	1210	1990	3030	1100	1900
		1	4820	2040	3120	4310	1530	2680	4090	1350	2360	4050	1290	2260	3860	1200	2100
	1-3/4	5/8	2310	1370	1630	1990	1160	1380	1860	1070	1270	1840	1060	1250	1760	1000	1180
		3/4	3060	1810	2110	2670	1550	1790	2510	1370	1660	2480	1310	1630	2370	1210	1550
		7/8	3940	2240	2640	3470	1680	2260	3270	1470	2100	3240	1410	2060	3110	1290	1930
		1	4960	2380	3240	4400	1790	2680	4170	1580	2360	4120	1510	2260	3970	1400	2100
	3-1/2	5/8	2590	1770	1770	2340	1560	1560	2240	1410	1460	2220	1390	1450	2150	1290	1390
		3/4	3730	2380	2480	3380	1910	2180	3220	1750	2050	3190	1700	1970	3090	1610	1810
		7/8	5080	2820	3290	4600	2330	2530	4390	2130	2210	4350	2070	2110	4130	1960	1930
		1	6630	3340	3570	5740	2780	2360	5330	2580	2360	5250	2520	2260	4990	2410	2100
5-1/2	1-1/2	5/8	2150	1310	1510	1870	1130	1290	1760	1040	1190	1740	1030	1170	1660	940	1110
		3/4	2890	1770	1980	2550	1330	1690	2400	1170	1580	2380	1130	1550	2280	1040	1480
		7/8	3780	1920	2520	3360	1440	2170	3180	1260	2030	3150	1210	1990	3030	1100	1900
		1	4820	2040	3120	4310	1530	2700	4090	1350	2480	4050	1290	2370	3860	1200	2200
	3-1/2	5/8	2590	1770	1770	2340	1560	1560	2240	1410	1460	2220	1390	1450	2150	1290	1390
		3/4	3730	2380	2480	3380	1910	2180	3220	1750	2050	3190	1700	2020	3090	1610	1900
		7/8	5080	2820	3290	4600	2330	2650	4390	2130	2310	4350	2070	2210	4130	1960	2020
		1	6630	3340	3740	5740	2780	2810	5330	2580	2480	5250	2520	2370	4990	2410	2200
7-1/2	1-1/2	5/8	2150	1310	1510	1870	1130	1290	1760	1040	1190	1740	1030	1170	1660	940	1110
		3/4	2890	1770	1980	2550	1330	1690	2400	1170	1580	2380	1130	1550	2280	1040	1480
		7/8	3780	1920	2520	3360	1440	2170	3180	1260	2030	3150	1210	1990	3030	1100	1900
		1	4820	2040	3120	4310	1530	2700	4090	1350	2530	4050	1290	2480	3860	1200	2390
	3-1/2	5/8	2590	1770	1770	2340	1560	1560	2240	1410	1460	2220	1390	1450	2150	1290	1390
		3/4	3730	2380	2480	3380	1910	2180	3220	1750	2050	3190	1700	2020	3090	1610	1940
		7/8	5080	2820	3290	4600	2330	2720	4390	2130	2720	4350	2070	2670	4130	1960	2560
		1	6630	3340	4190	5740	2780	3680	5330	2580	3380	5250	2520	3230	4990	2410	3000

1. Tabulated lateral design values (Z) for bolted connections shall be multiplied by all applicable adjustment factors (see Table 10.3.1).
2. Tabulated lateral design values (Z) are for "full diameter" bolts (see Appendix L) with bending yield strength (F_{yb}) of 45,000 psi.

Table 11F (Cont.) BOLTS: Reference Lateral Design Values (Z) for Double Shear (three member) Connections[1,2]

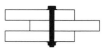

for sawn lumber or SCL with all members of identical specific gravity

Main Member t_m in.	Side Member t_s in.	Bolt Diameter D in.	G=0.43 Hem-Fir $Z_{||}$ lbs.	$Z_{s\perp}$ lbs.	$Z_{m\perp}$ lbs.	G=0.42 Spruce-Pine-Fir $Z_{||}$ lbs.	$Z_{s\perp}$ lbs.	$Z_{m\perp}$ lbs.	G=0.37 Redwood (open grain) $Z_{||}$ lbs.	$Z_{s\perp}$ lbs.	$Z_{m\perp}$ lbs.	G=0.36 Eastern Softwoods Spruce-Pine-Fir(S) Western Cedars Western Woods $Z_{||}$ lbs.	$Z_{s\perp}$ lbs.	$Z_{m\perp}$ lbs.	G=0.35 Northern Species $Z_{||}$ lbs.	$Z_{s\perp}$ lbs.	$Z_{m\perp}$ lbs.
1-1/2	1-1/2	1/2	900	650	380	880	640	370	780	580	310	760	560	290	730	550	290
		5/8	1130	840	420	1100	830	410	970	690	350	950	660	330	910	640	320
		3/4	1350	920	460	1320	900	450	1170	740	370	1140	720	360	1100	700	350
		7/8	1580	1000	500	1540	970	490	1360	810	410	1330	790	390	1280	740	370
		1	1800	1080	540	1760	1050	530	1560	870	440	1520	840	420	1460	810	410
1-3/4	1-3/4	1/2	1050	670	450	1030	660	430	910	590	360	890	580	340	850	570	330
		5/8	1310	950	490	1290	940	480	1130	810	400	1110	770	380	1070	740	370
		3/4	1580	1080	540	1540	1050	530	1360	870	430	1330	840	420	1280	810	410
		7/8	1840	1160	580	1800	1130	570	1590	950	470	1550	920	460	1490	860	430
		1	2100	1260	630	2060	1230	610	1820	1020	510	1770	980	490	1710	950	470
2-1/2	1-1/2	1/2	1100	650	640	1080	640	610	990	580	510	980	560	490	950	550	480
		5/8	1590	840	700	1570	830	690	1450	690	580	1430	660	550	1390	640	530
		3/4	2190	920	770	2160	900	750	1950	740	620	1900	720	600	1830	700	580
		7/8	2630	1000	830	2570	970	810	2270	810	680	2210	790	660	2130	740	610
		1	3000	1080	900	2940	1050	880	2590	870	730	2530	840	700	2440	810	680
3-1/2	1-1/2	1/2	1100	650	760	1080	640	740	990	580	670	980	560	660	950	550	640
		5/8	1590	840	980	1570	830	960	1450	690	810	1430	660	770	1390	640	740
		3/4	2190	920	1080	2160	900	1050	2010	740	870	1990	720	840	1940	700	810
		7/8	2920	1000	1160	2880	970	1130	2690	810	950	2660	790	920	2560	740	860
		1	3600	1080	1260	3530	1050	1230	3110	870	1020	3040	840	980	2930	810	950
3-1/2	1-3/4	1/2	1180	670	820	1160	660	800	1060	590	720	1040	580	680	1010	570	670
		5/8	1670	950	980	1650	940	960	1510	810	810	1490	770	770	1450	740	740
		3/4	2270	1080	1080	2240	1050	1050	2070	870	870	2040	840	840	1990	810	810
		7/8	2980	1160	1160	2950	1130	1130	2740	950	950	2700	920	920	2640	860	860
		1	3820	1260	1260	3770	1230	1230	3520	1020	1020	3480	980	980	3410	950	950
	3-1/2	1/2	1330	880	880	1310	870	860	1230	800	720	1220	780	680	1200	760	670
		5/8	2070	1190	980	2050	1170	960	1930	1030	810	1900	1000	770	1870	970	740
		3/4	2980	1490	1080	2950	1460	1050	2720	1290	870	2660	1270	840	2560	1240	810
		7/8	3680	1840	1160	3600	1810	1130	3180	1640	950	3100	1610	920	2990	1550	860
		1	4200	2280	1260	4110	2240	1230	3630	2030	1020	3540	1960	980	3410	1890	950
5-1/4	1-1/2	5/8	1590	840	1050	1570	830	1040	1450	690	940	1430	660	920	1390	640	900
		3/4	2190	920	1400	2160	900	1380	2010	740	1250	1990	720	1230	1940	700	1210
		7/8	2920	1000	1750	2880	970	1700	2690	810	1420	2660	790	1380	2560	740	1290
		1	3600	1080	1890	3530	1050	1840	3110	870	1520	3040	840	1470	2930	810	1420
	1-3/4	5/8	1670	950	1110	1650	940	1100	1510	810	990	1490	770	970	1450	740	940
		3/4	2270	1080	1460	2240	1050	1440	2070	870	1300	2040	840	1260	1990	810	1220
		7/8	2980	1160	1750	2950	1130	1700	2740	950	1420	2700	920	1380	2640	860	1290
		1	3820	1260	1890	3770	1230	1840	3520	1020	1520	3480	980	1470	3410	950	1420
	3-1/2	5/8	2070	1190	1320	2050	1170	1310	1930	1030	1210	1900	1000	1150	1870	970	1120
		3/4	2980	1490	1610	2950	1460	1580	2770	1290	1300	2740	1270	1260	2660	1240	1220
		7/8	3900	1840	1750	3840	1810	1700	3480	1640	1420	3410	1610	1380	3320	1550	1290
		1	4730	2280	1890	4660	2240	1840	4240	2030	1520	4170	1960	1470	4050	1890	1420
5-1/2	1-1/2	5/8	1590	840	1050	1570	830	1040	1450	690	940	1430	660	920	1390	640	900
		3/4	2190	920	1400	2160	900	1380	2010	740	1250	1990	720	1230	1940	700	1210
		7/8	2920	1000	1800	2880	970	1780	2690	810	1490	2660	790	1440	2560	740	1350
		1	3600	1080	1980	3530	1050	1930	3110	870	1600	3040	840	1540	2930	810	1490
	3-1/2	5/8	2070	1190	1320	2050	1170	1310	1930	1030	1210	1900	1000	1180	1870	970	1160
		3/4	2980	1490	1690	2950	1460	1650	2770	1290	1360	2740	1270	1320	2660	1240	1280
		7/8	3900	1840	1830	3840	1810	1780	3480	1640	1490	3410	1610	1440	3320	1550	1350
		1	4730	2280	1980	4660	2240	1930	4240	2030	1600	4170	1960	1540	4050	1890	1490
7-1/2	1-1/2	5/8	1590	840	1050	1570	830	1040	1450	690	940	1430	660	920	1390	640	900
		3/4	2190	920	1400	2160	900	1380	2010	740	1250	1990	720	1230	1940	700	1210
		7/8	2920	1000	1800	2880	970	1780	2690	810	1630	2660	790	1600	2560	740	1550
		1	3600	1080	2270	3530	1050	2240	3110	870	2040	3040	840	2010	2930	810	1970
	3-1/2	5/8	2070	1190	1320	2050	1170	1310	1930	1030	1210	1900	1000	1180	1870	970	1160
		3/4	2980	1490	1850	2950	1460	1820	2770	1290	1670	2740	1270	1650	2660	1240	1620
		7/8	3900	1840	2450	3840	1810	2420	3480	1640	2030	3410	1610	1970	3320	1550	1840
		1	4730	2280	2700	4660	2240	2630	4240	2030	2180	4170	1960	2100	4050	1890	2030

1. Tabulated lateral design values (Z) for bolted connections shall be multiplied by all applicable adjustment factors (see Table 10.3.1).
2. Tabulated lateral design values (Z) are for "full diameter" bolts (see Appendix L) with bending yield strength (F_{yb}) of 45,000 psi.

DOWEL-TYPE FASTENERS

11

Table 11G BOLTS: Reference Lateral Design Values (Z) for Double Shear (three member) Connections[1,2]

for sawn lumber or SCL with 1/4" ASTM A 36 steel side plate

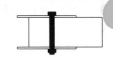

Main Member t_m in.	Side Member t_s in.	Bolt Diameter D in.	G=0.67 Red Oak $Z_{\parallel}$ lbs.	$Z_{\perp}$ lbs.	G=0.55 Mixed Maple Southern Pine $Z_{\parallel}$ lbs.	$Z_{\perp}$ lbs.	G=0.50 Douglas Fir-Larch $Z_{\parallel}$ lbs.	$Z_{\perp}$ lbs.	G=0.49 Douglas Fir-Larch (N) $Z_{\parallel}$ lbs.	$Z_{\perp}$ lbs.	G=0.46 Douglas Fir(S) Hem-Fir(N) $Z_{\parallel}$ lbs.	$Z_{\perp}$ lbs.	G=0.43 Hem-Fir $Z_{\parallel}$ lbs.	$Z_{\perp}$ lbs.	G=0.42 Spruce-Pine-Fir $Z_{\parallel}$ lbs.	$Z_{\perp}$ lbs.	G=0.37 Redwood (open grain) $Z_{\parallel}$ lbs.	$Z_{\perp}$ lbs.	G=0.36 Eastern Softwoods Spruce-Pine-Fir(S) Western Cedars Western Woods $Z_{\parallel}$ lbs.	$Z_{\perp}$ lbs.	G=0.35 Northern Species $Z_{\parallel}$ lbs.	$Z_{\perp}$ lbs.
1-1/2	1/4	1/2	1410	730	1150	550	1050	470	1030	460	970	420	900	380	880	370	780	310	760	290	730	290
		5/8	1760	810	1440	610	1310	530	1290	520	1210	470	1130	420	1100	410	970	350	950	330	910	320
		3/4	2110	890	1730	660	1580	590	1550	560	1450	520	1350	460	1320	450	1170	370	1140	360	1100	350
		7/8	2460	960	2020	720	1840	630	1800	600	1690	550	1580	500	1540	490	1360	410	1330	390	1280	370
		1	2810	1020	2310	770	2100	680	2060	650	1930	600	1800	540	1760	530	1560	440	1520	420	1460	410
1-3/4	1/4	1/2	1640	850	1350	640	1230	550	1200	530	1130	490	1050	450	1030	430	910	360	890	340	850	330
		5/8	2050	940	1680	710	1530	610	1500	600	1410	550	1310	490	1290	480	1130	400	1110	380	1070	370
		3/4	2460	1040	2020	770	1840	680	1800	660	1690	600	1580	540	1540	530	1360	430	1330	420	1280	410
		7/8	2870	1120	2350	840	2140	740	2110	700	1970	640	1840	580	1800	570	1590	470	1550	460	1490	430
		1	3280	1190	2690	890	2450	790	2410	750	2250	700	2100	630	2060	610	1820	510	1770	490	1710	470
2-1/2	1/4	1/2	1870	1210	1720	910	1650	790	1640	760	1590	700	1500	640	1470	610	1300	510	1270	490	1220	480
		5/8	2740	1340	2400	1020	2190	880	2150	860	2010	780	1880	700	1840	690	1620	580	1580	550	1520	530
		3/4	3520	1480	2880	1110	2630	980	2580	940	2410	860	2250	770	2200	750	1950	620	1900	600	1830	580
		7/8	4100	1600	3360	1200	3060	1050	3010	1010	2820	920	2630	830	2570	810	2270	680	2210	660	2130	610
		1	4690	1700	3840	1280	3500	1130	3440	1080	3220	1000	3000	900	2940	880	2590	730	2530	700	2440	680
3-1/2	1/4	1/2	1870	1240	1720	1030	1650	1030	1640	1010	1590	970	1540	890	1530	860	1450	720	1430	680	1410	670
		5/8	2740	1720	2510	1420	2410	1230	2390	1200	2330	1090	2260	980	2230	960	2110	810	2090	770	2060	740
		3/4	3800	2070	3480	1550	3340	1370	3320	1310	3220	1210	3120	1080	3080	1050	2720	870	2660	840	2560	810
		7/8	5060	2240	4630	1680	4290	1470	4210	1410	3940	1290	3680	1160	3600	1130	3180	950	3100	920	2990	860
		1	6520	2380	5380	1790	4900	1580	4810	1510	4510	1400	4200	1260	4110	1230	3630	1020	3540	980	3410	950
5-1/4	1/4	5/8	2740	1720	2510	1510	2410	1420	2390	1400	2330	1340	2260	1280	2230	1270	2110	1170	2090	1140	2060	1120
		3/4	3800	2290	3480	2000	3340	1890	3320	1850	3220	1780	3120	1610	3090	1580	2920	1300	2890	1260	2840	1220
		7/8	5060	2930	4630	2530	4440	2210	4410	2110	4280	1930	4150	1750	4110	1700	3880	1420	3840	1380	3770	1290
		1	6520	3570	5960	2680	5720	2360	5670	2260	5510	2100	5330	1890	5280	1840	4990	1520	4930	1470	4850	1420
5-1/2	1/4	5/8	2740	1720	2510	1510	2410	1420	2390	1400	2330	1340	2260	1280	2230	1270	2110	1170	2090	1140	2060	1120
		3/4	3800	2290	3480	2000	3340	1890	3320	1850	3220	1780	3120	1690	3090	1650	2920	1360	2890	1320	2840	1280
		7/8	5060	2930	4630	2570	4440	2310	4410	2210	4280	2020	4150	1830	4110	1780	3880	1490	3840	1440	3770	1350
		1	6520	3640	5960	2810	5720	2480	5670	2370	5510	2200	5330	1980	5280	1930	4990	1600	4930	1540	4850	1420
7-1/2	1/4	5/8	2740	1720	2510	1510	2410	1420	2390	1400	2330	1340	2260	1280	2230	1270	2110	1170	2090	1140	2060	1120
		3/4	3800	2290	3480	2000	3340	1890	3320	1850	3220	1780	3120	1690	3090	1670	2920	1530	2890	1500	2840	1480
		7/8	5060	2930	4630	2570	4440	2410	4410	2360	4280	2260	4150	2160	4110	2130	3880	1960	3840	1930	3770	1840
		1	6520	3640	5960	3180	5720	3000	5670	2940	5510	2840	5330	2700	5280	2630	4990	2180	4930	2100	4850	2030
9-1/2	1/4	3/4	3800	2290	3480	2000	3340	1890	3320	1850	3220	1780	3120	1690	3090	1670	2920	1530	2890	1500	2840	1480
		7/8	5060	2930	4630	2570	4440	2410	4410	2360	4280	2260	4150	2160	4110	2130	3880	1960	3840	1930	3770	1870
		1	6520	3640	5960	3180	5720	3000	5670	2940	5510	2840	5330	2700	5280	2660	4990	2440	4930	2400	4850	2350
11-1/2	1/4	7/8	5060	2930	4630	2570	4440	2410	4410	2360	4280	2260	4150	2160	4110	2130	3880	1960	3840	1930	3770	1870
		1	6520	3640	5960	3180	5720	3000	5670	2940	5510	2840	5330	2700	5280	2660	4990	2440	4930	2400	4850	2350
13-1/2	1/4	1	6520	3640	5960	3180	5720	3000	5670	2940	5510	2840	5330	2700	5280	2660	4990	2440	4930	2400	4850	2350

1. Tabulated lateral design values (Z) for bolted connections shall be multiplied by all applicable adjustment factors (see Table 10.3.1).

2. Tabulated lateral design values (Z) are for "full diameter" bolts (see Appendix L) with bending yield strength (F_{yb}) of 45,000 psi and a dowel bearing strength (F_e) of 87,000 psi for ASTM A 36 steel.

Table 11H BOLTS: Reference Lateral Design Values (Z) for Double Shear (three member) Connections[1,2]

for structural glued laminated timber main member with sawn lumber side member of identical species

Thickness			G=0.55 Southern Pine			G=0.50 Douglas Fir-Larch			G=0.46 Douglas Fir(S) Hem-Fir(N)			G=0.43 Hem-Fir			G=0.42 Spruce-Pine-Fir			G=0.36 Spruce-Pine-Fir(S) Western Woods		
Main Member	Side Member	Bolt Diameter																		
t_m in.	t_s in.	D in.	$Z_\parallel$ lbs.	$Z_{s\perp}$ lbs.	$Z_{m\perp}$ lbs.	$Z_\parallel$ lbs.	$Z_{s\perp}$ lbs.	$Z_{m\perp}$ lbs.	$Z_\parallel$ lbs.	$Z_{s\perp}$ lbs.	$Z_{m\perp}$ lbs.	$Z_\parallel$ lbs.	$Z_{s\perp}$ lbs.	$Z_{m\perp}$ lbs.	$Z_\parallel$ lbs.	$Z_{s\perp}$ lbs.	$Z_{m\perp}$ lbs.	$Z_\parallel$ lbs.	$Z_{s\perp}$ lbs.	$Z_{m\perp}$ lbs.
2-1/2	1-1/2	1/2	-	-	-	1230	730	790	1160	680	700	1100	650	640	1080	640	610	980	560	490
		5/8	-	-	-	1760	1040	880	1660	940	780	1590	840	700	1570	830	690	1430	660	550
		3/4	-	-	-	2400	1170	980	2280	1040	860	2190	920	770	2160	900	750	1900	720	600
		7/8	-	-	-	3060	1260	1050	2820	1100	920	2630	1000	830	2570	970	810	2210	790	660
		1	-	-	-	3500	1350	1130	3220	1200	1000	3000	1080	900	2940	1050	880	2530	840	700
3	1-1/2	1/2	1320	800	940	-	-	-	-	-	-	-	-	-	-	-	-	-	-	-
		5/8	1870	1130	1220	-	-	-	-	-	-	-	-	-	-	-	-	-	-	-
		3/4	2550	1330	1330	-	-	-	-	-	-	-	-	-	-	-	-	-	-	-
		7/8	3360	1440	1440	-	-	-	-	-	-	-	-	-	-	-	-	-	-	-
		1	4310	1530	1530	-	-	-	-	-	-	-	-	-	-	-	-	-	-	-
3-1/8	1-1/2	1/2	-	-	-	1230	730	860	1160	680	810	1100	650	760	1080	640	740	980	560	610
		5/8	-	-	-	1760	1040	1090	1660	940	980	1590	840	880	1570	830	860	1430	660	680
		3/4	-	-	-	2400	1170	1220	2280	1040	1080	2190	920	960	2160	900	940	1990	720	750
		7/8	-	-	-	3180	1260	1310	3030	1100	1150	2920	1000	1040	2880	970	1010	2660	790	820
		1	-	-	-	4090	1350	1410	3860	1200	1250	3600	1080	1130	3530	1050	1090	3040	840	880
5	1-1/2	5/8	1870	1130	1290	-	-	-	-	-	-	-	-	-	-	-	-	-	-	-
		3/4	2550	1330	1690	-	-	-	-	-	-	-	-	-	-	-	-	-	-	-
		7/8	3360	1440	2170	-	-	-	-	-	-	-	-	-	-	-	-	-	-	-
		1	4310	1530	2550	-	-	-	-	-	-	-	-	-	-	-	-	-	-	-
5-1/8	1-1/2	5/8	-	-	-	1760	1040	1190	1660	940	1110	1590	840	1050	1570	830	1040	1430	660	920
		3/4	-	-	-	2400	1170	1580	2280	1040	1480	2190	920	1400	2160	900	1380	1990	720	1230
		7/8	-	-	-	3180	1260	2030	3030	1100	1880	2920	1000	1700	2880	970	1660	2660	790	1350
		1	-	-	-	4090	1350	2310	3860	1200	2050	3600	1080	1850	3530	1050	1790	3040	840	1440
6-3/4	1-1/2	5/8	1870	1130	1290	1760	1040	1190	1660	940	1110	1590	840	1050	1570	830	1040	1430	660	920
		3/4	2550	1330	1690	2400	1170	1580	2280	1040	1480	2190	920	1400	2160	900	1380	1990	720	1230
		7/8	3360	1440	2170	3180	1260	2030	3030	1100	1900	2920	1000	1800	2880	970	1780	2660	790	1600
		1	4310	1530	2700	4090	1350	2530	3860	1200	2390	3600	1080	2270	3530	1050	2240	3040	840	1890

1. Tabulated lateral design values (Z) for bolted connections shall be multiplied by all applicable adjustment factors (see Table 10.3.1).
2. Tabulated lateral design values (Z) are for "full diameter" bolts (see Appendix L) with bending yield strength (F_{yb}) of 45,000 psi.

Table 11I BOLTS: Reference Lateral Design Values (Z) for Double Shear (three member) Connections[1,2]

for structural glued laminated timber with 1/4" ASTM A 36 steel side plate

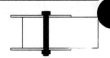

Main Member t_m in.	Side Member t_s in.	Bolt Diameter D in.	G=0.55 Southern Pine $Z_{\parallel}$ lbs.	$Z_{\perp}$ lbs.	G=0.50 Douglas Fir-Larch $Z_{\parallel}$ lbs.	$Z_{\perp}$ lbs.	G=0.46 Douglas Fir(S) Hem-Fir(N) $Z_{\parallel}$ lbs.	$Z_{\perp}$ lbs.	G=0.43 Hem-Fir $Z_{\parallel}$ lbs.	$Z_{\perp}$ lbs.	G=0.42 Spruce-Pine-Fir $Z_{\parallel}$ lbs.	$Z_{\perp}$ lbs.	G=0.36 Spruce-Pine-Fir(S) Western Woods $Z_{\parallel}$ lbs.	$Z_{\perp}$ lbs.
2-1/2	1/4	1/2	-	-	1650	790	1590	700	1500	640	1470	610	1270	490
		5/8	-	-	2190	880	2010	780	1880	700	1840	690	1580	550
		3/4	-	-	2630	980	2410	860	2250	770	2200	750	1900	600
		7/8	-	-	3060	1050	2820	920	2630	830	2570	810	2210	660
		1	-	-	3500	1130	3220	1000	3000	900	2940	880	2530	700
3	1/4	1/2	1720	1100	-	-	-	-	-	-	-	-	-	-
		5/8	2510	1220	-	-	-	-	-	-	-	-	-	-
		3/4	3460	1330	-	-	-	-	-	-	-	-	-	-
		7/8	4040	1440	-	-	-	-	-	-	-	-	-	-
		1	4610	1530	-	-	-	-	-	-	-	-	-	-
3-1/8	1/4	1/2	-	-	1650	980	1590	880	1540	800	1530	770	1430	610
		5/8	-	-	2410	1090	2330	980	2260	880	2230	860	1980	680
		3/4	-	-	3280	1220	3020	1080	2810	960	2750	940	2370	750
		7/8	-	-	3830	1310	3520	1150	3280	1040	3210	1010	2770	820
		1	-	-	4380	1410	4020	1250	3750	1130	3670	1090	3160	880
5	1/4	5/8	2510	1510	-	-	-	-	-	-	-	-	-	-
		3/4	3480	2000	-	-	-	-	-	-	-	-	-	-
		7/8	4630	2410	-	-	-	-	-	-	-	-	-	-
		1	5960	2550	-	-	-	-	-	-	-	-	-	-
5-1/8	1/4	5/8	-	-	2410	1420	2330	1340	2260	1280	2230	1270	2090	1120
		3/4	-	-	3340	1890	3220	1770	3120	1580	3090	1540	2890	1230
		7/8	-	-	4440	2150	4280	1880	4150	1700	4110	1660	3840	1350
		1	-	-	5720	2310	5510	2050	5330	1850	5280	1790	4930	1440
6-3/4	1/4	5/8	2510	1510	2410	1420	2330	1340	2260	1280	2230	1270	2090	1140
		3/4	3480	2000	3340	1890	3220	1780	3120	1690	3090	1670	2890	1500
		7/8	4630	2570	4440	2410	4280	2260	4150	2160	4110	2130	3840	1770
		1	5960	3180	5720	3000	5510	2700	5330	2430	5280	2360	4930	1890
8-1/2	1/4	3/4	3480	2000	-	-	-	-	-	-	-	-	-	-
		7/8	4630	2570	-	-	-	-	-	-	-	-	-	-
		1	5960	3180	-	-	-	-	-	-	-	-	-	-
8-3/4	1/4	3/4	-	-	3340	1890	3220	1780	3120	1690	3090	1670	2890	1500
		7/8	-	-	4440	2410	4280	2260	4150	2160	4110	2130	3840	1930
		1	-	-	5720	3000	5510	2840	5330	2700	5280	2660	4930	2400
10-1/2	1/4	7/8	4630	2570	-	-	-	-	-	-	-	-	-	-
		1	5960	3180	-	-	-	-	-	-	-	-	-	-
10-3/4	1/4	7/8	-	-	4440	2410	4280	2260	4150	2160	4110	2130	3840	1930
		1	-	-	5720	3000	5510	2840	5330	2700	5280	2660	4930	2400
12-1/4	1/4	7/8	-	-	4440	2410	4280	2260	4150	2160	4110	2130	3840	1930
		1	-	-	5720	3000	5510	2840	5330	2700	5280	2660	4930	2400
14-1/4	1/4	1	-	-	5720	3000	5510	2840	5330	2700	5280	2660	4930	2400

1. Tabulated lateral design values (Z) for bolted connections shall be multiplied by all applicable adjustment factors (see Table 10.3.1).
2. Tabulated lateral design values (Z) are for "full diameter" bolts (see Appendix L) with bending yield strength (F_{yb}) of 45,000 psi and dowel bearing strength (F_e) of 87,000 psi for ASTM A 36 steel.

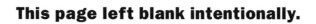

This page left blank intentionally.

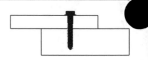

Table 11J LAG SCREWS: Reference Lateral Design Values (Z) for Single Shear (two member) Connections[1,2,3]

for sawn lumber or SCL with both members of identical specific gravity

Side Member Thickness	Lag Screw Diameter	G=0.67 Red Oak				G=0.55 Mixed Maple Southern Pine				G=0.50 Douglas Fir-Larch				G=0.49 Douglas Fir-Larch(N)				G=0.46 Douglas Fir(S) Hem-Fir(N)			
t_s	D	$Z_{\parallel}$	$Z_{s\perp}$	$Z_{m\perp}$	$Z_{\perp}$	$Z_{\parallel}$	$Z_{s\perp}$	$Z_{m\perp}$	$Z_{\perp}$	$Z_{\parallel}$	$Z_{s\perp}$	$Z_{m\perp}$	$Z_{\perp}$	$Z_{\parallel}$	$Z_{s\perp}$	$Z_{m\perp}$	$Z_{\perp}$	$Z_{\parallel}$	$Z_{s\perp}$	$Z_{m\perp}$	$Z_{\perp}$
in.	in.	lbs.	lbs.	lbs.	lbs.	lbs.	lbs.	lbs.	lbs.	lbs.	lbs.	lbs.	lbs.	lbs.	lbs.	lbs.	lbs.	lbs.	lbs.	lbs.	lbs.
1/2	1/4	150	110	110	110	130	90	100	90	120	90	90	80	120	90	90	80	110	80	90	80
	5/16	170	130	130	120	150	110	120	100	150	100	110	100	140	100	110	90	140	100	100	90
	3/8	180	130	130	120	160	110	110	100	150	100	110	90	150	90	110	90	140	90	100	90
5/8	1/4	160	120	130	120	140	100	110	100	130	90	100	90	130	90	100	90	120	90	90	80
	5/16	190	140	140	130	160	110	120	110	150	110	110	100	150	100	110	100	150	100	110	90
	3/8	190	130	140	120	170	110	120	100	160	100	110	100	160	100	110	90	150	100	110	90
3/4	1/4	180	140	140	130	150	110	110	110	140	100	110	100	140	100	110	90	130	90	100	90
	5/16	210	150	160	140	180	120	130	120	170	110	120	110	160	110	120	100	160	100	110	100
	3/8	210	140	160	130	180	120	130	110	170	110	120	100	170	110	120	100	160	110	110	90
1	1/4	180	140	140	140	160	120	120	120	150	120	120	110	150	110	110	110	150	110	110	100
	5/16	230	170	170	160	210	140	150	130	190	130	140	120	190	120	140	120	180	120	130	110
	3/8	230	160	170	160	210	130	150	120	200	120	140	110	190	120	140	110	180	110	130	100
1-1/4	1/4	180	140	140	140	160	120	120	120	150	120	120	110	150	110	110	110	150	110	110	100
	5/16	230	170	170	160	210	150	150	140	200	140	140	130	200	140	140	130	190	130	140	120
	3/8	230	170	170	160	210	150	150	140	200	140	140	130	200	130	140	120	190	120	140	120
1-1/2	1/4	180	140	140	140	160	120	120	120	150	120	120	110	150	110	110	110	150	110	110	100
	5/16	230	170	170	160	210	150	150	140	200	140	140	130	200	140	140	130	190	140	140	130
	3/8	230	170	170	160	210	150	150	140	200	140	140	130	200	140	140	130	190	140	140	120
	7/16	360	260	260	240	320	220	230	200	310	200	210	180	310	190	210	180	300	180	200	160
	1/2	460	310	320	280	410	250	290	230	390	220	270	200	390	220	260	200	370	210	250	190
	5/8	700	410	500	370	600	340	420	310	560	310	380	280	550	310	380	270	530	290	360	260
	3/4	950	550	660	490	830	470	560	410	770	440	510	380	760	430	510	370	730	400	480	360
	7/8	1240	720	830	630	1080	560	710	540	1020	490	660	490	1010	470	650	470	970	430	610	430
	1	1550	800	1010	780	1360	600	870	600	1290	530	810	530	1280	500	790	500	1230	470	760	470
1-3/4	1/4	180	140	140	140	160	120	120	120	150	120	120	110	150	110	110	110	150	110	110	100
	5/16	230	170	170	160	210	150	150	140	200	140	140	130	200	140	140	130	190	140	140	130
	3/8	230	170	170	160	210	150	150	140	200	140	140	130	200	140	140	130	190	140	140	120
	7/16	360	260	260	240	320	230	230	210	310	210	210	190	310	210	210	190	300	200	200	180
	1/2	460	320	320	290	410	270	290	250	390	240	270	220	390	240	260	220	380	220	250	200
	5/8	740	440	500	400	660	360	440	320	610	330	420	290	600	320	410	290	570	300	390	270
	3/4	1030	580	720	520	890	480	600	430	830	450	550	390	820	440	540	380	780	420	510	360
	7/8	1320	740	890	650	1150	630	750	550	1070	570	700	510	1060	550	680	490	1010	500	650	470
	1	1630	910	1070	790	1420	700	910	670	1340	610	850	610	1320	590	830	590	1270	550	790	550
2-1/2	1/4	180	140	140	140	160	120	120	120	150	120	120	110	150	110	110	110	150	110	110	100
	5/16	230	170	170	160	210	150	150	140	200	140	140	130	200	140	140	130	190	140	140	130
	3/8	230	170	170	160	210	150	150	140	200	140	140	130	200	140	140	130	190	140	140	120
	7/16	360	260	260	240	320	230	230	210	310	210	210	190	310	210	210	190	300	200	200	180
	1/2	460	320	320	290	410	290	290	250	390	270	270	240	390	260	260	230	380	250	250	220
	5/8	740	500	500	450	670	430	440	390	640	390	420	350	630	380	410	340	610	360	390	320
	3/4	1110	680	740	610	1010	550	650	490	960	500	610	450	950	490	600	430	920	460	580	410
	7/8	1550	830	1000	740	1370	690	880	600	1280	630	830	550	1260	620	810	530	1190	580	770	500
	1	1940	980	1270	860	1660	830	1080	720	1550	770	990	660	1520	750	970	640	1450	720	920	620
3-1/2	1/4	180	140	140	140	160	120	120	120	150	120	120	110	150	110	110	110	150	110	110	100
	5/16	230	170	170	160	210	150	150	140	200	140	140	130	200	140	140	130	190	140	140	130
	3/8	230	170	170	160	210	150	150	140	200	140	140	130	200	140	140	130	190	140	140	120
	7/16	360	260	260	240	320	230	230	210	310	210	210	190	310	210	210	190	300	200	200	180
	1/2	460	320	320	290	410	290	290	250	390	270	270	240	390	260	260	230	380	250	250	220
	5/8	740	500	500	450	670	440	440	390	640	420	420	360	630	410	410	360	610	390	390	340
	3/4	1110	740	740	650	1010	650	650	560	960	600	610	520	950	580	600	510	920	550	580	490
	7/8	1550	990	1000	860	1400	800	880	710	1340	720	830	640	1320	700	810	620	1280	660	780	570
	1	2020	1140	1270	1010	1830	930	1120	810	1740	850	1060	740	1730	830	1040	720	1670	790	1000	680

1. Tabulated lateral design values (Z) shall be multiplied by all applicable adjustment factors (see Table 10.3.1).
2. Tabulated lateral design values (Z) are for "reduced diameter body" lag screws (see Appendix L) inserted in side grain with screw axis perpendicular to wood fibers; minimum screw penetration, p, into the main member equal to 8D; screw bending yield strengths (F_{yb}): F_{yb} = 70,000 psi for D = 1/4"; F_{yb} = 60,000 psi for D = 5/16"; F_{yb} = 45,000 psi for D ≥ 3/8"
3. When 4D ≤ p < 8D, tabulated lateral design values (Z) shall be multiplied by p/8D.

Table 11J (Cont.) LAG SCREWS: Reference Lateral Design Values (Z) for Single Shear (two member) Connections[1,2,3]

for sawn lumber or SCL with both members of identical specific gravity

Side Member Thickness	Lag Screw Diameter	G=0.43 Hem-Fir				G=0.42 Spruce-Pine-Fir				G=0.37 Redwood (open grain)				G=0.36 Eastern Softwoods Spruce-Pine-Fir(S) Western Cedars Western Woods				G=0.35 Northern Species			
t_s	D	$Z_\parallel$	$Z_{s\perp}$	$Z_{m\perp}$	$Z_\perp$	$Z_\parallel$	$Z_{s\perp}$	$Z_{m\perp}$	$Z_\perp$	$Z_\parallel$	$Z_{s\perp}$	$Z_{m\perp}$	$Z_\perp$	$Z_\parallel$	$Z_{s\perp}$	$Z_{m\perp}$	$Z_\perp$	$Z_\parallel$	$Z_{s\perp}$	$Z_{m\perp}$	$Z_\perp$
in.	in.	lbs.	lbs.	lbs.	lbs.	lbs.	lbs.	lbs.	lbs.	lbs.	lbs.	lbs.	lbs.	lbs.	lbs.	lbs.	lbs.	lbs.	lbs.	lbs.	lbs.
1/2	1/4	110	80	80	70	110	80	80	70	100	70	70	60	100	70	70	60	90	70	70	60
	5/16	130	90	100	80	130	90	90	80	120	80	90	80	120	80	90	70	120	80	80	70
	3/8	140	80	100	80	130	80	90	80	120	60	90	60	120	60	80	60	120	60	80	60
5/8	1/4	120	80	90	80	110	80	90	70	110	70	80	70	100	70	80	60	100	70	70	60
	5/16	140	90	100	90	140	90	100	90	130	80	90	80	130	80	90	70	120	80	90	70
	3/8	140	90	100	80	140	90	100	80	130	80	90	70	130	70	90	70	120	70	70	70
3/4	1/4	130	90	100	80	120	80	90	80	110	80	80	70	110	70	80	70	110	70	80	70
	5/16	150	100	110	90	150	100	110	90	130	90	100	80	130	90	90	80	130	80	90	80
	3/8	150	100	110	90	150	90	110	90	140	90	100	80	130	80	90	70	130	80	90	70
1	1/4	140	100	110	90	140	100	100	90	130	90	100	80	130	80	90	80	130	80	90	70
	5/16	170	110	130	100	170	110	120	100	150	90	110	90	150	90	110	80	150	90	100	80
	3/8	170	100	120	100	170	100	120	90	150	90	110	80	150	90	110	80	150	90	100	80
1-1/4	1/4	140	110	110	100	140	100	100	100	130	100	100	90	130	90	90	90	130	90	90	80
	5/16	180	120	130	110	180	120	130	110	170	100	120	100	170	100	120	90	160	100	110	90
	3/8	190	110	130	110	180	110	130	100	170	100	120	90	170	100	120	90	170	90	110	90
1-1/2	1/4	140	110	110	100	140	100	100	100	130	100	100	90	130	90	90	90	130	90	90	80
	5/16	180	130	130	120	180	130	130	120	170	110	120	110	170	110	120	100	160	110	110	100
	3/8	190	130	130	120	180	130	130	110	170	110	120	100	170	110	120	100	170	100	110	90
	7/16	290	170	190	150	280	160	190	150	260	140	180	130	260	140	170	130	250	140	170	120
	1/2	350	190	240	180	350	190	240	170	310	170	210	150	310	160	210	150	300	160	200	140
	5/8	500	280	340	240	490	270	330	240	450	250	300	210	440	240	290	210	430	240	280	200
	3/4	700	360	450	330	690	350	440	330	630	290	400	290	620	280	390	280	610	270	380	270
	7/8	930	390	580	390	910	380	570	380	850	320	520	320	840	310	510	310	820	290	490	290
	1	1180	420	720	420	1160	410	710	410	1080	340	640	340	1070	330	630	330	1050	320	620	320
1-3/4	1/4	140	110	110	100	140	100	100	100	130	100	100	90	130	90	90	90	130	90	90	80
	5/16	180	130	130	120	180	130	130	120	170	120	120	110	170	120	120	110	160	110	110	100
	3/8	190	130	130	120	180	130	130	110	170	120	120	100	170	120	120	100	170	110	110	100
	7/16	290	180	190	160	280	180	190	160	270	160	180	140	260	150	170	140	260	140	170	130
	1/2	360	210	240	190	360	200	240	180	340	180	220	160	340	170	220	150	330	170	210	150
	5/8	540	290	360	250	530	280	360	250	480	250	320	220	480	250	310	210	460	240	300	210
	3/4	740	400	480	340	730	390	470	340	670	330	420	300	660	320	420	300	640	310	410	290
	7/8	970	450	610	440	950	440	600	440	880	370	540	370	870	360	530	360	850	330	520	330
	1	1210	490	750	490	1200	480	740	480	1110	400	670	400	1090	380	650	380	1070	370	640	370
2-1/2	1/4	140	110	110	100	140	100	100	100	130	100	100	90	130	90	90	90	130	90	90	80
	5/16	180	130	130	120	180	130	130	120	170	120	120	110	170	120	120	110	160	110	110	100
	3/8	190	130	130	120	180	130	130	110	170	120	120	100	170	120	120	100	170	110	110	100
	7/16	290	190	190	170	280	190	190	170	270	180	180	150	260	170	170	150	260	170	170	150
	1/2	360	240	240	210	360	240	240	210	340	220	220	190	340	210	220	190	330	200	210	180
	5/8	590	330	380	290	580	320	370	290	550	290	340	250	540	280	340	240	530	270	330	240
	3/4	890	430	550	380	880	420	540	370	800	380	500	320	780	370	490	320	760	360	480	310
	7/8	1130	550	730	470	1110	540	710	460	1010	490	640	420	990	480	620	410	970	470	600	390
	1	1380	680	870	580	1360	670	850	570	1240	570	760	510	1220	550	750	500	1190	530	730	490
3-1/2	1/4	140	110	110	100	140	100	100	100	130	100	100	90	130	90	90	90	130	90	90	80
	5/16	180	130	130	120	180	130	130	120	170	120	120	110	170	120	120	110	160	110	110	100
	3/8	190	130	130	120	180	130	130	110	170	120	120	100	170	120	120	100	170	110	110	100
	7/16	290	190	190	170	280	190	190	170	270	180	180	150	260	170	170	150	260	170	170	150
	1/2	360	240	240	210	360	240	240	210	340	220	220	190	340	220	220	190	330	210	210	180
	5/8	590	380	380	320	580	370	370	320	550	340	340	290	540	330	340	280	530	320	330	280
	3/4	890	500	550	440	880	490	540	430	830	430	500	370	820	420	490	370	800	410	480	360
	7/8	1240	610	750	530	1220	600	740	520	1150	530	680	460	1140	520	670	450	1110	500	650	430
	1	1610	740	950	630	1600	720	940	620	1480	650	860	550	1450	630	850	540	1410	620	830	520

1. Tabulated lateral design values (Z) shall be multiplied by all applicable adjustment factors (see Table 10.3.1).
2. Tabulated lateral design values (Z) are for "reduced diameter body" lag screws (see Appendix L) inserted in side grain with screw axis perpendicular to wood fibers; minimum screw penetration, p, into the main member equal to 8D; screw bending yield strengths (F_{yb}): F_{yb} = 70,000 psi for D = 1/4"; F_{yb} = 60,000 psi for D = 5/16"; F_{yb} = 45,000 psi for D ≥ 3/8"
3. When 4D ≤ p < 8D, tabulated lateral design values (Z) shall be multiplied by p/8D.

Table 11K LAG SCREWS: Reference Lateral Design Values (Z) for Single Shear (two member) Connections[1,2,3]

with 1/4" ASTM A 36 steel side plate, or ASTM A 653, Grade 33 steel side plate (for t_s < 1/4")

Side Member Thickness t_s (in.)	Lag Screw Diameter D (in.)	G=0.67 Red Oak $Z_\parallel$ (lbs.)	$Z_\perp$ (lbs.)	G=0.55 Mixed Maple Southern Pine $Z_\parallel$ (lbs.)	$Z_\perp$ (lbs.)	G=0.5 Douglas Fir-Larch $Z_\parallel$ (lbs.)	$Z_\perp$ (lbs.)	G=0.49 Douglas Fir-Larch (N) $Z_\parallel$ (lbs.)	$Z_\perp$ (lbs.)	G=0.46 Douglas Fir(S) Hem-Fir(N) $Z_\parallel$ (lbs.)	$Z_\perp$ (lbs.)	G=0.43 Hem-Fir $Z_\parallel$ (lbs.)	$Z_\perp$ (lbs.)	G=0.42 Spruce-Pine-Fir $Z_\parallel$ (lbs.)	$Z_\perp$ (lbs.)	G=0.37 Redwood (open grain) $Z_\parallel$ (lbs.)	$Z_\perp$ (lbs.)	G=0.36 Eastern Softwoods Spruce-Pine-Fir(S) Western Cedars Western Woods $Z_\parallel$ (lbs.)	$Z_\perp$ (lbs.)	G=0.35 Northern Species $Z_\parallel$ (lbs.)	$Z_\perp$ (lbs.)
0.075 (14 gage)	1/4	170	130	160	120	150	110	150	110	150	100	140	100	140	100	130	90	130	90	130	90
	5/16	220	160	200	140	190	130	190	130	190	130	180	120	180	120	170	110	170	110	160	100
	3/8	220	160	200	140	200	130	190	130	190	120	180	120	180	120	170	110	170	100	170	100
0.105 (12 gage)	1/4	180	140	170	130	160	120	160	120	160	110	150	110	150	110	140	100	140	100	140	90
	5/16	230	170	210	150	200	140	200	140	190	130	190	130	190	120	180	110	170	110	170	110
	3/8	230	160	210	140	200	140	200	130	200	130	190	120	190	120	180	110	180	110	170	110
0.120 (11 gage)	1/4	190	150	180	130	170	120	170	120	160	120	160	110	160	110	150	100	150	100	140	100
	5/16	230	170	210	150	210	140	200	140	200	140	190	130	190	130	180	120	180	110	180	110
	3/8	240	170	220	150	210	140	210	140	200	130	200	130	190	120	180	110	180	110	180	110
0.134 (10 gage)	1/4	200	150	180	140	180	130	170	130	170	120	160	120	160	110	150	110	150	100	150	100
	5/16	240	180	220	160	210	150	210	140	200	140	200	130	200	130	190	120	180	120	180	120
	3/8	240	170	220	150	220	140	210	140	210	140	200	130	200	130	190	120	190	120	180	110
0.179 (7 gage)	1/4	220	170	210	150	200	150	200	140	190	140	190	130	190	130	180	120	170	120	170	120
	5/16	260	190	240	170	230	160	230	160	230	150	220	150	220	150	210	130	200	130	200	130
	3/8	270	190	250	170	240	160	240	160	230	150	220	140	220	140	210	130	210	130	200	130
0.239 (3 gage)	1/4	240	180	220	160	210	150	210	150	200	140	200	140	190	130	180	120	180	120	180	120
	5/16	300	220	280	190	270	180	260	180	260	170	250	160	250	160	230	150	230	150	230	140
	3/8	310	220	280	190	270	180	270	180	260	170	250	160	250	160	240	140	230	140	230	140
	7/16	420	290	390	260	380	240	370	240	360	230	350	220	350	220	330	200	330	200	320	190
	1/2	510	340	470	300	460	290	450	280	440	270	430	260	420	260	400	240	400	230	390	230
	5/8	770	490	710	430	680	400	680	400	660	380	640	370	630	360	600	330	590	330	580	320
	3/4	1110	670	1020	590	980	560	970	550	950	530	920	500	910	500	860	450	850	450	840	440
	7/8	1510	880	1390	780	1330	730	1320	710	1280	690	1250	650	1230	650	1170	590	1160	590	1140	570
	1	1940	1100	1780	960	1710	910	1700	890	1650	860	1600	820	1590	810	1500	740	1480	730	1460	710
1/4	1/4	240	180	220	160	210	150	210	150	200	140	200	140	190	130	180	120	180	120	180	120
	5/16	310	220	280	200	270	180	270	180	260	170	250	170	250	160	230	150	230	150	230	140
	3/8	320	220	290	190	280	180	270	180	270	170	260	160	250	160	240	150	240	140	230	140
	7/16	480	320	440	280	420	270	420	260	410	250	390	240	390	230	370	220	360	210	360	210
	1/2	580	390	540	340	520	320	510	320	500	310	480	290	480	290	460	270	450	260	440	260
	5/8	850	530	780	470	750	440	740	440	720	420	700	400	690	400	660	370	650	360	640	350
	3/4	1200	730	1100	640	1060	600	1050	590	1020	570	990	540	980	530	930	490	920	480	900	470
	7/8	1600	930	1470	820	1410	770	1400	750	1360	720	1320	690	1310	680	1240	630	1220	620	1200	600
	1	2040	1150	1870	1000	1800	950	1780	930	1730	900	1680	850	1660	840	1570	770	1550	760	1530	740

1. Tabulated lateral design values (Z) shall be multiplied by all applicable adjustment factors (see Table 10.3.1).
2. Tabulated lateral design values (Z) are for "reduced body diameter" lag screws (see Appendix L) inserted in side grain with screw axis perpendicular to wood fibers; minimum screw penetration, p, into the main member equal to 8D; dowel bearing strengths (F_e) of 61,850 psi for ASTM A 653, Grade 33 steel and 87,000 psi for ASTM A 36 steel and screw bending yield strengths (F_{yb}): F_{yb} = 70,000 psi for D = 1/4"; F_{yb} = 60,000 psi for D = 5/16"; F_{yb} = 45,000 psi for D ≥ 3/8"
3. When 4D ≤ p < 8D, tabulated lateral design values (Z) shall be multiplied by p/8D.

Table 11L WOOD SCREWS: Reference Lateral Design Values (Z) for Single Shear (two member) Connections[1,2,3]

for sawn lumber or SCL with both members of identical specific gravity

Side Member Thickness t_s in.	Wood Screw Diameter D in.	Wood Screw Number	G=0.67 Red Oak lbs.	G=0.55 Mixed Maple Southern Pine lbs.	G=0.5 Douglas Fir-Larch lbs.	G=0.49 Douglas Fir-Larch(N) lbs.	G=0.46 Douglas Fir(S) Hem-Fir(N) lbs.	G=0.43 Hem-Fir lbs.	G=0.42 Spruce-Pine-Fir lbs.	G=0.37 Redwood (open grain) lbs.	G=0.36 Eastern Softwoods Spruce-Pine-Fir(S) Western Cedars Western Woods lbs.	G=0.35 Northern Species lbs.
1/2	0.138	6	88	67	59	57	53	49	47	41	40	38
	0.151	7	96	74	65	63	59	54	52	45	44	42
	0.164	8	107	82	73	71	66	61	59	51	50	48
	0.177	9	121	94	83	81	76	70	68	59	58	56
	0.190	10	130	101	90	87	82	75	73	64	63	60
	0.216	12	156	123	110	107	100	93	91	79	78	75
	0.242	14	168	133	120	117	110	102	99	87	86	83
5/8	0.138	6	94	76	66	64	59	53	52	44	43	41
	0.151	7	104	83	72	70	64	58	56	48	47	45
	0.164	8	120	92	80	77	72	65	63	54	53	51
	0.177	9	136	103	91	88	81	74	72	62	61	58
	0.190	10	146	111	97	94	88	80	78	67	65	63
	0.216	12	173	133	117	114	106	97	95	82	80	77
	0.242	14	184	142	126	123	115	106	103	89	87	84
3/4	0.138	6	94	79	72	71	65	58	57	47	46	44
	0.151	7	104	87	80	77	71	64	62	52	50	48
	0.164	8	120	101	88	85	78	71	69	58	56	54
	0.177	9	142	114	99	96	88	80	78	66	64	61
	0.190	10	153	122	107	103	95	86	83	71	69	66
	0.216	12	192	144	126	122	113	103	100	86	84	80
	0.242	14	203	154	135	131	122	111	108	93	91	87
1	0.138	6	94	79	72	71	67	63	61	55	54	51
	0.151	7	104	87	80	78	74	69	68	60	59	56
	0.164	8	120	101	92	90	85	80	78	67	65	62
	0.177	9	142	118	108	106	100	94	90	75	73	70
	0.190	10	153	128	117	114	108	101	97	81	78	75
	0.216	12	193	161	147	143	131	118	114	96	93	89
	0.242	14	213	178	157	152	139	126	122	102	100	95
1-1/4	0.138	6	94	79	72	71	67	63	61	55	54	52
	0.151	7	104	87	80	78	74	69	68	60	59	57
	0.164	8	120	101	92	90	85	80	78	70	68	66
	0.177	9	142	118	108	106	100	94	92	82	80	78
	0.190	10	153	128	117	114	108	101	99	88	87	84
	0.216	12	193	161	147	144	137	128	125	108	105	100
	0.242	14	213	178	163	159	151	141	138	115	111	106
1-1/2	0.138	6	94	79	72	71	67	63	61	55	54	52
	0.151	7	104	87	80	78	74	69	68	60	59	57
	0.164	8	120	101	92	90	85	80	78	70	68	66
	0.177	9	142	118	108	106	100	94	92	82	80	78
	0.190	10	153	128	117	114	108	101	99	88	87	84
	0.216	12	193	161	147	144	137	128	125	111	109	106
	0.242	14	213	178	163	159	151	141	138	123	120	117
1-3/4	0.138	6	94	79	72	71	67	63	61	55	54	52
	0.151	7	104	87	80	78	74	69	68	60	59	57
	0.164	8	120	101	92	90	85	80	78	70	68	66
	0.177	9	142	118	108	106	100	94	92	82	80	78
	0.190	10	153	128	117	114	108	101	99	88	87	84
	0.216	12	193	161	147	144	137	128	125	111	109	106
	0.242	14	213	178	163	159	151	141	138	123	120	117

1. Tabulated lateral design values (Z) shall be multiplied by all applicable adjustment factors (see Table 10.3.1).
2. Tabulated lateral design values (Z) are for rolled thread wood screws (see Appendix L) inserted in side grain with nail axis perpendicular to wood fibers; minimum screw penetration, p, into the main member equal to 10D; and screw bending yield strengths (F_{yb}): F_{yb} = 100,000 psi for 0.099" ≤ D ≤ 0.142"; F_{yb} = 90,000 psi for 0.142" < D ≤ 0.177"; F_{yb} = 80,000 psi for 0.177" < D ≤ 0.236"; F_{yb} = 70,000 psi for 0.236" < D ≤ 0.273"
3. When 6D ≤ p < 10D, tabulated lateral design values (Z) shall be multiplied by p/10D.

Table 11M WOOD SCREWS: Reference Lateral Design Values (Z) for Single Shear (two member) Connections[1,2,3]

with ASTM A 653, Grade 33 steel side plate

Side Member Thickness t_s (in.)	Wood Screw Diameter D (in.)	Wood Screw Number	G=0.67 Red Oak	G=0.55 Mixed Maple Southern Pine	G=0.5 Douglas Fir-Larch	G=0.49 Douglas Fir-Larch(N)	G=0.46 Douglas Fir(S) Hem-Fir(N)	G=0.43 Hem-Fir	G=0.42 Spruce-Pine-Fir	G=0.37 Redwood (open grain)	G=0.36 Eastern Softwoods Spruce-Pine-Fir(S) Western Cedars Western Woods	G=0.35 Northern Species
			lbs.	lbs.	lbs.	lbs.	lbs.	lbs.	lbs.	lbs.	lbs.	lbs.
0.036 (20 gage)	0.138	6	89	76	70	69	66	62	60	54	53	52
	0.151	7	99	84	78	76	72	68	67	60	59	57
	0.164	8	113	97	89	87	83	78	77	69	67	66
0.048 (18 gage)	0.138	6	90	77	71	70	67	63	61	55	54	53
	0.151	7	100	85	79	77	74	69	68	61	60	58
	0.164	8	114	98	90	89	84	79	78	70	69	67
0.060 (16 gage)	0.138	6	92	79	73	72	68	64	63	57	56	54
	0.151	7	101	87	81	79	75	71	70	63	61	60
	0.164	8	116	100	92	90	86	81	79	71	70	68
	0.177	9	136	116	107	105	100	94	93	83	82	79
	0.190	10	146	125	116	114	108	102	100	90	88	86
0.075 (14 gage)	0.138	6	95	82	76	75	71	67	66	59	58	57
	0.151	7	105	90	84	82	78	74	72	65	64	62
	0.164	8	119	103	95	93	89	84	82	74	73	71
	0.177	9	139	119	110	108	103	97	95	86	84	82
	0.190	10	150	128	119	117	111	105	103	92	91	88
	0.216	12	186	159	147	145	138	130	127	114	112	109
	0.242	14	204	175	162	158	151	142	139	125	123	120
0.105 (12 gage)	0.138	6	104	90	84	82	79	74	73	66	65	63
	0.151	7	114	99	92	90	86	81	80	72	71	69
	0.164	8	129	111	103	102	97	92	90	81	80	77
	0.177	9	148	128	119	116	111	105	103	93	91	89
	0.190	10	160	138	128	125	120	113	111	100	98	96
	0.216	12	196	168	156	153	146	138	135	122	120	116
	0.242	14	213	183	170	167	159	150	147	132	130	126
0.120 (11 gage)	0.138	6	110	95	89	87	83	79	77	70	68	67
	0.151	7	120	104	97	95	91	86	84	76	75	73
	0.164	8	135	117	109	107	102	96	94	85	84	82
	0.177	9	154	133	124	121	116	110	107	97	95	93
	0.190	10	166	144	133	131	125	118	116	104	103	100
	0.216	12	202	174	162	159	152	143	140	126	124	121
	0.242	14	219	189	175	172	164	155	152	137	134	131
0.134 (10 gage)	0.138	6	116	100	93	92	88	83	81	73	72	70
	0.151	7	126	110	102	100	96	91	89	80	79	77
	0.164	8	141	122	114	112	107	101	99	89	88	86
	0.177	9	160	139	129	127	121	114	112	101	100	97
	0.190	10	173	149	139	136	130	123	121	109	107	104
	0.216	12	209	180	167	164	157	148	145	131	129	126
	0.242	14	226	195	181	177	169	160	157	141	139	135
0.179 (7 gage)	0.138	6	126	107	99	97	92	86	84	76	74	72
	0.151	7	139	118	109	107	102	95	93	84	82	80
	0.164	8	160	136	126	123	117	110	108	96	95	92
	0.177	9	184	160	148	145	138	129	127	113	111	108
	0.190	10	198	172	159	156	149	140	137	122	120	117
	0.216	12	234	203	189	186	178	168	165	149	146	143
	0.242	14	251	217	202	198	190	179	176	159	156	152
0.239 (3 gage)	0.138	6	126	107	99	97	92	86	84	76	74	72
	0.151	7	139	118	109	107	102	95	93	84	82	80
	0.164	8	160	136	126	123	117	110	108	96	95	92
	0.177	9	188	160	148	145	138	129	127	113	111	108
	0.190	10	204	173	159	156	149	140	137	122	120	117
	0.216	12	256	218	201	197	187	176	172	154	151	147
	0.242	14	283	241	222	217	207	194	190	170	167	162

1. Tabulated lateral design values (Z) shall be multiplied by all applicable adjustment factors (see Table 10.3.1).
2. Tabulated lateral design values (Z) are for rolled thread wood screws (see Appendix L) inserted in side grain with screw axis perpendicular to wood fibers; minimum screw penetration, p, into the main member equal to 10D; dowel bearing strength (F_e) of 61,850 psi for ASTM A 653, Grade 33 steel and screw bending yield strengths (F_{yb}): $F_{yb} = 100,000$ psi for $0.099" \le D \le 0.142"$; $F_{yb} = 90,000$ psi for $0.142" < D \le 0.177"$; $F_{yb} = 80,000$ psi for $0.177" < D \le 0.236"$; $F_{yb} = 70,000$ psi for $0.236" < D \le 0.273"$
3. When $6D \le p < 10D$, tabulated lateral design values (Z) shall be multiplied by p/10D.

WOOD SCREWS

Table 11N COMMON WIRE, BOX, or SINKER NAILS: Reference Lateral Design Values (Z) for Single Shear (two member) Connections[1,2,3,4]

for sawn lumber or SCL with both members of identical specific gravity

Side Member Thickness t_s in.	Nail Diameter D in.	Common Wire Nail	Box Nail	Sinker Nail (Pennyweight)	G=0.67 Red Oak lbs.	G=0.55 Mixed Maple Southern Pine lbs.	G=0.5 Douglas Fir-Larch lbs.	G=0.49 Douglas Fir-Larch (N) lbs.	G=0.46 Douglas Fir(S) Hem-Fir(N) lbs.	G=0.43 Hem-Fir lbs.	G=0.42 Spruce-Pine-Fir lbs.	G=0.37 Redwood (open grain) lbs.	G=0.36 Eastern Softwoods Spruce-Pine-Fir(S) Western Cedars Western Woods lbs.	G=0.35 Northern Species lbs.
3/4	0.099	6d		7d	73	61	55	54	51	48	47	39	38	36
	0.113	6d	8d	8d	94	79	72	71	65	58	57	47	46	44
	0.120			10d	107	89	80	77	71	64	62	52	50	48
	0.128		10d		121	101	87	84	78	70	68	57	56	54
	0.131	8d			127	104	90	87	80	73	70	60	58	56
	0.135		16d	12d	135	108	94	91	84	76	74	63	61	58
	0.148	10d	20d	16d	154	121	105	102	94	85	83	70	69	66
	0.162	16d	40d		183	138	121	117	108	99	96	82	80	77
	0.177			20d	200	153	134	130	121	111	107	92	90	87
	0.192	20d		30d	206	157	138	134	125	114	111	96	93	90
	0.207	30d		40d	216	166	147	143	133	122	119	103	101	97
	0.225	40d			229	178	158	154	144	132	129	112	110	106
	0.244	50d		60d	234	182	162	158	147	136	132	115	113	109
1	0.099	6d		7d	73	61	55	54	51	48	47	42	41	40
	0.113	6d[4]	8d	8d	94	79	72	71	67	63	61	55	54	51
	0.120			10d	107	89	81	80	76	71	69	60	59	56
	0.128		10d		121	101	93	91	86	80	79	66	64	61
	0.131	8d			127	106	97	95	90	84	82	68	66	63
	0.135		16d	12d	135	113	103	101	96	89	86	71	69	66
	0.148	10d	20d	16d	154	128	118	115	109	99	96	80	77	74
	0.162	16d	40d		184	154	141	137	125	113	109	91	89	85
	0.177			20d	213	178	155	150	138	125	121	102	99	95
	0.192	20d		30d	222	183	159	154	142	128	124	105	102	98
	0.207	30d		40d	243	192	167	162	149	135	131	111	109	104
	0.225	40d			268	202	177	171	159	144	140	120	117	112
	0.244	50d		60d	274	207	181	175	162	148	143	123	120	115
1-1/4	0.099	6d[4]		7d[4]	73	61	55	54	51	48	47	42	41	40
	0.113	6d[4]	8d	8d[4]	94	79	72	71	67	63	61	55	54	52
	0.120			10d	107	89	81	80	76	71	69	62	60	59
	0.128		10d		121	101	93	91	86	80	79	70	69	67
	0.131	8d[4]			127	106	97	95	90	84	82	73	72	70
	0.135		16d	12d	135	113	103	101	96	89	88	78	76	74
	0.148	10d	20d	16d	154	128	118	115	109	102	100	89	87	84
	0.162	16d	40d		184	154	141	138	131	122	120	103	100	95
	0.177			20d	213	178	163	159	151	141	136	113	110	105
	0.192	20d		30d	222	185	170	166	157	145	140	116	113	108
	0.207	30d		40d	243	203	186	182	169	152	147	123	119	114
	0.225	40d			268	224	200	193	177	160	155	130	127	121
	0.244	50d		60d	276	230	204	197	181	163	158	133	129	124
1-1/2	0.099			7d[4]	73	61	55	54	51	48	47	42	41	40
	0.113		8d[4]	8d[4]	94	79	72	71	67	63	61	55	54	52
	0.120			10d	107	89	81	80	76	71	69	62	60	59
	0.128		10d		121	101	93	91	86	80	79	70	69	67
	0.131	8d[4]			127	106	97	95	90	84	82	73	72	70
	0.135		16d	12d	135	113	103	101	96	89	88	78	76	74
	0.148	10d	20d	16d	154	128	118	115	109	102	100	89	87	84
	0.162	16d	40d		184	154	141	138	131	122	120	106	104	101
	0.177			20d	213	178	163	159	151	141	138	123	121	117
	0.192	20d		30d	222	185	170	166	157	147	144	128	126	120
	0.207	30d		40d	243	203	186	182	172	161	158	135	131	125
	0.225	40d			268	224	205	201	190	178	172	143	138	132
	0.244	50d		60d	276	230	211	206	196	181	175	146	141	135
1-3/4	0.113		8d[4]		94	79	72	71	67	63	61	55	54	52
	0.120			10d[4]	107	89	81	80	76	71	69	62	60	59
	0.128		10d		121	101	93	91	86	80	79	70	69	67
	0.135		16d	12d	135	113	103	101	96	89	88	78	76	74
	0.148	10d[4]	20d	16d	154	128	118	115	109	102	100	89	87	84
	0.162	16d	40d		184	154	141	138	131	122	120	106	104	101
	0.177			20d	213	178	163	159	151	141	138	123	121	117
	0.192	20d		30d	222	185	170	166	157	147	144	128	126	122
	0.207	30d		40d	243	203	186	182	172	161	158	140	137	133
	0.225	40d			268	224	205	201	190	178	174	155	151	144
	0.244	50d		60d	276	230	211	206	196	183	179	159	154	147

1. Tabulated lateral design values (Z) shall be multiplied by all applicable adjustment factors (see Table 10.3.1).

2. Tabulated lateral design values (Z) are for common wire, box, and sinker nails (see Appendix L) inserted in side grain with nail axis perpendicular to wood fibers; minimum nail penetration, p, into the main member equal to 10D; and nail bending yield strengths (F_{yb}): F_{yb} = 100,000 psi for 0.099" $\leq$ D $\leq$ 0.142"; F_{yb} = 90,000 psi for 0.142" < D $\leq$ 0.177"; F_{yb} = 80,000 psi for 0.177" < D $\leq$ 0.236"; F_{yb} = 70,000 psi for 0.236" < D $\leq$ 0.273"

3. When 6D $\leq$ p < 10D, tabulated lateral design values (Z) shall be multiplied by p/10D.

4. Nail length is insufficient to provide 10D penetration. Tabulated lateral design values (Z) shall be adjusted per footnote 3.

Table 11P COMMON WIRE, BOX, or SINKER NAILS: Reference Lateral Design Values (Z) for Single Shear (two member) Connections[1,2,3]

with ASTM A 653, Grade 33 steel side plates

Side Member Thickness t_s in.	Nail Diameter D in.	Common Wire Nail	Box Nail	Sinker Nail	G=0.67 Red Oak lbs.	G=0.55 Mixed Maple Southern Pine lbs.	G=0.5 Douglas Fir-Larch lbs.	G=0.49 Douglas Fir-Larch (N) lbs.	G=0.46 Douglas Fir(S) Hem-Fir(N) lbs.	G=0.43 Hem-Fir lbs.	G=0.42 Spruce-Pine-Fir lbs.	G=0.37 Redwood (open grain) lbs.	G=0.36 Eastern Softwoods Spruce-Pine-Fir(S) Western Cedars Western Woods lbs.	G=0.35 Northern Species lbs.
0.036 (20 gage)	0.099		6d	7d	69	59	54	53	51	48	47	42	41	40
	0.113	6d	8d	8d	89	76	70	69	66	62	60	54	53	52
	0.120			10d	100	86	79	77	74	69	68	61	60	58
	0.128		10d		114	97	90	88	84	79	77	69	68	66
	0.131	8d			120	102	94	92	88	82	81	72	71	69
	0.135		16d	12d	127	108	100	98	93	87	86	77	75	73
	0.148	10d	20d	16d	145	123	114	111	106	100	98	87	86	83
0.048 (18 gage)	0.099		6d	7d	70	60	55	54	52	49	48	43	42	41
	0.113	6d	8d	8d	90	77	71	70	67	63	61	55	54	53
	0.120			10d	101	87	80	78	75	70	69	62	61	59
	0.128		10d		115	98	91	89	85	80	78	70	69	67
	0.131	8d			120	103	95	93	89	83	82	73	72	70
	0.135		16d	12d	128	109	101	99	94	88	87	78	76	74
	0.148	10d	20d	16d	145	124	115	112	107	101	99	88	87	84
	0.162	16d	40d		174	148	137	134	128	120	118	105	104	101
	0.177			20d	201	171	158	155	147	138	136	122	119	116
	0.192	20d	30d		209	178	164	161	153	144	141	126	124	121
	0.207	30d	40d		229	195	179	176	167	157	154	138	136	132
0.060 (16 gage)	0.099		6d	7d	72	62	57	56	54	51	50	45	44	43
	0.113	6d	8d	8d	92	79	73	72	68	64	63	57	56	54
	0.120			10d	103	88	82	80	76	72	71	63	62	61
	0.128		10d		117	100	92	91	86	81	80	72	70	68
	0.131	8d			122	104	97	95	90	85	83	75	73	71
	0.135		16d	12d	129	111	102	100	96	90	88	79	78	76
	0.148	10d	20d	16d	147	126	116	114	109	102	100	90	88	86
	0.162	16d	40d		175	150	138	135	129	121	119	107	105	102
	0.177			20d	202	172	159	156	149	140	137	123	121	117
	0.192	20d	30d		210	179	165	162	154	145	142	128	125	122
	0.207	30d	40d		229	195	180	177	168	158	155	139	137	133
	0.225	40d			253	215	199	195	185	174	171	153	150	146
	0.244	50d		60d	260	221	204	200	191	179	176	157	155	150
0.075 (14 gage)	0.099		6d	7d	75	65	60	59	56	53	52	47	46	45
	0.113	6d	8d	8d	95	82	76	75	71	67	66	59	58	57
	0.120			10d	106	91	85	83	79	75	73	66	65	63
	0.128		10d		120	103	95	93	89	84	82	74	73	71
	0.131	8d			125	107	99	97	93	88	86	77	76	74
	0.135		16d	12d	132	113	105	103	98	93	91	82	80	78
	0.148	10d	20d	16d	150	129	119	117	111	105	103	92	91	88
	0.162	16d	40d		178	152	141	138	132	124	122	109	107	104
	0.177			20d	204	175	162	158	151	142	139	125	123	120
	0.192	20d	30d		212	182	168	165	157	148	145	130	128	124
	0.207	30d	40d		231	198	183	179	171	161	157	141	139	135
	0.225	40d			254	217	201	197	187	176	173	155	152	148
	0.244	50d		60d	261	223	206	202	193	181	178	159	156	152
0.105 (12 gage)	0.099		6d	7d	84	73	68	67	64	60	59	53	53	51
	0.113	6d	8d	8d	104	90	84	82	79	74	73	66	65	63
	0.120			10d	115	100	93	91	87	82	80	73	71	69
	0.128		10d		129	111	103	101	97	91	90	81	79	77
	0.131	8d			134	116	107	105	101	95	93	84	82	80
	0.135		16d	12d	141	122	113	111	106	100	98	88	87	84
	0.148	10d	20d	16d	159	137	127	125	119	113	110	99	98	95
	0.162	16d	40d		187	161	149	146	140	132	129	116	114	111
	0.177			20d	213	183	169	166	159	149	147	132	130	126
	0.192	20d	30d		220	189	175	172	164	155	152	137	134	131
	0.207	30d	40d		238	205	190	186	177	167	164	147	145	141
	0.225	40d			260	223	207	203	193	182	179	161	158	153
	0.244	50d		60d	268	230	212	208	199	187	183	165	162	158

1. Tabulated lateral design values (Z) shall be multiplied by all applicable adjustment factors (see Table 10.3.1).
2. Tabulated lateral design values (Z) are for common wire, box, and sinker nails (see Appendix L) inserted in side grain with nail axis perpendicular to wood fibers; minimum nail penetration, p, into the main member equal to 10D; dowel bearing strength (F_e) of 61,850 psi for ASTM A 653, Grade 33 steel and nail bending yield strengths (F_{yb}): F_{yb} = 100,000 psi for 0.099" $\leq$ D $\leq$ 0.142"; F_{yb} = 90,000 psi for 0.142" < D $\leq$ 0.177"; F_{yb} = 80,000 psi for 0.177" < D $\leq$ 0.236"; F_{yb} = 70,000 psi for 0.236" < D $\leq$ 0.273"
3. When 6D $\leq$ p < 10D, tabulated lateral design values (Z) shall be multiplied by p/10D.

Table 11P (Cont.) COMMON WIRE, BOX, or SINKER NAILS: Reference Lateral Design Values (Z) for Single Shear (two member) Connections[1,2,3]

with ASTM A 653, Grade 33 steel side plates

Side Member Thickness t_s in.	Nail Diameter D in.	Common Wire Nail	Box Nail	Sinker Nail	G=0.67 Red Oak lbs.	G=0.55 Mixed Maple Southern Pine lbs.	G=0.5 Douglas Fir-Larch lbs.	G=0.49 Douglas Fir-Larch (N) lbs.	G=0.46 Douglas Fir(S) Hem-Fir(N) lbs.	G=0.43 Hem-Fir lbs.	G=0.42 Spruce-Pine-Fir lbs.	G=0.37 Redwood (open grain) lbs.	G=0.36 Eastern Softwoods Spruce-Pine-Fir(S) Western Cedars Western Woods lbs.	G=0.35 Northern Species lbs.
0.120 (11 gage)	0.099		6d	7d	90	78	72	71	68	64	63	57	56	53
	0.113	6d	8d	8d	110	95	89	87	83	79	77	70	68	66
	0.120			10d	121	105	97	96	91	86	85	76	75	73
	0.128		10d		134	116	108	106	101	96	94	85	83	81
	0.131	8d			140	121	112	110	105	99	97	88	86	84
	0.135		16d	12d	147	127	118	116	110	104	102	92	91	88
	0.148	10d	20d	16d	165	143	133	130	124	117	115	104	102	99
	0.162	16d	40d		193	166	154	152	145	137	134	121	119	115
	0.177			20d	218	188	174	171	163	154	151	136	134	130
	0.192	20d		30d	226	195	181	177	169	159	156	141	138	135
	0.207	30d		40d	244	210	194	191	182	172	168	151	149	145
	0.225	40d			265	228	211	207	198	186	183	164	161	157
	0.244	50d		60d	272	234	217	213	203	191	187	169	166	161
0.134 (10 gage)	0.099		6d	7d	95	82	76	74	71	66	65	58	56	54
	0.113	6d	8d	8d	116	100	93	92	88	83	81	73	72	69
	0.120			10d	127	110	102	100	96	91	89	80	79	76
	0.128		10d		140	122	113	111	106	100	98	89	87	85
	0.131	8d			146	126	117	115	110	104	102	92	90	88
	0.135		16d	12d	153	132	123	121	115	109	107	96	95	92
	0.148	10d	20d	16d	172	148	138	135	129	122	120	108	106	104
	0.162	16d	40d		199	172	160	157	150	142	139	125	123	120
	0.177			20d	224	194	180	176	169	159	156	141	138	135
	0.192	20d		30d	232	200	186	182	174	164	161	145	143	139
	0.207	30d		40d	249	215	199	196	187	176	173	156	153	149
	0.225	40d			270	233	216	212	202	191	187	168	165	161
	0.244	50d		60d	277	239	221	217	207	195	192	173	170	165
0.179 (7 gage)	0.099		6d	7d	97	82	76	74	71	66	65	58	56	54
	0.113	6d	8d	8d	126	107	99	97	92	86	84	76	74	70
	0.120			10d	142	121	111	109	104	97	95	85	83	79
	0.128		10d		161	137	126	124	118	111	108	97	94	90
	0.131	8d			168	144	132	130	123	116	114	102	99	94
	0.135		16d	12d	175	152	141	138	131	123	121	108	105	100
	0.148	10d	20d	16d	195	170	158	155	148	140	137	123	121	117
	0.162	16d	40d		224	194	180	177	169	160	157	142	140	136
	0.177			20d	249	215	200	197	188	178	174	157	155	151
	0.192	20d		30d	256	222	206	203	194	183	179	162	159	155
	0.207	30d		40d	272	236	219	215	205	194	190	172	169	164
	0.225	40d			292	252	234	230	220	207	203	184	180	176
	0.244	50d		60d	299	258	240	235	225	212	208	188	185	180
0.239 (3 gage)	0.099		6d	7d	97	82	76	74	71	66	65	58	56	54
	0.113	6d	8d	8d	126	107	99	97	92	86	84	76	74	70
	0.120			10d	142	121	111	109	104	97	95	85	83	79
	0.128		10d		161	137	126	124	118	111	108	97	94	90
	0.131	8d			169	144	132	130	123	116	114	102	99	94
	0.135		16d	12d	180	153	141	138	131	123	121	108	105	100
	0.148	10d	20d	16d	205	174	160	157	149	140	137	123	121	117
	0.162	16d	40d		245	209	192	188	179	168	165	147	145	140
	0.177			20d	284	241	222	218	207	195	191	170	167	162
	0.192	20d		30d	295	251	231	227	216	202	198	177	174	169
	0.207	30d		40d	310	270	251	246	236	222	217	194	191	185
	0.225	40d			328	285	265	260	249	235	231	209	205	200
	0.244	50d		60d	336	291	271	266	254	240	236	213	210	204

1. Tabulated lateral design values (Z) shall be multiplied by all applicable adjustment factors (see Table 10.3.1).

2. Tabulated lateral design values (Z) are for common wire, box, and sinker nails (see Appendix L) inserted in side grain with nail axis perpendicular to wood fibers; minimum nail penetration, p, into the main member equal to 10D; dowel bearing strength (F_e) of 61,850 psi for ASTM A 653, Grade 33 steel and nail bending yield strengths (F_{yb}): F_{yb} = 100,000 psi for 0.099" ≤ D ≤ 0.142"; F_{yb} = 90,000 psi for 0.142" < D ≤ 0.177"; F_{yb} = 80,000 psi for 0.177" < D ≤ 0.236"; F_{yb} = 70,000 psi for 0.236" < D ≤ 0.273"

3. When 6D ≤ p < 10D, tabulated lateral design values (Z) shall be multiplied by p/10D.

NAILS

DOWEL-TYPE FASTENERS

11

Table 11Q COMMON WIRE, BOX, or SINKER NAILS: Reference Lateral Design Values (Z) for Single Shear (two member) Connections[1,2,3,4]

with wood structural panel side members with an effective G = 0.50

Side Member Thickness t_s (in.)	Nail Diameter D (in.)	Common Wire Nail	Box Nail	Sinker Nail	G=0.67 Red Oak (lbs.)	G=0.55 Mixed Maple Southern Pine (lbs.)	G=0.5 Douglas Fir-Larch (lbs.)	G=0.49 Douglas Fir-Larch (N) (lbs.)	G=0.46 Douglas Fir(S) Hem-Fir(N) (lbs.)	G=0.43 Hem-Fir (lbs.)	G=0.42 Spruce-Pine-Fir (lbs.)	G=0.37 Redwood (open grain) (lbs.)	G=0.36 Eastern Softwoods Spruce-Pine-Fir(S) Western Cedars Western Woods (lbs.)	G=0.35 Northern Species (lbs.)
3/8	0.099		6d	7d	47	45	43	43	42	40	40	38	37	37
	0.113	6d	8d	8d	60	56	54	54	52	51	50	47	47	46
	0.120			10d	67	62	60	60	58	56	56	52	52	51
	0.128		10d		75	70	68	67	65	63	63	59	58	57
	0.131	8d			78	73	71	70	68	66	65	61	61	60
	0.135		16d	12d	83	78	75	74	72	70	69	65	64	63
	0.148	10d	20d	16d	94	88	85	84	82	79	78	73	72	71
7/16	0.099		6d	7d	50	47	45	45	44	43	42	40	40	39
	0.113	6d	8d	8d	62	58	56	56	55	53	52	49	49	48
	0.120			10d	69	65	63	62	60	59	58	55	54	53
	0.128		10d		77	72	70	69	68	66	65	61	60	59
	0.131	8d			80	75	73	72	70	68	67	63	63	62
	0.135		16d	12d	85	80	77	76	74	72	71	67	66	65
	0.148	10d	20d	16d	96	90	87	86	84	81	80	76	75	73
	0.162	16d	40d		114	106	102	101	99	96	95	89	88	86
15/32	0.099		6d	7d	51	48	47	46	45	44	44	41	41	40
	0.113	6d	8d	8d	64	60	58	57	56	54	54	51	50	49
	0.120			10d	70	66	64	63	62	60	59	56	55	54
	0.128		10d		78	74	71	71	69	67	66	62	62	61
	0.131	8d			82	77	74	73	72	70	69	65	64	63
	0.135		16d	12d	86	81	78	77	76	73	72	68	67	66
	0.148	10d	20d	16d	97	91	88	87	85	83	82	77	76	75
	0.162	16d	40d		115	108	104	103	100	97	96	90	89	88
19/32	0.099		6d	7d	58	55	53	53	51	50	50	47	46	46
	0.113	6d	8d	8d	70	66	64	64	62	61	60	57	56	55
	0.120			10d	77	73	70	70	68	66	66	62	61	60
	0.128		10d		85	80	78	77	75	73	72	68	68	67
	0.131	8d			88	83	80	80	78	76	75	71	70	69
	0.135		16d	12d	93	87	84	84	82	79	79	74	73	72
	0.148	10d	20d	16d	104	98	95	94	92	89	88	83	82	81
	0.162	16d	40d		121	114	110	109	107	103	102	96	95	94
	0.177			20d	137	128	124	123	120	116	115	108	107	105
	0.192	20d		30d	142	133	128	127	124	120	119	112	111	109
23/32	0.099		6d	7d	62	58	55	55	53	51	51	47	47	46
	0.113	6d	8d	8d	78	74	72	71	69	67	66	62	61	60
	0.120			10d	85	80	78	77	76	73	73	69	68	67
	0.128		10d		93	88	85	85	83	80	80	75	75	74
	0.131	8d			96	91	88	87	86	83	82	78	77	76
	0.135		16d	12d	101	95	92	91	89	87	86	81	81	79
	0.148	10d	20d	16d	113	106	103	102	100	97	96	91	90	89
	0.162	16d	40d		130	122	118	117	115	111	110	104	103	102
	0.177			20d	145	137	132	131	128	124	123	116	115	113
	0.192	20d		30d	150	141	136	135	132	128	127	120	118	116
1	0.099[5]		6d	7d	62	58	55	55	53	51	51	47	47	46
	0.113[5]	6d[4]	8d	8d	81	75	72	71	69	67	66	62	61	60
	0.120[5]			10d	92	85	81	81	78	76	75	69	69	67
	0.128		10d		104	97	93	92	89	86	85	79	78	77
	0.131	8d			109	101	97	96	93	90	89	83	82	80
	0.135		16d	12d	116	108	103	102	99	96	94	88	87	85
	0.148	10d	20d	16d	132	123	118	116	113	109	108	100	99	97
	0.162	16d	40d		154	146	141	139	135	131	129	120	119	116
	0.177			20d	169	160	155	154	151	146	145	137	136	134
	0.192	20d		30d	174	164	159	158	155	150	149	141	140	138
1-1/8	0.128[5]		10d		104	97	93	92	89	86	85	79	78	77
	0.131[5]	8d			109	101	97	96	93	90	89	83	82	80
	0.135[5]		16d	12d	116	108	103	102	99	96	94	88	87	85
	0.148[5]	10d	20d	16d	132	123	118	116	113	109	108	100	99	97
	0.162	16d	40d		158	147	141	139	135	131	129	120	119	116
	0.177			20d	181	170	163	161	157	151	149	139	137	135
	0.192	20d		30d	186	176	170	168	163	157	155	145	143	140
1-1/4	0.148	10d	20d	16d	132	123	118	116	113	109	108	100	99	97
	0.162	16d	40d		158	147	141	139	135	131	129	120	119	116
	0.177			20d	183	170	163	161	157	151	149	139	137	135
	0.192	20d		30d	191	177	170	168	163	157	155	145	143	140

1. Tabulated lateral design values (Z) shall be multiplied by all applicable adjustment factors (see Table 10.3.1).
2. Tabulated lateral design values (Z) are for common wire, box, and sinker nails (see Appendix L) inserted in side grain with nail axis perpendicular to wood fibers; minimum nail penetration, p, into the main member equal to 10D and nail bending yield strengths (F_{yb}): F_{yb} = 100,000 psi for 0.099" $\leq$ D $\leq$ 0.142"; F_{yb} = 90,000 psi for 0.142" < D $\leq$ 0.177"; F_{yb} = 80,000 psi for 0.177" < D $\leq$ 0.236"
3. When 6D $\leq$ p < 10D, tabulated lateral design values (Z) shall be multiplied by p/10D.
4. Nail length is insufficient to provide 10D penetration. Tabulated lateral design values (Z) shall be adjusted per footnote 3.
5. Tabulated lateral design values (Z) shall be permitted to apply for greater side member thickness when adjusted per footnote 3.

able 11R COMMON WIRE, BOX, or SINKER NAILS: Reference Lateral Design Values (Z) for Single Shear (two member) Connections[1,2,3,4]

with wood structural panel side members with an effective G = 0.42

Side Member Thickness t_s in.	Nail Diameter D in.	Common Wire Nail	Box Nail	Sinker Nail Pennyweight	G=0.67 Red Oak lbs.	G=0.55 Mixed Maple Southern Pine lbs.	G=0.5 Douglas Fir-Larch lbs.	G=0.49 Douglas Fir-Larch (N) lbs.	G=0.46 Douglas Fir(S) Hem-Fir(N) lbs.	G=0.43 Hem-Fir lbs.	G=0.42 Spruce-Pine-Fir lbs.	G=0.37 Redwood (open grain) lbs.	G=0.36 Eastern Softwoods Spruce-Pine-Fir(S) Western Cedars Western Woods lbs.	G=0.35 Northern Species lbs.
3/8	0.099		6d	7d	41	39	37	37	36	35	35	33	33	32
	0.113	6d	8d	8d	52	49	48	47	46	45	45	42	42	41
	0.120			10d	58	55	53	53	52	50	50	47	47	46
	0.128		10d		66	62	60	60	59	57	56	53	53	52
	0.131	8d			69	65	63	63	61	59	59	56	55	54
	0.135		16d	12d	73	69	67	66	65	63	62	59	58	57
	0.148	10d	20d	16d	84	79	76	76	74	72	71	67	66	65
7/16	0.099		6d	7d	42	40	39	38	38	37	36	35	34	34
	0.113	6d	8d	8d	53	50	49	48	48	46	46	43	43	42
	0.120			10d	59	56	54	54	53	51	51	48	48	47
	0.128		10d		67	63	61	61	60	58	57	54	54	53
	0.131	8d			70	66	64	64	62	60	60	57	56	55
	0.135		16d	12d	74	70	68	67	66	64	63	60	59	58
	0.148	10d	20d	16d	84	80	77	76	75	73	72	68	67	66
	0.162	16d	40d		100	95	92	91	89	86	85	81	80	78
15/32	0.099		6d	7d	43	41	40	39	39	38	37	35	35	35
	0.113	6d	8d	8d	54	51	50	49	48	47	47	44	44	43
	0.120			10d	60	57	55	55	54	52	52	49	49	48
	0.128		10d		68	64	62	62	60	59	58	55	55	54
	0.131	8d			70	67	65	64	63	61	61	57	57	56
	0.135		16d	12d	75	71	68	68	66	65	64	61	60	59
	0.148	10d	20d	16d	85	80	78	77	75	73	72	69	68	67
	0.162	16d	40d		101	95	92	91	89	87	86	81	80	79
19/32	0.099		6d	7d	47	45	44	43	43	41	41	39	39	38
	0.113	6d	8d	8d	58	55	54	53	52	51	50	48	48	47
	0.120			10d	64	61	59	59	58	56	56	53	52	52
	0.128		10d		71	68	66	65	64	62	62	59	58	57
	0.131	8d			74	70	68	68	67	65	64	61	61	60
	0.135		16d	12d	78	74	72	71	70	68	68	64	64	63
	0.148	10d	20d	16d	88	84	81	81	79	77	76	72	72	71
	0.162	16d	40d		103	98	95	94	93	90	89	85	84	83
	0.177			20d	118	112	108	108	105	102	101	96	95	94
	0.192	20d		30d	123	116	112	112	109	106	105	100	99	97
23/32	0.099		6d	7d	52	50	48	48	47	46	46	44	43	43
	0.113	6d	8d	8d	63	60	58	58	57	56	55	53	52	52
	0.120			10d	69	66	64	64	62	61	60	58	57	56
	0.128		10d		76	73	71	70	69	67	67	63	63	62
	0.131	8d			79	75	73	73	71	70	69	66	65	64
	0.135		16d	12d	83	79	77	76	75	73	72	69	68	67
	0.148	10d	20d	16d	93	89	86	86	84	82	81	77	77	76
	0.162	16d	40d		108	103	100	99	98	95	94	90	89	87
	0.177			20d	122	116	113	112	110	107	106	101	100	98
	0.192	20d		30d	127	120	117	117	114	111	110	104	103	102
1	0.099[5]		6d	7d	56	53	51	50	49	48	47	44	44	43
	0.113[5]	6d[4]	8d	8d	73	68	66	66	64	62	61	58	57	56
	0.120[5]			10d	82	77	75	74	72	70	69	65	64	63
	0.128		10d		91	87	85	84	82	80	79	74	73	72
	0.131	8d			93	89	87	87	85	83	82	77	77	75
	0.135		16d	12d	97	93	91	90	89	87	86	82	81	80
	0.148	10d	20d	16d	109	104	101	101	99	97	96	91	91	90
	0.162	16d	40d		124	118	115	115	113	110	109	104	103	102
	0.177			20d	137	131	128	127	125	122	121	115	114	112
	0.192	20d		30d	141	135	131	131	128	125	124	118	117	116
1-1/8	0.128[5]		10d		93	88	85	84	82	80	79	74	73	72
	0.131[5]	8d			98	92	89	88	86	83	82	77	77	75
	0.135[5]		16d	12d	104	98	94	94	91	88	88	82	81	80
	0.148[5]	10d	20d	16d	117	111	108	107	104	101	100	94	93	91
	0.162	16d	40d		132	127	123	123	120	118	117	111	110	109
	0.177			20d	146	139	136	135	132	129	128	122	121	120
	0.192	20d		30d	150	143	139	138	136	133	132	126	125	123
1-1/4	0.148	10d	20d	16d	118	111	108	107	104	101	100	94	93	91
	0.162	16d	40d		141	134	129	128	125	121	120	112	111	109
	0.177			20d	155	148	144	143	141	138	136	130	129	126
	0.192	20d		30d	159	152	148	147	144	141	140	134	133	131

1. Tabulated lateral design values (Z) shall be multiplied by all applicable adjustment factors (see Table 10.3.1).
2. Tabulated lateral design values (Z) are for common wire, box, and sinker nails (see Appendix L) inserted in side grain with nail axis perpendicular to wood fibers; minimum nail penetration, p, into the main member equal to 10D and nail bending yield strengths (F_{yb}): F_{yb} = 100,000 psi for 0.099" ≤ D ≤ 0.142"; F_{yb} = 90,000 psi for 0.142" < D ≤ 0.177"; F_{yb} = 80,000 psi for 0.177" < D ≤ 0.236"
3. When 6D ≤ p < 10D, tabulated lateral design values (Z) shall be multiplied by p/10D.
4. Nail length is insufficient to provide 10D penetration. Tabulated lateral design values (Z) shall be adjusted per footnote 3.
5. Tabulated lateral design values (Z) shall be permitted to apply for greater side member thickness when adjusted per footnote 3.

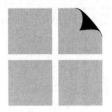

SPLIT RING AND SHEAR PLATE CONNECTORS

12

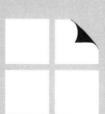

12.1 General

12.1.1 Terminology

A connector unit shall be defined as one of the following:

(a) One split ring with its bolt or lag screw in single shear (see Figure 12A).

(b) Two shear plates used back to back in the contact faces of a wood-to-wood connection with their bolt or lag screw in single shear (see Figures 12B and 12C).

(c) One shear plate with its bolt or lag screw in single shear used in conjunction with a steel strap or shape in a wood-to-metal connection (see Figures 12B and 12C).

Figure 12A   Split Ring Connector

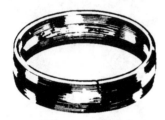

Figure 12B   Pressed Steel Shear Plate Connector

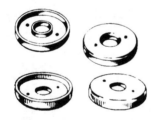

Figure 12C   Malleable Iron Shear Plate Connector

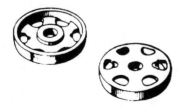

12.1.2 Quality of Split Ring and Shear Plate Connectors

12.1.2.1 Design provisions and reference design values herein apply to split ring and shear plate connectors of the following quality:

(a) Split rings manufactured from SAE 1010 hot rolled carbon steel (Reference 34). Each ring shall form a closed true circle with the principal axis of the cross section of the ring metal parallel to the geometric axis of the ring. The ring shall fit snugly in the precut groove. This shall be accomplished with a ring, the metal section of which is beveled from the central portion toward the edges to a thickness less than at midsection, or by any other method which will accomplish equivalent performance. It shall be cut through in one place in its circumference to form a tongue and slot (see Figure 12A).

(b) Shear plate connectors:

(1) 2-5/8" Pressed Steel Type—Pressed steel shear plates manufactured from SAE 1010 hot rolled carbon steel. Each plate shall be a true circle with a flange around the edge, extending at right angles to the face of the plate and extending from one face only, the plate portion having a central bolt hole, with an integral hub concentric to the hole or without an integral hub, and two small perforations on opposite sides of the hole and midway from the center and circumference (see Figure 12B).

(2) 4" Malleable Iron Type—Malleable iron shear plates manufactured according to Grade 32510 of ASTM Standard A47. Each casting shall consist of a perforated round plate with a flange around the edge extending at right angles to the face of the plate and projecting from one face only, the plate portion having a central bolt hole with an integral hub extending from the same face as the flange (see Figure 12C).

12.1.2.2 Dimensions for typical split ring and shear plate connectors are provided in Appendix K. Dimensional tolerances of split ring and shear plate connectors shall not be greater than those conforming to standard practices for the machine operations involved in manufacturing the connectors.

12.1.2.3 Bolts used with split ring and shear plate connectors shall conform to 11.1.2. The bolt shall have an unreduced nominal or shank (body) diameter in accordance with ANSI/ASME Standard B18.2.1.

12.1.2.4 When lag screws are used in place of bolts, the lag screws shall conform to 11.1.3 and the shank of the lag screw shall have the same diameter as the bolt specified for the split ring or shear plate connector (see Tables 12.2A and 12.2B). The lag screw shall have an unreduced nominal or shank (body) diameter and threads in accordance with ANSI/ASME Standard B18.2.1.

12.1.3 Fabrication and Assembly

12.1.3.1 The grooves, daps, and bolt holes specified in Appendix K shall be accurately cut or bored, and shall be oriented in contacting faces. Since split ring and shear plate connectors from different manufacturers differ slightly in shape and cross section, cutter heads shall be designed to produce daps and grooves conforming accurately to the dimensions and shape of the particular split ring or shear plate connectors used.

12.1.3.2 When lag screws are used in place of bolts, the hole for the unthreaded shank shall be the same diameter as the shank. The diameter of the hole for the threaded portion of the lag screw shall be approxi-mately 70% of the shank diameter, or as specified in 11.1.3.2.

12.1.3.3 In installation of split ring or shear plate connectors and bolts or lag screws, a nut shall be placed on each bolt, and washers, not smaller than the size specified in Appendix K, shall be placed between the outside wood member and the bolt or lag screw head and between the outside wood member and nut. When an outside member of a shear plate connection is a steel strap or shape, the washer is not required, except when a longer bolt or lag screw is used, in which case, the washer prevents the metal plate or shape from bearing on the threaded portion of the bolt or lag screw.

12.1.3.4 Reference design values for split ring and shear plate connectors are based on the assumption that the faces of the members are brought into contact when the connector units are installed, and allow for seasonal variations after the wood has reached the moisture content normal to the conditions of service. When split ring or shear plate connectors are installed in wood which is not seasoned to the moisture content normal to the conditions of service, the connections shall be tightened by turning down the nuts periodically until moisture equilibrium is reached.

12.2 Reference Design Values

12.2.1 Reference Design Values

12.2.1.1 Tables 12.2A and 12.2B contain reference design values for a single split ring or shear plate connector unit with bolt in single shear, installed in the side grain of two wood members (Table 12A) with sufficient member thicknesses, edge distances, end distances, and spacing to develop reference design values. Reference design values (P, Q) shall be multiplied by all applicable adjustment factors (see Table 10.3.1) to obtain adjusted design values (P', Q').

12.2.1.2 Adjusted design values (P', Q') for shear plate connectors shall not exceed the limiting reference design values specified in Footnote 2 of Table 12.2B. The limiting reference design values in Footnote 2 of Table 12.2B shall not be multiplied by adjustment factors in this Specification since they are based on strength of metal rather than strength of wood (see 10.2.3).

Table 12A   Species Groups for Split Ring and Shear Plate Connectors

Species Group	Specific Gravity, G
A	$G \geq 0.60$
B	$0.49 \leq G < 0.60$
C	$0.42 \leq G < 0.49$
D	$G < 0.42$

12.2.2 Thickness of Wood Members

12.2.2.1 Reference design values shall not be used for split ring or shear plate connectors installed in any piece of wood of a net thickness less than the minimum specified in Tables 12.2A and 12.2B.

12.2.2.2 Reference design values for split ring or shear plate connectors installed in any piece of wood of net thickness intermediate between the minimum thickness and that required for maximum reference design value, as specified in Tables 12.2A and 12.2B, shall be obtained by linear interpolation.

Table 12.2A Split Ring Connector Unit Reference Design Values

Tabulated design values[1] apply to ONE split ring and bolt in single shear.

Split ring diameter in.	Bolt diameter in.	Number of faces of member with connectors on same bolt	Net thickness of member in.	Loaded parallel to grain (0°) Design value, P, per connector unit and bolt, lbs.				Loaded perpendicular to grain (90°) Design value, Q, per connector unit and bolt, lbs.			
				Group A species	Group B species	Group C species	Group D species	Group A species	Group B species	Group C species	Group D species
2-1/2	1/2	1	1" minimum	2630	2270	1900	1640	1900	1620	1350	1160
			1-1/2" or thicker	3160	2730	2290	1960	2280	1940	1620	1390
		2	1-1/2" minimum	2430	2100	1760	1510	1750	1500	1250	1070
			2" or thicker	3160	2730	2290	1960	2280	1940	1620	1390
4	3/4	1	1" minimum	4090	3510	2920	2520	2840	2440	2040	1760
			1-1/2"	6020	5160	4280	3710	4180	3590	2990	2580
			1-5/8" or thicker	6140	5260	4380	3790	4270	3660	3050	2630
		2	1-1/2" minimum	4110	3520	2940	2540	2980	2450	2040	1760
			2"	4950	4250	3540	3050	3440	2960	2460	2120
			2-1/2"	5830	5000	4160	3600	4050	3480	2890	2500
			3" or thicker	6140	5260	4380	3790	4270	3660	3050	2630

1. Tabulated lateral design values (P,Q) for split ring connector units shall be multiplied to all applicable adjustment factors (see Table 10.3.1).

Table 12.2B Shear Plate Connector Unit Reference Design Values

Tabulated design values[1,2,3] apply to ONE shear plate and bolt in single shear.

Shear plate diameter in.	Bolt diameter in.	Number of faces of member with connectors on same bolt	Net thickness of member in.	Loaded parallel to grain (0°) Design value, P, per connector unit and bolt, lbs.				Loaded perpendicular to grain (90°) Design value, Q, per connector unit and bolt, lbs.			
				Group A species	Group B species	Group C species	Group D species	Group A species	Group B species	Group C species	Group D species
2-5/8	3/4	1	1-1/2" minimum	3110*	2670	2220	2010	2170	1860	1550	1330
		2	1-1/2" minimum	2420	2080	1730	1500	1690	1450	1210	1040
			2"	3190*	2730	2270	1960	2220	1910	1580	1370
			2-1/2" or thicker	3330*	2860	2380	2060	2320	1990	1650	1440
4	3/4 or 7/8	1	1-1/2" minimum	4370	3750	3130	2700	3040	2620	2170	1860
			1-3/4" or thicker	5090*	4360	3640	3140	3540	3040	2530	2200
		2	1-3/4" minimum	3390*	2910	2420	2090	2360	2020	1680	1410
			2"	3790	3240	2700	2330	2640	2260	1880	1630
			2-1/2"	4310	3690	3080	2660	3000	2550	2140	1850
			3"	4830*	4140	3450	2980	3360	2880	2400	2060
			3-1/2" or thicker	5030*	4320	3600	3110	3500	3000	2510	2160

1. Tabulated lateral design values (P,Q) for shear plate connector units shall be multiplied to all applicable adjustment factors (see Table 10.3.1).
2. Allowable design values for shear plate connector units shall not exceed the following:
   (a) 2-5/8" shear plate ....2900 pounds
   (b) 4" shear plate with 3/4" bolt ....4400 pounds
   (c) 4" shear plate with 7/8" bolt ....6000 pounds
   The design values in Footnote 2 shall be permitted to be increased in accordance with the American Institute of Steel Construction (AISC) Manual of Steel Construction, 9th edition, Section A5.2 ''Wind and Seismic Stresses'', except when design loads have already been reduced by load combination factors (see NDS 10.2.3).
3. Loads followed by an asterisk (*) exceed those permitted by Footnote 2, but are needed for determination of design values for other angles of load to grain. Footnote 2 limitations apply in all cases.

12.2.3 Penetration Depth Factor, C_d

When lag screws instead of bolts are used with split ring or shear plate connectors, reference design values shall be multiplied by the appropriate penetration depth factor, C_d, specified in Table 12.2.3. Lag screw penetration into the member receiving the point shall not be less than the minimum penetration specified in Table 12.2.3. When the actual lag screw penetration into the member receiving the point is greater than the minimum penetration, but less than the minimum penetration for $C_d = 1.0$, the penetration depth factor, C_d, shall be determined by linear interpolation. The penetration depth factor shall not exceed unity, $C_d \leq 1.0$.

12.2.4 Metal Side Plate Factor, C_{st}

When metal side members are used in place of wood side members, the reference design values parallel to grain, P, for 4" shear plate connectors shall be multiplied by the appropriate metal side plate factor specified in Table 12.2.4.

Table 12.2.4 Metal Side Plate Factors, C_{st}, for 4" Shear Plate Connectors Loaded Parallel to Grain

Species Group	C_{st}
A	1.18
B	1.11
C	1.05
D	1.00

The adjusted design values parallel to grain, P', shall not exceed the limiting reference design values given in Footnote 2 of Table 12.2B (see 12.2.1.2).

12.2.5 Load at Angle to Grain

12.2.5.1 When a load acts in the plane of the wood surface at an angle to grain other than 0° or 90°, the adjusted design value, N', for a split ring or shear plate connector unit shall be determined as follows (see Appendix J):

$$N' = \frac{P'Q'}{P' \sin^2 \theta + Q' \cos^2 \theta} \qquad (12.2-1)$$

where:

θ = angle between direction of load and direction of grain (longitudinal axis of member)

Table 12.2.3 Penetration Depth Factors, C_d, for Split Ring and Shear Plate Connectors Used with Lag Screws

	Side Member	Penetration	Penetration of Lag Screw into Main Member (number of shank diameters) Species Group (see Table 12A)				Penetration Depth Factor, C_d
			Group A	Group B	Group C	Group D	
2-1/2" Split Ring 4" Split Ring 4" Shear Plate	Wood or Metal	Minimum for $C_d = 1.0$	7	8	10	11	1.0
		Minimum for $C_d = 0.75$	3	3-1/2	4	4-1/2	0.75
2-5/8" Shear Plate	Wood	Minimum for $C_d = 1.0$	4	5	7	8	1.0
		Minimum for $C_d = 0.75$	3	3-1/2	4	4-1/2	0.75
	Metal	Minimum for $C_d = 1.0$	3	3-1/2	4	4-1/2	1.0

12.2.5.2 Adjusted design values at an angle to grain, N', for shear plate connectors shall not exceed the limiting reference design values specified in Footnote 2 of Table 12.2.B (see 12.2.1.2).

12.2.6 Split Ring and Shear Plate Connectors in End Grain

12.2.6.1 When split ring or shear plate connectors are installed in a surface that is not parallel to the general direction of the grain of the member, such as the end of a square-cut member, or the sloping surface of a member cut at an angle to its axis, or the surface of a structural glued laminated timber cut at an angle to the direction of the laminations, the following terminology shall apply:

- "Side grain surface" means a surface parallel to the general direction of the wood fibers ($\alpha = 0°$), such as the top, bottom, and sides of a straight beam.
- "Sloping surface" means a surface cut at an angle, α, other than 0° or 90° to the general direction of the wood fibers.
- "Square-cut surface" means a surface perpendicular to the general direction of the wood fibers ($\alpha = 90°$).
- "Axis of cut" defines the direction of a sloping surface relative to the general direction of the wood fibers. For a sloping cut symmetrical about one of the major axes of the member, as in Figures 12D, 12G, 12H, and 12I, the axis of cut is parallel to a major axis. For an asymmetrical sloping surface (i.e., one that slopes relative to both major axes of the member), the axis of cut is the direction of a line defining the intersection of the sloping surface with any plane that is both normal to the sloping surface and also is aligned with the general direction of the wood fibers (see Figure 12E).

   α = the least angle formed between a sloping surface and the general direction of the wood fibers (i.e., the acute angle between the axis of cut and the general direction of the fibers. Sometimes called the slope of the cut. See Figures 12D through 12I).

   φ = the angle between the direction of applied load and the axis of cut of a sloping surface, measured in the plane of the sloping surface (see Figure 12I).

   P' = adjusted design value for a split ring or shear plate connector unit in a side grain surface, loaded parallel to grain ($\alpha = 0°$, $\varphi = 0°$).

Q' = adjusted design value for a split ring or shear plate connector unit in a side grain surface, loaded perpendicular to grain ($\alpha = 0°$, $\varphi = 90°$).

Q'_{90} = adjusted design value for a split ring or shear plate connector unit in a square-cut surface, loaded in any direction in the plane of the surface ($\alpha = 90°$).

P'_{α} = adjusted design value for a split ring or shear plate connector unit in a sloping surface, loaded in a direction parallel to the axis of cut ($0° < \alpha < 90°$, $\varphi = 0°$).

Q'_{α} = adjusted design value for a split ring or shear plate connector unit in a sloping surface, loaded in a direction perpendicular to the axis of cut ($0° < \alpha < 90°$, $\varphi = 90°$).

N'_{α} = adjusted design value for a split ring or shear plate connector unit in a sloping surface, when direction of load is at an angle φ from the axis of cut.

Figure 12D Axis of Cut for Symmetrical Sloping End Cut

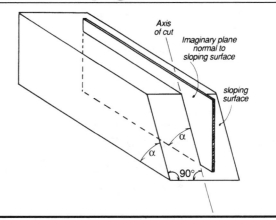

Figure 12E Axis of Cut for Asymmetrical Sloping End Cut

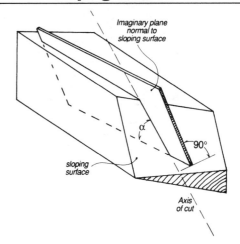

12.2.6.2 When split ring or shear plate connectors are installed in square-cut end grain or sloping surfaces, adjusted design values shall be determined as follows (see 10.2.2):

(a) Square-cut surface; loaded in any direction ($\alpha = 90°$, see Figure 12F).

$$Q_{90}' = 0.60Q'$$ (12.2-2)

Figure 12F Square End Cut

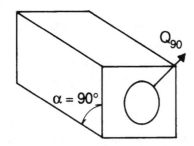

(b) Sloping surface; loaded parallel to axis of cut ($0° < \alpha < 90°$, $\varphi = 0°$, see Figure 12G).

$$P_\alpha' = \frac{P'Q_{90}'}{P' \sin^2 \alpha + Q_{90}' \cos^2 \alpha}$$ (12.2-3)

Figure 12G Sloping End Cut with Load Parallel to Axis of Cut ($\varphi = 0°$)

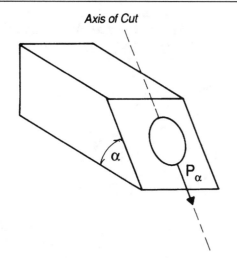

(c) Sloping surface; loaded perpendicular to axis of cut ($0° < \alpha < 90°$, $\varphi = 90°$, see Figure 12H).

$$Q_\alpha' = \frac{Q'Q_{90}'}{Q' \sin^2 \alpha + Q_{90}' \cos^2 \alpha}$$ (12.2-4)

Figure 12H Sloping End Cut with Load Perpendicular to Axis of Cut ($\varphi = 90°$)

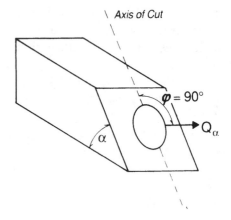

(d) Sloping surface; loaded at angle φ to axis of cut ($0° < \alpha < 90°$, $0° < \varphi < 90°$, see Figure 12I).

$$N_\alpha' = \frac{P_\alpha'Q_\alpha'}{P_\alpha' \sin^2 \varphi + Q_\alpha' \cos^2 \varphi}$$ (12.2-5)

Figure 12I Sloping End Cut with Load at an Angle φ to Axis of Cut

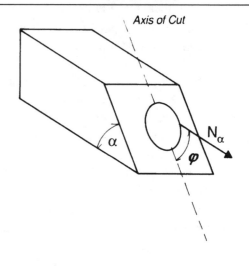

12.3 Placement of Split Ring and Shear Plate Connectors

12.3.1 Terminology

12.3.1.1 "Edge distance" is the distance from the edge of a member to the center of the nearest split ring or shear plate connector, measured perpendicular to grain. When a member is loaded perpendicular to grain, the loaded edge shall be defined as the edge toward which the load is acting. The unloaded edge shall be defined as the edge opposite the loaded edge (see Figure 12J).

12.3.1.2 "End distance" is the distance measured parallel to grain from the square-cut end of a member to the center of the nearest split ring or shear plate connector (see Figure 12J). If the end of a member is not cut at a right angle to its longitudinal axis, the end distance, measured parallel to the longitudinal axis from any point on the center half of the transverse connector diameter, shall not be less than the end distance required for a square-cut member. In no case shall the perpendicular distance from the center of a connector to the sloping end cut of a member, be less than the required edge distance (see Figure 12K).

Figure 12J Connection Geometry for Split Rings and Shear Plates

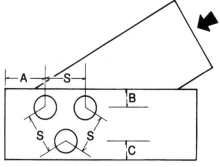

A = End Distance
B = Unloaded Edge Distance
C = Loaded Edge Distance
S = Spacing

12.3.1.3 "Spacing" is the distance between centers of split ring or shear plate connectors measured along a line joining their centers (see Figure 12J).

Figure 12K End Distance for Members with Sloping End Cut

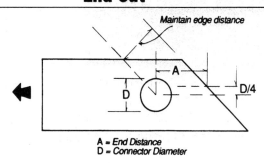

A = End Distance
D = Connector Diameter

12.3.2 Geometry Factor, C_Δ

Reference design values are for split ring and shear plate connectors with edge distance, end distance, and spacing greater than or equal to the minimum required for $C_\Delta = 1.0$. When the edge distance, end distance, or spacing provided is less than the minimum required $C_\Delta = 1.0$, reference design values shall be multiplied by the smallest applicable geometry factor, C_Δ, determined from the edge distance, end distance, and spacing requirements for split ring and shear plate connectors (see 12.3.3, 12.3.4, and 12.3.5). The smallest geometry factor for any split ring or shear plate connector in a group shall apply to all split ring and shear plate connectors in the group.

12.3.3 Edge Distance

12.3.3.1 Members Loaded Parallel or Perpendicular to Grain. Minimum edge distances and associated geometry factors, C_Δ, for split ring and shear plate connectors installed in side grain and loaded parallel or perpendicular to grain are provided in Table 12.3. When the actual loaded edge distance is greater than or equal to the minimum loaded edge distance, but less than the minimum loaded edge distance for $C_\Delta = 1.0$, the geometry factor, C_Δ, shall be determined by linear interpolation.

12.3.3.2 Members Loaded at Angle to Grain. When members are loaded at an angle to grain, θ, other than 0° or 90°, the minimum loaded edge distances and the minimum unloaded edge distances in Table 12.3 shall apply for all angles of load to grain. Minimum loaded edge distances for $C_\Delta = 1.0$ shall be determined as follows:

(a) When $45° \leq \theta \leq 90°$, the minimum loaded edge distance for $C_\Delta = 1.0$ for perpendicular to grain loading shall apply.

(b) When $0° \leq \theta < 45°$, the minimum loaded edge distance for $C_\Delta = 1.0$ shall be determined by linear interpolation between the minimum loaded edge distance and the minimum loaded edge distance for $C_\Delta = 1.0$ for perpendicular to grain loading.

When a member is loaded at an angle to grain, θ, other than $0°$ or $90°$, the geometry factor, C_Δ, based on edge distance requirements shall apply to both the reference parallel and perpendicular to grain design values (P, Q).

12.3.4 End Distance

12.3.4.1 Members Loaded Parallel or Perpendicular to Grain. Minimum end distances and associated geometry factors, C_Δ, for split ring and shear plate connectors installed in side grain and loaded parallel or perpendicular to grain are provided in Table 12.3. When the actual end distance is greater than or equal to the minimum end distance, but less than the minimum end distance for $C_\Delta = 1.0$, the geometry factor, C_Δ, shall be determined by linear interpolation.

12.3.4.2 Members Loaded at Angle to Grain. When members are loaded at an angle to grain, θ, other than $0°$ or $90°$, minimum end distances and minimum end distances for $C_\Delta = 1.0$ shall be determined by linear interpolation between tabulated end distances for parallel and perpendicular to grain loading.

12.3.5 Spacing

12.3.5.1 Members Loaded Parallel or Perpendicular to Grain. Minimum parallel and perpendicular to grain spacings and associated geometry factors, C_Δ, for split ring and shear plate connectors installed in side grain and loaded parallel or perpendicular to grain are provided in Table 12.3. When the line joining the centers of two adjacent split ring or shear plate connectors is at an angle to grain other than $0°$ or $90°$, the minimum spacing and the minimum spacing for $C_\Delta = 1.0$ shall be determined in accordance with the graphical method specified in References 47 and 48. When the actual spacing between split ring or shear plate connectors is greater than the minimum spacing, but less than the minimum spacing for $C_\Delta = 1.0$, the geometry factor, C_Δ, shall be determined by linear interpolation.

12.3.5.2 Members Loaded at Angle to Grain. When members are loaded at an angle to grain, θ, other than $0°$ or $90°$, the minimum spacing and minimum spacing for $C_\Delta = 1.0$ shall be determined in accordance with the graphical method specified in References 50 and 52.

12.3.6 Split Ring and Shear Plate Connectors in End Grain

12.3.6.1 The provisions for edge distance, end distance, and spacing given in 12.3.3, 12.3.4, and 12.3.5 for split ring and shear plate connectors installed in side grain shall apply to split ring and shear plate connectors installed in square-cut surfaces and sloping surfaces as follows (see 12.2.6 for definitions and terminology):

(a) Square-cut surface, loaded in any direction - apply provisions for perpendicular to grain loading.

(b) Sloping surface with α from $45°$ to $90°$, loaded in any direction - apply provisions for perpendicular to grain loading.

(c) Sloping surface with α less than $45°$, loaded parallel to axis of cut - apply provisions for parallel to grain loading.

(d) Sloping surface with α less than $45°$, loaded perpendicular to axis of cut - apply provisions for perpendicular to grain loading.

(e) Sloping surface with α less than $45°$, loaded at angle ϕ to axis of cut - apply provisions for members loaded at angles to grain other than $0°$ or $90°$.

12.3.6.2 When split ring or shear plate connectors are installed in end grain, the members shall be designed for shear parallel to grain in accordance with 3.4.3.3.

12.3.7 Multiple Split Ring or Shear Plate Connectors

12.3.7.1 When a connection contains two or more split ring or shear plate connector units which are in the same shear plane, are aligned in the direction of load, and on separate bolts or lag screws, the group action factor, C_g, shall be as specified in 10.3.6 and the total adjusted design value for the connection shall be as specified in 10.2.2.

12.3.7.2 If grooves for two sizes of split rings are cut concentric in the same wood surface, split ring connectors shall be installed in both grooves and the reference design value shall be taken as the reference design value for the larger split ring connector.

12.3.7.3 Local stresses in connections using multiple fasteners shall be evaluated in accordance with principles of engineering mechanics (see 10.1.2).

Table 12.3 Geometry Factors, C_Δ, for Split Ring and Shear Plate Connectors

		2-1/2" Split Ring Connectors & 2-5/8" Shear Plate Connectors				4" Split Ring Connectors & 4" Shear Plate Connectors			
		Parallel to grain loading		Perpendicular to grain loading		Parallel to grain loading		Perpendicular to grain loading	
		Minimum Value	Minimum for C_Δ = 1.0	Minimum Value	Minimum for C_Δ = 1.0	Minimum Value	Minimum for C_Δ = 1.0	Minimum Value	Minimum for C_Δ = 1.0
Edge Distance	Unloaded Edge C_Δ	1-3/4" 1.0	1-3/4" 1.0	1-3/4" 1.0	1-3/4" 1.0	2-3/4" 1.0	2-3/4" 1.0	2-3/4" 1.0	2-3/4" 1.0
	Loaded Edge C_Δ	1-3/4" 1.0	1-3/4" 1.0	1-3/4" 0.83	2-3/4" 1.0	2-3/4" 1.0	2-3/4" 1.0	2-3/4" 0.83	3-3/4" 1.0
End Distance	Tension Member C_Δ	2-3/4" 0.625	5-1/2" 1.0	2-3/4" 0.625	5-1/2" 1.0	3-1/2" 0.625	7" 1.0	3-1/2" 0.625	7" 1.0
	Compression Member C_Δ	2-1/2" 0.625	4" 1.0	2-3/4" 0.625	5-1/2" 1.0	3-1/4" 0.625	5-1/2" 1.0	3-1/2" 0.625	7" 1.0
Spacing	Spacing parallel to grain C_Δ	3-1/2" 0.5	6-3/4" 1.0	3-1/2" 1.0	3-1/2" 1.0	5" 0.5	9" 1.0	5" 1.0	5" 1.0
	Spacing perpendicular to grain C_Δ	3-1/2" 1.0	3-1/2" 1.0	3-1/2" 0.5	4-1/4" 1.0	5" 1.0	5" 1.0	5" 0.5	6" 1.0

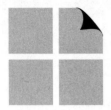

TIMBER RIVETS

13

13.1 General

Design criteria for timber rivet joints apply to timber rivets that satisfy the requirements of 13.1.1 loaded in single shear, with steel side plates on Douglas Fir-Larch or Southern Pine structural glued laminated timber manufactured in accordance with ANSI/AITC A190.1.

13.1.1 Quality of Rivets and Steel Side Plates

13.1.1.1 Design provisions and reference design values herein apply to timber rivets that are hot-dip galvanized in accordance with ASTM A 153 and manufactured from AISI 1035 steel to have the following properties tested in accordance with ASTM A 370:

Hardness	Ultimate tensile strength, F_u
Rockwell C32-39	145,000 psi, minimum

See Appendix M for rivet dimensions.

13.1.1.2 Steel side plates shall conform to ASTM Standard A 36 with a minimum 1/8" thickness. See Appendix M for steel side plate dimensions.

13.1.1.3 For wet service conditions, steel side plates shall be hot-dip galvanized in accordance with ASTM A 153.

13.1.2 Fabrication and Assembly

13.1.2.1 Each rivet shall, in all cases, be placed with its major cross-sectional dimension aligned paral-lel to the grain. Design criteria are based on rivets driven through circular holes in the side plates until the conical heads are firmly seated, but rivets shall not be driven flush. (Timber rivets at the perimeter of the group shall be driven first. Successive timber rivets shall be driven in a spiral pattern from the outside to the center of the group.)

13.1.2.2 The maximum penetration of any rivet shall be 70% of the thickness of the wood member. Except as permitted by 13.1.2.3, for joints with rivets driven from opposite faces of a wood member, the rivet length shall be such that the points do not overlap.

13.1.2.3 For joints where rivets are driven from opposite faces of a wood member such that their points overlap, the minimum spacing requirements of 13.3.1 shall apply to the distance between the rivets at their points and the maximum penetration requirement of 13.1.2.2 shall apply. The reference lateral design value of the connection shall be calculated in accordance with 13.2 considering the connection to be a one sided timber rivet joint, with:

(a) the number of rivets associated with the one plate equalling the total number of rivets at the joint, and

(b) s_p and s_q determined as the distances between the rivets at their points.

13.2 Reference Design Values

13.2.1 Parallel to Grain Loading

For timber rivet connections (one plate and rivets associated with it) where:

(a) the load acts perpendicular to the axis of the timber rivets

(b) member thicknesses, edge distances, end distances, and spacing are sufficient to develop full adjusted design values (see 13.3)

(c) timber rivets are installed in the side grain of wood members the reference design value per rivet joint parallel to grain, P, shall be calculated as the lesser of reference rivet capacity, P_r, and reference wood capacity, P_w:

$$P_r = 280 \, p^{0.32} \, n_R \, n_c \qquad (13.2-1)$$

P_w = reference wood capacity design values parallel to grain (Tables 13.2.1A through 13.2.1F) using wood member thickness for the member dimension in Tables 13.2.1A through 13.2.1F for connections with steel plates on opposite sides; and twice the wood member thickness for the member dimension in Tables 13.2.1A through 13.2.1F for connections having only one plate, lbs.

where:

p = depth of penetration of rivet in wood member (see Appendix M), in.

= rivet length – plate thickness – 1/8"

n_R = number of rows of rivets parallel to direction of load

n_c = number of rivets per row

Reference design values, P, for timber rivet connections parallel to grain shall be multiplied by all applicable adjustment factors (see Table 10.3.1) to obtain adjusted design values, P'.

13.2.2 Perpendicular to Grain Loading

For timber rivet connections (one plate and rivets associated with it) where:
(a) the load acts perpendicular to the axis of the timber rivets
(b) member thicknesses, edge distances, end distances, and spacing are sufficient to develop full adjusted design values (see 13.3)
(c) timber rivets are installed in the side grain of wood members the reference design value per rivet joint perpendicular to grain, Q, shall be calculated as the lesser of reference rivet capacity, Q_r, and reference wood capacity, Q_w.

$$Q_r = 160\, p^{0.32} n_R n_c \qquad (13.2\text{-}2)$$

$$Q_w = q_w\, p^{0.8} C_\Delta \qquad (13.2\text{-}3)$$

where:

p = depth of penetration of rivet in wood member (see Appendix M), in.

= rivet length – plate thickness – 1/8"

n_R = number of rows of rivets parallel to direction of load

n_c = number of rivets per row

q_w = value determined from Table 13.2.2A, lbs.

C_Δ = geometry factor determined from Table 13.2.2B

Reference design values, Q, for timber rivet connections perpendicular to grain shall be multiplied by all applicable adjustment factors (see Table 10.3.1) to obtain adjusted design values, Q'.

13.2.3 Metal Side Plate Factor, C_{st}

The reference design value parallel to grain, P, or perpendicular to grain, Q, for timber rivet connections, when reference rivet capacity (P_r, Q_r) controls, shall be multiplied by the appropriate metal side plate factor, C_{st}, specified in Table 13.2.3:

Table 13.2.3 Metal Side Plate Factor, C_{st}, for Timber Rivet Connections

Metal Side Plate Thickness, t_s	C_{st}
$t_s \geq 1/4"$	1.00
$3/16" \leq t_s < 1/4"$	0.90
$1/8" \leq t_s < 3/16"$	0.80

13.2.4 Load at Angle to Grain

When a load acts in the plane of the wood surface at an angle, θ, to grain other than 0° or 90°, the adjusted design value, N', for a timber rivet connection shall be determined as follows (see Appendix J):

$$N' = \frac{P'Q'}{P' \sin^2 \theta + Q' \cos^2 \theta} \qquad (13.2\text{-}4)$$

13.2.5 Timber Rivets in End Grain

When timber rivets are used in end grain, the factored lateral resistance of the joint shall be 50% of that for perpendicular to side grain applications when the slope of cut is 90° to the side grain. For sloping end cuts, these values can be increased linearly to 100% of the applicable parallel or perpendicular to side grain value.

13.2.6 Design of Metal Parts

Metal parts shall be designed in accordance with applicable metal design procedures (see 10.2.3).

13.3 Placement of Timber Rivets

13.3.1 Spacing Between Rivets

Minimum spacing of rivets shall be 1/2" perpendicular to grain, s_q, and 1" parallel to grain, s_p.

13.3.2 End and Edge Distance

Minimum values for end distance (a_p, a_q) and edge distance (e_p, e_q) as shown and noted in Figure 13A, are listed in Table 13.3.2.

Table 13.3.2 Minimum End and Edge Distances for Timber Rivet Joints

Number of rivet rows, n_R	Minimum end distance, a, in.		Minimum edge distance, e, in.	
	Load Parallel to grain, a_p	Load perpendicular to grain, a_q	Unloaded Edge e_p	Loaded edge e_q
1, 2	3	2	1	2
3 to 8	3	3	1	2
9, 10	4	3-1/8	1	2
11, 12	5	4	1	2
13, 14	6	4-3/4	1	2
15, 16	7	5-1/2	1	2
17 and greater	8	6-1/4	1	2

Note: End and edge distance requirements are shown in Figure 13A.

Figure 13A End and Edge Distance Requirements for Timber Rivet Joints

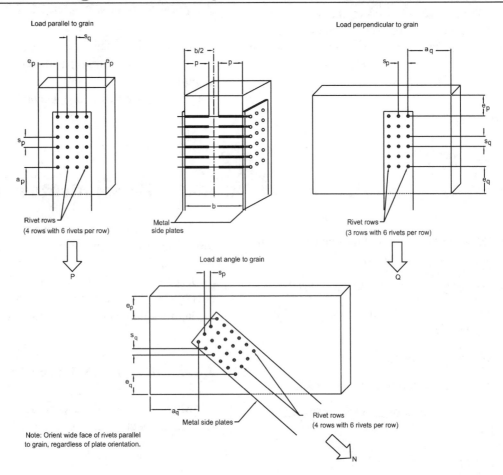

Load parallel to grain

Rivet rows (4 rows with 6 rivets per row)

P

Metal side plates

Load perpendicular to grain

Rivet rows (3 rows with 6 rivets per row)

Q

Load at angle to grain

Note: Orient wide face of rivets parallel to grain, regardless of plate orientation.

Metal side plates

Rivet rows (4 rows with 6 rivets per row)

N

Rivet Length = 1-1/2"   s$_p$ = 1"   s$_q$ = 1"

Member Thickness in.	Rivets per row	P$_w$ (lbs.) No. of rows per side									
		2	4	6	8	10	12	14	16	18	20
3	2	2050	4900	7650	10770	14100	17050	19760	22660	25690	28990
	4	3010	6460	9700	13530	17450	20840	23870	27020	30530	34460
	6	4040	8010	11770	16320	20870	24770	27950	31450	35710	40300
	8	5110	9480	13970	18840	23910	28230	31990	35760	40130	45290
	10	5900	10930	15880	21390	26940	32020	35660	40080	44830	50590
	12	6670	12100	17760	23980	29980	35010	39780	44480	49570	55940
	14	7310	13540	19400	26380	32740	38610	43090	48640	54720	61750
	16	7670	14960	21380	28260	35470	41670	46310	52870	59350	66970
	18	8520	16250	23290	30440	38010	44500	50050	56120	63840	70970
	20	9030	17770	24950	32300	40160	46880	52590	59800	66880	74300
5	2	2680	5160	5980	7250	9280	10860	12470	15150	19410	24260
	4	3930	6610	7610	9050	11460	13390	15110	17890	22090	26280
	6	5280	8190	9290	10890	13770	15870	18080	21120	25640	29870
	8	6690	9700	10940	12740	15950	18230	20580	23780	28450	32570
	10	7720	11160	12550	14550	18120	20600	23140	26550	31500	36850
	12	8730	12680	14170	16240	20100	23100	25410	29610	35000	40730
	14	9560	14160	15720	17980	22210	25460	27940	32450	38220	44250
	16	10030	15610	17330	19650	24200	27680	30320	35100	42230	48910
	18	11150	17020	18770	21450	26110	29780	33140	38370	46160	51900
	20	11800	18410	20310	23000	28270	32260	35900	41570	50030	56260
6.75	2	2930	4810	5550	6740	8630	10110	11610	14120	18080	22630
	4	4300	6170	7080	8420	10680	12490	14100	16700	20630	24570
	6	5780	7650	8640	10150	12840	14820	16890	19740	23980	27960
	8	7320	9060	10190	11880	14890	17040	19250	22240	26630	30510
	10	8440	10420	11690	13580	16920	19260	21640	24850	29500	34540
	12	9540	11850	13210	15150	18780	21610	23780	27730	32800	38200
	14	10450	13230	14650	16790	20760	23820	26170	30410	35830	41520
	16	10970	14590	16160	18350	22630	25910	28410	32900	39610	45910
	18	12190	15910	17510	20040	24420	27890	31050	35980	43310	48740
	20	12910	17210	18950	21490	26450	30210	33650	38990	46950	52860
8.5 and greater	2	2930	4740	5460	6630	8500	9950	11440	13900	17810	22290
	4	4300	6080	6970	8290	10520	12300	13890	16450	20330	24210
	6	5780	7530	8510	10000	12650	14600	16640	19460	23630	27560
	8	7320	8920	10030	11700	14670	16790	18970	21930	26250	30080
	10	8440	10270	11520	13370	16680	18980	21330	24500	29090	34060
	12	9540	11670	13010	14930	18510	21300	23450	27340	32340	37670
	14	10450	13040	14430	16540	20460	23480	25800	29980	35340	40960
	16	10970	14370	15920	18080	22310	25540	28010	32450	39060	45290
	18	12190	15670	17250	19750	24070	27490	30620	35480	42720	48090
	20	12910	16950	18670	21180	26070	29790	33190	38460	46310	52150

TIMBER RIVETS

13

Note: Member dimension is identified as "b" in Figure 13A for connections with steel side plates on opposite sides. For connections having only one plate, member dimension is twice the thickness of the wood member. Linear interpolation for intermediate values shall be permitted.

Table 13.2.1B   Reference Wood Capacity Design Values Parallel to Grain, P_w, for Timber Rivets

Rivet Length = 1-1/2" s_p = 1-1/2" s_q = 1"

Member Thickness in.	Rivets per row	P_w (lbs.) No. of rows per side									
		2	4	6	8	10	12	14	16	18	20
3	2	2320	5650	8790	12270	16000	19800	23200	26100	29360	33180
	4	3420	7450	11150	15420	19810	24200	28020	31130	34900	39430
	6	4580	9230	13530	18600	23690	28760	32810	36230	40810	46120
	8	5810	10920	16060	21480	27150	32780	37550	41200	45860	51830
	10	6700	12600	18250	24380	30590	37180	41870	46180	51230	57890
	12	7570	13940	20420	27340	34040	40650	46700	51250	56650	64020
	14	8290	15600	22310	30070	37180	44840	50590	56040	62540	70670
	16	8710	17250	24580	32220	40280	48400	54360	60910	67820	76650
	18	9680	18720	26770	34700	43150	51680	58750	64660	72960	81220
	20	10250	20480	28680	36820	45600	54450	61740	68900	76440	85030
5	2	3040	5360	6740	8600	11930	14870	18310	23450	32100	42850
	4	4470	7660	9560	11970	16430	20450	24740	30870	40740	51580
	6	5990	9910	12180	15050	20610	25320	30910	38070	49400	60320
	8	7590	12000	14680	18020	24440	29760	36020	43870	56110	67790
	10	8760	14010	17090	20880	28170	34120	41080	49700	63030	75720
	12	9900	16080	19480	23530	31570	38650	45570	55990	70740	83740
	14	10850	18080	21770	26240	35120	42890	50480	61810	77820	92440
	16	11390	20040	24140	28830	38490	46900	55080	67230	86450	100250
	18	12660	21950	26250	31620	41690	50680	60450	73800	94910	106230
	20	13400	23810	28500	34010	45310	55090	65720	80250	99970	111210
6.75	2	3320	5000	6260	8000	11110	13850	17060	21870	29940	39990
	4	4890	7150	8900	11150	15330	19090	23110	28850	38090	48440
	6	6560	9250	11340	14040	19240	23660	28900	35620	46240	57570
	8	8310	11210	13680	16810	22840	27840	33710	41080	52570	64320
	10	9580	13090	15930	19500	26330	31930	38470	46570	59100	73900
	12	10830	15020	18170	21980	29520	36180	42700	52490	66360	82550
	14	11860	16900	20310	24520	32860	40180	47320	57980	73030	90400
	16	12460	18730	22520	26950	36030	43940	51650	63090	81170	100510
	18	13840	20520	24500	29560	39040	47500	56710	69290	89150	107180
	20	14660	22270	26610	31810	42440	51650	61680	75360	96980	116640
8.5 and greater	2	3320	4930	6160	7880	10930	13640	16810	21540	29490	39400
	4	4890	7050	8760	10990	15100	18800	22770	28430	37540	47750
	6	6560	9110	11170	13830	18960	23310	28490	35110	45590	56770
	8	8310	11040	13480	16560	22510	27440	33230	40510	51840	63430
	10	9580	12890	15690	19210	25960	31480	37930	45920	58280	72900
	12	10830	14800	17900	21660	29100	35670	42110	51770	65450	81440
	14	11860	16650	20000	24170	32390	39610	46670	57190	72040	89190
	16	12460	18450	22190	26560	35520	43330	50940	62240	80080	99190
	18	13840	20220	24140	29140	38490	46850	55940	68350	87960	105780
	20	14660	21940	26220	31360	41840	50940	60840	74350	95690	115120

Note: Member dimension is identified as "b" in Figure 13A for connections with steel side plates on opposite sides. For connections having only one plate, member dimension is twice the thickness of the wood member. Linear interpolation for intermediate values shall be permitted.

Rivet Length = 2-1/2"   s$_p$ = 1"   s$_q$ = 1"

Member Thickness in.	Rivets per row	P$_w$ (lbs.) No. of rows per side									
		2	4	6	8	10	12	14	16	18	20
5	2	2340	5610	8750	12310	16120	19500	22600	25910	29380	33160
	4	3440	7390	11100	15470	19950	23830	27290	30900	34920	39400
	6	4620	9160	13460	18660	23860	28320	31970	35960	40830	46080
	8	5850	10840	15980	21550	27350	32280	36580	40900	45890	51790
	10	6750	12500	18160	24460	30810	36610	40780	45840	51260	57850
	12	7630	13830	20310	27420	34280	40030	45490	50870	56690	63970
	14	8360	15480	22190	30170	37450	44150	49280	55620	62580	70620
	16	8770	17110	24450	32320	40570	47660	52960	60450	67870	76590
	18	9750	18580	26630	34810	43460	50890	57230	64170	73010	81160
	20	10320	20320	28530	36940	45920	53610	60140	68380	76480	84960
6.75	2	2710	6490	10130	14260	18660	22570	26170	30000	34020	38390
	4	3980	8550	12850	17910	22580	26120	29190	34220	40420	45620
	6	5350	10600	15590	20390	25510	29030	32670	37760	45400	52330
	8	6770	12550	18500	22880	28260	31840	35470	40500	47980	54310
	10	7810	14480	21020	25280	30980	34680	38400	43540	51130	59140
	12	8830	16020	23510	27430	33360	37720	40900	47070	55050	63330
	14	9670	17920	25690	29640	35930	40500	43810	50240	58540	67000
	16	10160	19810	28310	31700	38300	43040	46460	53110	63200	72360
	18	11290	21510	30160	33950	40490	45390	49750	56870	67670	75240
	20	11950	23530	32140	35770	43070	48280	52920	60500	72000	80080
8.5	2	3070	7350	10580	13060	16620	19300	21990	26530	33760	41900
	4	4510	9690	12400	14710	18410	21240	23720	27810	34060	40180
	6	6060	12000	14390	16700	20790	23640	26610	30780	37040	42750
	8	7670	13920	16320	18720	23050	25970	28960	33100	39250	44510
	10	8850	15730	18150	20680	25290	28330	31420	35660	41930	48600
	12	10010	17590	19970	22430	27270	30870	33520	38630	45240	52180
	14	10960	19360	21660	24250	29400	33190	35960	41310	48200	55320
	16	11510	21050	23410	25950	31370	35320	38200	43740	52130	59860
	18	12790	22670	24900	27810	33200	37290	40960	46920	55920	62350
	20	13540	24220	26510	29310	35350	39720	43640	49990	59580	66480
10.5	2	3400	7730	9830	11980	15210	17650	20110	24260	30870	38340
	4	5000	9490	11460	13490	16860	19460	21740	25500	31230	36880
	6	6710	11400	13250	15310	19060	21690	24430	28270	34030	39320
	8	8490	13150	15020	17170	21150	23850	26610	30440	36110	41000
	10	9800	14810	16700	18980	23230	26040	28900	32840	38630	44830
	12	11080	16520	18360	20600	25060	28400	30870	35610	41730	48190
	14	12130	18140	19910	22280	27040	30560	33150	38110	44500	51140
	16	12740	19680	21520	23850	28870	32550	35240	40390	48170	55390
	18	14160	21160	22900	25570	30570	34390	37820	43350	51710	57750
	20	14990	22580	24380	26970	32570	36640	40310	46220	55140	61620
12.5 and greater	2	3540	7610	9540	11590	14710	17060	19440	23450	29840	37060
	4	5210	9300	11100	13040	16300	18820	21030	24670	30230	35700
	6	6990	11140	12840	14810	18440	20990	23650	27370	32960	38100
	8	8860	12840	14540	16620	20470	23090	25780	29490	35000	39750
	10	10220	14440	16160	18370	22490	25230	28010	31830	37450	43490
	12	11550	16090	17770	19940	24270	27520	29920	34530	40470	46760
	14	12650	17650	19270	21580	26190	29620	32150	36970	43180	49650
	16	13290	19140	20840	23100	27970	31560	34180	39190	46760	53800
	18	14760	20570	22170	24770	29630	33350	36690	42080	50210	56110
	20	15630	21940	23600	26130	31570	35550	39120	44880	53560	59880

Note: Member dimension is identified as "b" in Figure 13A for connections with steel side plates on opposite sides. For connections having only one plate, member dimension is twice the thickness of the wood member. Linear interpolation for intermediate values shall be permitted.

TIMBER RIVETS

13

Table 13.2.1D Reference Wood Capacity Design Values Parallel to Grain, P_w, for Timber Rivets

Rivet Length = 2-1/2" s_p = 1-1/2" s_q = 1"

Member Thickness in.	Rivets per row	P_w (lbs.) No. of rows per side									
		2	4	6	8	10	12	14	16	18	20
5	2	2660	6460	10050	14040	18300	22640	26530	29850	33580	37950
	4	3910	8520	12750	17640	22650	27670	32040	35600	39900	45090
	6	5240	10560	15480	21270	27090	32890	37530	41430	46670	52740
	8	6640	12490	18370	24560	31050	37490	42940	47120	52450	59270
	10	7660	14410	20870	27880	34980	42520	47880	52810	58580	66200
	12	8660	15950	23350	31260	38920	46490	53400	58610	64790	73210
	14	9480	17840	25510	34390	42520	51270	57850	64080	71520	80820
	16	9960	19720	28110	36850	46060	55340	62170	69650	77560	87650
	18	11070	21410	30610	39680	49350	59090	67180	73940	83440	92880
	20	11720	23420	32800	42110	52140	62260	70600	78790	87410	97230
6.75	2	3070	7480	11640	16250	21190	26210	30720	34560	38880	43930
	4	4520	9860	14770	20420	26230	32040	37100	41220	46200	52210
	6	6070	12220	17920	24630	31370	38080	43450	47970	54030	61060
	8	7690	14460	21260	28440	35950	43400	49720	54550	60720	68620
	10	8870	16690	24160	32280	40500	49230	55430	61150	67820	76650
	12	10030	18460	27030	36200	45060	53820	61830	67860	75010	84760
	14	10980	20660	29530	39820	49220	59360	66980	74190	82800	93570
	16	11530	22830	32550	42660	53320	64070	71980	80640	89800	101480
	18	12810	24790	35440	45940	57130	68420	77780	85600	96600	107530
	20	13560	27110	37970	48750	60370	72080	81740	91220	101200	112570
8.5	2	3480	8230	11610	14990	20600	25440	31030	39170	44060	49790
	4	5120	11170	14980	18590	25140	30870	36920	45610	52360	59170
	6	6880	13850	18020	21920	29500	35710	43060	52490	61230	69190
	8	8710	16390	20820	25060	33380	40030	47840	57640	68810	77760
	10	10050	18910	23430	28020	37080	44230	52570	62910	76860	86860
	12	11360	20920	25960	30640	40320	48610	56590	68770	85000	96060
	14	12440	23410	28300	33320	43740	52600	61110	74030	92320	106040
	16	13070	25860	30710	35810	46880	56250	65240	78780	100360	115000
	18	14520	27900	32770	38510	49810	59620	70230	84840	108100	121860
	20	15370	29860	34970	40700	53190	63690	75060	90690	114690	127580
10.5	2	3860	7930	10760	13740	18860	23280	28400	36090	48770	55110
	4	5670	10740	13810	17050	23050	28310	33880	41870	54800	65490
	6	7610	13360	16580	20110	27080	32800	39590	48290	62110	76590
	8	9640	15700	19140	23010	30670	36830	44050	53110	67340	81680
	10	11130	17870	21540	25740	34110	40740	48470	58060	72990	90530
	12	12580	20050	23860	28170	37130	44820	52230	63540	79580	98220
	14	13770	22110	26020	30660	40300	48540	56460	68470	85450	104980
	16	14460	24060	28240	32970	43240	51950	60330	72930	92990	114320
	18	16070	25920	30140	35470	45960	55110	65010	78610	100260	119710
	20	17020	27710	32170	37520	49120	58920	69530	84110	107290	128200
12.5 and greater	2	4020	7800	10440	13290	18230	22500	27450	34890	47430	57470
	4	5920	10500	13370	16490	22300	27390	32790	40540	53060	66920
	6	7940	13040	16050	19460	26210	31770	38350	46780	60200	74320
	8	10060	15300	18530	22270	29710	35680	42690	51500	65300	79260
	10	11600	17390	20850	24930	33050	39490	47000	56320	70830	87900
	12	13120	19490	23110	27290	35980	43460	50680	61670	77270	95420
	14	14370	21480	25200	29700	39080	47090	54800	66480	83000	102030
	16	15080	23370	27350	31950	41930	50420	58580	70850	90360	111160
	18	16760	25170	29200	34380	44590	53500	63140	76390	97460	116450
	20	17750	26900	31170	36380	47660	57220	67550	81760	104330	124740

Note: Member dimension is identified as "b" in Figure 13A for connections with steel side plates on opposite sides. For connections having only one plate, member dimension is twice the thickness of the wood member. Linear interpolation for intermediate values shall be permitted.

Table 13.2.1E   Reference Wood Capacity Design Values Parallel to Grain, P_w, for Timber Rivets

Rivet Length = 3-1/2" s_p = 1" s_q = 1"

Member Thickness in.	Rivets per row	P_w (lbs.) No. of rows per side									
		2	4	6	8	10	12	14	16	18	20
6.75	2	2440	5850	9130	12850	16820	20350	23590	27040	30670	34610
	4	3590	7710	11580	16150	20820	24870	28490	32250	36450	41130
	6	4820	9560	14050	19480	24910	29560	33370	37540	42620	48100
	8	6100	11310	16680	22490	28550	33700	38180	42690	47900	54060
	10	7040	13050	18950	25530	32160	38220	42570	47850	53510	60380
	12	7960	14440	21200	28630	35780	41780	47480	53100	59170	66770
	14	8720	16160	23160	31490	39090	46090	51440	58050	65320	73710
	16	9160	17860	25530	33740	42340	49740	55280	63100	70840	79940
	18	10170	19390	27790	36330	45370	53120	59740	66990	76210	84710
	20	10770	21210	29780	38560	47930	55960	62770	71380	79830	88680
8.5	2	2710	6490	10130	14250	18660	22570	26160	29990	34010	38380
	4	3980	8550	12840	17910	23090	27580	31600	35770	40420	45610
	6	5350	10600	15590	21600	27620	32790	37000	41630	47270	53350
	8	6770	12550	18500	24940	31660	37370	42350	47340	53120	59950
	10	7810	14480	21020	28320	35670	42390	47210	53060	59340	66970
	12	8830	16020	23510	31750	39680	46340	52660	58890	65620	74060
	14	9670	17920	25690	34920	43350	51110	57050	64390	72440	81750
	16	10160	19810	28310	37420	46960	55170	61310	69980	78560	88660
	18	11280	21510	30830	40300	50310	58910	66250	74290	84510	93950
	20	11950	23520	33030	42760	53160	62060	69620	79160	88540	98360
10.5	2	3020	7240	11300	15900	20820	25180	29190	33460	37940	42820
	4	4440	9540	14330	19980	25760	30770	35250	39900	45090	50890
	6	5960	11830	17390	24100	30820	36580	41280	46440	52740	59510
	8	7550	14000	20630	27830	35320	40570	44460	49980	58370	65230
	10	8720	16150	23450	31420	38000	41760	45450	50740	58770	67160
	12	9850	17870	26230	32850	39220	43470	46330	52530	60650	68990
	14	10790	19990	28660	34370	40770	45050	47920	54190	62370	70660
	16	11330	22100	31580	35730	42190	46510	49400	55710	65540	74330
	18	12590	23990	33750	37340	43510	47850	51650	58300	68630	75640
	20	13330	26240	35340	38490	45290	49850	53850	60830	71650	79050
12.5	2	3320	7960	12420	17490	22890	27690	32090	36790	41720	47090
	4	4890	10490	15760	21970	28330	33840	38760	43880	49590	55960
	6	6560	13010	19120	25230	31370	35100	38780	44070	52180	59340
	8	8310	15390	22350	26580	32170	35480	38780	43560	50870	56880
	10	9580	17760	24250	27850	33280	36450	39640	44260	51300	58690
	12	10830	19650	25950	28920	34280	37940	40440	45890	53030	60430
	14	11870	21990	27400	30150	35610	39340	41890	47420	54640	62020
	16	12460	24300	28890	31290	36860	40660	43240	48840	57520	65380
	18	13840	26360	30040	32670	38030	41880	45280	51190	60340	66660
	20	14660	28020	31320	33670	39620	43680	47270	53490	63100	69790
14.5 and greater	2	3580	8580	13390	18850	24670	29840	34590	39650	44970	50750
	4	5270	11020	16940	22830	29290	33640	37040	42730	51500	59860
	6	7070	13590	19540	23990	29520	32900	36290	41210	48800	55490
	8	8950	15930	21540	25060	30160	33200	36280	40760	47610	53260
	10	10330	18090	23150	26150	31160	34110	37110	41450	48060	55040
	12	11680	20230	24620	27120	32090	35530	37890	43020	49740	56740
	14	12790	22170	25890	28250	33350	36870	39280	44500	51310	58300
	16	13430	23950	27220	29310	34540	38120	40580	45870	54070	61530
	18	14920	25580	28250	30610	35650	39300	42530	48120	56770	62800
	20	15800	27070	29430	31550	37160	41020	44440	50330	59420	65810

Note: Member dimension is identified as "b" in Figure 13A for connections with steel side plates on opposite sides. For connections having only one plate, member dimension is twice the thickness of the wood member. Linear interpolation for intermediate values shall be permitted.

TIMBER RIVETS

13

Table 13.2.1F Reference Wood Capacity Design Values Parallel to Grain, P_w, for Timber Rivets

Rivet Length = 3-1/2" s_p = 1-1/2" s_q = 1"

Member Thickness in.	Rivets per row	P_w (lbs.) No. of rows per side									
		2	4	6	8	10	12	14	16	18	20
6.75	2	2770	6740	10490	14650	19100	23630	27690	31160	35050	39610
	4	4080	8890	13310	18410	23640	28880	33440	37160	41650	47070
	6	5470	11020	16160	22200	28280	34330	39170	43250	48710	55050
	8	6930	13040	19170	25640	32410	39130	44820	49180	54740	61860
	10	8000	15040	21780	29110	36510	44380	49970	55130	61150	69100
	12	9040	16640	24370	32630	40630	48520	55740	61180	67620	76420
	14	9900	18630	26630	35900	44380	53520	60390	66890	74650	84360
	16	10390	20590	29340	38460	48080	57770	64890	72710	80960	91490
	18	11550	22350	31950	41420	51510	61680	70130	77180	87090	96950
	20	12230	24450	34230	43960	54430	64990	73690	82240	91240	101490
8.5	2	3070	7480	11640	16250	21190	26210	30710	34560	38870	43930
	4	4520	9860	14760	20420	26220	32030	37090	41210	46190	52200
	6	6070	12220	17920	24630	31360	38080	43440	47960	54020	61050
	8	7690	14460	21260	28440	35950	43400	49710	54550	60710	68610
	10	8870	16680	24160	32280	40500	49220	55420	61140	67820	76640
	12	10020	18460	27030	36190	45060	53820	61820	67850	75000	84750
	14	10980	20660	29530	39810	49220	59360	66970	74180	82790	93560
	16	11530	22830	32540	42660	53320	64070	71970	80630	89790	101460
	18	12810	24790	35440	45940	57130	68410	77770	85600	96590	107520
	20	13560	27110	37970	48750	60360	72070	81730	91210	101190	112560
10.5	2	3430	8340	12980	18130	23640	29240	34260	38550	43360	49000
	4	5040	11000	16470	22780	29250	35740	41380	45980	51530	58240
	6	6770	13630	19990	27470	34990	42480	48460	53510	60270	68110
	8	8570	16130	23720	31720	40100	48420	55460	60850	67730	76540
	10	9890	18610	26950	36010	45180	54910	61830	68210	75660	85500
	12	11180	20590	30150	40380	50270	60040	68970	75690	83670	94550
	14	12250	23040	32940	43530	54910	65690	74710	82760	92360	104370
	16	12860	25470	36300	45490	58120	68370	78030	89950	100170	113190
	18	14290	27650	39530	47750	60310	70840	82200	95490	107750	119950
	20	15130	30250	42360	49450	63130	74240	86230	101750	112880	125570
12.5	2	3770	8940	14280	19930	25990	32150	37680	42390	47680	53890
	4	5550	12090	18110	25050	32170	39300	45500	50560	56670	64040
	6	7440	14990	21980	30210	38480	46710	53290	58840	66270	74890
	8	9430	17740	26080	32640	42400	49720	58300	66910	74480	84170
	10	10880	20470	29450	34550	44560	52030	60770	71680	83190	94020
	12	12300	22640	31480	36220	46470	54910	62900	75440	92000	103970
	14	13470	25340	33270	38080	48780	57570	65900	78860	97350	114770
	16	14140	28010	35150	39800	50920	60030	68660	81990	103470	124470
	18	15710	30410	36640	41810	52910	62310	72460	86620	109420	129590
	20	16640	33260	38300	43320	55450	65400	76150	91130	115220	136640
14.5 and greater	2	4060	8940	15370	21480	28010	34650	40610	45690	51390	58080
	4	5980	12730	19520	26990	34670	42350	49040	54490	61080	69020
	6	8020	16160	23590	28890	37960	44900	53060	63410	71430	80720
	8	10160	19120	25880	30610	39690	46550	54610	64800	80270	90710
	10	11720	21820	27800	32370	41740	48760	56990	67280	83550	101330
	12	13250	24280	29620	33930	43560	51520	59070	70900	87820	107340
	14	14520	26450	31250	35680	45760	54070	61960	74220	91690	111670
	16	15240	28390	32980	37310	47800	56430	64630	77250	97570	119050
	18	16940	30160	34370	39220	49710	58630	68270	81700	103290	122520
	20	17930	31770	35920	40670	52140	61590	71820	86040	108880	129320

Note: Member dimension is identified as "b" in Figure 13A for connections with steel side plates on opposite sides. For connections having only one plate, member dimension is twice the thickness of the wood member. Linear interpolation for intermediate values shall be permitted.

Table 13.2.2A Values of q_w (lbs.) Perpendicular to Grain for Timber Rivets

$$s_p = 1''$$

s_q in.	Rivets per row	Number of rows 2	4	6	8	10
	2	776	809	927	1089	1255
	3	768	806	910	1056	1202
	4	821	870	963	1098	1232
	5	874	923	1013	1147	1284
	6	959	1007	1094	1228	1371
	7	1048	1082	1163	1297	1436
	8	1173	1184	1256	1391	1525
	9	1237	1277	1345	1467	1624
	10	1318	1397	1460	1563	1752
1	11	1420	1486	1536	1663	1850
	12	1548	1597	1628	1786	1970
	13	1711	1690	1741	1882	2062
	14	1924	1802	1878	1997	2170
	15	2042	1937	1963	2099	2298
	16	2182	2102	2063	2218	2449
	17	2350	2223	2178	2313	2541
	18	2553	2365	2313	2422	2644
	19	2524	2432	2407	2548	2762
	20	2497	2506	2514	2692	2897
	2	1136	1097	1221	1414	1630
	3	1124	1093	1199	1371	1561
	4	1202	1180	1268	1426	1601
	5	1280	1251	1334	1490	1668
	6	1404	1366	1442	1595	1780
	7	1534	1467	1532	1685	1865
	8	1717	1606	1654	1806	1980
	9	1811	1731	1772	1905	2110
	10	1929	1894	1923	2030	2275
1-1/2	11	2078	2016	2023	2159	2403
	12	2265	2166	2145	2319	2559
	13	2504	2292	2293	2444	2678
	14	2817	2444	2473	2593	2818
	15	2989	2627	2586	2725	2984
	16	3193	2850	2717	2880	3181
	17	3439	3014	2869	3004	3300
	18	3737	3207	3047	3146	3434
	19	3695	3298	3171	3309	3588
	20	3655	3398	3311	3496	3762

Table 13.2.2B Geometry Factor, C_Δ, for Timber Rivet Connections Loaded Perpendicular to Grain

$\dfrac{e_p}{(n_c-1)S_q}$	C_Δ	$\dfrac{e_p}{(n_c-1)S_q}$	C_Δ
0.1	5.76	3.2	0.79
0.2	3.19	3.6	0.77
0.3	2.36	4.0	0.76
0.4	2.00	5.0	0.72
0.5	1.77	6.0	0.70
0.6	1.61	7.0	0.68
0.7	1.47	8.0	0.66
0.8	1.36	9.0	0.64
0.9	1.28	10.0	0.63
1.0	1.20	12.0	0.61
1.2	1.10	14.0	0.59
1.4	1.02	16.0	0.57
1.6	0.96	18.0	0.56
1.8	0.92	20.0	0.55
2.0	0.89	25.0	0.53
2.4	0.85	30.0	0.51
2.8	0.81		

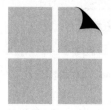

SHEAR WALLS AND DIAPHRAGMS

14

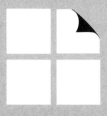

14.1 General

14.1.1 Application

Chapter 14 applies to the design of wood structural panel and lumber sheathed shear walls and diaphragms acting as elements of the lateral force-resisting system.

14.1.2 Definitions

14.1.2.1 The term "diaphragm" refers to a roof, floor, or other membrane or bracing system acting to transfer lateral forces to the vertical resisting elements.

14.1.2.2 The term "shear wall" refers to a wall designed to resist lateral forces parallel to the plane of the wall (sometimes referred to as a vertical diaphragm).

14.1.3 Framing Members

All framing including boundary members provided at shear wall and diaphragm perimeters, openings, and discontinuities and re-entrant corners shall be proportioned to resist the induced forces.

14.1.4 Fasteners

Values of fastener strength shall be determined in accordance with provisions of this standard.

14.1.5 Sheathing

Sheathing shall be proportioned to resist induced forces. The resistance of wood structural panel sheathing and lumber sheathing shall be investigated in accordance with the provisions of this standard.

14.2 Design Principles

Shear walls and diaphragms shall be designed according to a beam analogy with sheathing resisting in plane shear and framing members resisting axial forces or, alternate methods based on rational analysis. Design shall include consideration of sheathing, framing, fasteners, boundary members, and all required connections.

14.3 Shear Walls

14.3.1 Definitions

14.3.1.1 The term "shear wall height" refers to:
(1) The maximum clear height from the top of the foundation to the bottom of diaphragm framing above or,
(2) the maximum clear height from top of diaphragm below to the bottom of diaphragm framing above. Where the diaphragm framing is sloped, the average height to the diaphragm framing above may be used.

14.3.1.2 The term "shear wall width" refers to the dimension of a shear wall in the direction of application of force and is measured as the dimension between the boundary elements of the shear wall (in many cases, this will match the sheathed dimension).

14.3.1.3 The term "shear wall aspect ratio" refers to the ratio of height-to-width of a shear wall.

14.3.2 Shear Wall Anchorage

Connections shall be provided between the shear wall and attached components to transmit the induced forces.

14.3.3 Shear Force

The design shear force per unit length shall not exceed the adjusted shear wall shear resistance per unit length, $D \leq D'$.

14.3.4 Shear Resistance

The adjusted shear resistance, D', shall be determined by using principles of engineering mechanics using values of fastener strength and sheathing through-the-thickness shear resistance or, alternatively, from approved tables.

14.4 Diaphragms

14.4.1 Definitions

14.4.1.1 The term "collector" refers to a diaphragm element parallel and in line with the applied force that collects and transfers diaphragm shear forces to the vertical elements of the lateral-force-resisting system and/or distributes forces within the diaphragm.

14.4.1.2 The term "diaphragm chord" refers to a diaphragm boundary element perpendicular to the applied load that is assumed to take axial stresses due to the diaphragm moment.

14.4.1.3 The term "diaphragm length" (see Figure 14A) refers to the dimension of a diaphragm in the direction perpendicular to the application of force and is measured as the distance between vertical elements of the lateral-force-resisting system (in many cases, this will match the sheathed dimensions).

14.4.1.4 The term "diaphragm width" refers to the dimension of a diaphragm in the direction of application of force and is measured as the distance between diaphragm chords (in many cases, this will match the sheathed dimensions).

14.3.5 Shear Wall Deflection

When required in the design, the deflection of a shear wall shall be calculated in accordance with principles of engineering mechanics or by other approved methods.

14.4.1.5 The term "diaphragm aspect ratio" refers to the ratio of length to width of a diaphragm.

14.4.2 Shear Force

The design shear force per unit length shall not exceed the adjusted diaphragm shear resistance per unit length, $D \leq D'$.

14.4.3 Shear Resistance

The adjusted shear resistance, D', shall be determined by using principles of engineering mechanics using values of fastener strength and sheathing through-the-thickness shear resistance or, alternatively, from approved tables.

14.4.4 Diaphragm Deflection

When required in the design, the deflection of a diaphragm shall be calculated in accordance with principles of engineering mechanics or by other approved methods.

Figure 14A   Diaphragm Length and Width

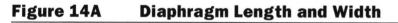

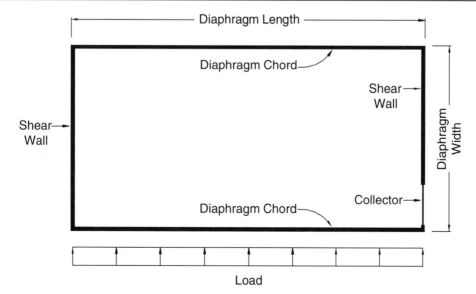

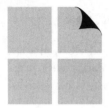

SPECIAL
LOADING
CONDITIONS

15

15.1 Lateral Distribution of a Concentrated Load

15.1.1 Lateral Distribution of a Concentrated Load for Moment

When a concentrated load at the center of the beam span is distributed to adjacent parallel beams by a wood or concrete-slab floor, the load on the beam nearest the point of application shall be determined by multiplying the load by the following factors:

Table 15.1.1 Lateral Distribution Factors for Moment

Kind of Floor	Load on Critical Beam (for one traffic lane[2])
2" plank	S/4.0[1]
4" nail laminated	S/4.5[1]
6" nail laminated	S/5.0[1]
Concrete, structurally designed	S/6.0[1]

1. S = average spacing of beams, ft. If S exceeds the denominator of the factor, the load on the two adjacent beams shall be the reactions of the load, with the assumption that the floor slab between the beams acts as a simple beam.
2. See Reference 48 for additional information concerning two or more traffic lanes.

15.1.2 Lateral Distribution of a Concentrated Load for Shear

When the load distribution for moment at the center of a beam is known or assumed to correspond to specific values in the first two columns of Table 15.1.2, the distribution to adjacent parallel beams when loaded at or near the quarter point (the approximate point of maximum shear) shall be assumed to be the corresponding values in the last two columns of Table 15.1.2.

Table 15.1.2 Lateral Distribution in Terms of Proportion of Total Load

Load Applied at Center of Span		Load Applied at 1/4 Point of Span	
Center Beam	Distribution to Side Beams	Center Beam	Distribution to Side Beams
1.00	0	1.00	0
0.90	0.10	0.94	0.06
0.80	0.20	0.87	0.13
0.70	0.30	0.79	0.21
0.60	0.40	0.69	0.31
0.50	0.50	0.58	0.42
0.40	0.60	0.44	0.56
0.33	0.67	0.33	0.67

15.2 Spaced Columns

15.2.1 General

15.2.1.1 The design load for a spaced column shall be the sum of the design loads for each of its individual members.

15.2.1.2 The increased load capacity of a spaced column due to the end-fixity developed by the split ring or shear plate connectors and end blocks is effective only in the direction perpendicular to the wide faces of the individual members (direction parallel to dimension d_1 in Figure 15A). The capacity of a spaced column in the direction parallel to the wide faces of the individual members (direction parallel to dimension d_2 in Figure 15A) shall be subject to the provisions for simple solid columns, as set forth in 15.2.3.

Figure 15A Spaced Column Joined by Split Ring or Shear Plate Connectors

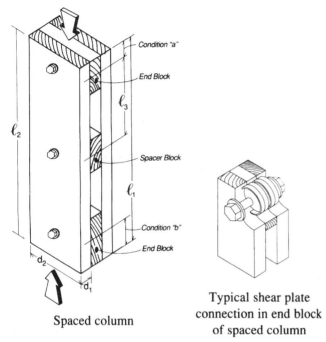

Spaced column

Typical shear plate connection in end block of spaced column

Condition "a": end distance $\leq \ell_1/20$

ℓ_1 and ℓ_2 = distances between points of lateral support in planes 1 and 2, measured from center to center of lateral supports for continuous spaced columns, and measured from end to end for simple spaced columns, inches.

ℓ_3 = Distance from center of spacer block to centroid of the group of split ring or shear plate connectors in end blocks, inches.

d_1 and d_2 = cross-sectional dimensions of individual rectangular compression members in planes of lateral support, inches.

Condition "b": $\ell_1/20 <$ end distance $\leq \ell_1/10$

15.2.2 Spacer and End Block Provisions

15.2.2.1 Spaced columns shall be classified as to end fixity either as condition "a" or condition "b" (see Figure 15A), as follows:

(a) For condition "a", the centroid of the split ring or shear plate connector, or the group of connectors, in the end block shall be within $\ell_1/20$ from the column end.

(b) For condition "b", the centroid of the split ring or shear plate connector, or the group of connectors, in the end block shall be between $\ell_1/20$ and $\ell_1/10$ from the column end.

15.2.2.2 When a single spacer block is located within the middle 1/10 of the column length, ℓ_1, split ring or shear plate connectors shall not be required for this block. If there are two or more spacer blocks, split

ring or shear plate connectors shall be required and the distance between two adjacent blocks shall not exceed ½ the distance between centers of split ring or shear plate connectors in the end blocks.

15.2.2.3 For spaced columns used as compression members of a truss, a panel point which is stayed laterally shall be considered as the end of the spaced column, and the portion of the web members, between the individual pieces making up a spaced column, shall be permitted to be considered as the end blocks.

15.2.2.4 Thickness of spacer and end blocks shall not be less than that of individual members of the spaced column nor shall thickness, width, and length of spacer and end blocks be less than required for split ring or shear plate connectors of a size and number capable of carrying the load computed in 15.2.2.5.

15.2.2.5 To obtain spaced column action the split ring or shear plate connectors in each mutually contacting surface of end block and individual member at each end of a spaced column shall be of a size and number to provide a load capacity in pounds equal to the required cross-sectional area in square inches of one of the individual members times the appropriate end spacer block constant, K_S, determined from the following equations:

Species Group	End Spacer Block Constant, K_S
A	$K_S = 9.55\,(\ell_1/d_1 - 11) \leq 468$
B	$K_S = 8.14\,(\ell_1/d_1 - 11) \leq 399$
C	$K_S = 6.73\,(\ell_1/d_1 - 11) \leq 330$
D	$K_S = 5.32\,(\ell_1/d_1 - 11) \leq 261$

If spaced columns are a part of a truss system or other similar framing, the split ring or shear plate connectors required by the connection provisions in Chapter 12 of this Specification shall be checked against the end spacer block constants, K_S, specified above.

15.2.3 Column Stability Factor, C_P

15.2.3.1 The effective column length, ℓ_e, for a spaced column shall be determined in accordance with principles of engineering mechanics. One method for determining effective column length, when end-fixity conditions are known, is to multiply actual column length by the appropriate effective length factor specified in Appendix G, $\ell_e = (K_e)(\ell)$, except that the effective column length, ℓ_e, shall not be less than the actual column length, ℓ.

SPECIAL LOADING CONDITIONS

15

15.2.3.2 For individual members of a spaced column (see Figure 15A):

(a) ℓ_1/d_1 shall not exceed 80, where ℓ_1 is the distance between lateral supports that provide restraint perpendicular to the wide faces of the individual members.

(b) ℓ_2/d_2 shall not exceed 50, where ℓ_2 is the distance between lateral supports that provide restraint in a direction parallel to the wide faces of the individual members.

(c) ℓ_3/d_1 shall not exceed 40, where ℓ_3 is the distance between the center of the spacer block and the centroid of the group of split ring or shear plate connectors in an end block.

15.2.3.3 The column stability factor shall be calculated as follows:

$$C_P = \frac{1+\left(F_{cE}/F_c^*\right)}{2c} - \sqrt{\left[\frac{1+\left(F_{cE}/F_c^*\right)}{2c}\right]^2 - \frac{F_{cE}/F_c^*}{c}} \quad (15.2\text{-}1)$$

where:

F_c^* = reference compression design value parallel to grain multiplied by all applicable adjustment factors except C_P (see 2.3)

$$F_{cE} = \frac{0.822\,K_x\,E_{min}'}{\left(\ell_e/d\right)^2}$$

K_x = 2.5 for fixity condition "a"

= 3.0 for fixity condition "b"

c = 0.8 for sawn lumber

= 0.9 for structural glued laminated timber or structural composite lumber

15.2.3.4 When individual members of a spaced column are of different species, grades, or thicknesses, the lesser adjusted compression parallel to grain design value, F_c', for the weaker member shall apply to both members.

15.2.3.5 The adjusted compression parallel to grain design value, F_c', for a spaced column shall not exceed the adjusted compression parallel to grain design value, F_c', for the individual members evaluated as solid columns without regard to fixity in accordance with 3.7 using the column slenderness ratio ℓ_2/d_2 (see Figure 15A).

15.2.3.6 For especially severe service conditions and/or extraordinary hazard, use of lower adjusted design values may be necessary. See Appendix H for background information concerning column stability calculations and Appendix F for information concerning coefficient of variation in modulus of elasticity (COV_E).

15.2.3.7 The equations in 3.9 for combined flexure and axial loading apply to spaced columns only for uniaxial bending in a direction parallel to the wide face of the individual member (dimension d_2 in Figure 15A).

15.3 Built-Up Columns

15.3.1 General

The following provisions apply to nailed or bolted built-up columns with 2 to 5 laminations in which:

(a) each lamination has a rectangular cross section and is at least 1-1/2" thick, $t \geq 1\text{-}1/2"$.

(b) all laminations have the same depth (face width), d

(c) faces of adjacent laminations are in contact.

(d) all laminations are full column length.

(e) the connection requirements in 15.3.3 or 15.3.4 are met.

Nailed or bolted built-up columns not meeting the preceding limitations shall have individual laminations designed in accordance with 3.6.3 and 3.7. When individual laminations are of different species, grades, or thicknesses, the lesser adjusted compression parallel to grain design value, F_c', and modulus of elasticity for beam and column stability, E_{min}', for the weakest lamination shall apply.

15.3.2 Column Stability Factor, C_P

15.3.2.1 The effective column length, ℓ_e, for a built-up column shall be determined in accordance with principles of engineering mechanics. One method for determining effective column length, when end-fixity conditions are known, is to multiply actual column length by the appropriate effective length factor specified in Appendix G, $\ell_e = (K_e)(\ell)$.

15.3.2.2 The slenderness ratios ℓ_{e1}/d_1 and ℓ_{e2}/d_2 (see Figure 15B) where each ratio has been adjusted by the appropriate buckling length coefficient, K_e, from Appendix G, shall be determined. Each ratio shall be used calculate a column stability factor, C_P, per section 5.3.2.4 and the smaller C_P shall be used in determining the adjusted compression design value parallel to grain, F_c', for the column. F_c' for built-up columns need not be less than F_c' for the individual laminations designed as individual solid columns per section 3.7.

15.3.2.3 The slenderness ratio, ℓ_e/d, for built-up columns shall not exceed 50, except that during construction ℓ_e/d shall not exceed 75.

15.3.2.4 The column stability factor shall be calculated as follows:

$$C_P = K_f \left[\frac{1+\left(F_{cE}/F_c^*\right)}{2c} - \sqrt{\left[\frac{1+\left(F_{cE}/F_c^*\right)}{2c}\right]^2 - \frac{F_{cE}/F_c^*}{c}} \right] \quad (15.3\text{-}1)$$

where:

F_c^* = reference compression design value parallel to grain multiplied by all applicable modification factors except C_P (see 2.3)

$$F_{cE} = \frac{0.822\,E_{min}'}{\left(\ell_e/d\right)^2}$$

K_f = 0.6 for built-up columns where ℓ_{e2}/d_2 is used to calculate F_{cE} and the built-up columns are nailed in accordance with 15.3.3

K_f = 0.75 for built-up columns where ℓ_{e2}/d_2 is used to calculate F_{cE} and the built-up columns are bolted in accordance with 15.3.4

K_f = 1.0 for built-up columns where ℓ_{e1}/d_1 is used to calculate F_{cE} and the built-up columns are either nailed or bolted in accordance with 15.3.3 or 15.3.4, respectively

c = 0.8 for sawn lumber

c = 0.9 for structural glued laminated timber or structural composite lumber

15.3.2.5 For especially severe service conditions and/or extraordinary hazard, use of lower adjusted design values may be necessary. See Appendix H for background information concerning column stability calculations and Appendix F for information concerning coefficient of variation in modulus of elasticity (COV_E).

Figure 15B Mechanically Laminated Built-Up Columns

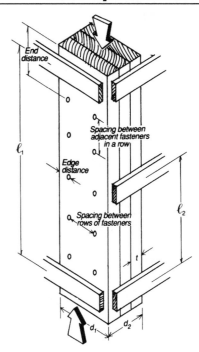

15.3.3 Nailed Built-Up Columns

15.3.3.1 The provisions in 15.3.1 and 15.3.2 apply to nailed built-up columns (see Figure 15C) in which:

(a) adjacent nails are driven from opposite sides of the column

(b) all nails penetrate at least 3/4 of the thickness of the last lamination

(c) $15D \le$ end distance $\le 18D$

(d) $20D \le$ spacing between adjacent nails in a row $\le 6t_{min}$

(e) $10D \le$ spacing between rows of nails $\le 20D$

(f) $5D \le$ edge distance $\le 20D$

(g) 2 or more longitudinal rows of nails are provided when $d > 3t_{min}$

where:

D = nail diameter

d = depth (face width) of individual lamination

t_{min} = thickness of thinnest lamination

When only one longitudinal row of nails is required, adjacent nails shall be staggered (see Figure 15C). When three or more longitudinal rows of nails are used, nails in adjacent rows shall be staggered.

SPECIAL LOADING CONDITIONS

15

Figure 15C   Typical Nailing Schedules for Built-Up Columns

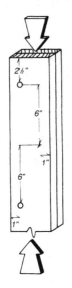

Two 2"x 4" laminations with one row of staggered 10d common wire nails (D = 0.148", L = 3")

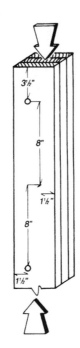

Three 2"x 4" laminations with one row of staggered 30d common wire nails (D = 0.207", L = 4-1/2")

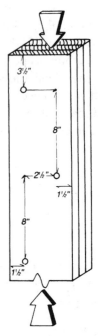

Three 2"x 6" laminations with two rows of 30d common wire nails (D = 0.207", L = 4-1/2")

15.3.4 Bolted Built-Up Columns

15.3.4.1 The provisions in 15.3.1 and 15.3.2 apply to bolted built-up columns in which:

(a) a metal plate or washer is provided between the wood and the bolt head, and between the wood and the nut

(b) nuts are tightened to insure that faces of adjacent laminations are in contact

(c) for softwoods: $7D \leq$ end distance $\leq 8.4D$
for hardwoods: $5D \leq$ end distance $\leq 6D$

(d) $4D \leq$ spacing between adjacent bolts in a row $\leq 6t_{min}$

(e) $1.5D \leq$ spacing between rows of bolts $\leq 10D$

(f) $1.5D \leq$ edge distance $\leq 10D$

(g) 2 or more longitudinal rows of bolts are provided when $d > 3t_{min}$

where:

D = bolt diameter

d = depth (face width) of individual lamination

t_{min} = thickness of thinnest lamination

15.3.4.2 Figure 15D provides an example of a bolting schedule which meets the preceding connection requirements.

Figure 15D Typical Bolting Schedules for Built-Up Columns

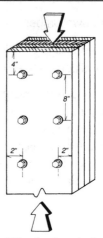

Four 2" x 8" laminations (softwoods) with two rows of ½" diameter bolts.

15.4 Wood Columns with Side Loads and Eccentricity

15.4.1 General Equations

One design method that allows calculation of the direct compression load that an eccentrically loaded column, or one with a side load, is capable of sustaining is as follows:

(a) Members subjected to a combination of bending from eccentricity and/or side loads about one or both principal axes, and axial compression, shall be proportioned so that:

$$\left(\frac{f_c}{F_c'}\right)^2 + \frac{f_{b1} + f_c(6e_1/d_1)[1+0.234(f_c/F_{cE1})]}{F_{b1}'\left[1-(f_c/F_{cE1})\right]} + \qquad (15.4\text{-}1)$$

$$\frac{f_{b2} + f_c(6e_2/d_2)\left\{1+0.234(f_c/F_{cE2})+0.234\left[\dfrac{f_{b1}+f_c(6e_1/d_1)}{F_{bE}}\right]^2\right\}}{F_{b2}'\left\{1-(f_c/F_{cE2})-\left[\dfrac{f_{b1}+f_c(6e_1/d_1)}{F_{bE}}\right]^2\right\}} \leq 1.0$$

(b) Members subjected to a combination of bending and compression from an eccentric axial load about one or both principal axes, shall be proportioned so that:

$$\left(\frac{f_c}{F_c'}\right)^2 + \frac{f_c(6e_1/d_1)[1+0.234(f_c/F_{cE1})]}{F_{b1}'\left[1-(f_c/F_{cE1})\right]} + \qquad (15.4\text{-}2)$$

$$\frac{f_c(6e_2/d_2)\left\{1+0.234(f_c/F_{cE2})+0.234\left[\dfrac{f_c(6e_1/d_1)}{F_{bE}}\right]^2\right\}}{F_{b2}'\left\{1-(f_c/F_{cE2})-\left[\dfrac{f_c(6e_1/d_1)}{F_{bE}}\right]^2\right\}} \leq 1.0$$

where:

$$f_c < F_{cE1} = \frac{0.822 E_{min}'}{\left(\ell_{e1}/d_1\right)^2} \quad \text{for either uniaxial edgewise bending or biaxial bending}$$

and

$$f_c < F_{cE2} = \frac{0.822 E_{min}'}{\left(\ell_{e2}/d_2\right)^2} \quad \text{for uniaxial flatwise bending or biaxial bending}$$

and

$$f_{b1} < F_{bE} = \frac{1.20 E_{min}'}{R_B^2} \quad \text{for biaxial bending}$$

f_c = compression stress parallel to grain due to axial load

f_{b1} = edgewise bending stress due to side loads on narrow face only

f_{b2} = flatwise bending stress due to side loads on wide face only

F_c' = adjusted compression design value parallel to grain that would be permitted if axial compressive stress only existed, determined in accordance with 2.3 and 3.7

F_{b1}' = adjusted edgewise bending design value that would be permitted if edgewise bending stress only existed, determined in accordance with 2.3 and 3.3.3

F_{b2}' = adjusted flatwise bending design value that would be permitted if flatwise bending stress only existed, determined in accordance with 2.3 and 3.3.3

R_B = slenderness ratio of bending member (see 3.3.3)

d_1 = wide face dimension

d_2 = narrow face dimension

e_1 = eccentricity, measured parallel to wide face from centerline of column to centerline of axial load

e_2 = eccentricity, measured parallel to narrow face from centerline of column to centerline of axial load

Effective column lengths, ℓ_{e1} and ℓ_{e2}, shall be determined in accordance with 3.7.1.2. F_{cE1} and F_{cE2} shall be determined in accordance with 3.7. F_{bE} shall be determined in accordance with 3.3.3.

15.4.2 Columns with Side Brackets

15.4.2.1 The formulas in 15.4.1 assume that the eccentric load is applied at the end of the column. One design method that allows calculation of the actual bending stress, f_b, if the eccentric load is applied by a bracket within the upper quarter of the length of the column is as follows.

5.4.2.2 Assume that a bracket load, P, at a distance, a, from the center of the column (Figure 15E), is replaced by the same load, P, centrally applied at the top of the column, plus a side load, P_s, applied at midheight. Calculate P_s from the following formula:

$$P_s = \frac{3P\,a\,\ell_p}{\ell^2} \qquad\qquad (15.4\text{-}3)$$

where:

    P = actual load on bracket, lbs.

    P_s = assumed horizontal side load placed at center of height of column, lbs.

    a = horizontal distance from load on bracket to center of column, in.

    ℓ = total length of column, in.

    ℓ_p = distance measured vertically from point of application of load on bracket to farther end of column, in.

The assumed centrally applied load, P, shall be added to other concentric column loads, and the calculated side load, P_s, shall be used to determine the actual bending stress, f_b, for use in the formula for concentric end and side loading.

Figure 15E   Eccentrically Loaded Column

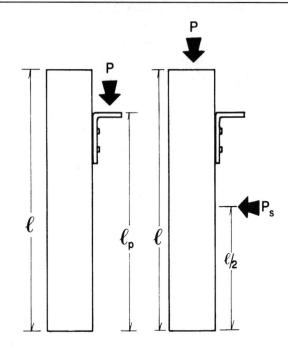

FIRE DESIGN OF WOOD MEMBERS

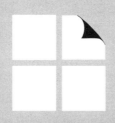

AMERICAN FOREST & PAPER ASSOCIATION

16.1 General

Chapter 16 establishes general fire design provisions that apply to all wood structural members and connections covered under this Specification, unless otherwise noted. Each wood member or connection shall be of sufficient size and capacity to carry the applied loads without exceeding the design provisions specified herein. Reference design values and specific design provisions applicable to particular wood products or connections to be used with the provisions of this Chapter are given in other Chapters of this Specification.

16.2 Design Procedures for Exposed Wood Members

The induced stress shall not exceed the resisting strength which have been adjusted for fire exposure. Wood member design provisions herein are limited to fire resistance calculations not exceeding 2 hours.

16.2.1 Char Rate

The effective char rate to be used in the this procedure can be estimated from published nominal 1-hour char rate data using the following equation:

$$\beta_{eff} = \frac{1.2\beta_n}{t^{0.187}} \qquad (16.2-1)$$

where:

β_{eff} = effective char rate (in./hr.), adjusted for exposure time, t

β_n = nominal char rate (in./hr.), linear char rate based on 1-hour exposure

t = exposure time (hrs.)

A nominal char rate, β_n, of 1.5 in./hr. is commonly assumed for solid sawn and structural glued laminated softwood members. For β_n = 1.5 in./hr., the effective char rates, β_{eff}, and effective char layer thicknesses, a_{char}, for each exposed surface are shown in Table 16.2.1.

Table 16.2.1 Effective Char Rates and Char Layer Thicknesses (for β_n = 1.5 in./hr.)

Required Fire Endurance (hr.)	Effective Char Rate, β_{eff} (in./hr.)	Effective Char Layer Thickness, a_{char} (in.)
1-Hour	1.8	1.8
1½-Hour	1.67	2.5
2-Hour	1.58	3.2

Section properties shall be calculated using standard equations for area, section modulus, and moment of inertia using the reduced cross-sectional dimensions. The dimensions are reduced by the effective char layer thickness, a_{char}, for each surface exposed to fire.

16.2.2 Member Strength

For solid sawn, structural glued laminated timber, and structural composite lumber wood members, the average member strength can be approximated by multiplying reference design values (F_b, F_t, F_c, F_{bE}, F_{cE}) by the adjustment factors specified in Table 16.2.2.

All member strength and cross-sectional properties shall be adjusted prior to use of the interaction calculations in 3.9 or 15.4.

16.2.3 Design of Members

The induced stress calculated using reduced section properties determined in 16.2.1 shall not exceed the member strength determined in 16.2.2.

6.2.4 Special Provisions for Structural Glued Laminated Timber Beams

For structural glued laminated timber bending members given in Table 5A and rated for 1-hour fire endurance, an outer tension lamination shall be substituted for a core lamination on the tension side for unbalanced beams and on both sides for balanced beams. For structural glued laminated timber bending members given in Table 5A and rated for 1½- or 2-hour fire endurance, 2 outer tension laminations shall be substituted for 2 core laminations on the tension side for unbalanced beams and on both sides for balanced beams.

16.2.5 Provisions for Timber Decks

Timber decks consist of planks that are at least 2" (actual) thick. The planks shall span the distance between supporting beams. Single and double tongue-and-groove (T&G) decking shall be designed as an assembly of wood beams fully exposed on one face. Butt-jointed decking shall be designed as an assembly of wood beams partially exposed on the sides and fully exposed on one face. To compute the effects of partial exposure of the decking on its sides, the char rate for this limited exposure shall be reduced to 33% of the effective char rate. These calculation procedures do not address thermal separation.

Table 16.2.2 Adjustment Factors for Fire Design[1]

			ASD					
			Design Stress to Member Strength Factor	Size Factor [2]	Volume Factor [2]	Flat Use Factor [2]	Beam Stability Factor [3]	Column Stability Factor [3]
Bending Strength	F_b	x	2.85	C_F	C_V	C_{fu}	C_L	-
Tensile Strength	F_t	x	2.85	C_F	-	-	-	-
Compression Strength	F_c	x	2.58	C_F	-	-	-	C_P
Beam Buckling Strength	F_{bE}	x	2.03	-	-	-	-	-
Column Buckling Strength	F_{cE}	x	2.03	-	-	-	-	-

1. See 4.3, 5.3 and 8.3 for applicability of adjustment factors for specific products.
2. Factor shall be based on initial cross-section dimensions.
3. Factor shall be based on reduced cross-section dimensions.

16.3 Wood Connections

Where fire endurance is required, connectors and fasteners shall be protected from fire exposure by wood, fire-rated gypsum board, or any coating approved for the required endurance time.

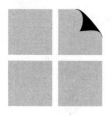

APPENDIX

Appendix A (Non-mandatory) Construction and Design Practices

A.1 Care of Material

Lumber shall be so handled and covered as to prevent marring and moisture absorption from snow or rain.

A.2 Foundations

A.2.1 Foundations shall be adequate to support the building or structure and any required loads, without excessive or unequal settlement or uplift.

A.2.2 Good construction practices generally eliminate decay or termite damage. Such practices are designed to prevent conditions which would be conducive to decay and insect attack. The building site shall be graded to provide drainage away from the structure. All roots and scraps of lumber shall be removed from the immediate vicinity of the building before backfilling.

A.3 Structural Design

Consideration shall be given in design to the possible effect of cross-grain dimensional changes which may occur in lumber fabricated or erected in a green condition (i.e., provisions shall be made in the design so that if dimensional changes caused by seasoning to moisture equilibrium occur, the structure will move as a whole, and the differential movement of similar parts and members meeting at connections will be a minimum).

A.4 Drainage

In exterior structures, the design shall be such as to minimize pockets in which moisture can accumulate, or adequate caps, drainage, and drips shall be provided.

A.5 Camber

Adequate camber in trusses to give proper appearance and to counteract any deflection from loading should be provided. For timber connector construction, such camber shall be permitted to be estimated from the formula:

$$\Delta = \frac{K_1 L^3 + K_2 L^2}{H} \qquad \text{(A-1)}$$

where:

Δ = camber at center of truss, in.

L = truss span, ft

H = truss height at center, ft

K_1 = 0.000032 for any type of truss

K_2 = 0.0028 for flat and pitched trusses

K_2 = 0.00063 for bowstring trusses (i.e., trusses without splices in upper chord)

A.6 Erection

A.6.1 Provision shall be made to prevent the overstressing of members or connections during erection.

A.6.2 Bolted connections shall be snugly tightened, but not to the extent of crushing wood under washers.

A.6.3 Adequate bracing shall be provided until permanent bracing and/or diaphragms are installed.

A.7 Inspection

Provision should be made for competent inspection of materials and workmanship.

A.8 Maintenance

There shall be competent inspection and tightening of bolts in connections of trusses and structural frames.

A.9 Wood Column Bracing

In buildings, for forces acting in a direction parallel to the truss or beam, column bracing shall be permitted to be provided by knee braces or, in the case of trusses, by extending the column to the top chord of the truss where the bottom and top chords are separated sufficiently to provide adequate bracing action. In a direction perpendicular to the truss or beam, bracing shall be permitted to be provided by wall construction, knee braces, or bracing between columns. Such bracing between columns should be installed preferably in the same bays as the bracing between trusses.

A.10 Truss Bracing

In buildings, truss bracing to resist lateral forces shall be permitted as follows:

(a) Diagonal lateral bracing between top chords of trusses shall be permitted to be omitted when the provisions of Appendix A.11 are followed or when the roof joists rest on and are securely fastened to the top chords of the trusses and are covered with wood sheathing. Where sheathing other than wood is applied, top chord diagonal lateral bracing should be installed.

(b) In all cases, vertical sway bracing should be installed in each third or fourth bay at intervals of approximately 35 feet measured parallel to trusses. Also, bottom chord lateral bracing should be installed in the same bays as the vertical sway bracing, where practical, and should extend from side wall to side wall. In addition, struts should be installed between bottom chords at the same truss panels as vertical sway bracing and should extend continuously from end wall to end wall. If the roof construction does not provide proper top chord strut action, separate additional members should be provided.

A.11 Lateral Support of Arches, Compression Chords of Trusses and Studs

A.11.1 When roof joists or purlins are used between arches or compression chords, or when roof joists or purlins are placed on top of an arch or compression chord, and are securely fastened to the arch or compression chord, the largest value of ℓ_e/d, calculated using the depth of the arch or compression chord or calculated using the breadth (least dimension) of the arch or compression chord between points of intermittent lateral support, shall be used. The roof joists or purlins should be placed to account for shrinkage (for example by placing the upper edges of unseasoned joists approximately 5% of the joist depth above the tops of the arch or chord), but also placed low enough to provide adequate lateral support.

A.11.2 When planks are placed on top of an arch or compression chord, and securely fastened to the arch or compression chord, or when sheathing is nailed properly to the top chord of trussed rafters, the depth rather than the breadth of the arch, compression chord, or trussed rafter shall be permitted to be used as the least dimension in determining ℓ_e/d.

A.11.3 When stud walls in light frame construction are adequately sheathed on at least one side, the depth, rather than breadth of the stud, shall be permitted to be taken as the least dimension in calculating the ℓ_e/d ratio. The sheathing shall be shown by experience to provide lateral support and shall be adequately fastened.

Appendix B (Non-mandatory) Load Duration (ASD Only)

B.1 Adjustment of Reference Design Values for Load Duration

B.1.1 Normal Load Duration. The reference design values in this Specification are for normal load duration. Normal load duration contemplates fully stressing a member to its allowable design value by the application of the full design load for a cumulative duration of approximately 10 years and/or the application of 90% of the full design load continuously throughout the remainder of the life of the structure, without encroaching on the factor of safety.

B.1.2 Other Load Durations. Since tests have shown that wood has the property of carrying substantially greater maximum loads for short durations than for long durations of loading, reference design values for normal load duration shall be multiplied by load duration factors, C_D, for other durations of load (see Figure B1). Load duration factors do not apply to reference modulus of elasticity design values, E, nor to reference compression design values perpendicular to grain, $F_{c\perp}$, based on a deformation limit.

(a) When the member is fully stressed to the adjusted design value by application of the full design load permanently, or for a cumulative total of more than 10 years, reference design values for normal load duration (except E and $F_{c\perp}$ based on a deformation limit) shall be multiplied by the load duration factor, $C_D = 0.90$.

(b) Likewise, when the duration of the full design load does not exceed the following durations, reference design values for normal load duration (except E and $F_{c\perp}$ based on a deformation limit) shall be multiplied by the following load duration factors:

C_D	Load Duration
1.15	two months duration
1.25	seven days duration
1.6	ten minutes duration
2.0	impact

(c) The 2 month load duration factor, $C_D = 1.15$, is applicable to design snow loads based on ASCE 7. Other load duration factors shall be permitted to be used where such adjustments are referenced to the duration of the design snow load in the specific location being considered.

(d) The 10 minutes load duration factor, $C_D = 1.6$, is applicable to design earthquake loads and design wind loads based on ASCE 7.

(e) Load duration factors greater than 1.6 shall not apply to structural members pressure-treated with water-borne preservatives (see Reference 30), or fire retardant chemicals. The impact load duration factor shall not apply to connections.

B.2 Combinations of Loads of Different Durations

When loads of different durations are applied simultaneously to members which have full lateral support to prevent buckling, the design of structural members and connections shall be based on the critical load combination determined from the following procedures:

(a) Determine the magnitude of each load that will occur on a structural member and accumulate subtotals of combinations of these loads. Design loads established by applicable building codes and standards may include load combination factors to adjust for probability of simultaneous occurrence of various loads (see Appendix B.4). Such load combination factors should be included in the load combination subtotals.

(b) Divide each subtotal by the load duration factor, C_D, for the shortest duration load in the combination of loads under consideration.

Shortest Load Duration in the Combination of Loads	Load Duration Factor, C_D
Permanent	0.9
Normal	1.0
Two Months	1.15
Seven Days	1.25
Ten Minutes	1.6
Impact	2.0

(c) The largest value thus obtained indicates the critical load combination to be used in designing the structural member or connection.

EXAMPLE: Determine the critical load combination for a structural member subjected to the following loads:

D = dead load established by applicable building code or standard

L = live load established by applicable building code or standard

S = snow load established by applicable building code or standard

W = wind load established by applicable building code or standard

The actual stress due to any combination of the above loads shall be less than or equal to the adjusted design value modified by the load duration factor, C_D, for the shortest duration load in that combination of loads:

Actual stress due to	(C_D)	x (Design value)
D	≤ (0.9)	x (design value)
D+L	≤ (1.0)	x (design value)
D+W	≤ (1.6)	x (design value)
D+L+S	≤ (1.15)	x (design value)
D+L+W	≤ (1.6)	x (design value)
D+S+W	≤ (1.6)	x (design value)
D+L+S+W	≤ (1.6)	x (design value)

The equations above may be specified by the applicable building code and shall be checked as required. Load combination factors specified by the applicable building code or standard should be included in the above equations, as specified in B.2(a).

B.3 Mechanical Connections

Load duration factors, $C_D \leq 1.6$, apply to reference design values for connections, except when connection capacity is based on design of metal parts (see 10.2.3).

B.4 Load Combination Reduction Factors

Reductions in total design load for certain combinations of loads account for the reduced probability of simultaneous occurrence of the various design loads. Load duration factors, C_D, account for the relationship between wood strength and time under load. Load duration factors, C_D, are independent of load combination reduction factors, and both may be used in design calculations (see 1.4.4).

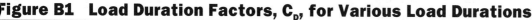

Figure B1   Load Duration Factors, C_D, for Various Load Durations

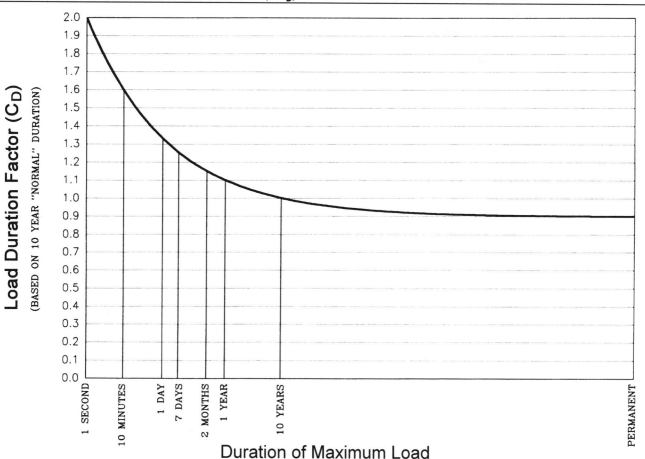

Appendix C (Non-mandatory) Temperature Effects

C.1

As wood is cooled below normal temperatures, its strength increases. When heated, its strength decreases. This temperature effect is immediate and its magnitude varies depending on the moisture content of the wood. Up to 150°F, the immediate effect is reversible. The member will recover essentially all its strength when the temperature is reduced to normal. Prolonged heating to temperatures above 150°F can cause a permanent loss of strength.

C.2

In some regions, structural members are periodically exposed to fairly elevated temperatures. However, the normal accompanying relative humidity generally is very low and, as a result, wood moisture contents also are low. The immediate effect of the periodic exposure to the elevated temperatures is less pronounced because of this dryness. Also, independently of temperature changes, wood strength properties generally increase with a decrease in moisture content. In recognition of these offsetting factors, it is traditional practice to use the reference design values from this Specification for ordinary temperature fluctuations and occasional short-term heating to temperatures up to 150°F.

C.3

When wood structural members are heated to temperatures up to 150°F for extended periods of time, adjustment of the reference design values in this Specification may be necessary (see 2.3.3 and 10.3.4). See Reference 53 for additional information concerning the effect of temperature on wood strength.

D.1

Slenderness ratios and related equations for adjusting reference bending design values for lateral buckling in 3.3.3 are based on theoretical analyses and beam verification tests.

D.2

Treatment of lateral buckling in beams parallels that for columns given in 3.7.1 and Appendix H. Beam stability calculations are based on slenderness ratio, R_B, defined as:

$$R_B = \sqrt{\frac{\ell_e d}{b^2}} \qquad (D\text{-}1)$$

with ℓ_e as specified in 3.3.3.

D.3

For beams with rectangular cross section where R_B does not exceed 50, adjusted bending design values are obtained by the equation (where $C_L \le C_V$):

$$F_b' = F_b^* \left[\frac{1 + \left(F_{bE}/F_b^*\right)}{1.9} - \sqrt{\left[\frac{1 + \left(F_{bE}/F_b^*\right)}{1.9}\right]^2 - \frac{F_{bE}/F_b^*}{0.95}} \right] \qquad (D\text{-}2)$$

where:

$$F_{bE} = \frac{1.20\,E_{min}'}{R_B^2} \qquad (D\text{-}3)$$

F_b^* = reference bending design value multiplied by all applicable adjustment factors except C_{fu}, C_V, and C_L (see 2.3)

D.4

Reference modulus of elasticity for beam and column stability, E_{min}, in Equation D-3 is based on the following equation:

$$E_{min} = E\,[1 - 1.645\,COV_E](1.03)/1.66 \qquad (D\text{-}4)$$

where:

E = reference modulus of elasticity

1.03 = adjustment factor to convert E values to a pure bending basis except that the factor is 1.05 for structural glued laminated timber

1.66 = factor of safety

COV_E = coefficient of variation in modulus of elasticity (see Appendix F)

E_{min} represents an approximate 5% lower exclusion value on pure bending modulus of elasticity, plus a 1.66 factor of safety.

D.5

For products with less E variability than visually graded sawn lumber, higher critical buckling design values (F_{bE}) may be calculated. For a product having a lower coefficient of variation in modulus of elasticity, use of Equations D-3 and D-4 will provide a 1.66 factor of safety at the 5% lower exclusion value.

Appendix E (Non-mandatory) Local Stresses in Fastener Groups

E.1 General

Where a fastener group is composed of closely spaced fasteners loaded parallel to grain, the capacity of the fastener group may be limited by wood failure at the net section or tear-out around the fasteners caused by local stresses. One method to evaluate member strength for local stresses around fastener groups is outlined in the following procedures.

E.1.1 Reference design values for timber rivet connections in Chapter 13 account for local stress effects and do not require further modification by procedures outlined in this Appendix.

E.1.2 The capacity of connections with closely spaced, large diameter bolts has been shown to be limited by the capacity of the wood surrounding the connection. Connections with groups of smaller diameter fasteners, such as typical nailed connections in wood-frame construction, may not be limited by wood capacity.

E.2 Net Section Tension Capacity

The adjusted tension capacity is calculated in accordance with provisions of 3.1.2 and 3.8.1 as follows:

$$Z_{NT}' = F_t' A_{net} \qquad (E.2\text{-}1)$$

where:

Z_{NT}' = adjusted tension capacity of net section area

F_t' = adjusted tension design value parallel to grain

A_{net} = net section area per 3.1.2

E.3 Row Tear-Out Capacity

The adjusted tear-out capacity of a row of fasteners can be estimated as follows:

$$Z_{RTi}' = n_i \frac{F_v' A_{critical}}{2} \qquad (E.3\text{-}1)$$

where:

Z_{RTi}' = adjusted row tear out capacity of row i

F_v' = adjusted shear design value parallel to grain

$A_{critical}$ = minimum shear area of any fastener in row i

n_i = number of fasteners in row i

E.3.1 Assuming one shear line on each side of bolts in a row (observed in tests of bolted connections), Equation E.3-1 becomes:

$$Z_{RTi}' = \frac{F_v' t}{2}\big[n_i s_{critical}\big](2 \text{ shear lines}) \qquad (E.3\text{-}2)$$

$$= n_i F_v' t s_{critical}$$

where:

$s_{critical}$ = minimum spacing in row i taken as the lesser of the end distance or the spacing between fasteners in row i

t = thickness of member

The total adjusted row tear-out capacity of multiple rows of fasteners can be estimated as:

$$Z_{RT}' = \sum_{i=1}^{n_{row}} Z_{RTi}' \qquad (E.3\text{-}3)$$

where:

Z_{RT}' = adjusted row tear out capacity of multiple rows

n_{row} = number of rows

E.3.2 In Equation E.3-1, it is assumed that the induced shear stress varies from a maximum value of $f_v = F_v'$ to a minimum value of $f_v = 0$ along each shear line between fasteners in a row and that the change in shear stress/strain is linear along each shear line. The resulting triangular stress distribution on each shear line between fasteners in a row establishes an apparent shear stress equal to half of the adjusted design shear stress, $F_v'/2$, as shown in Equation E.3-1. This assumption is combined with the critical area concept for evaluating stresses in fastener groups and provides good agreement with results from tests of bolted connections.

E3.3 Use of the minimum shear area of any fastener in a row for calculation of row tear-out capacity is based on the assumption that the smallest shear area between fasteners in a row will limit the capacity of the row of fasteners. Limited verification of this approach is provided from tests of bolted connections.

E.4 Group Tear-Out Capacity

The adjusted tear-out capacity of a group of "n" rows of fasteners can be estimated as:

$$Z_{GT}' = \frac{Z_{RT-1}'}{2} + \frac{Z_{RT-n}'}{2} + F_t'A_{group-net}$$ (E.4-1)

where:

Z_{GT}' = adjusted group tear-out capacity

Z_{RT-1}' = adjusted row tear-out capacity of row 1 of fasteners bounding the critical group area

Z_{RT-n}' = adjusted row tear-out capacity of row n of fasteners bounding the critical group area

$A_{group-net}$ = critical group net section area between row 1 and row n

E.4.1 For groups of fasteners with non-uniform spacing between rows of fasteners various definitions of critical group area should be checked for group tear-out in combination with row tear-out to determine the adjusted capacity of the critical section.

E.5 Effects of Fastener Placement

E 5.1 Modification of fastener placement within a fastener group can be used to increase row tear-out and group tear-out capacity limited by local stresses around the fastener group. Increased spacing between fasteners in a row is one way to increase row tear-out capacity. Increased spacing between rows of fasteners is one way to increase group tear-out capacity.

E 5.2 Footnote 2 to Table 11.5.1D limits the spacing between outer rows of fasteners paralleling the member on a single splice plate to 5 inches. This requirement is imposed to limit local stresses resulting from shrinkage of wood members. When special detailing is used to address shrinkage, such as the use of slotted holes, the 5-inch limit can be adjusted.

E.6 Sample Solution of Staggered Bolts

Calculate the net section area tension, row tear-out, and group tear-out ASD adjusted design capacities for the double-shear bolted connection in Figure E1.

Main Member:
Combination 3 Douglas fir 3-1/8 x 12 glued laminated timber member
F_t' = 1450 psi
F_v' = 240 psi
Main member thickness, t_m: 3.125 inches
Main member width, w: 12 inches

Side Member:
A36 steel plates on each side
Side plate thickness, t_s: 0.25 inches

Connection Details:
Bolt diameter, D: 1 inch
Bolt hole diameter, D_h: 1.0625 inches
Adjusted ASD bolt design value, $Z_{||}'$: 4380 lbs. (see NDS Table 11I. For this trial design, the group action factor, C_g, is taken as 1.0).
Spacing between rows: s_{row} = 2.5D

Adjusted ASD Connection Capacity, $nZ_{||}'$:

$nZ_{||}'$ = (8 bolts)(4,380 lbs.) = 35,040 lbs.

Figure E1 Staggered Rows of Bolts

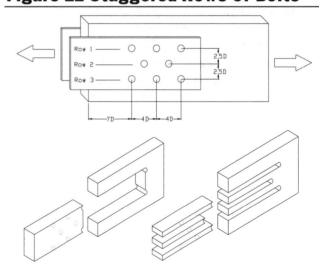

Adjusted ASD Net Section Area Tension Capacity, Z_{NT}':

$$Z_{NT}' = F_t't[w - n_{row}D_h]$$

$$\begin{aligned}
Z_{NT}' &= (1,450\ psi)(3.125")[12" - 3(1.0625")] \\
&= 39,930\ lbs.
\end{aligned}$$

Adjusted ASD Row Tear-Out Capacity, $Z_{RT}{}'$:

$$Z_{RTi}{}' = n_i F_v{}' t s_{critical}$$

$$
\begin{aligned}
Z_{RT\text{-}1}{}' &= 3(240 \text{ psi})(3.125")(4") = 9{,}000 \text{ lbs.}\\
Z_{RT\text{-}2}{}' &= 2(240 \text{ psi})(3.125")(4") = 6{,}000 \text{ lbs.}\\
Z_{RT\text{-}3}{}' &= 3(240 \text{ psi})(3.125")(4") = 9{,}000 \text{ lbs.}
\end{aligned}
$$

$$Z_{RT}{}' = \sum_{i=1}^{n_{row}} Z_{RTi}{}' = 9{,}000 + 6{,}000 + 9{,}000 = 24{,}000 \text{ lbs.}$$

Adjusted ASD Group Tear-Out Capacity, $Z_{GT}{}'$:

$$Z_{GT}{}' = \frac{Z_{RT\text{-}1}{}'}{2} + \frac{Z_{RT\text{-}3}{}'}{2} + F_t{}' t\big[(n_{row}-1)(s_{row}-D_h)\big]$$

$$
\begin{aligned}
Z_{GT}{}' &= (9{,}000 \text{ lbs.})/2 + (9{,}000 \text{ lbs.})/2 +\\
&\quad (1{,}450 \text{ psi})(3.125")[(3-1)(2.5"-1.0625")]\\
&= 22{,}030 \text{ lbs.}
\end{aligned}
$$

In this sample calculation, the adjusted ASD connection capacity is limited to 22,030 pounds by group tear-out, $Z_{GT}{}'$.

E.7 Sample Solution of Row of Bolts

Calculate the net section area tension and row tear-out adjusted ASD design capacities for the single-shear single-row bolted connection represented in Figure E2.

Main and Side Members:
#2 grade Hem-Fir 2x4 lumber
$F_t{}' = 788$ psi
$F_v{}' = 145$ psi
Main member thickness, t_m: 3.5 inches
Side member thickness, t_s: 1.5 inches
Main and side member width, w: 3.5 inches

Connection Details:
Bolt diameter, D: 1/2 inch
Bolt hole diameter, D_h: 0.5625 inches
Adjusted ASD bolt design value, $Z_\parallel{}'$: 550 lbs. (See NDS Table 11A. For this trial design, the group action factor, C_g, is taken as 1.0).

Adjusted ASD Connection Capacity, $nZ_\parallel{}'$:

$$nZ_\parallel{}' = (3 \text{ bolts})(550 \text{ lbs.}) = 1{,}650 \text{ lbs.}$$

Adjusted ASD Net Section Area Tension Capacity, $Z_{NT}{}'$:

$$Z_{NT}{}' = F_t{}' t\big[w - n_{row}D_h\big]$$

$$Z_{NT}{}' = (788 \text{ psi})(1.5")[3.5" - 1(0.5625")] = 3{,}470 \text{ lbs.}$$

Figure E2 Single Row of Bolts

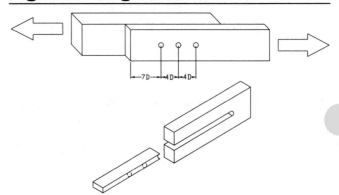

Adjusted ASD Row Tear-Out Capacity, $Z_{RT}{}'$:

$$Z_{RTi}{}' = n_i F_v{}' t s_{critical}$$

$$Z_{RT1}{}' = 3(145 \text{ psi})(1.5")(2") = 1{,}310 \text{ lbs.}$$

In this sample calculation, the adjusted ASD connection capacity is limited to 1,310 pounds by row tear-out, $Z_{RT}{}'$.

Calculate the net section area tension and row tear-out adjusted ASD design capacities for the single-shear single-row split ring connection represented in Figure E3.

Main and Side Members:
#2 grade Southern Pine 2x4 lumber
$F_t' = 825$ psi
$F_v' = 175$ psi
Main member thickness, t_m: 1.5 inches
Side member thickness, t_s: 1.5 inches
Main and side member width, w: 3.5 inches

Connection Details:
Split ring diameter, D: 2.5 inches (see Appendix K for connector dimensions)
Adjusted ASD split ring design value, P': 2,730 lbs. (see NDS Table 12.2A. For this trial design, the group action factor, C_g, is taken as 1.0).

Adjusted ASD Connection Capacity, nP':

$$nP' = (2 \text{ split rings})(2,730 \text{ lbs.}) = 5,460 \text{ lbs.}$$

Adjusted ASD Net Section Area Tension Capacity, Z_{NT}':

$$Z_{NT}' = F_t' A_{net}$$

$$Z_{NT}' = F_t' [A_{2x4} - A_{bolt-hole} - A_{split ring projected area}]$$

$$Z_{NT}' = (825 \text{ psi})[5.25 \text{ in.}^2 - 1.5'' (0.5625'') - 1.1 \text{ in.}^2]$$
$$= 2,728 \text{ lbs.}$$

Figure E3 Single Row of Split Ring Connectors

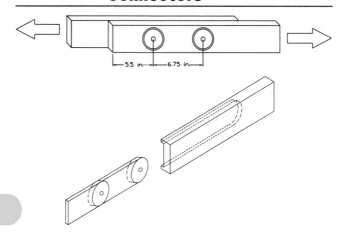

Adjusted ASD Row Tear-Out Capacity, Z_{RT}':

$$Z_{RTi}' = n_i \frac{F_v' A_{critical}}{2}$$

$$Z_{RT1}' = [(2 \text{ connectors})(175 \text{ psi})/2](21.735 \text{ in.}^2)$$
$$= 3,804 \text{ lbs.}$$

where:

$$A_{critical} = 21.735 \text{ in.}^2 \quad (\text{See Figure E4})$$

In this sample calculation, the adjusted ASD connection capacity is limited to 2,728 pounds by net section area tension capacity, Z_{NT}'.

Figure E4 $A_{critical}$ for Split Ring Connection

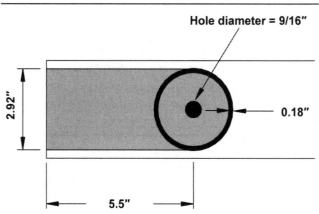

$$A_{critical} = A_{edge plane} + A_{bottom plane net}$$

$$= 21.735 \text{ in.}^2$$

$$A_{edge plane} = (2 \text{ shear lines}) (\text{groove depth})(s_{critical})$$

$$= (2 \text{ shear lines}) (0.375'')(5.5'') = 4.125 \text{ in.}^2$$

$$A_{bottom plane net} = (A_{bottom plane}) - (A_{split ring groove}) - (A_{bolt hole})$$

$$= [(5.5'')(2.92'') + (\pi)(2.92'')^2/8] - (\pi/4)[(2.92'')^2 - (2.92'' - 0.18'' - 0.18'')^2] - (\pi/4)(0.5625'')^2$$

$$= 17.61 \text{ in.}^2$$

Appendix F (Non-mandatory) Design for Creep and Critical Deflection Applications

F.1 Creep

F.1.1 Reference modulus of elasticity design values, E, in this Specification are intended for the calculation of immediate deformation under load. Under sustained loading, wood members exhibit additional time dependent deformation (creep) which usually develops at a slow but persistent rate over long periods of time. Creep rates are greater for members drying under load or exposed to varying temperature and relative humidity conditions than for members in a stable environment and at constant moisture content.

F.1.2 In certain bending applications, it may be necessary to limit deflection under long-term loading to specified levels. This can be done by applying an increase factor to the deflection due to long-term load. Total deflection is thus calculated as the immediate deflection due to the long-term component of the design load times the appropriate increase factor, plus the deflection due to the short-term or normal component of the design load.

F.2 Variation in Modulus of Elasticity

F.2.1 The reference modulus of elasticity design values, E, listed in Tables 4A, 4B, 4C, 4D, 4E, 4F, 5A, 5B, 5C, and 5D (published in the Supplement to this Specification) are average values and individual pieces having values both higher and lower than the averages will occur in all grades. The use of average modulus of elasticity values is customary practice for the design of normal wood structural members and assemblies. Field experience and tests have demonstrated that average values provide an adequate measure of the immediate deflection or deformation of these wood elements.

F.2.2 In certain applications where deflection may be critical, such as may occur in closely engineered, innovative structural components or systems, use of a reduced modulus of elasticity value may be deemed appropriate by the designer. The coefficient of variation in Table F1 shall be permitted to be used as a basis for modifying reference modulus of elasticity values listed in Tables 4A, 4B, 4C, 4D, 4E, 4F, 5A, 5B, 5C, and 5D to meet particular end use conditions.

F.2.3 Reducing reference average modulus of elasticity design values in this Specification by the product of the average value and 1.0 and 1.65 times the applicable coefficients of variation in Table F1 gives estimates of the level of modulus of elasticity exceeded by 84% and 95%, respectively, of the individual pieces, as specified in the following formulas:

$$E_{0.16} = E(1 - 1.0\,COV_E) \tag{F-1}$$

$$E_{0.05} = E(1 - 1.645\,COV_E) \tag{F-2}$$

Table F1 Coefficients of Variation in Modulus of Elasticity (COV_E) for Lumber and Structural Glued Laminated Timber

	COV_E
Visually graded sawn lumber (Tables 4A, 4B, 4D, 4E, and 4F)	0.25
Machine Evaluated Lumber (MEL) (Table 4C)	0.15
Machine Stress Rated (MSR) lumber (Table 4C)	0.11
Structural Glued laminated timber (Tables 5A, 5B, 5C, and 5D)	0.10[1]

1. The COV_E for structural glued laminated timber decreases as the number of laminations increases, and increases as the number of laminations decreases. $COV_E = 0.10$ is an approximate value for six or more laminations.

F.3 Shear Deflection

F.3.1 Reference modulus of elasticity design values, E, listed in Tables 4A, 4B, 4C, 4D, 4E, 4F, 5A, 5B, 5C, and 5D are apparent modulus of elasticity values and include a shear deflection component. For sawn lumber, the ratio of shear-free E to reference E is 1.03. For structural glued laminated timber, the ratio of shear-free E to reference E is 1.05.

F.3.2 In certain applications use of an adjusted modulus of elasticity to more accurately account for the shear component of the total deflection may be deemed appropriate by the designer. Standard methods for adjusting modulus of elasticity to other load and span-depth conditions are available (see Reference 54). When reference modulus of elasticity values have not been adjusted to include the effects of shear deformation, such as for pre-fabricated wood I-joists, consideration for the shear component of the total deflection is required.

F.3.3 The shear component of the total deflection of a beam is a function of beam geometry, modulus of elasticity, shear modulus, applied load and support conditions. The ratio of shear-free E to apparent E is 1.03 for the condition of a simply supported rectangular beam with uniform load, a span to depth ratio of 21:1, and elastic modulus to shear modulus ratio of 16:1. The ratio of shear-free E to apparent E is 1.05 for a similar beam with a span to depth ratio of 17:1. See Reference 53 for information concerning calculation of beam deflection for other span-depth and load conditions.

Appendix G (Non-mandatory) Effective Column Length

G.1

The effective column length of a compression member is the distance between two points along its length at which the member is assumed to buckle in the shape of a sine wave.

G.2

The effective column length is dependent on the values of end fixity and lateral translation (deflection) associated with the ends of columns and points of lateral support between the ends of column. It is recommended that the effective length of columns be determined in accordance with good engineering practice. Lower values of effective length will be associated with more end fixity and less lateral translation while higher values will be associated with less end fixity and more lateral translation.

G.3

In lieu of calculating the effective column length from available engineering experience and methodology, the buckling length coefficients, K_e, given in Table G1 shall be permitted to be multiplied by the actual column length, ℓ, or by the length of column between lateral supports to calculate the effective column length, ℓ_e.

G.4

Where the bending stiffness of the frame itself provides support against buckling, the buckling length coefficient, K_e, for an unbraced length of column, ℓ, is dependent upon the amount of bending stiffness provided by the other in-plane members entering the connection at each end of the unbraced segment. If the combined stiffness from these members is sufficiently small relative to that of the unbraced column segments, K_e could exceed the values given in Table G1.

Table G1 Buckling Length Coefficients, K_e

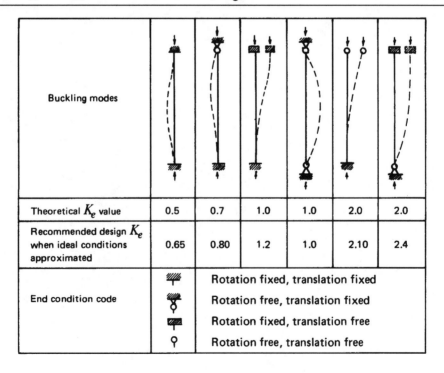

Buckling modes						
Theoretical K_e value	0.5	0.7	1.0	1.0	2.0	2.0
Recommended design K_e when ideal conditions approximated	0.65	0.80	1.2	1.0	2.10	2.4
End condition code		Rotation fixed, translation fixed				
		Rotation free, translation fixed				
		Rotation fixed, translation free				
		Rotation free, translation free				

Appendix H (Non-mandatory) Lateral Stability of Columns

H.1

Solid wood columns can be classified into three length classes, characterized by mode of failure at ultimate load. For short, rectangular columns with a small ratio of length to least cross-sectional dimension, ℓ_e/d, failure is by crushing. When there is an intermediate ℓ_e/d ratio, failure is generally a combination of crushing and buckling. At large ℓ_e/d ratios, long wood columns behave essentially as Euler columns and fail by lateral deflection or buckling. Design of these three length classes are represented by the single column Equation H-1.

H.2

For solid columns of rectangular cross section where the slenderness ratio, ℓ_e/d, does not exceed 50, adjusted compression design values parallel to grain are obtained by the equation:

$$F_c' = F_c^* \left[\frac{1 + \left(F_{cE}/F_c^*\right)}{2c} - \sqrt{\left[\frac{1 + \left(F_{cE}/F_c^*\right)}{2c}\right]^2 - \frac{F_{cE}/F_c^*}{c}} \right] \quad \text{(H-1)}$$

where:

$$F_{cE} = \frac{0.822 \, E_{min}'}{\left(\ell_e/d\right)^2} \quad \text{(H-2)}$$

F_c^* = reference compression design value parallel to grain multiplied by all applicable adjustment factors except C_p (see 2.3)

c = 0.8 for sawn lumber

c = 0.85 for round timber poles and piles

c = 0.9 for structural glued laminated timber or structural composite lumber

Equation H-2 is derived from the standard Euler equation, with radius of gyration, r, converted to the more convenient least cross-sectional dimension, d, of a rectangular column.

H.3

The equation for adjusted compression design value, F_c', in this Specification is for columns having rectangular cross sections. It may be used for other column shapes by substituting $r\sqrt{12}$ for d in the equations, where r is the applicable radius of gyration of the column cross section.

H.4

The 0.822 factor in Equation H-2 represents the Euler buckling coefficient for rectangular columns calculated as $\pi^2/12$. Modulus of elasticity for beam and column stability, E_{min}, in Equation H-2 represents an approximate 5% lower exclusion value on pure bending modulus of elasticity, plus a 1.66 factor of safety (see Appendix D.4).

H.5

Adjusted design values based on Equations H-1 and H-2 are customarily used for most sawn lumber column designs. Where unusual hazard exists, a larger reduction factor may be appropriate. Alternatively, in less critical end use, the designer may elect to use a smaller factor of safety.

H.6

For products with less E variability than visually graded sawn lumber, higher critical buckling design values may be calculated. For a product having a lower coefficient of variation (COV_E), use of Equation H-2 will provide a 1.66 factor of safety at the 5% lower exclusion value.

Appendix I (Non-mandatory) Yield Limit Equations for Connections

I.1 Yield Modes

The yield limit equations specified in 11.3.1 for dowel-type fasteners such as bolts, lag screws, wood screws, nails, and spikes represent four primary connection yield modes (see Figure I1). Modes I_m and I_s represent bearing-dominated yield of the wood fibers in contact with the fastener in either the main or side member(s), respectively. Mode II represents pivoting of the fastener at the shear plane of a single shear connection with localized crushing of wood fibers near the faces of the wood member(s). Modes III_m and III_s represent fastener yield in bending at one plastic hinge point per shear plane, and bearing-dominated yield of wood fibers in contact with the fastener in either the main or side member(s), respectively. Mode IV represents fastener yield in bending at two plastic hinge points per shear plane, with limited localized crushing of wood fibers near the shear plane(s).

I.2 Dowel Bearing Strength for Steel Members

Dowel bearing strength, F_e, for steel members shall be based on accepted steel design practices (see References 39, 40 and 41). Design values in Tables 11B, 11D, 11G, 11I, 11J, 11M, and 11N are for 1/4" ASTM A 36 steel plate or 3 gage and thinner ASTM A 653, Grade 33 steel plate with dowel bearing strength proportional to ultimate tensile strength. Bearing strengths used to calculate connection yield load represent nominal bearing strengths of 2.4 F_u and 2.2 F_u, respectively (based on design provisions in References 39, 40, and 41 for bearing strength of steel members at connections). To allow proper application of the load duration factor for these connections, the bearing strengths have been divided by 1.6.

I.3 Dowel Bearing Strength for Wood Members

Dowel bearing strength, F_e, for wood members may be determined in accordance with ASTM D 5764.

I.4 Fastener Bending Yield Strength, F_{yb}

In the absence of published standards which specify fastener strength properties, the designer should contact fastener manufacturers to determine fastener bending yield strength for connection design. ASTM F 1575 provides a standard method for testing bending yield strength of nails.

Fastener bending yield strength (F_{yb}) shall be determined by the 5% diameter (0.05D) offset method of analyzing load-displacement curves developed from fastener bending tests. However, for short, large diameter fasteners for which direct bending tests are impractical, test data from tension tests such as those specified in ASTM F 606 shall be evaluated to estimate F_{yb}.

Research indicates that F_{yb} for bolts is approximately equivalent to the average of bolt tensile yield strength and bolt tensile ultimate strength, $F_{yb} = F_y/2 + F_u/2$. Based on this approximation, 48,000 psi $\leq F_{yb} \leq$ 140,000 psi for various grades of SAE J429 bolts. Thus, the aforementioned research indicates that $F_{yb} = 45,000$ psi is reasonable for many commonly available bolts. Tests of limited samples of lag screws indicate that $F_{yb} = 45,000$ psi is also reasonable for many commonly available lag screws with D $\geq$ 3/8".

Tests of a limited sample of box nails and common wire nails from twelve U.S. nail manufacturers indicate that F_{yb} increases with decreasing nail diameter, and may exceed 100,000 psi for very small diameter nails. These tests indicate that the F_{yb} values used in Tables 11N through 11R are reasonable for many commonly available box nails and small diameter common wire nails (D < 0.2"). Design values for large diameter common wire nails (D > 0.2") are based on extrapolated estimates of F_{yb} from the aforementioned limited study. For hardened-steel nails, F_{yb} is assumed to be approximately 30% higher than for the same diameter common wire nails. Design values in Tables 11J through 11M for wood screws and small diameter lag screws (D < 3/8") are based on estimates of F_{yb} for common wire nails of the same diameter. Table I1 provides values of F_{yb} based on fastener type and diameter.

Single Shear Connections

Double Shear Connections

Mode I$_m$

Mode I$_s$

Mode II   (not applicable)

Mode III$_m$ (not applicable)

Mode III$_s$

Mode IV

I.5 Threaded Fasteners

The reduced moment resistance in the threaded portion of dowel-type fasteners can be accounted for by use of root diameter, D_r, in calculation of reference lateral design values. Use of diameter, D, is permitted when the threaded portion of the fastener is sufficiently far away from the connection shear plane(s). For example, diameter, D, may be used when the length of thread bearing in the main member of a two member connection does not exceed 1/4 of the total bearing length in the main member (member holding the threads). For a connection with three or more members, diameter, D, may be used when the length of thread bearing in the outermost member does not exceed 1/4 of the total bearing length in the outermost member (member holding the threads). Use of diameter, D, is permitted when full body diameter bolts defined in 11.1.2 are used since thread bearing lengths are typically small in the member holding the threads. For thread lengths greater than 1/4 of the total bearing length in the member holding the threads, the effect of reduced moment resistance of bolts defined in 11.1.2 is small when evaluated with a more detailed analysis.

Reference lateral design values for reduced body diameter lag screw and rolled thread wood screw connections are based on root diameter, D_r to account for the reduced diameter of these fasteners. These values may also be applicable for full-body diameter lag screws and cut thread wood screws since the length of threads for these fasteners is generally not known and/or the thread bearing length based on typical dimensions exceeds 1/4 the total bearing length in the member holding the threads. For bolted connections, reference lateral design values are based on diameter, D.

One alternate method of accounting for the moment and bearing resistance of the threaded portion of the fastener and moment acting along the length of the fastener is provided in AF&PA's *Technical Report 12 - General Dowel Equations for Calculating Lateral Connection Values* (see Reference 51). A general set of equations permits use of different fastener diameters for bearing resistance and moment resistance in each member.

Table I1   Fastener Bending Yield Strengths, F_{yb}

Fastener Type	F_{yb} (psi)
Bolt, lag screw (with D ≥ 3/8"), drift pin (SAE J429 Grade 1 - F_y = 36,000 psi and F_u = 60,000 psi)	45,000
Common, box, or sinker nail, spike, lag screw, wood screw (low to medium carbon steel)	
0.099" ≤ D ≤ 0.142"	100,000
0.142" < D ≤ 0.177"	90,000
0.177" < D ≤ 0.236"	80,000
0.236" < D ≤ 0.273"	70,000
0.273" < D ≤ 0.344"	60,000
0.344" < D ≤ 0.375"	45,000
Hardened steel nail (medium carbon steel)	
0.120" ≤ D ≤ 0.142"	130,000
0.142" < D ≤ 0.192"	115,000
0.192" < D ≤ 0.207"	100,000

Appendix J (Non-mandatory) Solution of Hankinson Formula

J.1

When members are loaded in bearing at an angle to grain between 0° and 90°, or when split ring or shear plate connectors, bolts, or lag screws are loaded at an angle to grain between 0° and 90°, design values at an angle to grain shall be determined using the Hankinson formula.

J.2

The Hankinson formula is for the condition where the loaded surface is perpendicular to the direction of the applied load.

J.3

When the resultant force is not perpendicular to the surface under consideration, the angle θ is the angle between the direction of grain and the direction of the force component which is perpendicular to the surface.

J.4

The bearing surface for a split ring or shear plate connector, bolt or lag screw is assumed perpendicular to the applied lateral load.

J.5

The bearing strength of wood depends upon the direction of grain with respect to the direction of the applied load. Wood is stronger in compression parallel to grain than in compression perpendicular to grain. The variation in strength at various angles to grain between 0° and 90° shall be determined by the Hankinson formula as follows:

$$F_\theta' = \frac{F_c^* F_{c\perp}'}{F_c^* \sin^2 \theta + F_{c\perp}' \cos^2 \theta} \tag{J-1}$$

where:

F_c^* = adjusted compression design value parallel to grain multiplied by all applicable adjustment factors except the column stability factor

$F_{c\perp}'$ = adjusted compression design value perpendicular to grain

F_θ' = adjusted bearing design value at an angle to grain

θ = angle between direction of load and direction of grain (longitudinal axis of member)

When determining dowel bearing design values at an angle to grain for bolt or lag screw connections, the Hankinson formula takes the following form:

$$F_{e\theta} = \frac{F_{e\|} F_{e\perp}}{F_{e\|} \sin^2 \theta + F_{e\perp} \cos^2 \theta} \tag{J-2}$$

where:

$F_{e\|}$ = dowel bearing strength parallel to grain

$F_{e\perp}$ = dowel bearing strength perpendicular to grain

$F_{e\theta}$ = dowel bearing strength at an angle to grain

When determining adjusted design values for bolt or lag screw wood-to-metal connections or wood-to-wood connections with the main or side member(s) loaded parallel to grain, the following form of the Hankinson formula provides an alternate solution:

$$Z_\theta' = \frac{Z_\|' Z_\perp'}{Z_\|' \sin^2 \theta + Z_\perp' \cos^2 \theta} \tag{J-3}$$

For wood-to-wood connections with side member(s) loaded parallel to grain,

$Z_\|'$ = adjusted lateral design value for a single bolt or lag screw connection with the main and side wood members loaded parallel to grain, $Z_\|$

$Z_\perp'$ = adjusted lateral design value for a single bolt or lag screw connection with the side member(s) loaded parallel to grain and main member loaded perpendicular to grain, $Z_{m\perp}$

For wood-to-wood connections with the main member loaded parallel to grain,

$Z_{\parallel}'$ = adjusted lateral design value for a single bolt or lag screw connection with the main and side wood members loaded parallel to grain, $Z_{\parallel}$

$Z_{\perp}'$ = adjusted lateral design value for a single bolt or lag screw connection with the main member loaded parallel to grain and side member(s) loaded perpendicular to grain, $Z_{s\perp}$

For wood-to-metal connections,

$Z_{\parallel}'$ = adjusted lateral design value for a single bolt or lag screw connection with the wood member loaded parallel to grain, $Z_{\parallel}$

$Z_{\perp}'$ = adjusted lateral design value for a single bolt or lag screw connection with the wood member loaded perpendicular to grain, $Z_{\perp}$

When determining adjusted design values for split ring or shear plate connectors or timber rivets, the Hankinson formula takes the following form:

$$N' = \frac{P'Q'}{P'\sin^2\theta + Q'\cos^2\theta} \qquad (J\text{-}4)$$

where:

P' = adjusted lateral design value parallel to grain for a single split ring connector unit or shear plate connector unit

Q' = adjusted lateral design value perpendicular to grain for a single split ring connector unit or shear plate connector unit

N' = adjusted lateral design value at an angle to grain for a single split ring connector unit or shear plate connector unit

The nomographs presented in Figure J1 provide a graphical solution of the Hankinson formula.

Figure J1 Solution of Hankinson Formula

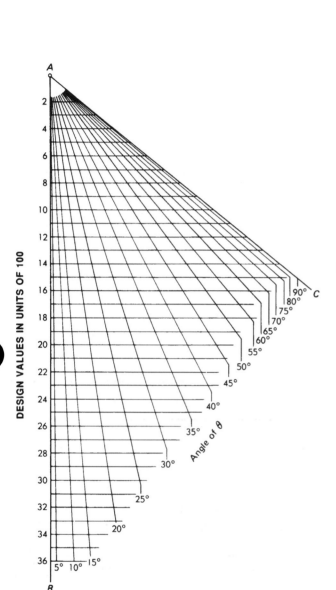

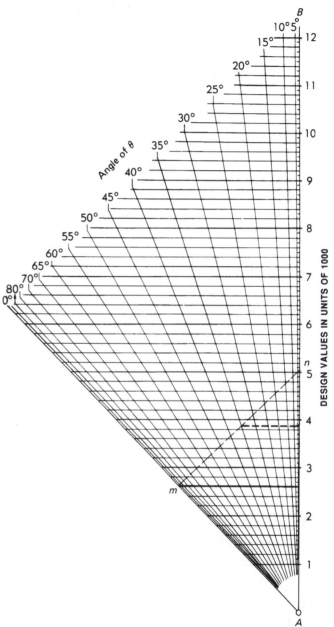

Figure J2 Connection Loaded at an Angle to Grain

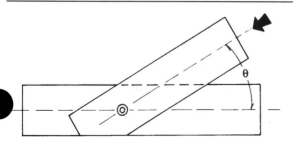

Sample Solution for Split Ring or Shear Plate Connection:

Assume that P' = 5,030 lbs., Q' = 2,620 lbs., and θ = 35° in Figure J2. On line A-B in Figure J1, locate 5,030 lbs. at point n. On the same line A-B, locate 2,620 lbs. and project to point m on line A-C. Where line m-n intersects the radial line for 35°, project to line A-B and read the ASD adjusted design value, N' = 3,870 lbs.

Appendix K (Non-mandatory) Typical Dimensions for Split Ring and Shear Plate Connectors

SPLIT RINGS[1]	2-1/2"	4"
Split Ring		
Inside diameter at center when closed	2.500"	4.000"
Thickness of metal at center	0.163"	0.193"
Depth of metal (width of ring)	0.750"	1.000"
Groove		
Inside diameter	2.56"	4.08"
Width	0.18"	0.21"
Depth	0.375"	0.50"
Bolt hole diameter in timber members	9/16"	13/16"
Washers, standard		
Round, cast or malleable iron, diameter	2-1/8"	3"
Round, wrought iron (minimum)		
Diameter	1-3/8"	2"
Thickness	3/32"	5/32"
Square plate		
Length of side	2"	3"
Thickness	1/8"	3/16"
Projected area: portion of one split ring within member	1.10 in.[2]	2.24 in.[2]

1. Courtesy of Cleveland Steel Specialty Co.

SHEAR PLATES	2-5/8"	2-5/8"	4"	4"
Shear plate[1]	Pressed	Malleable	Malleable	Malleable
Material	steel	cast iron	cast iron	cast iron
Plate diameter	2.62"	2.62"	4.02"	4.02"
Bolt hole diameter	0.81"	0.81"	0.81"	0.93"
Plate thickness	0.172"	0.172"	0.20"	0.20"
Plate depth	0.42"	0.42"	0.62"	0.62"
Bolt hole diameter in timber members and metal side plates[2]	13/16"	13/16"	13/16"	15/16"
Washers, standard				
Round, cast or malleable iron, diameter	3"	3"	3"	3-1/2"
Round, wrought iron (minimum)				
Diameter	2"	2"	2"	2-1/4"
Thickness	5/32"	5/32"	5/32"	11/64"
Square plate				
Length of side	3"	3"	3"	3"
Thickness	1/4"	1/4"	1/4"	1/4"
Projected area: portion of one shear plate within member	1.18 in.[2]	1.00 in.[2]	2.58 in.[2]	2.58 in.[2]

1. ASTM D 5933.
2. Steel straps or shapes used as metal side plates shall be designed in accordance with accepted metal practices (see 10.2.3).

Appendix L (Non-mandatory) Typical Dimensions for Dowel-Type Fasteners[1]

Table L1 Standard Hex Bolts

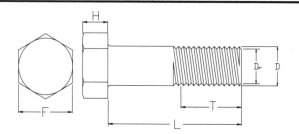

D = diameter
D_r = root diameter
T = thread length
L = bolt length
F = width of head across flats
H = height of head

		Diameter, D							
		1/4"	5/16"	3/8"	1/2"	5/8"	3/4"	7/8"	1"
D_r		0.189"	0.245"	0.298"	0.406"	0.514"	0.627"	0.739"	0.847"
F		7/16"	1/2"	9/16"	3/4"	15/16"	1-1/8"	1-5/16"	1-1/2"
H		11/64"	7/32"	1/4"	11/32"	27/64"	1/2"	37/64"	43/64"
T	L ≤ 6 in.	3/4"	7/8"	1"	1-1/4"	1-1/2"	1-3/4"	2"	2-1/4"
	L > 6 in.	1"	1-1/8"	1-1/4"	1-1/2"	1-3/4"	2"	2-1/4"	2-1/2"

1. Tolerances specified in ANSI B 18.2.1. Full body diameter bolt is shown. Root diameter based on UNC (coarse) thread series (see ANSI B1.1).

Table L2 Standard Hex Lag Screws[1]

D = diameter
D_r = root diameter
S = unthreaded shank length
T = minimum thread length[2]

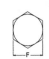
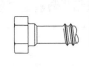
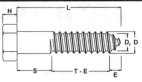

E = length of tapered tip
N = number of threads/inch
F = width of head across flats
H = height of head

Reduced Body Diameter — Full Body Diameter

HEX LAG SCREWS

Length, L		Diameter, D										
		1/4"	5/16"	3/8"	7/16"	1/2"	5/8"	3/4"	7/8"	1"	1-1/8"	1-1/4"
	D_r	0.173"	0.227"	0.265"	0.328"	0.371"	0.471"	0.579"	0.683"	0.780"	0.887"	1.012"
	E	5/32"	3/16"	7/32"	9/32"	5/16"	13/32"	1/2"	19/32"	11/16"	25/32"	7/8"
	H	11/64"	7/32"	1/4"	19/64"	11/32"	27/64"	1/2"	37/64"	43/64"	3/4"	27/32"
	F	7/16"	1/2"	9/16"	5/8"	3/4"	15/16"	1-1/8"	1-5/16"	1-1/2"	1-11/16"	1-7/8"
	N	10	9	7	7	6	5	4-1/2	4	3-1/2	3-1/4	3-1/4
1"	S	1/4"	1/4"	1/4"	1/4"	1/4"						
	T	3/4"	3/4"	3/4"	3/4"	3/4"						
	T-E	19/32"	9/16"	17/32"	15/32"	7/16"						
1-1/2"	S	1/4"	1/4"	1/4"	1/4"	1/4"						
	T	1-1/4"	1-1/4"	1-1/4"	1-1/4"	1-1/4"						
	T-E	1-3/32"	1-1/16"	1-1/32"	31/32"	15/16"						
2"	S	1/2"	1/2"	1/2"	1/2"	1/2"	1/2"					
	T	1-1/2"	1-1/2"	1-1/2"	1-1/2"	1-1/2"	1-1/2"					
	T-E	1-11/32"	1-5/16"	1-9/32"	1-7/32"	1-3/16"	1-3/32"					
2-1/2"	S	3/4"	3/4"	3/4"	3/4"	3/4"	3/4"					
	T	1-3/4"	1-3/4"	1-3/4"	1-3/4"	1-3/4"	1-3/4"					
	T-E	1-19/32"	1-9/16"	1-17/32"	1-15/32"	1-7/16"	1-11/32"					
3	S	1"	1"	1"	1"	1"	1"	1"	1"	1"		
	T	2"	2"	2"	2"	2"	2"	2"	2"	2"		
	T-E	1-27/32"	1-13/16"	1-25/32"	1-23/32"	1-11/16"	1-19/32"	1-1/2"	1-13/32"	1-5/16"		
4"	S	1-1/2"	1-1/2"	1-1/2"	1-1/2"	1-1/2"	1-1/2"	1-1/2"	1-1/2"	1-1/2"	1-1/2"	1-1/2"
	T	2-1/2"	2-1/2"	2-1/2"	2-1/2"	2-1/2"	2-1/2"	2-1/2"	2-1/2"	2-1/2"	2-1/2"	2-1/2"
	T-E	2-11/32"	2-5/16"	2-9/32"	2-7/32"	2-3/16"	2-3/32"	2"	1-29/32"	1-13/16"	1-23/32"	1-5/8"
5"	S	2"	2"	2"	2"	2"	2"	2"	2"	2"	2"	2"
	T	3"	3"	3"	3"	3"	3"	3"	3"	3"	3"	3"
	T-E	2-27/32"	2-13/16"	2-25/32"	2-23/32"	2-11/16"	2-19/32"	2-1/2"	2-13/32"	2-5/16"	2-7/32"	2-1/8"
6"	S	2-1/2"	2-1/2"	2-1/2"	2-1/2"	2-1/2"	2-1/2"	2-1/2"	2-1/2"	2-1/2"	2-1/2"	2-1/2"
	T	3-1/2"	3-1/2"	3-1/2"	3-1/2"	3-1/2"	3-1/2"	3-1/2"	3-1/2"	3-1/2"	3-1/2"	3-1/2"
	T-E	3-11/32"	3-5/16"	3-9/32"	3-7/32"	3-3/16"	3-3/32"	3"	2-29/32"	2-13/16"	2-23/32"	2-5/8"
7"	S	3"	3"	3"	3"	3"	3"	3"	3"	3"	3"	3"
	T	4"	4"	4"	4"	4"	4"	4"	4"	4"	4"	4"
	T-E	3-27/32"	3-13/16"	3-25/32"	3-23/32"	3-11/16"	3-19/32"	3-1/2"	3-13/32"	3-5/16"	3-7/32"	3-1/8"
8"	S	3-1/2"	3-1/2"	3-1/2"	3-1/2"	3-1/2"	3-1/2"	3-1/2"	3-1/2"	3-1/2"	3-1/2"	3-1/2"
	T	4-1/2"	4-1/2"	4-1/2"	4-1/2"	4-1/2"	4-1/2"	4-1/2"	4-1/2"	4-1/2"	4-1/2"	4-1/2"
	T-E	4-11/32"	4-5/16"	4-9/32"	4-7/32"	4-3/16"	4-3/32"	4"	3-29/32"	3-13/16"	3-23/32"	3-5/8"
9"	S	4"	4"	4"	4"	4"	4"	4"	4"	4"	4"	4"
	T	5"	5"	5"	5"	5"	5"	5"	5"	5"	5"	5"
	T-E	4-27/32"	4-13/16"	4-25/32"	4-23/32"	4-11/16"	4-19/32"	4-1/2"	4-13/32"	4-5/16"	4-7/32"	4-1/8"
10"	S	4-1/2"	4-1/2"	4-1/2"	4-1/2"	4-1/2"	4-1/2"	4-1/2"	4-1/2"	4-1/2"	4-1/2"	4-1/2"
	T	5-1/2"	5-1/2"	5-1/2"	5-1/2"	5-1/2"	5-1/2"	5-1/2"	5-1/2"	5-1/2"	5-1/2"	5-1/2"
	T-E	5-11/32"	5-5/16"	5-9/32"	5-7/32"	5-3/16"	5-3/32"	5"	4-29/32"	4-13/16"	4-23/32"	4-5/8"
11"	S	5"	5"	5"	5"	5"	5"	5"	5"	5"	5"	5"
	T	6"	6"	6"	6"	6"	6"	6"	6"	6"	6"	6"
	T-E	5-27/32"	5-13/16"	5-25/32"	5-23/32"	5-11/16"	5-19/32"	5-1/2"	5-13/32"	5-5/16"	5-7/32"	5-1/8"
12"	S	6"	6"	6"	6"	6"	6"	6"	6"	6"	6"	6"
	T	6"	6"	6"	6"	6"	6"	6"	6"	6"	6"	6"
	T-E	5-27/32"	5-13/16"	5-25/32"	5-23/32"	5-11/16"	5-19/32"	5-1/2"	5-13/32"	5-5/16"	5-7/32"	5-1/8"

1. Tolerances specified in ANSI B18.2.1. Full body diameter and reduced body diameter lag screws are shown. For reduced body diameter lag screws, the unthreaded shank diameter may be reduced to approximately the root diameter, D_r.
2. Minimum thread length (T) for lag screw lengths (L) is 6" or 1/2 the lag screw length plus 0.5", whichever is less. Thread lengths may exceed these minimums up to the full lag screw length (L).

Table L3   Standard Wood Screws[1]

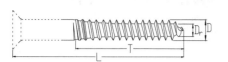

Cut Thread[2]

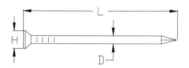

Rolled Thread[3]

D = diameter
D_r = root diameter
L = screw length
T = thread length

	Wood Screw Number										
	6	7	8	9	10	12	14	16	18	20	24
D	0.138"	0.151"	0.164"	0.177"	0.19"	0.216"	0.242"	0.268"	0.294"	0.32"	0.372"
D_r[4]	0.113"	0.122"	0.131"	0.142"	0.152"	0.171"	0.196"	0.209"	0.232"	0.255"	0.298"

1. Tolerances specified in ANSI B18.6.1
2. Thread length on cut thread wood screws is approximately 2/3 of the screw length.
3. Single lead thread shown. Thread length is at least four times the screw diameter or 2/3 of the screw length, whichever is greater. Screws which are too short to accommodate the minimum thread length, have threads extending as close to the underside of the head as practicable.
4. Taken as the average of the specified maximum and minimum limits for body diameter of rolled thread wood screws.

Table L4   Standard Common, Box, and Sinker Nails[1]

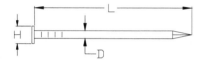

Common or Box

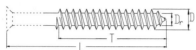

Sinker

D = diameter
L = length
H = head diameter

Type		Pennyweight										
		6d	7d	8d	10d	12d	16d	20d	30d	40d	50d	60d
Common	L	2"	2-1/4"	2-1/2"	3"	3-1/4"	3-1/2"	4"	4-1/2"	5"	5-1/2"	6"
	D	0.113"	0.113"	0.131"	0.148"	0.148"	0.162"	0.192"	0.207"	0.225"	0.244"	0.263"
	H	0.266"	0.266"	0.281"	0.312"	0.312"	0.344"	0.406"	0.438"	0.469"	0.5"	0.531"
Box	L	2"	2-1/4"	2-1/2"	3"	3-1/4"	3-1/2"	4"	4-1/2"	5"		
	D	0.099"	0.099"	0.113"	0.128"	0.128"	0.135"	0.148"	0.148"	0.162"		
	H	0.266"	0.266"	0.297"	0.312"	0.312"	0.344"	0.375"	0.375"	0.406"		
Sinker	L	1-7/8"	2-1/8"	2-3/8"	2-7/8"	3-1/8"	3-1/4"	3-3/4"	4-1/4"	4-3/4"		5-3/4"
	D	0.092"	0.099"	0.113"	0.12"	0.135"	0.148"	0.177"	0.192"	0.207"		0.244"
	H	0.234"	0.250"	0.266"	0.281"	0.312"	0.344"	0.375"	0.406"	0.438"		0.5"

1. Tolerances specified in ASTM F 1667. Typical shape of common, box, and sinker nails shown. See ASTM F 1667 for other nail types.

Appendix M (Non-mandatory) Manufacturing Tolerances for Rivets and Steel Side Plates for Timber Rivet Connections

Rivet dimensions are taken from ASTM F 1667.

Rivet Dimensions

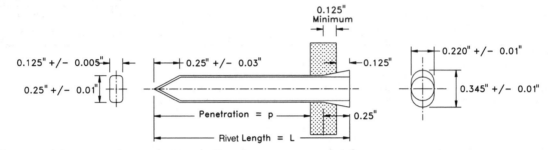

Steel Side Plate Dimensions

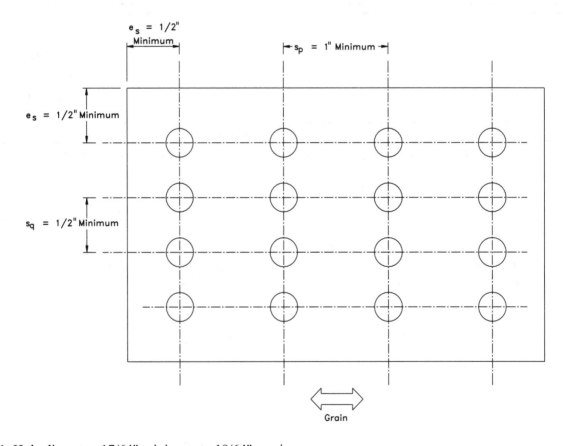

Notes:

1. Hole diameter: 17/64" minimum to 18/64" maximum.
2. Tolerences in location of holes: 1/8" maximum in any direction.
3. All dimensions are prior to galvanizing in inches.
4. s_p and s_q are defined in 13.3.
5. e_s is the end and edge distance as defined by the steel.
6. Orient wide face of rivets parallel to grain, regardless of plate orientation.

Appendix N (Mandatory) Load and Resistance Factor Design (LRFD)

N.1 General

N.1.1 Application

LRFD designs shall be made in accordance with Appendix N and all applicable provisions of this Specification. Applicable loads and load combinations, and adjustment of design values unique to LRFD are specified herein.

N.1.2 Loads and Load Combinations

Nominal loads and load combinations shall be those required by the applicable building code. In the absence of a governing building code, the nominal loads and associated load combinations shall be those specified in ASCE 7.

N.2 Design Values

N.2.1 Design Values

Adjusted LRFD design values for members and connections shall be determined in accordance with ASTM Specification D 5457 and design provisions in this Specification or in accordance with N.2.2 and N.2.3. Where LRFD design values are determined by the reliability normalization factor method in ASTM D 5457, the format conversion factor shall not apply (see N.3.1).

N.2.2 Member Design Values

Reference member design values in this Specification shall be adjusted in accordance with 4.3, 5.3, 6.3, 7.3, 8.3, and 9.3 for sawn lumber, structural glued laminated timber, poles and piles, prefabricated wood I-joists, structural composite lumber, and panel products, respectively, to determine the adjusted LRFD design value.

N.2.3 Connection Design Values

Reference connection design values in this Specification shall be adjusted in accordance with Table 10.3 to determine the adjusted LRFD design value.

N.3 Adjustment of Reference Design Values

N.3.1 Format Conversion Factor, K_F (LRFD Only)

Reference design values shall be multiplied by the format conversion factor, K_F, as specified in Table N1. Format conversion factors in Table N1 adjust reference ASD design values (based on normal duration) to the LRFD reference resistances (see Reference 55). Format conversion factors shall not apply where LRFD reference resistances are determined in accordance with the reliability normalization factor method in ASTM D 5457.

Table N1 Format Conversion Factor, K_F (LRFD Only)

Application	Property	K_F
Member	F_b, F_t, F_v, F_c, F_{rt}, F_s	$2.16/\phi$
	$F_{c\perp}$	$1.875/\phi$
	E_{min}	$1.5/\phi$
Connections	(all connections in the *NDS*)	$2.16/\phi$

N.3.2 Resistance Factor, ϕ (LRFD Only)

Reference design values shall be multiplied by the resistance factor, ϕ, as specified in Table N2 (see Reference 55).

Table N2 Resistance Factor, ϕ (LRFD Only)

Application	Property	Symbol	Value
Member	F_b	ϕ_b	0.85
	F_t	ϕ_t	0.80
	F_v, F_{rt}, F_s	ϕ_v	0.75
	F_c, $F_{c\perp}$	ϕ_c	0.90
	E_{min}	ϕ_s	0.85
Connections	(all)	ϕ_z	0.65

N.3.3 Time Effect Factor, λ (LRFD Only)

Reference design values shall be multiplied by the time effect factor, λ, as specified in Table N3.

Table N3 Time Effect Factor, λ (LRFD Only)

Load Combination[2]	λ
1.4(D+F)	0.6
1.2(D+F) + 1.6(H) + 0.5(L_r or S or R)	0.6
1.2(D+F) + 1.6(L+H) + 0.5(L_r or S or R)	0.7 when L is from storage 0.8 when L is from occupancy 1.25 when L is from impact[1]
1.2D + 1.6(L_r or S or R) + (L or 0.8W)	0.8
1.2D + 1.6W + L + 0.5(L_r or S or R)	1.0
1.2D + 1.0E + L + 0.2S	1.0
0.9D + 1.6W + 1.6H	1.0
0.9D + 1.0E + 1.6H	1.0

1. Time effect factors, λ, greater than 1.0 shall not apply to connections or to structural members pressure-treated with water-borne preservatives (see Reference 30) or fire retardant chemicals.
2. Load combinations and load factors consistent with ASCE 7-02 are listed for ease of reference. Nominal loads shall be in accordance with N.1.2.

REFERENCES

R

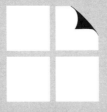

1. ACI 318-02 Building Code Requirements for Structural Concrete, American Concrete Institute, Farmington Hills, MI, 2002.

2. ACI 530-99/ASCE 5-99/TMS 402-99 Building Code Requirements for Masonry Structures, American Concrete Institute, Farmington Hills, MI, 1999.

3. AISI 1035 Standard Steels, American Iron and Steel Institute, Washington, DC, 1985.

4. ANSI/AITC Standard A190.1-2002, Structural Glued Laminated Timber, American Institute of Timber Construction, Vancouver, WA, 1992.

5. ANSI/ASCE Standard 7-02, Minimum Design Loads for Buildings and Other Structures, American Society of Civil Engineers, Reston, VA, 2003.

6. ANSI/ASME Standard B1.1-1989, Unified Inch Screw Threads UN and UNR Thread Form, American Society of Mechanical Engineers, New York, NY, 1989.

7. ANSI/ASME Standard B18.2.1-1996, Square and Hex Bolts and Screws (Inch Series), American Society of Mechanical Engineers, New York, NY, 1997.

8. ANSI/ASME Standard B18.6.1-1981 (Reaffirmed 1997), Wood Screws (Inch Series), American Society of Mechanical Engineers, New York, NY, 1982.

9. ANSI/TPI 1-2002 National Design Standard for Metal Plate Connected Wood Trusses, Truss Plate Institute, 2002.

10. ASTM Standard A 36-04, Specification for Standard Structural Steel, ASTM, West Conshohocken, PA, 2004.

11. ASTM Standard A 47-99, Specification for Ferritic Malleable Iron Castings, ASTM, West Conshohocken, PA, 1999.

12. ASTM A 153-03, Specification for Zinc Coating (Hot-Dip) on Iron and Steel Hardware, ASTM, West Conshohocken, PA, 2003.

13. ASTM A 370-03a, Standard Test Methods and Definitions for Mechanical Testing of Steel Products, ASTM, West Conshohocken, PA, 2003.

14. ASTM Standard A 653-03, Specification for Steel Sheet, Zinc-Coated (Galvanized) or Zinc-Iron Alloy-Coated (Galvannealed) by the Hot-Dip Process, 2003.

15. ASTM Standard D 25-91, Round Timber Piles, ASTM, West Conshohocken, PA, 1991.

16. ASTM Standard D 245-00$^{\varepsilon 1}$ (2002), Establishing Structural Grades and Related Allowable Properties for Visually Graded Lumber, ASTM, West Conshohocken, PA, 2002.

17. ASTM Standard D 1760-01, Pressure Treatment of Timber Products, ASTM, West Conshohocken, PA, 2001.

18. ASTM Standard D 1990-00$^{\varepsilon 1}$ (2002), Establishing Allowable Properties for Visually Graded Dimension Lumber from In-Grade Tests of Full-Size Specimens, ASTM, West Conshohocken, PA, 2002.

19. ASTM Standard D 2555-98$^{\varepsilon 1}$, Establishing Clear Wood Strength Values, ASTM, West Conshohocken, PA, 1998.

20. ASTM Standard D 2899-95, Establishing Design Stresses for Round Timber Piles, ASTM, West Conshohocken, PA, 1995.

21. ASTM Standard D 3200-74(2000), Establishing Recommended Design Stresses for Round Timber Construction Poles, ASTM, West Conshohocken, PA, 2000.

22. ASTM Standard D 3737-03, Establishing Stresses for Structural Glued Laminated Timber (Glulam), ASTM, West Conshohocken, PA, 2003.

23. ASTM Standard D 5055-04, Establishing and Monitoring Structural Capacities of Prefabricated Wood I-Joists, ASTM, West Conshohocken, PA, 2004.

24. ASTM Standard D 5456-03, Evaluation of Structural Composite Lumber Products, ASTM, West Conshohocken, PA, 2003.

25. ASTM Standard D 5764-97a (2002), Test Method for Evaluating Dowel Bearing Strength of Wood and Wood-Base Products, ASTM, West Conshohocken, PA, 2002.

26. ASTM Standard D 5933-96 (2001), Standard Specification for 2-5/8 in. and 4 in. Diameter Metal Shear Plates for Use in Wood Construction, ASTM, West Conshohocken, PA, 2001.

27. ASTM Standard F 606-02$^{\varepsilon1}$, Determining the Mechanical Properties of Externally and Internally Threaded Fasteners, Washers, and Rivets, ASTM, West Conshohocken, PA, 2002.

28. ASTM Standard F 1575-03, Standard Test Method for Determining Bending Yield Moment of Nails, ASTM, West Conshohocken, PA, 2003.

29. ASTM Standard F 1667-03, Standard for Driven Fasteners: Nails, Spikes, and Staples, ASTM, West Conshohocken, PA, 2003.

30. AWPA Book of Standards, American Wood Preservers' Association, Selma, AL, 2003.

31. American Softwood Lumber Standard, Voluntary Product Standard PS 20-99, National Institute of Standards and Technology, U.S. Department of Commerce, 1999.

32. Design/Construction Guide-Diaphragms and Shear Walls, Form L350, APA-The Engineered Wood Association, Tacoma, WA, 2001.

33. Engineered Wood Construction Guide, Form E30, APA-The Engineered Wood Association, Tacoma, WA, 2001.

34. Plywood Design Specification and Supplements, Form Y510, APA-The Engineered Wood Association, Tacoma, WA, 1997.

35. PS1-95, Construction and Industrial Plywood, United States Department of Commerce, National Institute of Standards and Technology, Gaithersburg, MD, 1995.

36. PS2-92, Performance Standard for Wood-Based Structural-Use Panels, United States Department of Commerce, National Institute of Standards and Technology, Gaithersburg, MD, 1992.

37. SAE J412, General Characteristics and Heat Treatment of Steels, Society of Automotive Engineers, Warrendale, PA, 1995.

38. SAE J429, Mechanical and Material Requirements for Externally Threaded Fasteners, Society of Automotive Engineers, Warrendale, PA, 1999.

39. Specification for Structural Joints Using ASTM A325 or A490 Bolts, American Institute of Steel Construction (AISC), Chicago, IL, 1985.

40. Specification for Structural Steel Buildings–Allowable Stress Design and Plastic Design, American Institute of Steel Construction (AISC), Chicago, IL, 1989.

41. Specification for the Design of Cold-Formed Steel Structural Members, American Iron and Steel Institute (AISI), Washington, DC, 1996.

42. Standard Grading Rules for Canadian Lumber, National Lumber Grades Authority (NLGA), New Westminster, BC, Canada, 2003.

43. Standard Grading Rules for Northeastern Lumber, Northeastern Lumber Manufacturers Association (NELMA), Cumberland Center, ME, 2003.

44. Standard Grading Rules for Northern and Eastern Lumber, Northern Softwood Lumber Bureau (NSLB), Cumberland Center, ME, 1993.

45. Standard Grading Rules for Southern Pine Lumber, Southern Pine Inspection Bureau (SPIB), Pensacola, FL, 2002.

46. Standard Grading Rules for West Coast Lumber, West Coast Lumber Inspection Bureau (WCLIB), Portland, OR, 2004.

47. Standard Specifications for Grades of California Redwood Lumber, Redwood Inspection Service (RIS), Novato, CA, 2000.

48. Standard Specifications for Highway Bridges, American Association of State Highway and Transportation Officials (AASHTO), Washington, DC, 1987.

49. Western Lumber Grading Rules, Western Wood Products Association (WWPA), Portland, OR, 2005.

50. Design Manual for TECO Timber Connectors Construction, TECO/Lumberlok, Colliers, WV, 1973.

51. Technical Report 12 General Dowel Equations for Calculating Lateral Connection Values, American Forest & Paper Association (AF&PA), Washington, DC, 1999.

52. Timber Construction Manual, American Institute of Timber Construction (AITC), John Wiley & Sons, 2004.

53. Wood Handbook: Wood as an Engineering Material, General Technical Report 113, Forest Products Laboratory, U.S. Department of Agriculture, 1999.

54. ASTM Standard D 2915-03, Standard Practice for Evaluating Allowable Properties for Grades of Structural Lumber, ASTM West Conshohocken, PA, 2003.

55. ASTM Standard D 5457-04, Standard Specification for Computing the Reference Resistance of Wood-Based Materials and Structural Connections for Load and Resistance Factor Design, ASTM, West Conshohocken, PA, 2004.

The *National Design Specification® for Wood Construction (NDS®)* was first issued in 1944 as the *National Design Specification for Stress-Grade Lumber and Its Fastenings*. In 1977 the title of the Specification was changed to its present form. The 2005 edition is the fourteenth edition of the publication.

The Commentary presented herein is intended to respond to user needs for background information and interpretive discussion of the provisions of the Specification. The Commentary follows the same subject matter organization as the Specification itself. Discussion of a particular provision in the Specification is identified in the Commentary by the same section or subsection number assigned to that provision in the Specification. The Commentary on each provision addressed consists of one or more of the following: background, interpretation and example. Information presented under background is intended to give the reader an understanding of the data and/or experience on which the provision is based. References containing more detailed information on the subject are included. Interpretive discussion of how a provision should be applied is given where users have suggested the intent of a requirement is ambiguous.

It is intended that this NDS Commentary be used in conjunction with competent engineering design, accurate fabrication, and adequate supervision of construction. AF&PA does not assume any responsibility for errors or omissions in the document, nor for engineering designs, plans, or construction prepared from it. Particular attention is directed to Section C2.1.2, relating to the designer's responsibility to make adjustments for particular end uses of structures.

Those using this document assume all liability arising from its use. The design of engineered structures is within the scope of expertise of licensed engineers, architects, or other licensed professionals for applications to a particular structure.

Inquiries, comments, and suggestions from the readers of this document are invited.

American Forest & Paper Association

C

COMMENTARY

C1 GENERAL REQUIREMENTS FOR STRUCTURAL DESIGN

C1.1 Scope

C1.1.1 Practice Defined

C1.1.1.1 This Specification defines a national standard of practice for the structural design of wood elements and their connections.

C1.1.1.2 Where the structural performance of assemblies utilizing panel products are dependent upon the capacity of the connections between the materials, such as in shear walls or diaphragms, the design provisions for mechanical connections in the Specification may be used for such assemblies when such application is based on accepted engineering practice or when experience has demonstrated such application provides for satisfactory performance in service.

C1.1.1.3 The data and engineering judgments on which the Specification are founded are based on principles of engineering mechanics and satisfactory performance in service. However, they are not intended to preclude the use of other products or design procedures where it can be demonstrated that these products or design procedures provide for satisfactory performance in the intended application. Other criteria for demonstrating satisfactory performance may be proprietary or specialized design standards applicable to a particular component type. The appropriateness and acceptability of alternate criteria are determined by the designer and the code authority having jurisdiction.

C1.1.2 Competent Supervision

There are several areas in which competent supervision should be required such as joint details and placement of fasteners. Special attention should be given to end details of columns and beam-columns to assure that design assumptions related to load eccentricity are met.

C1.2 General Requirements

C1.2.1 Conformance with Standards

The provisions of this Specification assume conformance with the standards specified.

C1.2.2 Framing and Bracing

Unless otherwise specified in the Specification, all reference design values assume that members are adequately framed, anchored, tied, and braced. Adequate bracing and anchorage of trusses and truss members to assure appropriate resistance to lateral loads is particularly important. Good practice recommendations (142) for installation between trusses of vertical sway (cross) bracing, continuous horizontal bottom chord struts and bottom chord cross bracing are given in NDS Appendix A.10.

In addition to providing adequate permanent bracing and bridging in the structure to resist wind and other racking forces, sufficient temporary bracing of load-carrying members should be used during construction to assure such members will withstand wind and temporary construction loads before adjacent members and cladding materials required by the design are installed.

C1.3 Standard as a Whole

The provisions of this Specification are intended to be used together. Unless otherwise noted, pertinent provisions from each chapter apply to every other chapter.

C1.4 Design Procedures

The Specification addresses both allowable stress design (ASD) and load and resistance factor design (LRFD) formats for design with wood structural members and their connections. In general, design of elements throughout a structure will utilize either the ASD or LRFD format; however, specific requirements to use a single design format for all elements within a structure are not included in this Specification. The suitability of mixing formats within a structure is the responsibility of the designer. Consideration should be given to building code limitations, where available. ASCE 7 – *Minimum Design Loads for Buildings and Other Structures* (3), referenced in building codes, limits mixing of design formats to cases where there are changes in materials.

C1.4.1 Loading Assumptions

The design provisions in the Specification assume adequacy of specified design loads.

C1.4.2 Governed by Codes

Design loads shall be based on the building code or other recognized minimum design loads such as ASCE 7 – *Minimum Design Loads for Buildings and Other Structures* (3).

C1.4.3 Loads Included

This section identifies types of loads to consider in design but is not intended to provide a comprehensive list of required loading considerations.

C1.4.4 Load Combinations

The reduced probability of the simultaneous occurrence of combinations of various loads on a structure, such as dead, live, wind, snow, and earthquake, is recognized for both ASD and LRFD in the model building codes and ASCE 7 (3). Specific load reductions for ASD or load combinations for LRFD apply when multiple transient loads act simultaneously.

For ASD, some codes provide for a reduction in design load for wind or earthquake even when both are not considered to act simultaneously. This particular load reduction is accounted for in such codes by allowing all materials a 1/3 increase in allowable stress for these loading conditions. Because individual jurisdictions and code regions may account for load combinations differently, the building code governing the structural design should be consulted to determine the proper method.

All modifications for load combinations are entirely separate from adjustments for load duration, C_D, or time effect, λ, which are directly applicable to wood design values (see C2.3.2 and C2.3.7). It should be emphasized that reduction of design loads to account for the probability of simultaneous occurrence of loads and the adjustment of wood resistances to account for the effect of the duration of the applied loads are independent of each other and both adjustments are applicable in the design calculation.

C1.5 Specifications and Plans

C1.5.1 Sizes

To assure that the building is constructed of members with the capacity and stiffness intended by the designer, the basis of the sizes of wood products given in the plans and specifications should be clearly referenced in these documents. The use of nominal dimensions in the distribution and sale of lumber and panel products has been a source of confusion to some designers, particularly those unfamiliar with wood structural design practices. The standard nominal sizes and the standard net sizes for sawn lumber are established for each product in national product standards (152). For proprietary or made-to-order products, special sizes should be specified.

C1.6 Notation

The system of notation used in the Specification helps to identify the meaning of certain frequently used symbols. Adjustment factors, identified by the symbol "C", modify reference design values for conditions of use, geometry, or stability. The subscripts "D", "F", "L", etc., are used to distinguish between different adjustment factors. In certain cases, upper and lower case subscripts of the same letter ("D" and "d") are used to denote two different adjustments (load duration factor and penetration depth factor for split ring and shear plate connections, respectively). There is no particular significance to the use of the same letter with different cases for different adjustment factors. The symbols "F" and "F$'$" denote reference and adjusted design values, respectively; where adjusted design values represent reference design values multiplied by all applicable adjustment factors. The symbol "f" indicates the actual or induced stress caused by the applied loads. The subscripts "b", "t", "c", "v", and "c$\perp$" indicate bending, tension parallel to grain, compression parallel to grain, shear, and compression perpendicular to grain stress, respectively.

C2 DESIGN VALUES FOR STRUCTURAL MEMBERS

C2.1 General

C2.1.1 General Requirement

The Specification addresses both ASD and LRFD formats for structural design with wood products (see 1.4).

C2.1.2 Responsibility of Designer to Adjust for Conditions of Use

The Specification identifies adjustments to reference design values for service conditions generally encountered in wood construction. However, this Specification does not address all possible design applications or conditions of use.

The designer has the final responsibility for determining the proper adjustment of design values for specific loading and exposure conditions. Particular attention is required to those uses where two or more extreme conditions of service converge. An example of such a use is one where it is known that the full design load will be applied continuously, that the structural members will be consistently exposed to water at elevated temperatures, and that the structural connections will be subjected to biaxial forces and moments. Assessment of the consequences of a failure of an individual member in the structure is an integral part of the designer's responsibility of relating design assumptions and design values.

C2.2 Reference Design Values

Reference design values used in this Specification and tabulated in the NDS Supplement are ASD values based on normal load duration and moisture conditions specified.

C2.3 Adjustment of Reference Design Values

C2.3.1 Applicability of Adjustment Factors

The Specification requires adjustment of reference design values for specific conditions of use, geometry and stability. Such modifications are made through application of adjustment factors. The adjustment factors are cumulative except where otherwise indicated. In addition to the adjustment factors given in this section, other adjustments of reference design values for special conditions of use may be required. Such additional adjustments may include modifications for creep effects, variability in modulus of elasticity, and fire retardant treatment.

C2.3.2 Load Duration Factor, C_D (ASD Only)

C2.3.2.1 Load duration factors, C_D, are applicable to all reference design values except modulus of elasticity

and compression perpendicular to grain. Exclusion of modulus of elasticity from load duration adjustment has been a provision of the Specification since the first edition. Load duration factors are based on the effect of time under load on ultimate load-carrying capacity. Increased deflection or deformation is a separate consideration, independent of ultimate strength. Compression perpendicular to grain design values were subject to adjustment for load duration when such values were based on proportional limit test values. For compression perpendicular to grain design values that are based on a deformation limit, the load duration factor does not apply.

Table 2.3.2 Frequently Used Load Duration Factors

Permanent Loads. In addition to construction dead loads due to materials, foundation soil loads and concentrated loads from equipment designed as part of the structure should be considered long-term loads that will

C

be applied continuously or cumulatively for more than 10 years. Special continuous loadings related to the particular purpose or use of the structure, such as water loads in cooling towers or heavy machinery in industrial buildings, also may be associated with durations exceeding 10 years.

Ten Year or Normal Loading. Loads traditionally characterized as normal are code specified floor loads, either uniform live or concentrated, which include furniture, furnishings, movable appliances and equipment, all types of storage loads, and all people loads. Although maximum human traffic loads may be infrequent and of short duration, such as those occurring on balconies, exterior walkways and stairways, this type of loading is considered normal loading.

Two Month Loads. A 2 month load duration adjustment factor of 1.15 was used for all code specified snow loads prior to 1986. Maximum snow loads published in ASCE 7 (3) based on probability of occurrence are significantly greater in some high snow regions than the loads previously used in those areas. Evaluation of annual snow load records available for some of these areas shows that the duration of the maximum snow load specified in ASCE 7 is much shorter than the 2 month duration previously assumed for all snow loads. The Specification provides for use of a larger snow load adjustment than 1.15 when information is available on the duration of the design snow load for a specific area.

Seven Day Loads. Where the minimum roof uniform load specified by the applicable building code exceeds the design snow load for the area and the specific building design, it is conventional practice to consider this load a construction type load for which a 7 day or 1.25 load duration factor is applicable. If the roof snow load is less than 92 percent of the minimum roof load specified, the latter will be the limiting of the two load conditions.

One Day Loads. Prior to 1987, a 1 day or 1.33 factor was used as the load duration adjustment for wind and earthquake loads. In the current Specification, the load duration factor for these loads has been based on a 10 minute load duration.

Ten Minute Loads. The 10 minute or 1.6 load duration factor is to be used with wind and earthquake loads in the current Specification. The wind loads in the model building codes and ASCE 7 are maximum loads expected to occur less than once in 50 years and to have durations of from 1 to 10 seconds. Peak earthquake loads are known to have cumulative durations less than 5 minutes rather than the 1 day duration traditionally assigned. The 10 minute load duration factor is conservatively estimated as the adjustment for the cumulative effect of these two load conditions.

Impact Loads. Loads in this category are considered to be those in which the load duration is 1 second or less. Such a duration is associated with an adjustment factor of 2.0 based on the general relationship between strength and load duration (see NDS Appendix B). Pressure treatment of wood with preservatives or fire retardant chemicals may reduce energy absorbing capacity as measured by work-to-maximum-load in bending; therefore, use of the 2.0 load duration factor in these applications is not permitted. Connections are also not permitted to use the 2.0 load duration factor (173).

C2.3.2.2 Design of structural members is based on the critical combination of loads representing different durations and resistances adjusted for these different durations. Note that load duration adjustments are not applicable to modulus of elasticity (see C2.3.2.1), hence, a member subject to buckling should be analyzed for the critical load combination after the critical buckling design value has been calculated.

C2.3.2.3 Reduction of design loads to account for the probability of simultaneous occurrence of loads and the adjustment of wood resistances to account for the effect of the duration of the applied loads are independent of each other and both adjustments are applicable in the design calculation (see C1.4.4).

C2.3.3 Temperature Factor, C_t

Temperature adjustments in the Specification apply when structural members are exposed to temperatures between 100°F and 150°F for extended periods of time, such as in industrial applications in which structural members are in close proximity to or in contact with heated fluids used in manufacturing processes. In general, adjustment of reference design values in the Specification for temperature should be considered for applications involving sustained heavy dead or equipment loads, or water immersion, or wet or high moisture content service conditions, when sustained or frequent extended exposure to elevated temperatures up to 150°F will occur.

Use of lumber or structural glued laminated timber members in applications involving prolonged exposure to temperatures over 150°F should be avoided. Where such exposures do occur, adjustments for both immediate and permanent strength reductions should be made. Permanent effects should be based on the cumulative time the members will be exposed to temperature levels over 150°F during the life of the structure and the strength losses associated with these levels (183). Roof systems and other assemblies subject to diurnal temperature fluctuations from solar radiation are not applications that normally require adjustment of reference design values for temperature.

Reversible Effects at or Below 150°F. The increase in the strength properties of wood when cooled below normal temperatures and the decrease in these properties when it is heated up to 150°F are immediate and generally reversible. When the temperature of the wood returns to normal temperature levels, it recovers its original properties. In general, these reversible effects are linear with temperature for a given moisture content (51). The magnitude of the increase or decrease, however, varies with moisture content. The higher the moisture content, the larger the increase in wood strength properties with decreasing temperature and the larger the decrease in wood strength properties with increasing temperature.

Permanent Effects Over 150°F. Prolonged exposure to temperatures over 150°F can cause a permanent loss in strength when cooled and tested at normal temperatures. The permanent effect is in addition to the immediate or reversible effect that occurs at the exposure temperature. Permanent losses in strength resulting from exposures over 212°F are greater for heating in steam than in water (183). For temperatures over 150°F, permanent decreases in strength are greater for heating in water than in dry air.

The use of 150°F as a nominal threshold for the beginning of permanent strength loss is substantiated by available test data showing an approximate 10 percent loss in bending strength (modulus of rupture) for material exposed for 300 days in water at 150°F and then tested at room temperature (183). Exposure in air at the same temperature would result in a smaller permanent strength loss.

Cold Temperatures. Adjustments for increasing reference design values for cooling below normal temperatures are difficult to establish in building design because of the variable nature of low temperature environments. Structural members that might be exposed to below freezing temperatures continuously for up to several months also are exposed to normal temperatures during periods of the year when the full design load might be resisted. For special applications such as arctic construction or transportation of cryogenic materials where the design load is always associated with low temperature environments, data from other sources may be used to make appropriate adjustments of design values (183, 51).

Elevated Temperatures Encountered in Normal Service. Temperatures higher than ambient can be reached in roof systems as a result of solar radiation. The temperatures reached in such systems are a function of many variables, including hour of day, season of year, cloud cover, wind speed, color of roofing, orientation, ventilation rate, presence of insulation, and thickness of sheathing. Measurements of roof system temperatures in actual buildings (64) show that structural framing members

in such roofs seldom if ever reach a temperature of 150°F, and when such levels are reached the duration is very short and is confined to the face of the member on which the sheathing is attached. Even in the severest of radiation and design conditions, the temperature of structural beams, rafters, and truss members in wood roofs generally do not reach 140°F. Normal temperature environments return as the sun sets.

The foregoing considerations and successful field experience are the basis for the long standing practice of applying the reference design values tabulated in the Specification without adjustment for temperature to structural wood roof members in systems designed to meet building code ventilation requirements. Reference design values also are appropriate for use with wood members directly exposed to solar radiation but otherwise surrounded by ambient air, such as members used in bridges, exterior balconies and stairways, and exterior vertical and horizontal structural framing.

C2.3.4 Fire Retardant Treatment

Fire retardant treatments are proprietary and chemical formulations vary between manufacturers. The fire retardant treatment manufacturers have established design values for wood products treated with their commercial formulations. It should be noted that use of individual company design value recommendations for fire retardant treated wood products is subject to approval of the authority having jurisdiction.

C2.3.5 Format Conversion Factor, K_F (LRFD Only)

Format conversion factors convert reference design values (allowable stress design values based on normal load duration) to LRFD reference resistances as described in ASTM D5457 (17). Specified format conversion factors, K_F, in NDS Table N1 are based on similar factors contained in ASTM D5457.

The LRFD reference resistance is a strength level design value for short-term loading conditions. Consequently, the format conversion factor includes: 1) a conversion factor to adjust an allowable design value to a higher strength level design value, 2) a conversion factor to adjust from a 10 year to a 10 minute (short-term) load basis, and 3) a conversion factor to adjust for a specified resistance factor, ϕ.

The term, LRFD reference resistance, is not specifically defined or calculated in the Specification but is included as part of the LRFD adjusted design value which includes all applicable adjustments to the reference design value. Because format conversion factors are based on calibrating ASD and LRFD formats for certain reference conditions, they apply only to reference design values in this Specification and should not apply where LRFD reference resistances are determined in accordance with the reliability normalization factor method in ASTM D5457.

C2.3.6 Resistance Factor, ϕ (LRFD Only)

Specified resistance factors, ϕ, in NDS Table N2 are based on resistance factors defined in ASTM D5457 (17). Resistance factors are assigned to various wood properties with only one factor assigned to each stress mode (i.e., bending, shear, compression, tension, and stability). In general, the magnitude of the resistance factor is considered to, in part, reflect relative variability of wood product properties. Actual differences in product variability are accounted for in the derivation of reference design values.

C2.3.7 Time Effect Factor, λ (LRFD Only)

The time effect factor, λ (LRFD counterpart to the ASD load duration factor, C_D, varies by load combination and is intended to establish a consistent target reliability

index for load scenarios represented by applicable load combinations. With the exception of the load combination for dead load only, each load combination can be viewed as addressing load scenarios involving peak values of one or more "primary" loads in combination with other transient loads. Specific time effect factors for various ASCE 7 (3) load combinations are largely dependant on the magnitude, duration, and variation of the primary load in each combination. For example, a time effect factor of 0.8 is associated with the load combination $1.2D + 1.6$ (L_r or S or R) + (L or 0.8W) to account for the duration and variation of the primary loads in that combination (roof live, snow, or rain water, or ice loads). The effect of transient loads in a particular load combination or even changes in the load factors within a given combination is considered to be small relative to the effect of the primary load on the load duration response of the wood. Consequently, specific time effect factors need not change to address load factor or load combination changes over time. Footnote 2 of NDS Table N3 provides clarification that the specific load factors shown are for reference only and are intended to provide flexibility in assignment of the time effect factor in the event of changes to specified load factors.

C3 DESIGN PROVISIONS AND EQUATIONS

C3.1 General

C3.1.1 Scope

This Chapter provides general design provisions for structural wood members and connections. Product-specific adjustments to these provisions are included in product Chapters 4 through 9 of the Specification. Specific connection design provisions are addressed in NDS Chapters 10 through 13.

C3.1.2 Net Section Area

C3.1.2.1 These provisions direct the designer to take into account the effects of removing material from the cross-sectional area. Specific provisions pertaining to notches in bending members are given in 3.2.3. Provisions for calculation of shear strength in notched bending members are given in 3.4.3. For compression parallel to grain, C3.6.3 provides for the use of gross section area when the reduced section of a column does not occur in the critical part of the length that is most subject to potential buckling.

C3.1.2.2 To avoid possible misapplication when non-uniform patterns are used, the provision requires staggered or offset fasteners in adjacent rows to be considered in the same critical section if the parallel to grain distance between them is less than four diameters.

C3.1.2.3 Where the parallel to grain distance between staggered split ring or shear plate connectors is less than or equal to one diameter, they should be considered to occur in the same critical section and used to determine net area. The limit should be applied to the parallel to grain offset or stagger of split rings or shear plates in adjacent rows.

C3.1.3 Connections

Particular attention should be given to the design of joints involving multiple fasteners and to those subject to moment forces. Only fastener types having the same general load-slip or stiffness characteristics should be employed in the same joint (see C10.1.4).

The provisions are intended to ensure each member in the joint carries its portion of the design load and that symmetrical members and fasteners are used unless the induced moments are taken into account. A lapped joint is an example of an unsymmetrical connection where the induced bending moments need to be considered.

C3.1.4 Time Dependent Deformations

Consideration of time dependent deformations in built-up members should provide for equal inelastic deformation of the components. One application addressed by this section is the use of a flange member to strengthen or stiffen a single main member in a truss without increasing the size of other members in the same plane (142). Because component connections in these built-up systems do not provide full composite action, judgment must be used to establish the level of contribution of these components and the time dependent effects on these connections. Member creep effects should also be considered in making this assessment.

C3.1.5 Composite Construction

Structural composites of lumber and other materials utilize the characteristics of each to obtain desirable structural efficiencies and/or extended service life. Timber-concrete bridge decks, timber-steel flitch beams, and plywood-lumber stress-skin panels and box beams are such composites. Proven design procedures for timber-concrete beams and timber-steel members are available in wood engineering handbooks and textbooks (58, 142). Detailed design and fabrication information for plywood-lumber structural components are available from APA – The Engineered Wood Association (106). The American Institute of Timber Construction provides design information for composites involving structural glued laminated timber (140).

C3.2 Bending Members - General

C3.2.1 Span of Bending Members

The design span length for simple, continuous, and cantilevered bending members is defined as the clear span plus 1/2 the required bearing length at each reaction to avoid unrealistic moment determinations where supports are wider than the required bearing.

C3.2.2 Lateral Distribution of Concentrated Load

Lateral distribution of concentrated loads to adjacent parallel bending members can be estimated using accepted engineering practice (See C15.1).

C3.2.3 Notches

C3.2.3.1 Notches are a special problem in bending members due to the stress concentrations occurring at the corners and the difficulty of calculating the effects of shear and perpendicular to grain stresses occurring at such locations. These stress concentrations can be reduced by using gradually tapered rather than square corner notches (181).

C3.2.3.2 The assumption that a notch having a depth of up to 1/6 the bending member depth and a length up to 1/3 the bending member depth has little practical effect on bending member stiffness (184, 181).

C3.3 Bending Members - Flexure

C3.3.3 Beam Stability Factor, C_L

The beam stability factor, C_L, adjusts the reference bending design value for the effects of lateral-torsional buckling. Lateral-torsional buckling is a limit state where beam deformation includes in-plane deformation, out-of-plane deformation and twisting. The load causing lateral instability is called the elastic lateral-torsional buckling load and is influenced by many factors such as loading and support conditions, member cross section, and unbraced length. In the 2005 and earlier versions of the NDS, the limit state of lateral-torsional buckling is addressed using an effective length format whereby unbraced lengths are adjusted to account for load and support conditions that influence the lateral-torsional buckling load. Another common format uses an equivalent moment factor to account for these conditions. AF&PA Technical Report 14 (138) describes the basis of the current effective length approach used in the NDS and summarizes the equivalent moment factor approach and provides a comparison between the two approaches.

It is common to assume buckling is not an issue in designing load-bearing beams used as headers over openings. However, long span header beams of slender cross sections demand particular attention to stability issues. An example would be dropped garage door headers in which the load is transferred into the beam through a cripple wall that does not provide lateral support to the beam. In this instance, raising the beam in the wall and attaching it directly to the top plate which is braced by a horizontal floor or ceiling diaphragm can be assumed to provide effective lateral support. Alternatively, the beam can be braced at points of bearing and designed as an unbraced member in accordance with NDS 3.3.3.

C3.3.3.1 For rectangular members, lateral-torsional buckling does not occur where the breadth of the bending member is equal to or greater than the depth and the load is applied in the plane of the member depth (184, 60). Note that lateral-torsional buckling does not occur in circular members.

C3.3.3.2 The rules for determining lateral support requirements based on depth to breadth ratios for sawn lumber bending members given in NDS 4.4.1 are alternate provisions to those of NDS 3.3.3. Specific span and loading conditions may be checked to compare the relative restrictiveness of the respective provisions.

C3.3.3.3 When the compression edge of a bending member is continuously supported along its length and bearing points are restrained against rotation and lateral displacement, lateral-torsional buckling under loads inducing compressive stresses in the supported edge are generally not a concern. However, the possibility of stress reversal, such as that associated with wind loading, should be considered to assure that the tension side of the bending member under the predominant loading case is adequately supported to carry any expected compressive forces. Also, bending members with large depth to breadth ratios should be braced on the tension edges.

C3.3.3.4 Where load is applied to the compression edge of a bending member using uniformly spaced purlins that are adequately attached to the compression edge, the unsupported length, ℓ_u, of the bending member is the distance between purlins (61). The bending member must also be braced at points of bearing.

C3.3.3.5 Formulas are provided for determining the effective span length, ℓ_e, from the unsupported length, ℓ_u, for different loading and support conditions (138). The ℓ_e values for small span-to-depth ratios, $\ell_u/d < 7$ are limited to address unrealistically large ℓ_e values that otherwise would be calculated for these short, deep bending members (60).

The constants in the formulas for effective length in NDS Table 3.3.3 include a 15 percent increase in ℓ_u to account for the possibility of imperfect torsional restraint at lateral supports. The formulas given in the table are applicable where loads are applied to the compression edge of the bending member, the most conservative loading case. Formulas given in the footnote for load conditions not covered by the formulas in the body of the table represent the most limiting formula for the ℓ_u/d range from those given

for specified load conditions. For more information on the derivation of these formulas, see TR14 (138).

C3.3.3.6 The beam slenderness ratio, R_B, is comparable to the slenderness ratio for solid columns, ℓ_e/d, in terms of its effect on bending member design strength.

C3.3.3.7 Limiting the beam slenderness ratio, R_B, to a maximum value of 50 is a good practice recommendation intended to preclude design of bending members with high buckling potential. This limit parallels the limit on slenderness ratio for columns, ℓ_e/d (60).

C3.3.3.8 The beam stability factor equation is applicable to all beam slenderness ratios, R_B. This equation provides a means of combining the bending design stress, F_b^*, with the critical buckling design stress, F_{bE}, to estimate an "effective" bending design value.

C3.3.3.10 See C3.9.2 on biaxial bending.

C3.4 Bending Members - Shear

C3.4.1 Strength in Shear Parallel to Grain (Horizontal Shear)

C3.4.1.1 Shear strength perpendicular to the grain, also referred to as cross-grain or vertical shear, refers to shear stresses in the radial-tangential plane tending to cut the wood fibers perpendicular to their long axis. The strength of wood in this plane is very high relative to shear strength parallel to grain, or horizontal shear, which refers to shear stresses in the longitudinal-radial or longitudinal-tangential plane tending to slide one fiber past another along their long axes. As both parallel and perpendicular to grain shear occur simultaneously, parallel to grain shear strength is always the limiting case. Therefore, reference shear design values, F_v, are horizontal or parallel to grain shear stresses.

Shear in the tangential-longitudinal or radial-longitudinal plane tending to roll one fiber over another perpendicular to their long axes is termed rolling shear. Rolling shear, which occurs in structural plywood applications as shear in the plane of the plies, is not a design consideration in most lumber or timber product applications.

C3.4.1.2 Shear design provisions in NDS 3.4 are limited to solid flexural members such as sawn lumber, structural glued laminated timber, structural composite lumber, and mechanically laminated timber. Built-up components, such as trusses, are specifically excluded because of field experience that indicated the procedures might not be adequate for shear design of top-hung parallel chord trusses and similar components that contained load-bearing web and top chord connections near points of support.

Shear design of built-up components is required to be based on testing, theoretical analysis, and/or documented experience due to the complexity of determining the effects of stress concentrations, the influence of embedded metal connectors, and questions regarding the applicability of the general practice of ignoring loads close to supports.

C3.4.2 Shear Design Equations

Actual shear stress parallel to grain, f_v, in a circular bending member may be determined as:

$$f_v = \frac{4V}{3A} \qquad (C3.4.2-1)$$

where:

V = shear force

A = cross-sectional area of circular member

C3.4.3 Shear Design

C3.4.3.1 (a) For purposes of calculating shear forces, ignoring uniform loads within a distance equal to the bending member depth, "d", of the support face assumes such loads are carried directly to the support by diagonal compression through the member depth. Concentrated loads within a distance "d" may be reduced proportionally to the distance from the face of the support. Where a member is loaded with a series of closely spaced framing members (such as a girder loaded by floor joists), a uniform load condition may be assumed even though the framing members can be viewed as individual point loads.

C3.4.3.1 (b) Placement of the critical moving load is assumed to be one beam depth from the support. Other loads within a distance, d, of the support are permitted to be ignored similar to the provisions of NDS 3.4.3.1(a).

C3.4.3.1 (c) Placement of two or more moving loads should be evaluated to determine the location that provides the maximum shear stress. Other loads within a distance, d, of the support are permitted to be ignored similar to the provisions of NDS 3.4.3.1(a).

C3.4.3.2 (a) The equation for determining the adjusted design shear of a tension-side notched member reduces the effective shear capacity by the square of the ratio of the remaining member depth, d_n, to the unnotched member depth, d. This relationship has been verified by tests of bending members at various depths (115) and is related to the concentration of tension and shear stresses occurring at the reentrant corner of the notch.

C3.4.3.2 (b) The equation for calculating the adjusted shear in members of circular cross section end-notched on the tension face parallels that for end-notched rectangular bending members. The area of the circular member, A_n, at the notch replaces the width, b, and depth at the notch, d_n, in the equation for the rectangular beam. It has been shown that maximum shear stresses near the neutral axis of an unnotched circular member calculated using $(VQ)/(Ib)$, or $(4V)/(3A)$, are within 5 percent of actual stresses (108).

Therefore, the adjusted design shear of a tension-side notched circular member is conservatively estimated using the factor 2/3 rather than 3/4 in the equation.

C3.4.3.2 (c) Procedures used to calculate the adjusted shear in bending members of other than rectangular or circular cross section containing end notches on the tension face should account for any effects of stress concentrations that may occur at reentrant corners.

C3.4.3.2 (d) Use of gradual tapered cuts rather than squared corner notches have been shown by test to greatly reduce stress concentrations at reentrant corners (see C3.2.3.1).

C3.4.3.2 (e) Shear strength of bending members is less affected by end notches on the compression face than on the tension face (181).

C3.4.3.3 (a) An equation for calculating the shear resistance at connections located less than five times the depth of the member from its end is similar to that for end-notched rectangular bending members where the ratio d_e/d is comparable to the factor d_n/d.

C3.4.3.3 (b) For connections that are at least five times the member depth from the end, net section is permitted to be used for calculating shear resistance.

C3.4.3.3 (c) Bending members supported by concealed or partially hidden hangers whose installation involves kerfing or notching of the member are designed for shear using the notched bending member provisions of 3.4.3.2.

C3.5 Bending Members - Deflection

C3.5.1 Deflection Calculations

Reference modulus of elasticity design values, E, in the Specification for wood bending members are average values. Individual pieces will have modulus of elasticity values higher or lower than the reference average value.

For solid rectangular and circular bending members, reference modulus of elasticity values are considered to contain a shear deflection component equivalent to that occurring in a rectangular bending member on a span-depth ratio of between 17 and 21 under uniformly distributed load. Assuming a modulus of elasticity to modulus of rigidity ratio (E/G) of 16, shear-free modulus of elasticity may be taken as 1.03 and 1.05 times the reference value for sawn lumber and structural glued laminated timber, respectively. Standard methods for adjusting modulus of elasticity to other load and span-depth conditions are available (4).

Experience has shown that use of average modulus of elasticity values provide an adequate measure of the immediate deflection of bending members used in normal wood structural applications. It should be noted that the reduced modulus of elasticity value, E_{min}, is used in beam stability analyses and contains both a statistical and a safety level reduction.

C3.5.2 Long-Term Loading

The reference modulus of elasticity values provide a measure of the immediate deflection of a member that occurs when a load is applied. If the load is sustained, the member will exhibit a slow but continual increase in deflection over time, otherwise known as creep. At moderate to low levels of sustained stress and under stable environmental conditions, the rate of creep will decrease over time (52, 62).

Where creep is decreasing over time, total creep occurring in a specific period of time is approximately proportional to the stress level (123, 185). Total bending creep increases with an increase in moisture content (34,

139) and temperature (112) and is greater under variable compared to constant relative humidity conditions (112). Creep deflection that is increasing at a constant rate should be considered a possible danger signal; and when creep deflection is increasing at an increasing rate, imminent failure is indicated (8, 139, 185).

Code specified maximum wind, snow, and live loads are pulse-type loadings with low frequency of occurrence. Thus creep deflection is not a significant factor in most situations. Where dead loads or sustained live loads represent a relatively high percentage of the total design load, creep may be a design consideration. In such situations, total deflection from long-term loading, Δ_T, is estimated by increasing the immediate deflection, Δ_{LT}, associated with the long-term load component by the time dependent deformation factor, K_{cr}, provided in the Specification.

C3.6 Compression Members – General

C3.6.2 Column Classifications

C3.6.2.1 Simple solid columns are defined as single piece members or those made of pieces glued together to form a single member. Such glued members are considered to have the grain of all component pieces oriented in the same direction and to be made with a phenolic, resorcinol, or other rigid adhesive. The performance of columns made using elastomeric adhesives are not covered by the provisions of the Specification except where it has been established that the adhesive being used possesses strength and creep properties comparable to those of standard rigid adhesives.

C3.6.2.2 Design provisions for spaced columns are covered in NDS 15.2.

C3.6.2.3 Mechanically laminated built-up columns are not designed as solid columns. Design provisions for these built-up columns are covered in NDS 15.3.

C3.6.3 Strength in Compression Parallel to Grain

In reduced section members, the actual compression stress parallel to grain, f_c, shall be checked as follows:

1. When the reduced section occurs in the critical buckling zone, the net section area shall be used to calculate $f_{c(net)}$, and $f_{c(net)} \leq F_c'$.
2. When the reduced section occurs outside the critical buckling zone, the gross section area shall be used to calculate $f_{c(gross)}$ and $f_{c(gross)} \leq F_c'$. In addition, the net section area shall be used to check for crushing, $f_{c(net)} \leq F_c^*$.

C3.6.4 Compression Members Bearing End to End

Compression design values parallel to grain, F_c^*, are applicable for bearing stresses occurring at the ends of compression members. See C3.10.1.

C3.6.5 Eccentric Loading or Combined Stresses

See C3.9 and C.15.4.

C3.6.6 Column Bracing

Column bracing should be designed using accepted engineering practice. Design of bracing systems is beyond the scope of the Specification; however, prescriptive recommendations are provided in NDS Appendix A.

C3.6.7 Lateral Support of Arches, Studs, and Compression Chords of Trusses

Where roof joists or purlins are used between arches or compression chords, the column stability factor, C_P, should be calculated using the larger of:

(i)   the slenderness ratio, ℓ_{e1}/d_1, based on distance between points of lateral support and the depth of the arch or chord (NDS Figure 3F).

(ii) the slenderness ratio, ℓ_{e2}/d_2, based on the distance between purlins or joists and the breadth of the arch or chord (NDS Figure 3F).

When continuous decking or sheathing is attached to the top of the arch or compression chord, it is common practice to assume that the slenderness ratio is the length between points of lateral support divided by the depth of the arch or chord, ℓ_{e1}/d_1.

Use of the depth of the stud as the least dimension in calculating the slenderness ratio in determining the axial load-carrying capacity of sheathed or clad light-frame wall systems is a long standing practice. Experience has shown that wood structural panels, fiberboard, hardboard, gypsum board, or other sheathing materials provide adequate lateral support of the stud across its thickness when properly fastened.

C3.7 Solid Columns

C3.7.1 Column Stability Factor, C_P

C3.7.1.2 In general, the effective length of a column is the distance between points of support that prevent lateral displacement of the member in the plane of buckling. It is common practice in wood construction to assume most column end conditions to be pin connected (translation fixed, rotation free) even though in many cases some partial rotational fixity is present. Where the end conditions in the plane of buckling are significantly different from the pinned assumption, recommended coefficients, K_e, for adjustment of column lengths are provided in NDS Appendix G.

As shown in Table G1 of NDS Appendix G, the recommended coefficients are larger than the theoretical values for all cases where rotational restraint of one or both ends of the column is assumed. This conservatism is introduced in recognition that full fixity is generally not realized in practice. The recommended values of K_e are the same as those used in steel design (125) except for the sixth case (rotation and translation fixed one end, rotation free and translation fixed other end) where a more conservative coefficient (20 percent larger than the theoretical value) is specified based on the ratio of theoretical/recommended value in the third case.

C3.7.1.4 The limitation on the slenderness ratio of solid columns to 50 precludes the use of column designs susceptible to potential buckling. The ℓ_e/d limit of 50 is comparable to the $K\ell/r$ limit of 200 (ℓ_e/d of 58) used in steel design (125).

Allowing a temporary ℓ_e/d ratio of 75 during construction is based on satisfactory experience with temporary bracing of trusses installed in accordance with truss industry standards (148); recognition that in most cases the assembly will carry only dead loads until load distributing and racking resisting sheathing elements are installed; and experience with a similar provision in steel design. In the latter regard, a $K\ell/r$ limit of 300 (ℓ_e/d of 87) is permitted during construction with cold-formed steel structural members (126). The critical buckling design load of a column with an ℓ_e/d ratio of 75 is approximately 45 percent that of a column with an equivalent cross section and an ℓ_e/d ratio of 50.

C3.7.1.5 The column stability factor equation is applicable to all column slenderness ratios (ℓ_e/d). This equation provides a means of combining the compression design stress, F_c^*, with the critical buckling design stress, F_{cE}, to estimate an "effective" compression design value (30, 68, 81, 97, 191).

The parameter "c" was empirically established from the stress-strain relationship of very short columns (ℓ_e/d of

2.5). The column stability factor equation provides a good approximation of column strength if the short column tests adequately characterize the properties and non-uniformities of the longer columns (101). By empirically fitting the column stability factor equation to column strength data, estimates of "c" closely predicted test results at all ℓ_e/d ratios (189, 191, 190). A significant advantage of the methodology is that by selecting column test material representative of the non-uniform properties across the cross section and along the length that are associated with permitted grade characteristics, such as knots, slope of grain, and warp, the combined effects of these variables on column behavior are included in the resultant value of "c" (190).

C3.7.1.6 Continuous exposure to elevated temperature and moisture in combination with continuous application of full design loads is an example of a severe service condition. Particularly when such design environments are coupled with design uncertainties, such as end fixity or stiffness of unsupported spliced connections, use of a reduced K_{cE} value should be considered. Included in such evaluations should be the possibility of eccentric application of the axial load and the need to design the member as a beam-column (see NDS 15.4).

C3.7.2 Tapered Columns

Analyses showed the general 1/3 rule (NDS Equation 3.7-3) was conservative for some end support conditions but unconservative for others (36). The use of a dimension taken at 1/3 the length from the smaller end underestimated the buckling load by 35 percent for a tapered column fixed at the large end and unsupported at the small end and by 16 percent for a tapered column simply supported (translation fixed) at both ends. Alternatively, the 1/3 rule was shown to overestimate the buckling load by 13 percent for a tapered column fixed at the small end and unsupported at the large end. These estimates were for a minimum to maximum diameter (dimension) ratio of 0.70. For these specific support conditions, NDS Equation 3.7-2 provides more realistic estimates of column strength. NDS Equation 3.7-3 remains applicable for other support conditions.

The one end fixed-one end unsupported or simply supported conditions referenced in NDS 3.7.2 correspond to the fifth and sixth buckling mode cases in NDS Appendix Table G1. The condition of both ends simply supported corresponds to the fourth case. Values for the constant "a" given under "Support Conditions" in NDS 3.7.2, are considered applicable when the ratio of minimum to maximum diameter equals or exceeds 1/3 (36).

The effective length factor, K_e, from NDS Appendix G is used in conjunction with the representative dimension (equivalent prism) when determining the stability factor, C_P, for tapered columns. It is to be noted that the actual compression stress parallel to grain, f_c, based on the minimum dimension of the column is not to exceed F_c^*.

C3.7.3 Round Columns

Round columns are designed as square columns of equivalent cross-sectional area and taper since the solid column provisions and equations in NDS 3.7.1 have been derived in terms of rectangular cross sections. A more generic form of the equations in NDS 3.7.1, applicable to nonrectangular cross sections, is given as:

$$C_p = \frac{1+\alpha}{2c} - \sqrt{\left[\frac{1+\alpha}{2c}\right]^2 - \frac{\alpha}{c}} \qquad (C3.7.3\text{-}1)$$

where:

$$\alpha = \frac{P_{cE}}{P_c^*}$$

$$P_c^* = F_c^* A$$

$$P_{cE} = \frac{\pi^2 E'_{min} I}{\ell_e^2}$$

All terms are as defined in the Specification.

C3.8 Tension Members

C3.8.2 Tension Perpendicular to Grain

Average strength values for tension perpendicular to grain that are available in reference documents (181, 183) apply to small, clear specimens that are free of shakes, checks, and other seasoning defects. Such information indicates that tension design values perpendicular to grain of clear, check- and shake-free wood may be considered to be about 1/3 the shear design value parallel to grain of comparable quality material of the same species (9). Because of undetectable ring shakes, checking and splitting can occur as a result of drying in service, therefore, very low strength values for the property can be encountered in commercial grades of lumber. For this reason, no sawn lumber tension design values perpendicular to grain have been published in the Specification. Cautionary provisions have been provided to alert the designer to avoid design configurations that induce tension perpendicular to grain stresses wherever possible. Connections where moderate to heavy loads are acting through the tension side of a bending member (see NDS Table 11.5.1A, footnote 2) should be avoided. These connections should be designed to ensure that perpendicular to grain loads are applied through the compression side of the bending member, either through direct connections or top-bearing connectors.

If perpendicular to grain tension stresses are not avoidable, use of stitch bolts or other mechanical reinforcement to resist these loads should be considered. When such a solution is used, care should be taken to ensure that the reinforcement itself does not cause splitting of the member as a result of drying in service (140). Ultimately, the designer is responsible for avoiding tension perpendicular to grain stresses or for assuring that mechanical reinforcing methods are adequate.

Radial stresses are induced in curved, pitch tapered, and certain other shapes of structural glued laminated timber beams. Radial tension design values perpendicular to grain are given in NDS 5.2.2 and have been shown to be adequate by both test (23, 24, 113) and experience.

C3.9 Combined Bending and Axial Loading

C3.9.1 Bending and Axial Tension

Theoretical analyses and experimental results show the linear interaction equation for combined bending and tension stresses yields conservative results (189). It can be shown that the effect of moment magnification, which is not included in the equation, serves to reduce the effective bending ratio rather than increase it.

Where eccentric axial tension loading is involved, the moment associated with the axial load, $(6Pe)/(bd^2)$, should be added to the actual bending stress when applying the interaction equation. The eccentricity, e, should carry the sign appropriate to the direction of eccentricity: positive when the moment associated with the axial load is increasing the moment due to the bending load and negative when it is reducing the moment.

Where biaxial bending occurs with axial tension, the equation should be expanded to:

$$\frac{f_t}{F_t^{'}} + \frac{f_{b1}}{F_{b1}^{*}} + \frac{f_{b2}}{F_{b2}^{*}} \leq 1.0 \qquad \text{(C3.9.2-1)}$$

where the subscripts indicate the principle axes.

Reference bending design values, F_b, are not adjusted for slenderness, C_L, in NDS Equation 3.9-1 because the tension load acts to reduce the buckling stress and the combined stress is not the critical buckling condition. Critical buckling is checked separately using NDS Equation 3.9-2.

C3.9.2 Bending and Axial Compression

The interaction equation given in NDS 3.9.2 (NDS Equation 3.9-3) addresses effects of beam buckling and bending about both principal axes, and closely matches beam-column test data for in-grade lumber as well as similar earlier data for clear wood material (189, 187).

The ratio of actual (induced) to adjusted compression stress in NDS Equation 3.9-3 is squared based on tests of short beam-columns made from various species of 2x4 and 2x6 lumber (68, 193, 189).

The moment magnification adjustment for edgewise bending in NDS Equation 3.9-3 is $(1 - f_c/F_{cE1})$. This adjustment is consistent with similar adjustments for other structural materials, and is based on theoretical analysis, confirmed by tests of intermediate and long wood beam-columns (189, 187).

The moment magnification adjustment for flatwise bending in NDS Equation 3.9-3 is $[1 - (f_c/F_{cE2}) - (f_{b1}/F_{bE})^2]$. The first term, $(1 - f_c/F_{cE1})$, is consistent with the adjustment for edgewise bending discussed previously. The second term, $(f_{b1}/F_{bE})^2$, represents the amplification of f_{b2} from f_{b1}. This second term is based on theoretical analysis (187) and has been verified using beam-column tests made on clear Sitka spruce (99, 187). The biaxial bending calculations in NDS Equation 3.9-3 conservatively model cantilever and multi-span beam-columns subject to biaxial loads (192).

C3.10 Design for Bearing

C3.10.1 Bearing Parallel to Grain

Where end grain bearing is a design consideration, the actual compression stress parallel to grain, f_c, shall not exceed the compression design value parallel to grain, F_c^{*}. For purposes of this section, the term "actual compressive bearing stress parallel to grain" and the term "compression stress parallel to grain," f_c, are synonymous.

Examples of end grain bearing configurations are end-to-end compression chord segments laterally supported by splice plates, butt end-bearing joints in individual laminations of mechanically laminated truss chords, roof-tied arch heel connections, notched chord truss heel joints, and columns supporting beams. Where the actual compression stress parallel to grain at the point of bearing is less than or equal to 75 percent of the compression design value parallel to grain ($f_c \leq 0.75\, F_c^{*}$), direct end-to-end bearing of wood surfaces is permitted provided that abutting end surfaces are parallel and appropriate lateral support is provided. The required use of a metal bearing plate or equivalently durable, rigid, homogeneous material in highly loaded end-to-end bearing joints ($f_c > 0.75\, F_c^{*}$) is to assure a uniform distribution of load from one member to another.

C3.10.2 Bearing Perpendicular to Grain

Ignoring any non-uniform distribution of bearing stress that may occur at the supports of a bending member as a result of the deflection or curvature of that member under load is long standing design practice.

C3.10.3 Bearing at an Angle to Grain

NDS Equation 3.10-1 for calculating the compressive stress at an angle to grain was developed from tests on Sitka spruce and verified for general applicability by tests on other species (184, 54, 59). The equation applies when the inclined or loaded surface is at right angles to the direction of load. The equation is limited to F_c' when the angle between direction of grain and direction of load, θ, is $0°$ and $F_{c\perp}'$ when this angle is $90°$. Stresses on both inclined surfaces in a notched member should be checked if the limiting case is not apparent.

C3.10.4 Bearing Area Factor, C_b

Provisions for increasing reference compression perpendicular design values for length of bearing are based on the results of test procedures in ASTM D143 (5) which involve loading a 2" wide steel plate bearing on a 2" wide by 2" deep by 6" long specimen. Research at the USDA Forest Products Laboratory on proportional limit stresses associated with bolt and washer loads showed that the smaller the width of the plate or bearing area relative to the length of the test specimen, the higher the proportional limit stress (146, 178). Early research conducted in Australia and Czechoslovakia confirmed the nature and magnitude of the bearing length effect (178).

The effect of length of bearing is attributed to the resisting bending and tension parallel to grain strengths in the fibers at the edges of the bearing plate (84, 178). Because of the localized nature of the edge effect, the contribution provided decreases as the length of the area under compressive load increases. When the bearing plate covers the entire surface of the supporting specimen (full bearing), test values will be lower than those obtained in the standard 2" plate test. For the case of complete surface or full bearing (bearing length equals supporting member length), such as may occur in a pressing operation, compression perpendicular to grain is approximately 75 percent of the reference compression perpendicular to grain design value. Deformation will also exceed that associated with the standard test.

Note that potential buckling perpendicular to grain is a design consideration that is not evaluated as part of the ASTM D143 (5) test procedures. One method of checking for buckling perpendicular to grain would be to use the provisions for column buckling parallel to grain in NDS 3.7.1 with mechanical properties from approved sources.

Bearing adjustment factors are useful in special cases such as highly loaded washers, metal supporting straps or hangers on wood beams, or highly loaded foundation studs bearing on wood plates and crossing wood members. See C4.2.6 for discussion of deformation occurring in this support condition relative to metal or end-grain bearing on side or face grain.

C4 SAWN LUMBER

C4.1 General

C4.1.1 Application

The design requirements given in Chapters 1 through 3 of the Specification are applicable to sawn lumber except where otherwise indicated. Chapter 4 of the Specification contains provisions which are particular to sawn lumber.

C4.1.2 Identification of Lumber

C4.1.2.1 The design provisions of the Specification applicable to sawn lumber are based on (i) use of lumber that displays the official grading mark of an agency that has been certified by the Board of Review of the American Lumber Standard Committee, established under the U.S. Department of Commerce's Voluntary Product Standard PS 20 (152); and (ii) use of design values tabulated in the Specification which have been taken from grading rules approved by the Board of Review (152). Those agencies publishing approved grading rules and design values are given in the Design Value Supplement to the Specification under "List of Sawn Lumber Grading Agencies." It is the responsibility of the designer to assure that the design values given in the Specification are applicable to the material so identified. If design values other than those tabulated in the Specification are used, it is the designer's responsibility to assure that the reliability and adequacy of the assignments are such that they may be used safely with the design provisions of the Specification.

The requirement that glued lumber products bear a distinct grademark indicating that the joint integrity is subject to qualification and quality control clarifies that the bond strength of the joint itself is to be monitored on a continuous basis under an inspection program.

C4.1.3 Definitions

C4.1.3.2 Categories and grades of "Dimension" lumber are standardized under the National Grading Rule for Softwood Dimension Lumber which was authorized by the American Softwood Lumber Standard PS 20 (152). The rule provides standard use categories, grade names, and grade descriptions. The National Grading Rule includes allowable knot sizes based on the strength ratio concept. Under this concept, the effect of a knot or other permitted strength reducing characteristic is expressed as the ratio of the assumed strength of the piece containing the char-

acteristic to the strength of clear, straight-grain wood of the same species (8).

Grades established under the National Grading Rule are:

Structural Light Framing 2" - 4" thick, 2" - 4" wide
> Select Structural
> No. 1
> No. 2
> No. 3

Light Framing 2" - 4" thick, 2"- 4" wide
> Construction
> Standard
> Utility

Studs 2" - 4" thick, 2" - 6" wide
> Stud

Structural Joists and Planks 2" - 4" thick, 5" and wider
> Select Structural
> No. 1
> No. 2
> No. 3

Design values for dimension lumber are based on in-grade tests of full-size pieces. Design values for Structural Light Framing and Structural Joists and Planks are consolidated under the common grade names (Select Structural, No. 1, No. 2, and No. 3) and separate width adjustments or values by width are provided (see NDS Supplement Tables 4A and 4B). There has been no change in the visual descriptions or maximum size of knots and other characteristics permitted in each width class of the grades established under the National Grading Rule.

C4.1.3.3 "Beams and Stringers" are uniformly defined in certified grading rules as lumber that is 5" (nominal) or more in thickness, with width more than 2" greater than thickness. Such members, for example 6x10, 6x12, 8x12, 8x16, and 10x14, are designed for use on edge as bending members. Grades for which design values are given in this Specification (NDS Supplement Table 4D) are:

Select Structural
> No. 1
> No. 2

C4.1.3.4 "Posts and Timbers" are defined as lumber that is 5" (nominal) or more in thickness and width not more than 2" greater than thickness. These members, such as 6x6, 6x8, 8x10, and 12x12, are designed to support axial column loads. Grades of lumber in this classification are the same as those for "Beams and Stringers." Posts and Timbers also may be used as beams; however, other grades and sections may be more efficient where strength in bending is a major consideration.

C4.1.4 Moisture Service Condition of Lumber

Design values tabulated in the Specification for sawn lumber apply to material surfaced in any condition and used in dry conditions of service. Such conditions are those in which the moisture content in use will not exceed a maximum of 19 percent. Adjustment factors, C_M, are provided in NDS Supplement Tables 4A through 4F for uses where this limit will be exceeded for a sustained period of time or for repeated periods.

Applications in which the structural members are regularly exposed directly to rain and other sources of moisture are typically considered wet conditions of service. Members that are protected from the weather by roofs or other means but are occasionally subjected to wind blown moisture are generally considered dry (moisture content 19 percent or less) applications. The designer has final responsibility for determining the appropriate moisture content basis for the design.

Design values tabulated for southern pine timbers and mixed southern pine timbers in NDS Supplement Table 4D have already been adjusted for use in wet service conditions. These values also apply when these species are used in dry service conditions.

C4.1.5 Lumber Sizes

C4.1.5.1 The minimum lumber sizes given in NDS Supplement Table 1A are minimum dressed sizes established in the American Softwood Lumber Standard, PS 20 (152).

C4.1.5.2 Dry net sizes are used in engineering computations for dimension lumber surfaced in any condition. When lumber is surfaced in the Green condition, it is oversized to allow for shrinkage (152).

C4.1.5.3 Beams and Stringers and Posts and Timbers are manufactured in the Green condition to standard Green dimensions (152). The reference design values for such lumber, which are applicable to dry conditions of service, include adjustments for the effects of shrinkage. Standard Green sizes, therefore, are to be used in engineering computations with these grades.

C4.1.6 End-Jointed or Edge-Glued Lumber

Design values tabulated in the Specification apply to end-jointed lumber of the same species and grade as unjointed sawn lumber when such material is identified by the grademark or inspection certificate of an approved agency (see C4.1.2.1). This identification indicates the glued product is subject to ongoing quality monitoring, including joint strength evaluation, by the agency.

End-jointed, face-glued, and edge-glued lumber may be used interchangeably with sawn lumber members of the same grade and species. The limitation on the use of finger-jointed lumber marked "STUD USE ONLY" or "VERTICAL USE ONLY" to those applications where any induced bending or tension stresses are of short duration is a provision to minimize possible joint creep associated with long-term loads. Bending and tension stresses associated with wind loads and seismic loads are examples of short duration stresses permitted in finger-jointed lumber marked for "STUD USE ONLY" or "VERTICAL USE ONLY."

C4.1.7 Resawn or Remanufactured Lumber

Material that has been regraded after resawing qualifies for design values tabulated in the Specification only when identified by the grademark or inspection certificate of an approved agency (see C4.1.2.1).

C4.2 Reference Design Values

C4.2.1 Reference Design Values

Design values tabulated in NDS Supplement Tables 4A through 4F have been taken from grading rules that have been certified by the Board of Review of the American Lumber Standard Committee as conforming to the provisions of the American Softwood Lumber Standard, PS 20 (152). Such grading rules may be obtained from the rules writing agencies listed in the NDS Supplement. Information on stress-rated board grades applicable to the various species is available from the respective grading rules agencies.

C4.2.2 Other Species and Grades

Where design values other than those tabulated in the Specification are to be used, it is the designer's responsibility to assure the technical adequacy of such assignments and the appropriateness of using them with the design provisions of the Specification (see C4.1.2.1).

C4.2.3 Basis for Reference Design Values

C4.2.3.2 Visually Graded Lumber
Dimension

In 1977, the softwood lumber industry in North America and the USDA Forest Products Laboratory began a testing program to evaluate the strength properties of in-grade full-size pieces of visually graded dimension lumber made from the most commercially important species in North America (65). The testing program, conducted over an 8-year period, involved the destructive testing of over 70,000 pieces of lumber from 33 species or species groups. The test method standard, ASTM D4761, covers the mechanical test methods used in the program (14). The standard practice, ASTM D1990, provides the procedures for establishing design values for visually graded dimension lumber from test results obtained from in-grade test programs (7).

Design values for bending, F_b, tension parallel to grain, F_t, compression parallel to grain, F_c, and modulus of elasticity, E, for 14 species or species combinations listed in Tables 4A and 4B of the NDS Supplement are based on in-grade test results. Further, the grade and size models developed under ASTM D1990 have been employed to establish grade and size relationships for those species whose index strengths are established by D245 methods. All design values for shear parallel to grain, F_v, and compression perpendicular to the grain, $F_{c\perp}$, in these tables are based on ASTM D245 provisions (8).

Timbers

Design values and adjustment factors for size, wet service, and shear stress given in NDS Supplement Table 4D for Beams and Stringers and Posts and Timbers are based on the provisions of ASTM D245 (8).

Decking

Design values for Decking in NDS Supplement Table 4E are based on ASTM D245 provisions except for the wet service factor, C_M, for F_b which is based on ASTM D1990. Reference bending design values, F_b, in Table 4E for all species and species combinations except Redwood are based on a 4" thickness. A 10-percent increase in these values applies when 2" decking is used (see C_F adjustment factor in the table).

C4.2.3.3 Machine Stress Rated (MSR) Lumber and Machine Evaluated Lumber (MEL)

Design values for F_b, F_t, F_c, and E given in NDS Supplement Table 4C for mechanically graded dimension lumber apply to material that meets the qualification and quality control requirements of the grading agency whose grademark appears on the piece. Stiffness-based stress-rating machines are set so that pieces passing through the machine will have the average E desired. For these machines, values of F_b are based on correlations established between minimum bending strength for lumber loaded on edge and E. Similarly, F_t and F_c values are based on test results for lumber in each F_b-E grade. Density-based grading machines operate under similar principles, using various density-based algorithms as the basis for grading decisions. For both machine types, machine settings are monitored and routinely verified through periodic stiffness and strength testing. Mechanically graded lumber also is required to meet certain visual grading requirements which include limitations on the size of edge knots and distorted grain on the wide face. Such limitations, expressed as a maximum proportion of the cross section occupied by the characteristics, generally range from 1/2 to 1/6 depending on the level of F_b.

Machine Stress Rated (MSR) lumber is material that is categorized in classes of regularly increasing strength (F_b, F_t, and F_c) and E assignments. As F_b values increase, F_t values increase at a greater rate, starting from 0.39 of the F_b value for the 900f grade to 0.80 of the F_b value for the 2400f and higher grades. Alternatively, F_c values increase at a lower rate than F_b values, starting from 1.17 of the F_b value for the 900f grade to 0.70 of the F_b value for the 3300f grade.

F_b, F_t, and E values for MSR lumber in NDS Supplement Table 4C are essentially the same as those published in the 1986 edition. Previously, F_c values were taken as 80 percent of the corresponding F_b value. As noted, these assignments now vary depending on level of F_b.

Design values for Machine Evaluated Lumber (MEL) are characterized by several different levels of E, F_t, or F_c for each level of F_b rather than assignment of qualifying material to specific stress classes, each of which has a generally unique assignment for each property. The MEL approach allows a greater percentage of total lumber production from a mill to be mechanically rated than is possible under the MSR classification system.

C4.2.4 Modulus of Elasticity, E

Design values for modulus of elasticity, E, are estimates of the average values for the species and grade of material. Reference modulus of elasticity for beam and column stability, E_{min}, is based on the following equation:

$$E_{min} = E[1 - 1.645COV_E](1.03)/1.66 \qquad (C4.2.4-1)$$

where:

$\qquad E$ = reference modulus of elasticity

$\qquad 1.03$ = adjustment factor to convert E values to a pure bending basis

$\qquad 1.66$ = factor of safety

$\qquad COV_E$ = coefficient of variation in modulus of elasticity (see NDS Appendix F)

E_{min} represents an approximate 5 percent lower exclusion value on pure bending modulus of elasticity, plus a 1.66 factor of safety. For more discussion, see NDS Appendix D.

C4.2.5 Bending, F_b

C4.2.5.1 When reference F_b values for dimension grades are applied to members with the load applied to the wide face, the flat use factor, C_{fu}, is to be used (see C4.3.7).

C4.2.5.4 Grade requirements for Beams and Stringers do not consider the effects of allowable knots and other permitted characteristics on the bending strength of the member under loads applied to the wide face. Therefore, reference bending design values, F_b, for Beams and Stringers in NDS Supplement Table 4D used to check loads applied on the wide face, should be adjusted by the applicable size factor in Table 4D. Posts and Timbers are graded for bending in both directions and can be used in biaxial bending design situations.

C4.2.6 Compression Perpendicular to Grain, F_c⊥

Reference compression design values perpendicular to grain in the 1977 and earlier editions of the Specification were based on proportional limit stresses and were adjusted for load duration. This practice changed when ASTM D245 provisions were revised to recognize compression perpendicular to grain as a serviceability limit state where the property is used as a measure of bearing deformation (8). Since 1982, lumber $F_{c\perp}$ values referenced in the Specification have been based on a uniform 0.04" deformation level for the condition of a steel plate on wood bearing condition. Such values are not adjusted for load duration.

The change in the basis of compression design values perpendicular to grain was an outgrowth of the introduction of ASTM D2555 in 1966. This standard gave new clear wood property information for western species and prescribed strict criteria for assignment of properties to combinations of species (see C4.2.3.2). Implementation of this information and the grouping criteria through ASTM D245 in 1971 resulted in a significant reduction in the $F_{c\perp}$ design value for a commercially important species group. The reduction caused bearing stress to become the limiting design property for the group in truss and other structural applications even though lumber of the group in these uses had performed satisfactorily at the previous higher bearing stress level for over 25 years.

Subsequent evaluation indicated that bearing perpendicular to the grain loads are not associated with structural failure and that deformation levels at proportional limit stresses could vary 100 percent between species in the standard ASTM D143 test. This test consists of loading a 2" wide steel plate bearing on the middle of a 2" by 2" by 6" long wood specimen (5). It was concluded that a uniform deformation limit was the preferred basis for establishing design loads concerned with bearing perpendicular to the grain. New methodology was developed to enable the stress at any deformation level to be estimated for any species based on its proportional limit stress (26, 27). This methodology was coupled with field experience to establish a deformation limit of 0.04" in the standard 2" specimen as an appropriate design stress base for applied loads of any duration. Stresses at 0.04" deformation for individual species were subsequently published in ASTM D2555 and provisions for basing compression design values perpendicular to grain on a deformation limit were introduced into ASTM D245.

In view of the outward load redistribution that occurs through the thickness of a member not subjected to a uniform bearing load along its length, and taking into account the effects of bearing deformation on the structure, establishment of a deformation limit state in terms of strain rate (deformation divided by member thickness) was not considered appropriate. On the basis of field experience, bearing stresses and deformations derived from the standard test of steel plate on 2" deep wood member are judged applicable to all lumber sizes. For the same stress, deformation of a joint consisting of two wood members both loaded perpendicular to grain will be approximately 2.5 times that of a metal to wood joint. The $F_{c\perp}$ values given in the 1982 edition of the Specification and continued in the present edition are about 60 percent greater than the proportional limit–normal load-based values published in earlier editions, but are applicable to wind, earthquake snow, and other load durations without adjustment.

The equation given in NDS 4.2.6 for adjusting reference $F_{c\perp}$ values to a 0.02" deformation limit is based on regression equations relating proportional limit mean stress to deformation at the 0.04 and the 0.02 levels (27). Use of this reduced compression design value perpendicular to grain may be appropriate where bearing deformations could affect load distribution or where total deflections of members must be closely controlled. Bearing deformation is not a significant factor in most lumber designs.

C4.3 Adjustment of Reference Design Values

C4.3.1 General

Applicable adjustment factors for sawn lumber are specified in NDS Table 4.3.1.

C4.3.2 Load Duration Factor, C_D (ASD Only)

See C2.3.2.

C4.3.3 Wet Service Factor, C_M

The wet service reduction value, C_M, for F_b, F_t, F_c, and E in NDS Supplement Tables 4A and 4B are based on provisions of ASTM D1990 (7). For F_v and $F_{c\perp}$, the values of C_M are based on ASTM D245. The wet service factors account for the increase in cross-section dimensions associated with this exposure.

C4.3.4 Temperature Factor, C_t

See C2.3.3.

C4.3.5 Beam Stability Factor, C_L

See C3.3.3.

C4.3.6 Size Factor, C_F

C4.3.6.1 Design values for F_b, F_t, and F_c in NDS Supplement Table 4A for all species and species combinations are adjusted for size using the size factors, C_F, referenced at the begining of the table. These factors and those used to develop the size specific values given in NDS Supplement Table 4B for certain species combinations are based on the adjustment equation for geometry given in ASTM D1990 (7). This equation, based on in-grade test data, accounts for differences in F_b, F_t, and F_c related to width and for differences in F_b and F_t related to length (test span). Reference values in Tables 4A and 4B for F_b and F_t are based on the following standardized lengths:

Width, in.	Length, ft
2 to 6	12
8 to 10	16
12 and wider	20

For constant length, the ASTM D1990 size equation provides for significantly greater reductions in bending design values, F_b, as width increases than comparable previous adjustments for this property. Width adjustments for tension design values parallel to grain, F_t, and compression design values parallel to grain, F_c, in the equation are applicable. Additionally, the modification of F_b and F_t for length is presented in the D1990 equation. Based on the total conservatism of these combined adjustments relative to past practice, use of design values in NDS Supplement Tables 4A and 4B for any member span length is considered appropriate.

C4.3.6.2 Bending design values for Beams and Stringers and Posts and Timbers in NDS Supplement Table 4D apply to a 12" depth. The NDS size factor equation for adjusting these values to deeper members is based on the formula given in ASTM D245.

C4.3.6.3 Beams of circular cross section (see C4.3.6.2).

C4.3.6.4 Values of F_b referenced for decking in NDS Supplement Table 4E are for members 4" thick. The increases of 10 percent and 4 percent allowed for 2" and 3" decking, respectively, are based on the NDS size equation in 4.3.6.2.

C4.3.7 Flat Use Factor, C_{fu}

Adjustment factors for flat use of bending members are based on the 1/9 power size equation discussed in C4.3.6.2 and C4.3.6.4. Relative to the test results that are available, the ASTM D245 equation gives conservative C_{fu} values. The flat use factor, C_{fu}, is to be used cumulatively with the size factor, C_F.

C4.3.8 Incising Factor, C_i

Incising involves making shallow, slit-like holes parallel to the grain in the surfaces of material to be preservative treated in order to obtain deeper and more uniform penetration of preservatives. It is used to improve the effectiveness of treatment of members having heartwood surfaces and of species which tend to be resistant to side penetration of preservative solution, such as Douglas fir, Engelmann spruce, and hemlock.

The effect of the incising process has been found to be dependent on depth and length of individual incisions and number of incisions (density) per square foot of surface area (105, 74, 174). The incising adjustment factors for E, F_b, F_t, F_v, and F_c given in NDS Table 4.3.8 are limited to patterns in which the incisions are not deeper than 0.4" and no more than 1100 per square foot in number. Where these limits are exceeded, it is the designer's responsibility to determine, by calculation or tests, the incising adjustment factors that should be used with the structural material being specified.

Adjustments given in NDS Table 4.3.8 are based on reductions observed for incised dimension lumber (e.g., 2" and 4" nominal thickness). A summary of early testing (105) of timbers and railway ties indicates that a slight decrease in strength properties for timbers may be expected. In some cases, no strength reductions were reported. Reductions provided in NDS Table 4.3.8 are not applicable to larger members such as solid sawn timbers.

C4.3.9 Repetitive Member Factor, C_r

The 15 percent repetitive member increase in reference bending design values, F_b, for lumber 2" to 4" thick is based on provisions in ASTM D245 (8) and D6555 (19). It is based on the increase in load-carrying capacity and stiffness obtained when multiple framing members are

fastened together or appropriately joined by transverse load distributing elements. Such an increase has been demonstrated by both analysis and test (28, 107, 149, 194). It reflects two interactions: load-sharing or redistribution of load among framing members and partial composite action of the framing member and the covering materials (149). Application of the C_r adjustment requires no assumption as to which of the two types of interaction is involved or predominates. A C_r value of 15 percent is generally considered to be conservative for sawn lumber assemblies (111, 177, 179).

The criteria for use of the repetitive member increase are three or more members in contact or spaced not more than 24" and joined by transverse load distributing elements such that the group of members performs as a unit rather than as separate pieces. The members may be any piece of dimension lumber loaded in bending, including studs, rafters, truss chords, and decking, as well as joists.

The repetitive member increase also applies to an assembly of three or more essentially parallel members of equal size and of the same orientation which are in direct contact with each other (28). In this case the transverse elements may be mechanical fasteners such as nails, nail gluing, tongue and groove joints, or bearing plates. The required condition is that the three or more members act together to resist the applied moment.

C4.3.10 Column Stability Factor, C_P

See C3.7.1.

C4.3.11 Buckling Stiffness Factor, C_T

See C4.4.2.

C4.3.12 Bearing Area Factor, C_b

See C3.10.4.

C4.3.13 Pressure-Preservative Treatment

The provision in the Specification for use of reference design values with lumber that has been preservative treated (170, 169, 168, 171, 172, 175) is applicable to material that has been treated and redried in accordance with AWPA Standards. In AWPA Standards, the maximum temperature for kiln-drying material after treatment is 165°F (22).

C4.3.14 Format Conversion Factor, K_F (LRFD Only)

See C2.3.5.

C4.3.15 Resistance Factor, ϕ (LRFD Only)

See C2.3.6.

C4.3.16 Time Effect Factor, λ (LRFD Only)

See C2.3.7.

C4.4 Special Design Considerations

C4.4.1 Stability of Bending Members

C4.4.1.1 Bending design values, F_b, given in NDS Supplement Tables 4A through 4F are based on a bending member having a compression edge supported throughout its length or having a depth to breadth ratio of 1 or less. When these conditions do not exist, F_b values are to be adjusted by the beam stability factor, C_L, calculated in accordance with the procedures of NDS 3.3.3. As an alternative method, bracing rules provided in NDS 4.4.1.2 are an acceptable method for providing restraint to prevent lateral displacement or rotation of lumber bending members (181).

C4.4.1.2 Sheathing, subflooring, or decking attached with two or more fasteners per piece provide acceptable edge restraint for a joist, rafter, or beam loaded through these load distributing elements. The requirement for bridging in the form of diagonal cross bracing or solid blocking in NDS 4.4.1.2(d) and the requirement for both edges to be supported in NDS 4.4.1.2(e) address: (i) redistribution of concentrated loads from long span members to adjacent members, and (ii) localized eccentricities due to cupping or twisting of deep members as a result of drying in service. Intermittent bridging specified in NDS 4.4.1.2(d) is not required in combination with tension and compression edge bracing specified in NDS 4.4.1.2(e).

The approximate rules of NDS 4.4.1.2(c) are equivalent to the beam stability provisions of NDS 3.3.3.3. For larger depth to breadth ratios the NDS 4.4.1.2 bracing rules are more restrictive than provisions of NDS 3.3.3.3. For smaller ratios the NDS 4.4.1.2 bracing rules are less restrictive, with the difference between effective bending stress based on the two methods increasing as F_b increases and E decreases.

C4.4.1.3 Tests of heavily stressed biaxial beam-columns showed that the bracing members could buckle as a result of the combination of loads applied directly on the bracing member and the loads induced by the beam-column as it buckles (147). Bracing members providing lateral support to a beam-column will typically have only one edge braced (such as a sheathed purlin bracing a rafter). The bracing member should have sufficient capacity to carry the additional compression load produced by the beam-column as it tends to buckle.

C4.4.2 Wood Trusses

C4.4.2.1 These provisions recognize the contribution of plywood sheathing to the buckling resistance of compression truss chords (in the plane of the chord depth). Quantification of the increase in chord buckling resistance from plywood sheathing was based on research (53, 55) involving stiffness tests of sheathed 2x4 members, nail slip tests, use of existing methodology for estimating the nail slip modulus of combinations of materials (155, 159), and application of a finite element analysis program for layered wood systems (149). It was found that the sheathing contribution increases with decrease in modulus of elasticity of the chord, with increase in span, and with increase in fastener slip modulus. Effects of plywood thickness and chord specific gravity were found to be of lesser significance.

The difference between the two K_M factors reflects the effect of drying on the nail load-slip modulus. The equations apply to chord lengths up to 96", 2x4 or smaller chords in trusses spaced 24" or less, and 3/8" or thicker plywood nailed to the narrow face of the chord using recommended schedules (38).

The analyses on which the equations are based assumed nails adjacent to joints between panel edges were located 1" from the panel edge, a chord specific gravity (ovendry volume basis) of 0.42, and an open joint without H-clips between sheathing panels. Clips were estimated to increase the C_T factor by 5 percent (53).

Because the buckling stiffness factor decreases with an increase in chord modulus of elasticity, the 1977 equations were based on the 5 percent exclusion value of E for the visually graded lumber species and grade having the highest reference design value. The 5 percent value was used because this is the basis for the E value used to establish the Euler column buckling load. It should be noted that the decrease in the relative contribution of sheathing that occurs as chord E increases above the 5 percent exclusion level is more than offset by the increase in the E of the chord itself.

C4.4.3 Notches

Prior to 1977, the Specification provided for the use of the net section at the notch for determining the bending strength of a notched bending member. This provision was based on early research which indicated that use of the net section at the notch was a sufficiently conservative design basis for commercial grades of sawn lumber (184, 181). It was recognized even at that time that stress concentrations at the corners of the notch caused lower proportional limit loads and caused failure to begin at lower loads than those expected from an unnotched bending member having a depth equal to the net depth of the notched bending member (184, 181).

In the 1977 edition, as a result of field experience and new research related to crack propagation, the use of the net section procedure for determining induced bending moment in notched bending members was discontinued and specific notch limitations were established for different bending member sizes. These new provisions were continued in the 1986 and 1991 editions. The field performance history considered included: (i) large bending members end-notched to the quarter points of the span which exhibited splitting and tension perpendicular to grain separations at relatively low loads; and (ii) the long record of satisfactory performance of light-frame construction joists notched using good practice recommendations. Fracture mechanics research also confirmed and quantified the propensity of cracks to develop at square-cornered notches at relatively low bending loads (92, 91, 132). Narrow slit notches (3/32"

long) were found to cause greater strength reductions than wide (greater than 2" long) notches of the same depth. The interaction of size and crack propagation has been characterized with crack initiation increasing in proportion to the square root of the bending member depth for a given relative notch depth and constant induced bending and shear stress (183).

C4.4.3.1 Tension perpendicular to grain stresses occur with shear stresses at end notches to make a bending member more susceptible to splitting at the corner of such notches. The limitation on end notches in sawn lumber bending members to 1/4 or less the bending member depth is a good practice recommendation that also reflects experience and the effects of shrinkage stresses.

C4.4.3.2 The allowance of notches on both the tension and compression sides of 2" and 3" thick sawn lumber bending members up to 1/6 the depth of the member in the outer thirds of a single span is consistent with good practice recommendations for light-frame construction (180). The satisfactory field performance of notched joists meeting these limitations, without use of the net section at the notch to determine actual stress, is attributed in part to the fact that reference bending design values, F_b, for the dimension grades of lumber already include section reductions for edge knots ranging from 1/6 to 1/2 the depth of the member. The restriction on interior notches in the tension side of nominal 4" and thicker sawn lumber bending members is based on experience with larger bending members and fracture mechanics analyses, as well as consideration of the shrinkage stresses that occur in such members when seasoning in service. Such stresses contribute to the perpendicular to grain stress conditions existing at the notch corners.

C4.4.3.3 The design provisions for shear in notched bending members given in NDS 3.4.3 include a magnification factor to account for tension perpendicular to grain stresses that occur with shear stresses making a bending member more susceptible to splitting at the corner of such notches.

COMMENTARY: SAWN LUMBER

C5 STRUCTURAL GLUED LAMINATED TIMBER

C5.1 General

Structural glued laminated timber, consisting of multiple layers of wood glued together with the grain of all layers approximately parallel, began its growth as a significant structural material in the United States in the 1930s. Technology developed in the formulation and use of casein glues to fabricate structural members in wood aircraft during and after World War I was extended to the construction of larger structural framing members used in buildings (181). The resistance of these glues to elevated relative humidities coupled with the use of pressing systems that could provide continuous pressure to all glue lines enabled the manufacture of large beams, arches, and other curved shapes with assured durability. The subsequent development of resorcinol and other synthetic resin glues with high moisture resistance expanded the uses of structural glued laminated timber to bridges, marine construction, and other applications involving direct exposure to the weather.

Glued laminated members are made of dry lumber laminations in which the location and frequency of knots and other strength reducing characteristics can be controlled. The result is a structural product in which splits, checks, and loosening of fasteners associated with drying in service are greatly reduced and relatively high strength is achieved.

The early development of design values for structural glued laminated timber paralleled that for visually graded lumber. In 1934, methods published in the USDA's Miscellaneous Publication 185 for the grading and determination of working stresses for structural timbers (167) were also applied to structural glued laminated timber. Under these procedures, strength values for small, clear, straight grain wood were reduced for load duration, variability, size, and factor of safety to basic stresses; and then these stresses were further reduced to account for the effects of knots, slope of grain, and other characteristics permitted in the grade of lumber being used as laminations. These design values were assigned by the manufacturers to the species and grades of structural glued laminated timber being produced.

The earliest comprehensive procedures for establishing design values that were specifically developed for structural glued laminated timber were published in 1939 in USDA Technical Bulletin 691 (166). These procedures

provided for the use of lower grades of lumber in the inner laminations than in the outer laminations. A simplified method of establishing design values from basic stresses also was given which was based on use of only two grades of lumber: one allowing knots up to 1/4 the width of the piece and one allowing up to 1/8 the width of the piece.

Design procedures for structural glued laminated timber were codified as national standards of practice in 1943 as part of the War Production Board's Directive No. 29 (153) and then in 1944 as part of the first edition of the *National Design Specification* (96). Design values established in the first edition were the same as those for the grade of sawn lumber used (based on the procedures in Miscellaneous Publication 185) except that increases for seasoning were permitted in compression parallel to grain and for all properties except shear parallel to grain when lumber 2" or less in thickness was used. In addition, increases were permitted for constructions in which knot limitations were twice as restrictive as those applicable to inner laminations. The procedures published in 1939 in Technical Bulletin 691 also were allowed as alternative methods.

The regional lumber rules writing agencies used the new Forest Products Laboratory procedures (49) to establish specifications for the design and fabrication of structural glued laminated lumber which provided design values for various species and lamination grade combinations. Design values established by these regional agencies were published in the Specification from 1951 through the 1968 editions.

A national consensus product standard covering minimum requirements for the production of structural glued laminated timber was promulgated as Commercial Standard CS253-63 by the U.S. Department of Commerce in 1963 (133).

In 1970, the American Institute of Timber Construction (AITC) assumed responsibility for developing laminating combinations and related design values for structural glued laminated timber. Beginning with the 1971 edition of the Specification, the design values established by AITC (130, 131) have been those published in the Specification.

In 1973, The CS253 standard was revised and re-promulgated by the U.S. Department of Commerce as Voluntary Product Standard PS 56-73 (134). In 1983, the standard was adopted as an American National Standard through American National Standards Institute's (ANSI) consensus process; it is now published as ANSI/AITC A190.1 (2). This product standard includes requirements for sizes, grade combinations, adhesives, inspection, testing, and certification of structural glued laminated timber products. Under A190.1, the grade combinations and related design values for structural glued laminated timber are required to be developed in accordance with ASTM D3737 or shall be obtained by performance testing and analysis in accordance with recognized standards. Procedures embodied in this ASTM standard, first published in 1978, reflect the previously used methodology (49) as modified by data from a succession of more recent full-scale test programs (2).

C5.1.1 Application

C5.1.1.1 The design requirements given in Chapters 1 through 3 of the Specification are applicable to structural glued laminated timber except where otherwise indicated. Chapter 5 of the Specification contains provisions which are particular to structural glued laminated timber.

The provisions of Chapter 5 contain only the basic requirements applicable to engineering design of structural glued laminated timber. Specific detailed requirements, such as those for curved and tapered members and connection details, are available from the American Institute of Timber Construction (140) and APA – The Engineered Wood Association.

C5.1.1.2 Where design values other than those given in NDS Supplement Tables 5A, 5B, 5C, and 5D, or as provided in the adjustments and footnotes of these tables are used, it shall be the designer's responsibility to assure that the values have been developed in accordance with all applicable provisions of ASTM D3737 and ANSI/AITC A190.1.

The design provisions in the Specification for structural glued laminated timber apply only to material certified by an approved agency as conforming to ANSI/AITC A190.1. The local building code body having jurisdiction over the structural design is the final authority as to the competency of the certifying agency and the acceptability of its grademarks.

C5.1.2 Definition

Laminations of structural glued laminated timber are usually made of sawn lumber. Laminated veneer lumber, consisting of graded veneers bonded together with grain parallel longitudinally, and manufactured lumber, lumber of two or more pieces glued together, may be used for tension laminations where high tensile strength is required (2).

Adhesives and glued joints in structural glued laminated timber members are required to meet the testing and related requirements of ANSI/AITC A190.1.

C5.1.3 Standard Sizes

C5.1.3.1 The finished widths of structural glued laminated timber members are typically less than the dimensions of surfaced lumber from which it is made in order to allow for removal of excess adhesive from the edges of the laminations and preparation of a smooth surface. This is done by removing from 3/8" to 1/2" of the width from the original lumber width by planing or sanding.

For applications where appearance is not important, structural glued laminated timbers having a finished width matching the dimensions of standard framing lumber widths are available in a Framing appearance grade. This appearance grade is not generally suitable for members which will be exposed to view (128).

Where necessary, widths other than standard sizes can be specified. These special widths require use of larger nominal lumber which may result in significant waste. For example, a 7" glued laminated beam would require the use of 2x10 (9.25") lumber laminations, while a 6-3/4" beam would require 2x8 (7.25") lumber laminations.

C5.1.3.2 The sizes of structural glued laminated timber are designated by the actual size after manufacture. Depths are usually produced in increments of the thickness of the lamination used. For straight or slightly curved members, this is a multiple of 1-1/2" for western species and 1-3/8" for southern pine. The faces of southern pine lumber generally are resurfaced prior to gluing, thereby reducing the thickness of this material an additional 1/8". For sharply curved members, nominal 1" rather than 2" thick lumber is used (140).

When members are tapered, the depth at the beginning and the end of the taper should be designated. In all cases, the length and net cross-section dimensions of all members should be specified.

C5.1.4 Specification

C5.1.4.1 It is the responsibility of the designer to specify the moisture content condition to which the members will be exposed during service (see C5.1.5). Grades of structural glued laminated timber are specified in terms of stress class, laminating combination, or the design values required.

C5.1.4.2 For glued laminated members made with hardwood species intended to be loaded primarily in bending about the x-x axis (load applied perpendicular to the wide face of the laminations), reference design values given in NDS Supplement Table 5C should be used. For glued laminated members made with hardwood species intended to be used to primarily resist axial loads (tension or compression), or bending loads about the y-y axis (loads applied parallel to the wide face of the laminations), reference design values given in NDS Supplement Table 5D should be used.

C5.1.5 Service Conditions

C5.1.5.1 When the equilibrium moisture content of members in service is less than 16 percent, the dry service design values tabulated in NDS Supplement Tables 5A, 5B, 5C, and 5D apply. A dry service condition for structural glued laminated timber prevails in most covered structures. However, members used in interior locations of high humidity, such as may occur in certain industrial operations or over unventilated swimming pools, may reach an equilibrium moisture content of 16 percent or

more. In such conditions, wet service factors should be applied to reference design values.

C5.1.5.2 Glued laminated members used in exterior exposures that are not protected from the weather by a roof, overhang, or eave and are subject to water exposure for a sustained period of time are generally considered wet conditions of use. Adjustment factors, C_M, are provided in NDS Supplement Tables 5A through 5D for uses where this limit will be exceeded. Bridges, towers, and loading docks represent typical wet service applications. Uses in which the member is in contact with the ground should be considered wet use for those portions of the member that will attain a moisture content of 16 percent or more. Where wet service conditions apply, the susceptibility of the member to decay and the need for preservative treatment (see C5.3.11) should also be considered.

C5.2 Reference Design Values

C5.2.1 Reference Design Values

Reference design values in NDS Supplement Tables 5A (and Table 5A Expanded) and 5B are for members made with softwood species. Reference design values in NDS Supplement Tables 5C and 5D are for members made with hardwood species. Because of the mixing of grades to provide maximum efficiency, values for a given property may vary with orientation of the loads on the member.

NDS Supplement Table 5A. Reference design values in this table are for softwood laminating combinations that have been optimized for members stressed in bending about the x-x axis (loads applied perpendicular to the wide face of the laminations). These values apply to members having four or more laminations. The stress class in the first column represents multiple laminating combinations, which have at least the indicated design properties. The stress class system was developed to simplify the design and specification of structural glued laminated timbers and to allow the manufacturer to supply laminate timbers which meet the stress class requirements, while making the most efficient use of available resources. Specification of a particular laminating combination from NDS Supplement Table 5A Expanded is also permissible.

NDS Supplement Table 5A Expanded. Reference design values in this table are for softwood laminating combinations that have been optimized for members stressed in bending about the x-x axis (loads applied perpendicular to the wide face of the laminations). These

values apply to members having four or more laminations and are divided into western species/visually graded, western species/E-rated, southern pine/visually graded and southern pine/E-rated. The combination symbol in the first column designates a specific combination and lay-up of grades of lumber. For example, 16F-V6 indicates a combination with a bending design value, F_{bx}, of 1600 psi (column 3 - tension zone stressed in tension) made with visually graded lumber (V). In the same format, 24F-E1 indicates an F_{bx} of 2400 psi (column 3 - tension zone stressed in tension) made with E-rated lumber. The second column of NDS Supplement Table 5A Expanded gives a two letter code indicating the species used for the outer laminations and for the core laminations of the member. For example, DF/HF indicates Douglas fir-Larch is used for the outer laminations and Hem-Fir is used for the core laminations.

NDS Supplement Table 5B. Reference design values in this table are for softwood laminating combinations that have been optimized for stresses due to axial loading or to bending about the y-y axis (loads applied parallel to the wide face of the laminations). Each combination consists of a single grade of one species of lumber. The grade associated with each numbered combination can be obtained from AITC 117 (131).

NDS Supplement Table 5C. Reference design values in this table are for hardwood laminating combinations that have been optimized for members stressed in bending about the x-x axis (loads applied perpendicular to the wide face of the laminations). These values apply to members having four or more laminations. The combination symbol in the first column designates a specific combination and lay-up of grades of lumber. For example, 16F-V1 indicates a combination with a bending design value, F_{bx}, of 1600 psi (column 2 - tension zone stressed in tension) made with visually graded lumber (V). In the same format, 24F-E2 indicates an F_{bx} of 2400 psi (column 2 - tension zone stressed in tension) made with E-rated lumber.

NDS Supplement Table 5D. Reference design values in this table are for hardwood laminating combinations that have been optimized for stresses due to axial loading or to bending about the y-y axis (loads applied parallel to the wide face of the laminations). Each combination consists of a single grade of one species of lumber. The grade associated with each numbered combination can be obtained from the AITC 119 (130).

C5.2.2 Radial Tension, F_{rt}

Radial tension stresses are induced in curved bending members when bending loads tend to flatten out the curve or increase the radius of curvature. In earlier editions, radial tension design values perpendicular to grain were established as 1/3 the corresponding shear design value parallel to grain for all species. This provision was based on strength data for small, clear specimens free of checks and other seasoning effects (9). It is important to note that the factor of 1/3 applies to the shear value for non-prismatic members as referenced in the footnotes to NDS Supplement Tables 5A, 5A-Expanded, and 5B. As a result of field experience, the radial tension design value perpendicular to grain for Douglas fir-Larch was limited to 15 psi except for conditions created by wind and earthquake loading. In 1991, this limit was expanded to all western species.

C5.2.3 Other Species and Grades

See C5.1.1.2.

C5.3 Adjustment of Reference Design Values

C5.3.1 General

Applicable adjustment factors for structural glued laminated timbers are specified in NDS Table 5.3.1.

C5.3.2 Load Duration Factor, C_D (ASD Only)

See C2.3.2.

C5.3.3 Wet Service Factor, C_M

The wet service reduction value, C_M, for F_b, F_t, F_v, $F_{c\perp}$, F_c, and E in NDS Supplement Tables 5A, 5B, 5C, and 5D are based on provisions of ASTM D3737 (13). The wet service factors account for both the decrease in mechanical properties and the increase in cross-section dimensions associated with this exposure.

C5.3.4 Temperature Factor, C_t

See C2.3.3.

C5.3.5 Beam Stability Factor, C_L

See C3.3.3.

C5.3.6 Volume Factor, C_V

The volume factor adjustment for structural glued laminated timber beams includes terms for the effects of width, length, and depth. The volume factor, C_V, equation (NDS Equation 5.3-1) is based on research involving tests of beams 5-1/8" and 8-3/4" wide, 6" to 48" deep, and 10 to 68 feet in length (90). This equation is based on the volume effect equation given in ASTM D3737 (13). The volume factor, C_V, applies when structural glued laminated timber bending members are loaded perpendicular to the wide face of the laminations.

As indicated in Footnote 1 of NDS Table 5.3.1, the volume factor, C_V, is not applied simultaneously with the beam stability factor, C_L. The smaller of the two adjustment factors applies. This provision is a continuation of the practice of considering beam stability and bending size modifications separately. The practice is based on design experience and the position that beam buckling is associated with stresses on the compression side of the beam, whereas bending design values and the effect of volume on such values are related primarily to the properties of the laminations stressed in tension.

C5.3.7 Flat Use Factor, C_fu

The flat use factor, C_{fu}, applies when structural glued laminated timber bending members are loaded parallel to the wide face of the laminations. The C_{fu} factors given in NDS Supplement Tables 5A, 5B, 5C, and 5D are applied only to the tabulated F_{byy} design values in these tables and cover only those members which are less than 12" in dimension parallel to the wide face of the laminations. For bending members loaded parallel to the wide face of the laminations with the dimension of the member in this direction greater than 12", a flat use factor based on NDS Equation 4.3-1 should be used.

C5.3.8 Curvature Factor, C_c

When the individual laminations of structural glued laminated timber members are bent to shape in curved forms, bending stresses are induced in each lamination that remain after gluing. In addition, the distribution of stresses about the neutral axis of curved members is not linear. The curvature factor, C_c, is an adjustment of reference bending design values, F_b, to account for the effects of these two conditions.

The curvature factor equation given in NDS 5.3.8 is based on early tests (166). The limits on the ratio of lamination thickness to radius of curvature of 1/100 for southern pine and hardwoods and 1/125 for other softwood species are imposed to avoid overstressing or possible breaking of the laminations.

Radii of curvature used in practice generally are larger than those allowed by the specified minimum thickness/radius of curvature ratios. For nominal 1" thick laminations (3/4" net), radii of curvature of 7 feet and 9.3 feet are typically used with southern pine and other softwood species, respectively. For nominal 2" laminations (1-1/2"

net), a radius of curvature of 27.5 feet is commonly used for all species.

C5.3.9 Column Stability Factor, C_P

See C3.7.1.

C5.3.10 Bearing Area Factor, C_b

See C3.10.4.

C5.3.11 Pressure–Preservative Treatment

The provision in the NDS for use of reference design values with structural glued laminated timber that has been preservative treated is applicable to material that has been treated and redried in accordance with AWPA Standards. In AWPA Standards, the maximum temperature for kiln-drying material after treatment is 165°F (22).

C5.3.12 Format Conversion Factor, K_F (LRFD Only)

See C2.3.5.

C5.3.13 Resistance Factor, φ (LRFD Only)

See C2.3.6.

C5.3.14 Time Effect Factor, λ (LRFD Only)

See C2.3.7.

C5.4 Special Design Considerations

C5.4.1 Radial Stress

C5.4.1.1 The equation for determining actual radial stress in a curved member of constant rectangular cross section is based on research published in 1939 (166). Radial stresses in curved members having variable cross section are determined by different procedures (46, 56). Complete design procedures for such members are available from other recognized sources (140).

C5.4.1.2 When the bending moment acts to reduce curvature, the actual radial stress is to be checked against

the adjusted radial tension design value perpendicular to grain, F_{rt}' (see C5.2.2). When mechanical reinforcing is provided which is sufficient to resist all induced radial stresses, the actual radial stress is still limited to no more than $(1/3) F_v'$.

C5.4.1.3 When the bending moment acts to increase curvature, the actual radial stress is to be checked against the adjusted compression design value perpendicular to grain. The appropriate compression perpendicular-to-grain design value for use is the value corresponding to the lamination grades used in the core of the beam, $F_{c\perp}$.

C5.4.2 Lateral Stability for Structural Glued Laminated Timber

C5.4.2.1 Reference bending design values, F_b, given in NDS Supplement Tables 5A, 5B, 5C, and 5D are based on members having a compression edge supported throughout its length or having a depth to breadth ratio of one or less. When these conditions do not exist, F_b values are to be adjusted by the beam stability factor, C_L, calculated in accordance with the procedures of NDS 3.3.3. As the tendency of the compression portion of the beam to buckle is a function of beam stiffness about the y-y axis (bending due to loading parallel to the wide face of the laminations), all glued laminated beam stability factor calculations are to be made with values of modulus of elasticity for bending about the y-y axis, E_{ymin}, modified by all applicable adjustment factors.

In determining the adequacy of lateral support, decking or subflooring applied directly to a beam with two or more fasteners per piece is acceptable edge restraint for a beam loaded through such decking or subflooring. Rafters, joists, or purlins attached 2 feet or less on center to the side of a beam and stabilized through the attachment of sheathing or subflooring are acceptable edge restraint for a beam that is loaded through such rafters, joists, or purlins. Recent research has shown that the bottom edges of rafters, joists, or purlins attached to the sides of beams by strap hangers or similar means do not have to be fixed to provide adequate lateral support to the beam if their top edges are restrained (164, 165).

C5.4.2.2 The depth to breadth limitations for laterally supported arches are good practice recommendations based on field experience over many years.

C5.4.3 Deflection

See C3.5.

C5.4.4 Notches

The designer has the responsibility of determining if structural glued laminated timber bending members should be notched and how load-carrying capacity should be calculated. Current good engineering practice is to avoid all notching of such bending members on the tension side except where end notching at the supports is necessary. This end notching is limited to the lesser of 1/10 of the bending member depth or 3" (140). The methods of NDS 3.4.3 are used to calculate shear force of end notches in structural glued laminated timber members (140).

COMMENTARY: STRUCTURAL GLUED LAMINATED TIMBER

C6 ROUND TIMBER POLES AND PILES

C6.1 General

Round timber piles have been widely used in the United States in the construction of railroads, highways, harbors, and dams, as well as for building foundations, since the middle of the 18th century. In addition to availability and cost, the natural taper of round timber piles makes them relatively easy to drive, compacts the soil around the pile during driving, and provides a larger diameter butt end capable of withstanding driving forces and supporting loads from other structural members (176).

The earliest standardization effort involving timber piles was the establishment of uniform size and grade characteristics in ASTM D25, Standard Specification for Round Timber Piles (10). First developed in 1915, the current edition of this standard includes specifications for minimum butt and tip sizes for various pile lengths, establishes limits on crook and knot sizes, and sets minimum rate of growth and percent summerwood quality requirements.

The establishment of standard physical characteristics for timber piles in ASTM D25 was subsequently followed by the development of standard requirements for preservative treatment. Such specifications were available from the American Wood-Preservers' Association (AWPA) since well before World War II (184). This Association's Standard C3, Piles-Preservative Treatment by Pressure Processes, establishes conditioning, pressure, temperature, retention, and penetration limitations and requirements for various preservative treatments by species and pile use (22). Because of the effect treatment processes can have on strength properties, standardization of the processes used are an important element in the specification and use of timber piles.

Engineering design with timber piles in the early years was largely based on experience, observation of the performance of piles under similar loading conditions, and the results of static loading tests. Piles were considered to fall into two groups: those in which the pile tip bears on a solid layer and were designed as columns and those in which the pile receives most of its support from soil friction on the sides and were designed from driving records or empirical formulas (184). Standard design procedures were not available.

To meet the growing need for uniform design recommendations, the American Association of State Highway Officials (AASHTO) began to specify allowable pile compression design values of 1200 psi for Douglas fir and slightly lower values for other species in the 1940s (176). However, maximum pile loads in the order of 36,000 to 50,000 pounds per pile also were specified which generally was the limiting criterion.

In the 1950s, AASHTO, the American Railway Engineering Association, and other user groups began to establish pile design values using the procedures of ASTM D245, Standard Methods for Establishing Structural Grades of Lumber (176) (see C4.2.3.2). Building codes also began to establish allowable pile stresses using basic stresses and other information given in ASTM D245 (161).

Uniform national standards for development of strength values for timber piles became available in 1970 with the publication of ASTM D2899, Standard Method for Establishing Design Stresses for Round Timber Piles (11). This consensus standard provides for the establishment of stresses for piles of any species meeting the size and quality requirements of ASTM D25. Under D2899, clear wood property information from ASTM D2555 (9) are adjusted for grade, relation of pile tip strength to clear wood strength, variability of pile strength to that of small clear specimens, load duration, and treatment conditioning effects. Compression design values parallel to grain established under D2899 are of the same general magnitude as those previously specified earlier by user and code groups.

A table of design values for round timber piles made of Douglas fir, southern pine, red pine, and red oak as recommended by the American Wood Preservers Institute was included in the 1971 edition of the Specification. A new timber piling section was introduced as Part X of the Specification in the 1973 edition which included a revised table of design values based on the methods of ASTM D2899. Covering the same species as were included in the 1971 edition, the 1973 design values were limited to piles conforming to the size and quality provisions of ASTM D25 and to the treating provisions of AWPA Standard C3.

In 1977, provisions for round timber piles in the specification were redesignated as Part VI and expanded to reference AWPA Standard C18 (Marine Use) and to include information on modification of design values for size and other factors, including adjustment of values for piles acting singly rather than in clusters. Reference design values were not changed from the 1973 edition.

Timber pile provisions of the 1977 edition, including reference design values, have been carried forward. In 1997, reference design values were added for construction poles based on ASTM D3200.

C6.1.1 Application

C6.1.1.2 The provisions of Chapter 6 of the Specification relate solely to the properties of round timber poles and piles. It is the responsibility of the designer to determine soil loads, such as frictional forces from subsiding soils and fills, the adequacy of the surrounding soil or water to provide sufficient lateral bracing, the method of pole or pile placement that will preclude damage to the wood member, the bearing capacity of the strata at the pile tip, and the effects of any other surrounding environmental factors on the supporting or loading of poles or piles.

C6.1.2 Specifications

C6.1.2.1 In addition to setting standard pile sizes, ASTM D25 (10) establishes minimum quality requirements, straightness criteria, and knot limitations. All pile tips are required to have an average rate of growth of six or more rings per inch and percent summerwood of 33 percent or more in the outer 50 percent of the radius; except less than six rings per inch growth rate is acceptable if the summerwood percentage is 50 percent or more in the outer 50 percent of the tip radius. Thus, 75 percent of the cross-sectional area of pile tips conforming to ASTM D25 essentially meet lumber requirements for dense material (8).

Knots in piles are limited by ASTM D25 to a diameter of not more than 1/6 of the circumference of the pile at the point where they occur. The sum of knot diameters in any 1 foot length of pile is limited to 1/3 or less of the circumference.

ASTM D3200 establishes standard sizes and minimum grades for construction poles based on ASTM D25 for piles.

C6.1.2.2 Preservative treatment requirements and limitations differ depending upon where the piles are to be used. Designation of the applicable treatment standard and use condition defines the treatment desired by the specifier.

C6.1.3 Standard Sizes

Standard sizes (10) for round timber piles range from 7" to 18" in diameter measured 3 feet from the butt. Pile lengths range from 20 to 85 feet for southern pine and to 120 feet for Douglas fir and other species. Pile taper is controlled by establishing a minimum tip circumference associated with a minimum circumference 3 feet from the butt for each length class; or by establishing a minimum circumference 3 feet from the butt associated with a minimum tip circumference for each length class. This provides a known tip area for use in engineering design as well as a conservative estimate of the area at any point along the length of the pile.

Standard sizes (12) for round timber construction poles range from 5" to 12" in diameter measured at the tip. Pole lengths range from 10 to 40 feet.

C6.1.4 Preservative Treatment

C6.1.4.1 Green timber piles are generally conditioned prior to pressure treatment (22). For southern pine the conditioning usually involves steaming under pressure to obtain a temperature of 245°F and then applying a vacuum. The process results in water being forced out of the outer part of the pile, but does not dry it to a seasoned condition (181, 63). Conditioning of Douglas fir is usually done by the Boulton or boiling-under-a-vacuum-process. This method of conditioning, which partially seasons the sapwood portion of the pile, involves heating the material in the preservative oil under a vacuum at temperatures up to 220°F (181, 63). The Boulton process also is used with hardwood species.

Both the steaming and Boulton conditioning processes affect pile strength properties (11, 176). These effects are accounted for in pile design values given in NDS Table 6A. In the 1991 edition, conditioning by kiln-drying is classified with the Boulton process for purposes of establishing design values (161, 176).

C6.1.4.2 Decay does not occur in softwood species and in most hardwoods that are completely saturated and an air supply is not available (63, 127). Permanently submerged piles meet these conditions.

C6.2 Reference Design Values

C6.2.1 Reference Design Values

C6.2.1.1 Reference design values for round timber piles given in NDS Table 6A are based on ASTM D2899 (11). All values are derived from the properties of small clear specimens of the applicable species as given in ASTM D2555 (9) adjusted as appropriate for the specific property for variability, load duration, grade, lower strength of pile tip, and lower variability of piles compared to small clear specimens (160). Pile bending design values include an adjustment relating the results of strength tests of full-size piles to the results of tests of small clear rectangular specimens selected from the same piles. Thus the effect of form is included in the reference design values.

Reference compression design values parallel to grain, F_c, include a 10 percent reduction for pile grade, a 10 percent reduction to adjust average small clear values for the whole tree to the tips of the piles, a conservative 10 percent reduction in standard deviation of small clear values to account for the reduced variability of tree size piles, a reduction for conditioning, and the standard adjustment of short-term test values for the property to a normal load duration. The combined factor applied to the nominal 5th percent exclusion value for small clear wood specimens of the species is 1/1.88 exclusive of the conditioning adjustment (160).

Similar adjustments are used for reference bending design values, F_b: 10 percent reduction for grade, 12 percent reduction to adjust average tree values to tip values, a conservative 12 percent reduction in standard deviation to account for the reduced variability of pile bending strength values, the conditioning adjustment, and the load duration adjustment for the property. The combined factor applied to the 5th percentile small clear strength value is 1/2.04 exclusive of the conditioning adjustment (160).

Reference shear design values parallel to the grain, F_v, are based on the 5th percentile clear wood strength value reduced for load duration and stress concentrations using the factor applied to lumber for these effects (8), a 25 percent reduction for possible splits and checks, and a conditioning adjustment. The combined factor on the clear wood 5th percentile value is 1/5.47 exclusive of the conditioning adjustment (160).

Reference compression design values perpendicular to grain, $F_{c\perp}$, in NDS Table 6A represent the average proportional limit stress for small clear specimens reduced 1/1.5 for ring orientation and an adjustment for conditioning. No adjustments are made to average clear wood modulus of elasticity values for application to piles.

Reference design values, except modulus of elasticity, for Pacific Coast Douglas fir, red oak, and red pine in NDS Table 6A contain a 10 percent reduction for conditioning treatment. This factor is based on the Boulton process adjustment in ASTM D2899. Comparable values for southern pine contain a 15 percent reduction for conditioning, the factor for steam conditioning in D2899.

The species designation Pacific Coast Douglas fir listed in NDS Table 6A refers to Douglas fir growing west of the summit of the Cascade Mountains in Washington, Oregon, and northern California and west of the summit of the Sierra Nevada Mountains in other areas of California (6). Values for red oak in NDS Table 6A apply only to the species northern red oak (*Quercus rubra*) and southern red oak (*Quercus falcata*).

C6.2.1.2 Design values for round timber poles given in NDS Table 6B are based on ASTM D3200 which uses provisions from ASTM D2899 (11) with similar adjustments used for round timber piles.

C6.2.2 Other Species or Grades

Where piles of species other than those listed in NDS Table 6A are used, it is the designer's responsibility to assure that the methods of ASTM D2899 for establishing design values are properly applied, including appropriate adjustments for conditioning process.

C6.3 Adjustment of Reference Design Values

C6.3.1 Applicability of Adjustment Factors

Applicable adjustment factors for round timber poles and piles are specified in NDS Table 6.3.1.

C6.3.2 Load Duration Factor, C_D (ASD Only)

See C2.3.2. As shown in NDS Table 6.3.1, the load duration factor, C_D, is applicable to compression design values perpendicular to grain, $F_{c\perp}$ for round timber piles and is not applicable to compression values perpendicular to grain, $F_{c\perp}$ for round timber poles. Pile design values for $F_{c\perp}$ in this Specification are based on proportional limit stresses and, in accordance with ASTM D245 (8), are subject to load duration adjustments.

Pressure impregnation of waterborne preservatives or fire retardant chemicals to retentions of 2.0 pcf or more may significantly reduce energy absorbing ability as measured by work-to-maximum-load in bending. For this reason, the impact load duration adjustment is not to be applied to members pressure treated with preservative oxides for salt water exposure or those pressure treated with fire retardant chemicals. These exclusions were introduced in the 1977 NDS for preservative oxides and the 1982 NDS for fire retardant chemicals.

C6.3.4 Temperature Factor, C_t

See C2.3.3.

C6.3.5 Untreated Factor, C_u

Increases to reference design values for poles and piles that are air-dried before treating or are used untreated (see C6.1.4.2) represent removal of the conditioning adjustments that are incorporated in the values for all properties except modulus of elasticity.

Reference design values in NDS Table 6A for Pacific Coast Douglas fir, red oak, and red pine contain a 10 percent reduction (1/1.11) for conditioning, assumed to be the Boulton or boiling-under-vacuum process. These values also are applied to piles that have been kiln-dried prior to treatment. Reference design values for southern pine piles contain a 15 percent reduction (1/1.18) for conditioning which is assumed to be by the steaming-and-vacuum process.

C6.3.6 Beam Stability Factor, C_L

A round member can be considered to have a d/b ratio of 1 and therefore, in accordance with NDS 3.3.3.1, C_L equals 1.0.

C6.3.7 Size Factor, C_F

Bending design values, F_b, for round timber poles and piles that are larger than 13.5" in diameter at the critical section in bending are adjusted for size using the same equation used to make size adjustments with sawn lumber Beams and Stringers and Posts and Timbers (see NDS 4.3.6.3 and C4.3.6.2). When applied to round timbers, NDS Equation 4.3-1 is entered with a d equal to the depth of a square beam having the same cross-sectional area as that of the round member. The equivalency of the load-carrying capacity of a circular member and a conventionally loaded square member of the cross-sectional area has long been recognized (98).

C6.3.8 Column Stability Factor, C_P

See C3.7.1. Column stability provisions from NDS 3.7.1 can be used for round timber poles and piles by substituting for the depth, d, in the equations, where r is the applicable radius of gyration of the column cross section.

C6.3.9 Critical Section Factor, C_{cs}

The critical section factor, C_{cs}, accounts for the effect of tree height on compression design values parallel to grain. The specific adjustment, applicable to Douglas fir and southern pine, provides for an increase in the design value as the critical section moves from the pile tip toward the pile butt. The factor is limited to 10 percent as this is the adjustment for tip end location used in the establishment of compression design values parallel to grain, F_c, for softwood species. As only limited data are available for red pine, the C_{cs} adjustment is not applied to this specie. The compression design value parallel to grain for red oak does not decrease with an increase in height in the tree and the 10 percent tip end adjustment factor is not used in the establishment of F_c values for this species group (11).

C6.3.10 Bearing Area Factor, C$_b$

See C3.10.4.

C6.3.11 Single Pile Factor, C$_{sp}$

Reference design values in NDS Table 6A are considered applicable to piles used in clusters. Where piles are used such that each pile is expected to carry its full portion of the design load, multiplication of reference compression design values parallel to grain, F_c, and bending design values, F_b, by a C_{sp} factor of 0.80 (1/1.25) and 0.77 (1.30), respectively.

Reference design values for round timber poles in NDS Table 6B have already been reduced to single pole values; therefore, this factor does not apply to these values.

C6.3.12 Format Conversion Factor K$_F$ (LRFD Only)

See C2.3.5.

C6.3.13 Resistance Factor, ϕ (LRFD Only)

See C2.3.6.

C6.3.14 Time Effect Factor, λ (LRFD Only)

See C2.3.7.

C7 PREFABRICATED WOOD I-JOISTS

C7.1 General

Prefabricated wood I-joists utilize the geometry of the cross section and high strength components to maximize the strength and stiffness of the wood fiber. Flanges are manufactured from solid sawn lumber or structural composite lumber, while webs typically consist of plywood or oriented strand board. Wood I-joists are generally produced as proprietary products. Acceptance reports and product literature should be consulted for current design information.

C7.1.1 Application

The general requirements given in Chapters 1, 2, and 3 of the Specification are applicable to prefabricated wood I-joists except where otherwise indicated. Chapter 7 of the Specification contains provisions which specifically apply to prefabricated wood I-joists manufactured and evaluated in accordance with ASTM D5055 (15). The provisions of NDS Chapter 7 contain only the basic requirements applicable to engineering design of prefabricated wood I-joists. Specific detailed requirements, such as those for bearing, web stiffeners, web holes, and notches, are available in the prefabricated wood I-joist manufacturer's literature and code evaluation reports.

C7.1.2 Definition

Prefabricated wood I-joists are specialized products, manufactured with specially designed equipment. Expertise in adhesives, wood products, manufacturing, and quality assurance are necessary ingredients for the fabrication of high-quality prefabricated wood I-joists.

Standard Sizes

Prefabricated wood I-joists are available in a range of sizes to handle a variety of applications. Common I-joist depths for residential flooring applications are 9.5", 11.875", 14", and 16". These sizes do not match standard sawn lumber depths to minimize the combined use of sawn lumber with wood I-joists in the same floor system. Mixing I-joists and sawn lumber in the same system is not recommended because differences in dimensional change between sawn lumber and wood I-joists can affect load distribution as the products reach equilibrium moisture content.

C7.1.3 Identification

Prefabricated wood I-joists are typically identified by product series and company name, plant location or number, qualified agency name or logo, code evaluation report numbers, and a means for establishing the date of manufacture.

C7.1.4 Service Conditions

Prefabricated wood I-joists are typically used in dry service conditions (less than 16 percent). For other conditions, the I-joist manufacturer should be consulted.

C7.2 Reference Design Values

Prefabricated wood I-joists are proprietary products and reference design values vary among manufacturers and product lines. Reference design values are obtained from the manufacturer through the manufacturer's literature or code evaluation report.

C7.3 Adjustment of Reference Design Values

C7.3.1 General

Applicable adjustment factors for prefabricated wood I-joists are specified in NDS Table 7.3.1. Volume effects are accounted for either directly in testing or indirectly in analysis as detailed in ASTM D5055 (15) and need not be considered in design.

C7.3.2 Load Duration Factor, C_D (ASD Only)

See C2.3.2. Duration of load effects in NDS 2.3.2 apply to all prefabricated wood I-joist design values except for those relating to stiffness, EI, EI_{min}, and K.

C7.3.3 Wet Service Factor, C_M

Prefabricated wood I-joists are limited to use in dry service conditions unless specifically allowed by the manufacturer (see NDS 7.1.4). I-joists are assembled with exterior adhesives and can tolerate the environmental conditions of typical jobsites. Care should be taken, however, to follow the manufacturer's recommendations for proper jobsite storage to minimize dimensional changes associated with changes in moisture content.

C7.3.4 Temperature Factor, C_t

See C2.3.3. Prefabricated wood I-joist reference design values are adjusted by the same temperature adjustment factors as other wood products (see Table C7.3-1).

C7.3.5 Beam Stability Factor, C_L

Bending design values provided in manufacturers' code evaluation reports are based on the I-joist having the compression edge supported throughout its entire length. This should be ensured by direct attachment of sheathing to the I-joist.

C7.3.6 Repetitive Member Factor, C_r

The repetitive member factor varies with composite action across a range of I-joist depths and series, I-joist stiffness variability, sheathing types, sheathing stiffnesses, and sheathing attachment. For several technical reasons, the magnitude of the repetitive member factor is typically much smaller than for sawn lumber. To provide a factor that could be applied across all applications, this factor was set at 1.0 in ASTM D5055 (15) and D6555 (19).

C7.3.7 Pressure-Preservative Treatment

Common treatments associated with I-joists include light solvent based preservatives offering protection against wood destroying fungi or insects. Any treatment of I-joists that require high pressure or harsh drying cycles should be avoided. Manufacturers should be consulted for any applications that require preservative treatment.

C7.3.8 Format Conversion Factor, K_F (LRFD Only)

See C2.3.5.

C7.3.9 Resistance Factor, ϕ (LRFD Only)

See C2.3.6.

C7.3.10 Time Effect Factor, λ (LRFD Only)

See C2.3.7.

Table C7.3-1 Temperature Factor, C_t, for Prefabricated Wood I-Joists

Reference Design Values	In-Service Moisture Conditions[1]	C_t		
		T≤100°F	100°F<T≤125°F	125°F<T≤150°F
EI, EI$_{min}$	Wet or Dry	1.0	0.9	0.9
M$_r$, V$_r$, R$_r$, and K	Dry	1.0	0.8	0.7
	Wet	1.0	0.7	0.5

1. Wet and dry service conditions for wood I-joists are specified in NDS 7.1.4.

7.4 Special Design Considerations

C7.4.1 Bearing

The end conditions of an I-joist require specific attention by the designer when considering the differences of designing with an "I" shape versus rectangular sections. The limit states at the bearing of an I-joist include the I-joist reaction (integrity of the web/flange rout), flange compression, compression of the support, reaction hardware (hangers), and shear.

The manufacturer's literature or code evaluation reports should be consulted for design assumptions at end conditions. Reaction capacity, R_r, and shear capacity, V_r, are typically published separately and should be checked independently. Published reaction capacity is based on testing conducted at one or more bearing lengths. Extrapolation beyond tested conditions is not appropriate. For end bearing, the minimum bearing length is typically 1-3/4", but never less than 1-1/2". The reaction capacity may or may not include the compression of the flange or bearing plate. The published capacities of joist hangers only include the capacity of the hanger. A complete design would include checking the I-joist capacity for the bearing length of the particular joist hanger.

C7.4.2 Load Application

The manufacturer's literature or code evaluation reports should be consulted for design assumptions where loads are not applied to the top flange or where concentrated loads or other non-uniform loads are applied to the I-joist.

C7.4.3 Web Holes

The manufacturer's literature or code evaluation reports should be consulted for the effect of web holes on strength and stiffness.

C7.4.4 Notches

The manufacturer's literature or code evaluation reports should be consulted when notching of the flange is being considered. However, as a general rule, flange notching is not permitted.

C7.4.5 Deflection

I-joist stiffness is presented as the product of the material modulus of elasticity and the effective moment of inertia (EI). I-joist floor systems are typically designed to L/480 deflection limits rather than the code minimum of L/360. Consideration of creep deflection for unique applications, such as those with heavy dead loads, may be in accordance with NDS 3.5.2.

C7.4.6 Vertical Load Transfer

See C7.4.2.

C7.4.7 Shear

See C7.4.1 and C7.4.2.

COMMENTARY: PREFABRICATED WOOD I-JOISTS

C8 STRUCTURAL COMPOSITE LUMBER

C8.1 General

Structural composite lumber (SCL) is manufactured from strips or full sheets of veneer. The process typically includes alignment of stress-graded fiber, application of adhesive, and pressing the material together under heat and pressure. By redistributing natural growth characteristics and monitoring manufacturing through quality control procedures, the resulting material has consistent quality and maximizes the strength and stiffness of the wood fiber.

Structural composite lumber is typically produced in a long length continuous or fixed press in a billet form. This is then resawn into required dimensions for use. Material is available in a variety of depths typically from 4-3/8" to 24" and thicknesses from 3/4" to 7".

C8.1.1 Application

The general requirements given in Chapters 1, 2, and 3 of the Specification are applicable to structural composite lumber except where otherwise indicated. Chapter 8 of the Specification contains provisions which are particular to structural composite lumber. The provisions of NDS Chapter 8 contain only the basic requirements applicable to engineering design of structural composite lumber manufactured in accordance with ASTM D5456 (16).

Specific detailed requirements, such as those for notches, are available from structural composite lumber manufacturers' literature or code evaluation reports.

C8.1.2 Definitions

Definitions for structural composite lumber, including laminated veneer lumber and parallel strand lumber, are based on definitions in ASTM D5456 (16).

C8.1.3 Identification

Structural composite lumber is typically identified by product grade and company name, plant location or number, quality assurance agency name or logo, code evaluation report numbers, and a means for establishing the date of manufacture.

C8.1.4 Service Conditions

Structural composite lumber is typically used in dry service conditions (less than 16 percent). For other conditions, the manufacturer should be consulted.

C8.2 Reference Design Values

Structural composite lumber is a proprietary product and design values vary among manufacturers and product lines. Reference design values should be obtained from the manufacturer through the manufacturer's literature or code evaluation report.

C8.3 Adjustment of Reference Design Values

C8.3.1 General

Applicable adjustment factors for structural composite lumber are specified in NDS Table 8.3.1.

C8.3.2 Load Duration Factor, C_D (ASD Only)

See C2.3.2.

C8.3.3 Wet Service Factor, C_M

Structural composite lumber is limited to use in dry service conditions unless specifically allowed by the manufacturer (see NDS 8.1.4).

C8.3.4 Temperature Factor, C_t

See C2.3.3.

C8.3.5 Beam Stability, C_L

See C3.3.3.

C8.3.6 Volume Factor, C_V

Volume effects of SCL beams are two dimensional in that increasing the width does not result in a strength reduction. Further, since SCL properties are established based on testing at a constant span-to-depth ratio, the only adjustment for volume required in design is an adjustment based on member depth that uses an exponent unique to each manufacturer (based on variability of the product).

C8.3.7 Repetitive Member Factor, C_r

The repetitive member factor for SCL is based on assumptions used to develop the repetitive member factor for sawn lumber (see C4.3.9), except that lower strength and stiffness variability limits the magnitude of the factor.

C8.3.8 Column Stability Factor, C_P

See C3.7.1.

C8.3.9 Bearing Area Factor, C_b

See C3.10.4.

C8.3.10 Pressure-Preservative Treatment

Per NDS 8.1.4, structural composite lumber is limited to use in dry service conditions unless specifically allowed by the manufacturer. Manufacturers should be consulted for any applications that require preservative treatment.

C8.3.11 Format Conversion Factor, K_F (LRFD Only)

See C2.3.5.

C8.3.12 Resistance Factor, ϕ (LRFD Only)

See C2.3.6.

C8.3.13 Time Effect Factor, λ (LRFD Only)

See C2.3.7.

C8.4 Special Design Considerations

C8.4.1 Notches

The designer has the responsibility of determining if structural composite lumber bending members should be notched and how load-carrying capacity should be calculated. Current good engineering practice is to avoid all notching of such bending members on the tension side except where end notching at the supports is necessary. This end notching is limited to 1/10 of the bending member depth, similar to structural glued laminated timber (140). The methods of NDS 3.4.3, used to calculate shear force at end notches in sawn lumber and structural glued laminated timber members, are permitted for structural composite lumber under the same design assumptions. Where different assumptions are made, the manufacturer should be consulted.

C9 WOOD STRUCTURAL PANELS

C9.1 General

C9.1.1 Application

The general requirements given in Chapters 1, 2, and 3 of the Specification are applicable to wood structural panels except where otherwise indicated. Chapter 9 of the Specification contains provisions that specifically apply to wood structural panels manufactured in accordance with USDOC PS 1 (150) or PS 2 (151). The provisions of NDS Chapter 9 contain only the basic requirements applicable to engineering design of wood structural panels. Specific requirements, such as the wet service factor, the Grade and Construction factor, and the panel size factor are available from the wood structural panel manufacturer or the qualified agency.

C9.1.2 Identification

C9.1.2.1 Panel grades for plywood manufactured in conformance with USDOC PS 1 (150), *Construction & Industrial Plywood,* are designated by the grade of the face and back veneers (e.g., C-D, C-C, A-C, etc.) or by intended end-use (e.g., Underlayment, Marine, Concrete Form, etc.). Corresponding grade names in PS 1 for Sheathing, Structural I Sheathing, and Single Floor are C-D, Structural I C-D, and Underlayment, respectively.

Panel grades for products manufactured in conformance with USDOC PS 2 *Performance Standard for Wood-Based Structural-Use Panels* (151), are identified by intended end-use and include: Sheathing, Structural I Sheathing, and Single Floor.

Sheathing grade panels are intended for use as structural covering material for roofs, subfloors, and walls. Structural I sheathing panels meet increased requirements for cross-panel strength and stiffness and are typically used in panelized roof systems, diaphragms, and shear walls. Single Floor grade panels are used as a combination subfloor and underlayment and may be used under several different types of finish flooring as well as subflooring in a two-layer floor system with underlayment.

Bond classification is related to the moisture resistance of the glue bond under intended end-use conditions and does not relate to the physical (i.e., erosion, ultraviolet) or biological (i.e., mold, fungal decay, insect) resistance of the panel. Structural-use panels manufactured in conformance with PS 1 or PS 2 must meet the bond classification requirements for *Exterior* or *Exposure 1.*

Exterior is defined in PS 1 and PS 2 as a bond classification for panels that are suitable for repeated wetting and redrying or long-term exposure to weather or other conditions of similar severity. *Exterior* plywood is manufactured with a minimum C-grade veneer.

Exposure 1 is defined in PS 1 and PS 2 as a bond classification for panels that are suitable for uses not permanently exposed to the weather. Panels classified as *Exposure 1* are intended to resist the effects of moisture on structural performance due to construction delays or other conditions of similar severity.

C9.1.2.2 Span ratings indicate the maximum on center spacing of supports, in inches, over which the panels should be placed for specific applications. The span rating system is intended for panels that are applied with the strength axis across two or more spans. The strength axis is typically the axis parallel to the orientation of oriented strand board (OSB) face strands or plywood face veneer grain and is the long dimension of the panel unless indicated otherwise by the manufacturer.

The span rating for Sheathing grade panels is provided as two numbers separated by a slash (e.g., 32/16 or 48/24). The first number is the maximum recommended on center (oc) support spacing in inches for roof applications. The second number is the maximum recommended on center support spacing when the panel is used for subflooring in residential and many light commercial applications. For example, a panel with a span rating of 32/16 may be used for roof sheathing over supports spaced up to 32" oc or as a subfloor over supports spaced up to 16" oc. Recommendations for use of Sheathing grade panels also include wall applications. Panels with roof span ratings of 16 oc or 2(oc may be installed with their strength axis either paralle or perpendicular to the wall studs space at 16" or less oc. Similarly, panels with roof span ratings of 24 oc maximum may be installed with their strength axis either parallel or perpendicular to the wall studs spaced at 24" or less oc.

Sheathing grade panels may also be used in wall applications, according to manufacturers' recommendations, both parallel and perpendicular to studs. Sheathing panels with span ratings of Wall-16 or Wall-24 are for use only as wall sheathing. The numerical index (16 or 24) corresponds to the maximum on center spacing of the studs. Wall sheathing panels are typically performance tested with the strength axis parallel to the studs. For this reason, wall sheathing panels may be applied with either the strength axis parallel to the supports or perpendicular to the supports.

The span rating for Single Floor grade panels appears as a single number and represents the maximum recommended on center support spacing in inches. Typical span ratings for Single Floor products are 20 oc and 24 oc, although 16 oc, 32 oc, and 48 oc panels are also available.

C9.1.3 Definitions

C9.1.3.3 Oriented strand board (OSB) was first commercially introduced in the early 1980s succeeding "waferboard." Waferboard is a mat-formed panel product that utilizes random distribution of rectangular wafers, whereas OSB is a mat-formed panel product with oriented layers resulting in directional properties.

C9.1.3.4 The term "ply" refers to the individual sheets of veneer used to construct plywood. A "layer" is defined as a single ply of veneer or two or more adjacent plies with grain oriented in the same direction. Veneer is classified into the following six grades:

N: Highest grade level. No knots, restricted patches.

A: Higher grade level. No knots, allows more patches than N-grade but quantity of patches is also restricted.

B: Solid surface - Small round knots. Patches and round plugs are allowed.

C Plugged: Special improved C grade.

C: Small knots, knotholes, patches. Lowest grade allowed in Exterior plywood.

D: Larger knots, knotholes, some limited white pocket in sheathing grades.

C9.1.4 Service Conditions

C9.1.4.1. When the equilibrium moisture content of wood structural panels in service is less than 16 percent (including either Exposure 1 or Exterior bond classification), the dry service design values apply. A dry service condition prevails in most covered structures. However, members used in interior locations subject to high humidity, such as may occur in certain industrial operations or over unventilated swimming pools, may reach an equilibrium moisture content of 16 percent or more. In such conditions, wet service factors (see C9.3.3) should be applied to reference design values. However, preservative treated panels should be used where there is a potential for wood decay such as when panels maintain an in-service moisture content of 19 percent or more, either from sustained high humidity levels or prolonged exposure to moisture.

Exterior exposures that are not protected from the weather are generally considered wet conditions of use. Wet service adjustment factors, C_M, are provided in Table C9.3.3 for uses where this limit will be exceeded for a sustained period of time or for repeated periods. Uses in which the panel is in contact with the ground should be considered wet use for those portions of the panel that will attain a moisture content of 16 percent or more. Where wet service conditions apply, the need for preservative treatment should be considered, as untreated panels used in these conditions are susceptible to degradation from fungal decay.

C9.2 Reference Design Values

C9.2.1 Panel Stiffness and Strength

C9.2.1.1 Minimum design stress values for wood structural panels are available from the panel manufacturer or the qualified agency for the panel grade and span rating. These unit design stress values, where provided, can be combined with the design section properties (see C9.2.4) to calculate panel stiffness and strength design capacities.

Panel stiffness and strength design capacities for specific panels may be available from the panel manufacturer.

C9.2.1.2 Structural panels have a strength axis direction, and a cross panel direction (see Figure C9.2.1). The direction of the strength axis is defined as the axis parallel to the orientation of OSB face strands or plywood face veneer grain and is the long dimension of the panel unless otherwise indicated by the manufacturer.

Figure C9.2.1 Structural Panel with Strength Direction Across Supports

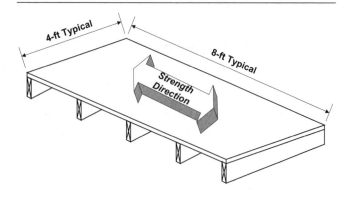

4-ft Typical

8-ft Typical

Strength Direction

C9.2.2 Strength and Elastic Properties

Reference strength and stiffness design values are available from the panel manufacturer (see C9.2.1.1).

C9.2.3 Design Thickness

Section properties associated with the nominal panel thickness should be used in design calculations (see C9.2.4), unless otherwise indicated. The relationship between the the span rating and the nominal panel thickness is provided in Table C9.2.3.

Table C9.2.3 Relationship Between Span Rating and Nominal Thickness

Span Rating	3/8	7/16	15/32	1/2	19/32	5/8	23/32	3/4	7/8	1	1-1/8
					Nominal Thickness (in.)						
Sheathing											
24/0	P	A	A	A							
24/16		P	A	A							
32/16			P	A	A	A					
40/20					P	A	A	A			
48/24							P	A	A		
Single Floor											
16 oc					P	A					
20 oc					P	A					
24 oc							P	A			
32 oc									P	A	
48 oc											P

P = Predominant nominal thickness for each span rating.
A = Alternative nominal thickness that may be available for each span rating. Check with suppliers regarding availability.

C9.2.4 Design Section Properties

The section properties associated with the nominal panel thickness and span rating are provided in Table C9.2.4. These values should be used with the panel stiffness and strength design stress values. Alternatively, these values can be combined with the panel stiffness and strength design stress values to provide panel stiffness and strength design capacities (see C9.2.1.1).

Table C9.2.4 Panel Section Properties[a]

Nominal Thickness (in.)	Approximate Weight[b] (psf)	Thickness t (in.)	Area A (in.²/ft.)	Moment of Inertia I (in.⁴/ft.)	Section Modulus S (in.³/ft.)	Statical Moment Q (in.³/ft.)	Shear Constant Ib/Q (in.²/ft.)
3/8	1.1	0.375	4.500	0.053	0.281	0.211	3.000
7/16	1.3	0.437	5.250	0.084	0.383	0.287	3.500
15/32	1.4	0.469	5.625	0.103	0.440	0.330	3.750
1/2	1.5	0.500	6.000	0.125	0.500	0.375	4.000
19/32	1.8	0.594	7.125	0.209	0.705	0.529	4.750
5/8	1.9	0.625	7.500	0.244	0.781	0.586	5.000
23/32	2.2	0.719	8.625	0.371	1.033	0.775	5.750
3/4	2.3	0.750	9.000	0.422	1.125	0.844	6.000
7/8	2.6	0.875	10.500	0.670	1.531	1.148	7.000
1	3.0	1.000	12.000	1.000	2.000	1.500	8.000
1-1/8	3.3	1.125	13.500	1.424	2.531	1.898	9.000

a. Properties based on rectangular cross section of 1-ft. width.
b. Approximate plywood weight for calculating actual dead loads. For OSB and COM-PLY panels, increase tabulated weights by 10%.

C9.3 Adjustment of Reference Design Values

C9.3.1 General

Applicable adjustment factors for wood structural panels are specified in NDS Table 9.3.1.

C9.3.2 Load Duration Factor, C_D (ASD Only)

See C2.3.2.

C9.3.3 Wet Service Factor, C_M, and Temperature Factor, C_t

Wet Service Factor

Design capacities for panels can be used without adjustment for moisture effects where the panel moisture content in service is expected to be less than 16 percent (see C9.1.4). Adjustment factors for conditions where the panel moisture content in service is expected to be 16 percent or greater should be obtained from the manufacturer, industry associations, or third-party inspection agency. Wet service adjustment factors traditionally used include

Table C9.3.3 Wet Service Factor, C_M

Reference Design Capacity	C_M
Strength (F_bS, F_tA, F_cA, $F_s(Ib/Q)$, F_vt_v)	0.75
Stiffness (EI, EA, G_vt_v)	0.85

Wood structural panels used in structural applications such as roof and wall sheathing, subfloors, diaphragms, and built-up members must be manufactured with either an "Exposure 1" or "Exterior" bond classification (see C9.1.2).

Temperature Factor

The temperature factor, C_t, shall be applied when wood structural panels are exposed to in-service sustained temperatures in excess of 100°F (see C2.3.3). In the range of 100°F to 200°F, the temperature factor is applicable only when the moisture content of the wood structural panels can be expected to remain at or above 12 percent. The rationale behind the latter recommendation is that the strength increases due to panel drying under the higher temperature is sufficient to offset the strength decreases due to the temperature itself. The temperature factor can be estimated using the following equation:

$$C_t = 1.0 - 0.005 \, (T - 100) \tag{C9.3-1}$$

where:

T = temperature (°F)

C9.3.4 Grade and Construction Factor, C_G, and Panel Size Factor, C_s

Reference design capacities available from the manufacturer (see C9.2.1.1) represent minimum design values for each listed grade and construction. These values can be adjusted to design capacities for other specific constructions and grades using Grade and Construction Factors, C_G. Alternatively, the reference design capacity for the specific construction and grade are obtained from the manufacturer.

Strength capacities for bending and axial tension are appropriate for panels 24" or greater in width (i.e., dimension perpendicular to the applied stress). For panels less than 24" in width, the capacities should be reduced by applying the appropriate panel size adjustment factor in Table C9.3.4. Single strips less than 8" wide used in stressed applications should be chosen such that they are relatively free of surface defects.

Table C9.3.4 Panel Size Factor, C_s

Panel Strip Width, w	C_s
w ≤ 8 in.	0.5
8 in. < w < 24 in.	(8+w)/32
w ≥ 24 in.	1.0

C9.4 Design Considerations

C9.4.1 Flatwise Bending

Special care should be taken to ensure that the section properties associated with the proper strength axis are used to calculate the bending capacity of the panel (see Figure C9.4.1).

Figure C9.4.1 Example of Structural Panel in Bending

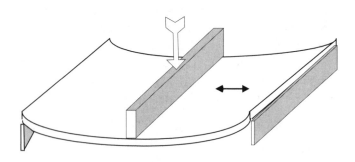

C9.4.2 Tension in the Plane of the Panel

Special care should be taken to ensure that the section properties associated with the proper strength axis are used to calculate the tensile capacity of the panel.

C9.3.5 Format Conversion Factor, K_F (LRFD Only)

See C2.3.5.

C9.3.6 Resistance Factor, ϕ (LRFD Only)

See C2.3.6.

C9.3.7 Time Effect Factor, λ (LRFD Only)

See C2.3.7.

C9.4.3 Compression in the Plane of the Panel

Special care should be taken to ensure that the section properties associated with the proper strength axis are used to calculate the compression capacity of the panel (see Figure C9.4.3).

Figure C9.4.3 Structural Panel with Axial Compression Load in Plane of the Panel

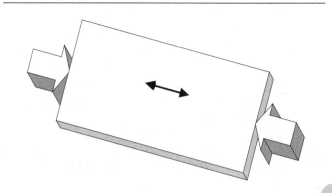

C9.4.4 Planar (Rolling) Shear

Special care should be taken to ensure that the section properties associated with the proper strength axis is used to calculate the planar shear (also called shear-in-the-plane or rolling shear) capacity of the panel (see Figure C9.4.4).

Figure C9.4.4 Planar (Rolling Shear) or Shear-in-the-Plane for Wood Structural Panels

Planar (Rolling) Shear

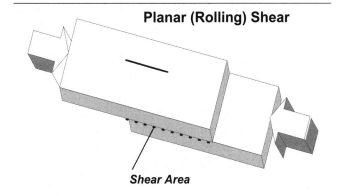

Shear Area

C9.4.5 Through-the-Thickness Shear

The section property for shear-through-the-thickness is the same both along the panel axis and across the panel axis (see Figure C9.4.5).

Figure C9.4.5 Through-the-Thickness Shear for Wood Structural Panels

Through-the-Thickness Shear

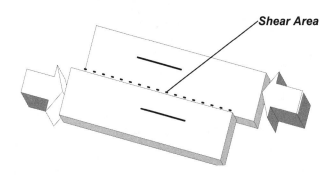

Shear Area

C9.4.6 Bearing

The design bearing stress on the panel face is independent of panel axis orientation.

C10 MECHANICAL CONNECTIONS

C10.1 General

C10.1.1 Scope

C10.1.1.2 See C3.1.3, C3.1.4, and C3.1.5.

C10.1.1.3 The adequacy of alternate methods or procedures for designing and verifying the reference design values of connections that differ from those in the Specification is the responsibility of the designer or the authority accepting or approving such alternate methods or procedures. This responsibility includes providing for appropriate margins of safety; assuring the applicability of load duration, wet service, and other adjustment factors in the Specification; and confirming the applicability of test results to field fabrication and service conditions (see C1.1.1.3).

C10.1.2 Stresses in Members at Connections

All connection designs should be checked for conformance of structural members to the net section area requirements of NDS 3.1.2 and the shear design provisions of NDS 3.4.3 (see C3.1.2 and C3.4.3). All single shear or lapped joints also should be checked to determine the adequacy of the member to resist the additional stresses induced by the eccentric transfer of load at the joint (see NDS 3.1.3). Often this will involve bending and compression or bending and tension interaction where the bending moment induced by the eccentric load at the joint results in bending about the weak axis of the member.

Where multiple fasteners are used, the capacity of the fastener group may be limited by wood failure at the net section or by tear-out around the fasteners caused by local stresses. One method for evaluating member strength for local stresses around fastener groups is outlined in NDS Appendix E.

C10.1.3 Eccentric Connections

Fastener eccentricity that induces tension perpendicular to grain stresses in the main wood member at the connection should be avoided. Where multiple fasteners occur with eccentricity, fasteners are to be placed, insofar as possible, such that the wood between them is placed in compression rather than in tension (see NDS Figure 10A).

In 1948, provisions for shear design of bending members at connections were introduced in an attempt to limit tension perpendicular to grain stresses at eccentric connections. In 1982, a provision was added prohibiting eccentric connections that induce tension perpendicular to grain stresses unless it has been shown by analysis or testing that such joints can safely carry all applied loads. The determination of the type and extent of the analysis and/or testing required to demonstrate the adequacy of eccentric connections that induce tension perpendicular to grain stresses in the wood members is the responsibility of the designer. Use of stitch bolts or plates to resist such stresses when they can not be avoided is a common practice.

It is to be emphasized that tension design values perpendicular to grain are not given in the Specification (see C3.8.2).

C10.1.4 Mixed Fastener Connections

The individual fasteners in a connection should generally be of the same size to assure comparable load-slip or stiffness characteristics. Such equivalency is required to obtain appropriate distribution of load among fasteners in the connection and is a condition for use of the group action factor, C_g, of NDS 10.3.6.

It is recognized that some designers have used different fastener types in the same connection where the addition of one or more fasteners of the type being used is precluded by area restrictions or is considered uneconomical. Such mixed-type connections, for example, the use of a single 1/2" bolt with three split ring connectors or the use of a 16d nail with two 1/2" bolts, are not covered by the design provisions of the Specification. Because of the different load-slip behavior of different fastener types, the allowable load on such connections can not be assumed to be the sum of the allowable loads for each fastener type, even when the different types are in different rows.

Allowable loads for connections employing more than one type or size of fastener shall be based on analyses that account for different connection stiffnesses, on test results, or on field experience (see C1.1.1.3). It is the designer's responsibility to assure that load capacities assigned to such connections contain adequate margins of safety and are achievable under field conditions.

C10.1.5 Connection Fabrication

Design values for connection joints have been applied to connections having both tight and loose nuts. This provision is based on the original bolted joint tests used to establish design values in which the nuts were intentionally not tightened in order to simulate the additional shrinkage that can occur during service (146). It is to be noted that these provisions only apply to the loosening of nuts that may occur from shrinkage and not the effects of moisture on bearing strength or the effects of checks and cracks that may occur from seasoning after fabrication. Reduction of connection design values for these factors is required when connections are assembled with wet or partially seasoned wood (see NDS 10.3.3).

C10.2 Reference Design Values

C10.2.1 Single Fastener Connections

Reference lateral design values for dowel-type fasteners (bolts, lag screws, wood screws, nails, and spikes) are based on a yield limit model which specifically accounts for the different ways these connections can behave under load. These behavior patterns or modes (see NDS Appendix I) are uniform bearing in the wood under the fastener, rotation of the fastener in the joint without dowel bending, and development of one or more plastic hinges in the fastener (67, 122). Equations have been developed for each mode relating the joint load to the maximum stresses in the wood members and in the fastener (67, 121). The capacity of the connection under each yield mode is keyed to the bearing strength of the wood under the fastener and the bending strength of the fastener, with the lowest capacity calculated for the various modes being taken as the design value for the connection.

The yield limit model provides a consistent basis for establishing the relative effects of side and main member thickness and bearing strength, and fastener bending strength on the load-carrying capacity of connections involving dowel-type fasteners. Because the yield strength of a wood connection is not well defined on the load-deformation curve for a connection, the limiting wood stresses used in the yield model are based on the load at which the load-deformation curve from a fastener embedment test intersects a line represented by the initial tangent modulus offset 5 percent of the fastener diameter (120). This nominal yield point is intermediate between the proportional limit and maximum load for the material and for the connection.

Reference lateral design values for connections in previous editions of the Specification represented nominal proportional limit values. For purposes of transition and to build on the long record of satisfactory performance obtained with these previous values, short-term design values based on direct application of the yield limit equations have been reduced to design levels published in previous editions for connections made with equivalent species and member sizes. This calibration was accomplished by establishing average ratios of previous Specification design values to yield limit model design values for each yield mode and direction of loading (parallel and perpendicular to grain). This soft conversion procedure retained historical safety levels while resulting in some design values for each fastener type being somewhat higher and some lower than previous values depending upon the fastener diameter and the thickness of main and side member.

C10.2.2 Multiple Fastener Connections

The reference design value for a connection containing two or more fasteners is obtained by summing the reference design values for each individual fastener. It is to be understood that this provision requires application of the group action factor of NDS 10.3.6 to the individual fastener reference design value wherever a row of two or more split ring connectors, shear plate connectors, or dowel-type fasteners are involved.

Summation of individual fastener reference design values to obtain a total reference design value for a connection containing two or more fasteners is limited to designs involving the same type and the same size of fastener (see C10.1.4). Fasteners of the same type, diameter, and length joining the same members and resisting load in the same shear plane may be assumed to exhibit the same yield mode.

C10.2.3 Design of Metal Parts

Metal parts, including fasteners, are to be designed in accordance with national standards of practice and specifications applicable to the material. Tension stresses in fasteners as a result of withdrawal loads, shear in cross sections of fasteners, bearing of fasteners on metal side plates, tension and shear of plates, and buckling of plates and rods are included under this provision.

Standard metal design practices are not to be used to account for bending stresses occurring in dowel-type fasteners in wood connections subject to lateral loads. These stresses are accounted for in this Specification under the provisions for the particular fastener type involved. Where the design value for a connection involving metal fasteners is limited by the provisions of this Specification, the adjustment factors of NDS 10.3 are to be applied. Where the design value of the connection is limited by the strength of the metal fastener or part, the adjustment factors of NDS 10.3 are not to be applied.

C10.2.4 Design of Concrete or Masonry Parts

Concrete or masonry parts are to be designed in accordance with national standards of practice and specifications applicable to the material.

C10.3 Adjustment of Reference Design Values

C10.3.1 Applicability of Adjustment Factors

Applicable adjustment factors for connections are specified in NDS Table 10.3.1.

C10.3.2 Load Duration Factor, C_D (ASD Only)

See C2.3.2. Reference design values for wood connections derived from the results of standard short-term tests (5 to 10 minute duration) and/or calculated using properties derived from short-term tests include a 1.6 reduction to account for the potential effects of long-term loading. When wood connections are used to resist short-term loads, the reference design values can be increased by a factor of up to 1.6 based on the provisions of NDS 2.3.2. Load duration factors greater than 1.6, including the impact load duration factor of 2.0, are not to be applied to design loads for connections.

C10.3.3 Wet Service Factor, C_M

The wet service factors in NDS Table 10.3.3 for bolts and lag screws, split ring and shear plate connectors, wood screws, and nails were recommended as part of early research on wood connections (184, 181).

The 0.80 factor for metal plate connectors installed in partially seasoned or wet lumber is based on the results of both truss and tension in-line joint tests (1, 109, 195).

The factor of 0.40 in NDS Table 10.3.3 for multiple rows of dowel fasteners installed in partially seasoned wood used in dry conditions of service is based on limited tests of connections fabricated with unseasoned members joined at right angles to each other and tested after drying (181).

C10.3.4 Temperature Factor, C_t

The temperature adjustment factors for connections in NDS Table 10.3.4 are equivalent to those for bending, compression, and shear design values in NDS 2.3.3 (see C2.3.3). Bearing under metal fasteners is closely correlated with compression parallel to grain or compression perpendicular to grain properties.

C10.3.5 Fire Retardant Treatment

See C2.3.4.

C10.3.6 Group Action Factor, C_g

Modification factors for two or more split ring connectors, shear plate connectors, or dowel-type fasteners in a row were added to the Specification in the 1973 edition. Earlier tests of bolted and shear plate connector joints had shown that the load capacity of connections containing multiple fasteners in a row was not directly proportional to the number of fasteners, with those located near the ends of the row carrying a greater proportion of the applied load than those located in the interior of the row (35, 39, 40, 66, 72).

The tables of factors included in the 1973 edition to account for the non-uniform loads on a row of fasteners was based on a linear analysis wherein the direct stresses in the main and side members of the connection were assumed to be uniformly distributed across their cross section, and the relationship between fastener slip and fastener load was assumed to be linear (77). This analytical procedure showed that the transfer of load from side to main members and the proportion of the total load carried by each fastener were determined by the modulii of elasticity, E, and cross-sectional areas of the side and main members, the number of fasteners in a row, the spacing between fasteners, and the joint load-slip modulus.

Two tables of modification factors for joints containing two or more fasteners in a row were developed using the linear analysis: one for connections with wood side plates and one for connections with metal side plates. For purposes of simplicity, factors were tabulated only in terms of the number of fasteners in the row and the cross-sectional areas of the members being joined. Other variables were assumed to have the following values (156):

Wood to wood connections:

E of side and main members	1,800,000 psi
Load-slip fastener modulus	220,000 lb/in.
Spacing between fasteners	6.5 inches

Wood to metal connections:

E of main member	1,400,000 psi
Load-slip fastener modulus	330,000 lb/in.
Spacing between fasteners	5.75 inches

With the foregoing constant values, the analytical procedure was used to calculate modification factors for three to eight fasteners in a row and then results were extrapolated up to 12 fasteners and down to two fasteners in a row

(156). The resulting tables of factors, ranging from 1.00 for two fasteners in a row to as low as 0.34 and 0.15 for 12 fasteners in a row in joints made with wood and metal side plates, respectively, were continued essentially unchanged through the 1986 edition. The group action factor equation given in NDS 10.3.6 consolidated the analytical procedure used to establish the modification factors given in previous editions (188). Concurrent with the development of the compact single equation for accounting for group action, more recent load-slip data for bolted joints and split ring and shear plate connectors have been used to establish new representative load-slip modulii for different types of connections (188).

It is to be noted that the variable A_s in the group action equation (NDS Equation 10.3-1) represents the sum of the cross-sectional area of the side members. Thus the equation accounts for single shear as well as double shear connections. For a connection with four or more members, each shear plane is evaluated as a single shear connection (see NDS 11.3.8). Where such a connection contains two or more fasteners in a row, a group action factor is calculated for each shear plane using an A_s based on the thinnest member adjacent to the plane being considered.

Perpendicular to Grain Loading. The number of fasteners in a row perpendicular to grain are generally limited in order to avoid splitting that can occur as a result of drying (see C10.3.3). When a row of multiple fasteners are used perpendicular to grain, it is standard practice to use the same group action factor as that for fasteners aligned parallel to grain. This practice is based on the assumption that use of the member and connection stiffnesses perpendicular to grain ($E_\perp$ and $\gamma_\perp$) in NDS Equation 10.3-1 would result in similar group action factors.

C11 DOWEL-TYPE FASTENERS

C11.1 General

C11.1.2 Bolts

C11.1.2.1 ANSI/ASME Standard B18.2.1 *Square and Hex Bolts and Screws (Inch Series)* is the quality reference standard for bolts. Bolt design provisions and tabulated bolt design values apply only to bolts having diameters of 1" or less. This limit was in response to reported field problems with connections involving large diameter bolts in structural glued laminated timber members and the results of research (31, 135). The latter showed drying in service, workmanship variables, and perpendicular to grain load components could interact to affect the capacity of connections made with multiple large diameter, relatively stiff bolts. Use of these procedures to establish reference design values for large diameter bolted connections is the sole responsibility of the designer.

C11.1.2.2 Generally, smaller diameter bolts will use the smaller oversize hole value and larger bolts the larger oversize value. The same target oversize is to be used for all holes in the same connection. Proper alignment, especially in groups of fasteners, is required to properly distribute the load into each fastener. Forcible driving of the fastener can damage the wood-bearing surface and reduce the capacity of the connection.

C11.1.2.3 Use of washers or equivalent metal parts under the head and nut prevent localized crushing of the wood at bolt holes.

C11.1.2.4 Edge distance, end distance, and fastener spacing requirements have been consolidated for dowel-type fasteners in NDS 11.5.

C11.1.3 Lag Screws

C11.1.3.1 ANSI/ASME Standard B18.2.1 *Square and Hex Bolts and Screws (Inch Series)* is the quality reference standard for lag screws. It provides standard lag screw dimensions (see NDS Appendix L) but does not specify metal having specific strength properties. The designer is responsible for specifying the metal strength of the lag screws that are to be used. Bending yield strength of the lag screw (see NDS Appendix I) is a required input variable to the yield equations of NDS 11.3.1. Additionally, the actual tensile stress in the lag screw at the root diameter must be checked when designing lag screw connections for withdrawal (see NDS 10.2.3).

C11.1.3.2 Lead hole requirements for three specific gravity classes are based on early lag screw research involving tests of Douglas fir, southern pine, white oak, redwood, and northern white pine (100).

C11.1.3.3 Provision for allowing 3/8" and smaller diameter lag screws loaded primarily in withdrawal to be inserted without a lead hole in wood of medium to low specific gravity was added to address the use of small lag screws. On the basis of field experience, early lag screw research (100), and information on the withdrawal resistance of tapping screws inserted with different size lead holes (163), use of small lag screws without lead holes were deemed acceptable when the following conditions are met:

1. The lag screws are being loaded primarily in withdrawal.
2. The lag screws are inserted in wood with specific gravity, $G \leq 0.5$.
3. Placement of lag screws avoids excessive splitting.

A lag screw subjected to both combined withdrawal and lateral loading may be considered loaded primarily in withdrawal when the axis of the screw is at angle of 75° or more to the grain of the wood member holding the threaded portion of the screw. The requirement that unusual splitting be avoided when lead holes are not used is to be considered a performance requirement that (i) is related to the ability of the screw to hold the cleat or side member to the main or foundation member and (ii) is applicable to both members being joined.

C11.1.3.5 A lubricant is sometimes used to facilitate lag screw insertion even when small diameter lag screws are inserted without the use of lead holes.

C11.1.3.6 Minimum penetration requirements are provided to ensure that fasteners can achieve the design value calculated using the yield equations in NDS 11.3.1.

C11.1.3.7 Edge distance, end distance, and fastener spacing requirements have been consolidated for dowel-type fasteners in NDS 11.5.

C11.1.4 Wood Screws

C11.1.4.1 ANSI/ASME Standard B18.6.1 is the quality reference standard for wood screws. It provides standard wood screw dimensions (see NDS Appendix L) but does not specify metal having specific strength properties. The designer is responsible for specifying the metal strength of the wood screws that are to be used. Bending yield strength of the wood screw (see NDS Appendix I) is a required input variable to the lateral design value yield limit equations of NDS 11.3.1. Additionally, the actual tensile stress in the wood screw at the root diameter must be checked when designing wood screw connections for withdrawal (see NDS 10.2.3).

C11.1.4.2 Lead hole requirements for wood screws are based on early research involving flat head wood screws up to 24 gage and 5" in length in seven species, including southern pine, cypress, and oak (43).

The provision allowing the insertion of wood screws without a lead hole in species with $G \leq 0.5$ when the screw was subject to withdrawal loads parallels that made for 3/8" and smaller diameter lag screws (see C11.1.3.3).

C11.1.4.3 Wood screws resisting lateral loads are required to have shank and threaded portion lead holes based on early lateral load tests of wood screws (184, 181, 70). Lead holes are required for all wood screws subject to lateral loads regardless of wood specific gravity.

C11.1.4.4 Wood screws tests (43, 181, 70) are based on inserting the screw by turning rather than driving with a hammer.

C11.1.4.5 A lubricant is sometimes used to facilitate screw insertion and avoid screw damage. Tests have shown that the lubricant has no significant effect on reference design values (43, 184, 70).

C11.1.4.6 Minimum penetration requirements are provided to ensure that fasteners can achieve the reference design value calculated using the yield equations in NDS 11.3.1.

C11.1.4.7 Edge distance, end distance, and fastener spacing requirements have been consolidated across all diameters for dowel-type fasteners in NDS Table 11.5.1. For diameters less than 1/4", specific requirements are not provided; however Table C11.1.4.7 may be used to establish wood screw placement recommendations. Designers should note that wood specie type, moisture content, and grain orientation will impact spacing effects between fasteners in a row.

Table C11.1.4.7 Wood Screw Minimum Spacing Tables

	Wood Side Members	
	Not Prebored	Prebored
Edge distance	2.5d	2.5d
End distance		
- tension load parallel to grain	15d	10d
- compression load parallel to grain	10d	5d
Spacing (pitch) between fasteners in a row		
- parallel to grain	15d	10d
- perpendicular to grain	10d	5d
Spacing (gage) between rows of fasteners		
- in-line	5d	3d
- staggered	2.5d	2.5d
	Steel Side Members	
	Not Prebored	Prebored
Edge distance	2.5d	2.5d
End distance		
- tension load parallel to grain	10d	5d
- compression load parallel to grain	5d	3d
Spacing (pitch) between fasteners in a row		
- parallel to grain	10d	5d
- perpendicular to grain	5d	2.5d
Spacing (gage) between rows of fasteners		
- in line	3d	2.5d
- staggered	2.5d	2.5d

C11.1.5 Nails and Spikes

C11.1.5.1 ASTM F 1667 provides standard nail and spike dimensions (see NDS Appendix L) but does not specify metal of particular strength properties. The designer is responsible for specifying the metal strength of the nails or spikes that are to be used. Bending yield strength of the nail or spike (see NDS Appendix I) is a required input variable to the lateral design value yield limit equations of NDS 11.3.1. Additionally, the actual tensile stress in the nail or spike must be checked when designing nailed connections for withdrawal (see NDS 10.2.3).

C11.1.5.4 Toe-nailing procedures consisting of slant driving of nails at a 30° angle from the face of the attached member with an end distance (distance between end of side member and initial point of entry) of 1/3 the nail length are based on lateral and withdrawal tests of nailed joints in frame wall construction (181, 118). The toe-nail factors of NDS 11.5.4.1 and NDS 11.5.4.2 presume use of these driving procedures and the absence of excessive splitting. If such splitting does occur, predrilling or a smaller nail should be used. The vertically projected length is used as the side member bearing length in yield limit equations when calculating lateral capacity of a toe-nailed connection.

C11.1.5.5 Minimum penetration requirements are provided to ensure that fasteners can achieve the design value calculated using the yield equations in NDS 11.3.1.

C11.1.5.6 Edge distance, end distance, and fastener spacing requirements have been consolidated across all diameters for dowel-type fasteners in NDS Table 11.5.1A through 11.5.1E. For diameters less than 1/4", specific requirements are not provided; however Table C11.1.5.6 may be used to establish nail placement recommendations. Designers should note that wood specie type, moisture content, and grain orientation will impact spacing effects between fasteners in a row.

Table C11.1.5.6 Nail Minimum Spacing Tables

| | Wood Side Members | |
	Not Prebored	Prebored
Edge distance	2.5d	2.5d
End distance		
- tension load parallel to grain	15d	10d
- compression load parallel to grain	10d	5d
Spacing (pitch) between fasteners in a row		
- parallel to grain	15d	10d
- perpendicular to grain	10d	5d
Spacing (gage) between rows of fasteners		
- in-line	5d	3d
- staggered	2.5d	2.5d
	Steel Side Members	
	Not Prebored	Prebored
Edge distance	2.5d	2.5d
End distance		
- tension load parallel to grain	10d	5d
- compression load parallel to grain	5d	3d
Spacing (pitch) between fasteners in a row		
- parallel to grain	10d	5d
- perpendicular to grain	5d	2.5d
Spacing (gage) between rows of fasteners		
- in line	3d	2.5d
- staggered	2.5d	2.5d

C11.1.6 Drift Bolts and Drift Pins

C11.1.6.1 Drift bolts and drift pins are unthreaded rods used to join large structural members where a smooth surface without protruding metal parts is desired. The designer is responsible for specifying the metal strength of the drift bolt or pin that is to be used. Bending yield strength of the drift bolt or pin (see NDS Appendix I) is a required input variable to the reference lateral design value yield limit equations of NDS 11.3.1.

C11.1.6.2 Additional penetration into the members is required to resist withdrawal of the drift bolt or pin.

C11.1.6.3 Edge distance, end distance, and fastener spacing requirements have been consolidated across all diameters for dowel-type fasteners in NDS Table 11.5.1A through 11.5.1E.

C11.1.7 Other Dowel-Type Fasteners

While specific installation instructions are not provided for all types of dowel-type fasteners, the generic yield equations in NDS 11.3 apply. The designer is responsible for determining the proper installation requirements and for specifying the metal strength of these fasteners.

C11.2 Reference Withdrawal Design Values

C11.2.1 Lag Screws

C11.2.1.1 NDS Equation 11.2-1 was used to establish the lag screw reference withdrawal design values given in NDS Table 11.2A. This equation was derived from the following equation based on research (181, 100):

$$W = K_W G^{\frac{3}{2}} D^{\frac{3}{4}} \qquad \text{(C11.2.1-1)}$$

where:

W = reference withdrawal design value per inch of thread penetration into main member, lbs

K_W = 1800

G = specific gravity of main member based on ovendry weight and volume, where $0.31 \leq G \leq 0.73$

D = lag screw thread diameter (equivalent to unthreaded shank diameter for full body diameter lag screws), in., where $0.25 \leq D \leq 1.25$

The value of K_W represents approximately 1/4 (1/5 increased by 20 percent) of the average constant at ovendry weight and volume obtained from ultimate load tests of joints made with five different species and seven sizes of lag screw (100), increased by 20 percent; or

$$K_W = 1.2 \left(\frac{7500}{5} \right) \qquad \text{(C11.2.1-2)}$$

The 20 percent increase was introduced as part of the World War II emergency increase in wood design values, and then subsequently codified as 10 percent for the change from permanent to normal loading and 10 percent for experience (see C2.3.2).

When the reference withdrawal capacity of a lag screw is determined by multiplying the reference unit design value by the length of penetration of the threaded portion into the side grain of the main member, the length of the tapered tip of the screw is not to be included. This tapered portion at the tip of the lag screw was not considered as part of the effective penetration depth in the original joint tests (100). In addition, the thickness of any washer used between the lag screw head and the cleat or side member should be taken into account when determining the length of penetration of the threaded portion in the main member. Standard lag screw dimensions, including minimum thread length and length of tapered tip, are given in NDS Appendix L.

C11.2.1.2 Reference withdrawal design values for lag screws are reduced 25 percent when the screw is inserted in the end grain (radial-tangential plane) of the main member rather than the side grain (radial-longitudinal or tangential-longitudinal plane) based on lag screw joint tests (100). Because of the greater possibility of splitting when subject to lateral load, it has been recommended that insertion of lag screws in end grain surfaces be avoided (181, 96).

C11.2.1.3 See C10.2.3.

C11.2.2 Wood Screws

C11.2.2.1 NDS Equation 11.2-2 was used to establish the wood screw reference withdrawal design values given in NDS Table 11.2B. This equation was based on testing of cut thread wood screws in seven wood species (43):

$$W = K_W G^2 D \qquad \text{(C11.2.2-1)}$$

where:

W = reference withdrawal design value per inch of thread penetration in the main member, lbs

K_W = 2850

G = specific gravity of main member based on ovendry weight and volume, where $0.31 \leq G \leq 0.73$

D = wood screw thread diameter, in., where $0.138 \leq D \leq 0.372$

The value of K_W represents 1/5 (1/6 increased by 20 percent) of the average constant at ovendry weight and volume obtained from ultimate load tests of joints (43) made with seven different species and cut-thread wood screw; or

$$K_W = 1.2 \left(\frac{14250}{6} \right) \qquad \text{(C11.2.2-2)}$$

The 20 percent increase was introduced as part of the World War II emergency increase in wood design values, and then subsequently codified as 10 percent for the change from permanent to normal loading and 10 percent for experience (see C2.3.2).

Wood screw reference withdrawal design values are based on tests of cut thread wood screws. The shank or body diameter of a cut thread screw is the same as the outside diameter of the thread. The shank or body diameter of the rolled thread screw is the same as the root diameter. For the same nominal diameter of screw, both screw thread types have the same threads per inch, the same outside thread diameter, and the same thread depth. If the tensile strength of the screw is adequate and the lead hole provisions based on root diameter are used, the withdrawal resistance of rolled thread screws is considered equivalent to that of cut thread screws (182, 163).

The ANSI/ASME B18.6.1 standard states that the thread length is approximately 2/3 of the nominal screw length.

C11.2.2.2 Early tests of wood screws in withdrawal from end grain surfaces of oak, southern pine, maple, and cypress gave somewhat erratic results relative to those for withdrawal from side grain (43). These irregular results were attributed to the tendency of the screw to split the wood in the end grain configuration. Average ratios of end grain withdrawal resistance to side grain withdrawal resistance ranged from 52 to 108 percent (43). Because of this variability, structural loading of wood screws in withdrawal from end grain has been prohibited.

C11.2.2.3 See C10.2.3.

C11.2.3 Nails and Spikes

C11.2.3.1 NDS Equation 11.2-3 was used to establish the nail and spike reference withdrawal design values given in NDS Table 11.2C. This equation was based on research (94, 95):

$$W = K_W G^{\frac{5}{2}} D \qquad \text{(C11.2.3-1)}$$

where:

W = nail or spike withdrawal design value per inch of penetration in main member, lbs

K_W = 1380

G = specific gravity of main member based on ovendry weight and volume, where $0.31 \leq G \leq 0.73$

D = shank diameter of the nail or spike, in., where $0.099 \leq D \leq 0.375$

The value of K_W represents 1/5 (1/6 increased by 20 percent) of the average constant at ovendry weight and volume obtained from ultimate load tests (184), increased by 20 percent; or

$$K_W = 1.2 \left(\frac{6900}{6} \right) \qquad \text{(C11.2.3-2)}$$

The 20 percent increase was introduced as part of the World War II emergency increase in wood design values, and then subsequently codified as 10 percent for the change from permanent to normal loading and 10 percent for experience (see C2.3.2).

For 8d, 10d, 16d, and 20d threaded hardened nails, reference withdrawal design values are the same as those for common wire nails of the same pennyweight class, although the wire diameters are slightly different (0.120", 0.135", 0.148", and 0.177" for threaded hardened nails versus 0.131", 0.148", 0.162", and 0.192" for common nails, respectively). Threaded hardened nail sizes of 20d, 30d, 40d, 50d, and 60d all have the same diameter (0.177") and, therefore, use the same reference withdrawal design value. Threaded hardened nail sizes of 70d, 80d, and 90d all have the same diameter (0.207") and use the same reference withdrawal design value as a 40d common nail.

Clinching. Withdrawal resistance of smooth-shank nails can be significantly increased by clinching (29).

C11.2.3.2 Reduction of withdrawal design values up to 50 percent have been reported for nails driven in end grain surfaces (radial-tangential plane) as compared to side grain (radial-longitudinal or tangential-longitudinal planes) surfaces (184, 118). When coupled with the effects of seasoning in service after fabrication, such reduction are considered too great for reliable design. On this basis, structural loading of nails in withdrawal from end grain has been prohibited.

C11.2.4 Drift Bolts and Drift Pins

C11.2.4.1 While specific provisions for determining withdrawal design values for round drift bolts or pins are not included in the Specification, the following equation has been used where friction and workmanship can be maintained (184, 181):

$$W = 1200 G^2 D \qquad \text{(C11.2.4-1)}$$

where:

W = drift bolt or drift pin reference withdrawal design value per inch of penetration, lbs

G = specific gravity based on ovendry weight and volume

D = drift bolt or drift pin diameter, in.

Equation C11.2.4-1 assumes the fastener is driven into a prebored hole having a diameter 1/8" less than the fastener diameter (184). The reference withdrawal design values calculated with Equation C11.2.4-1 are approximately 1/5 average ultimate test values (184, 181).

C11.3 Reference Lateral Design Values

Reference lateral design values for dowel-type fasteners (bolts, lag screws, wood screws, nails, and spikes) are based on a yield limit model which specifically accounts for the different ways these connections can behave under load. These behavior patterns or modes (see NDS Appendix I) are uniform bearing in the wood under the fastener, rotation of the fastener in the joint without bending, and development of one or more plastic hinges in the fastener (67, 122). Equations have been developed for each mode relating the joint load to the maximum stresses in the wood members and in the fastener (67, 121). The capacity of the connection under each yield mode is keyed to the bearing strength of the wood under the fastener and the bending strength of the fastener, with the lowest capacity calculated for the various modes being taken as the reference design value for the connection.

Although the yield limit model represents significantly different methodology than that used previously to establish fastener design values, the relative effects of various joint variables shown by both procedures are generally similar (85, 86, 89, 121). Short-term design values obtained from application of the yield limit equations have been reduced to the average design value levels published in previous editions of the Specifications for connections made with the same species and member sizes.

Bolts: Reference design values for bolted connections are indexed to proportional limit estimates from bolted connection tests (44, 57, 146, 162) at reference conditions (seasoned dry, normal load duration).

Lag Screws: Reference design values for lag screw connections are indexed to average proportional limit estimates from short-term tests (100) divided by 1.875. The 1.875 factor is based on an original reduction factor of 2.25, increased 20 percent for normal loading and experience. The 20 percent increase was introduced as part of the World War II emergency increase in wood design values, and then subsequently codified as 10 percent for the change from permanent to normal loading and 10 percent for experience (see C2.3.2).

Wood Screws: Reference design values for wood screw connections are indexed to average short-term proportional limit test values (184, 70) divided by 1.33. The 1.33 factor is based on an original reduction factor of 1.6, increased 20 percent for normal loading and experience. The 20 percent increase was introduced as part of the World War II emergency increase in wood design values, and then subsequently codified as 10 percent for the change from permanent to normal loading and 10 percent for experience (see C2.3.2). Lateral design values for wood screw connections at reference conditions (seasoned dry,

normal load duration) are about 1/5 of maximum tested capacities (184).

Nails and Spikes: Reference design values for nailed connections are indexed to average short-term proportional limit test values (184, 50) divided by 1.33. The 1.33 factor is based on an original reduction factor of 1.6, increased 20 percent for normal loading and experience. The 20 percent increase was introduced as part of the World War II emergency increase in wood design values, and then subsequently codified as 10 percent for the change from permanent to normal loading and 10 percent for experience (see C2.3.2). Lateral design values for nail connections at reference conditions (seasoned dry, normal load duration) are about 1/5 of maximum tested capacities for softwoods and 1/9 of maximum tested capacities for hardwoods (184, 50).

C11.3.1 Yield Limit Equations

The yield limit equations for single shear connections (NDS Equations 11.3-1 to 11.3-6) and for double shear connections (NDS Equations 11.3-7 to 11.3-10) were developed from European research (121, 78) and have been confirmed by tests on domestic species (21, 20, 88, 120, 121, 122). The limiting yield modes covered by these equations are bearing in the main or side members (Mode I), fastener rotation without bending (Mode II), development of a plastic hinge in the fastener in main or side member (Mode III), and development of plastic hinges in the fastener in both main and side members (Mode IV) (see NDS Appendix I).

The reduction term, R_d, in NDS Equations 11.3-1 through 11.3-10, reduces the values calculated using the yield limit equations to approximate estimates of the nominal proportional limit design values in previous editions of the Specification (157). For fasteners loaded perpendicular to grain with diameters equal to or greater than 0.25", the reduction term is increased 25 percent ($K_\theta = 1.25$) to match previous design values for perpendicular to grain loaded connections.

For detailed technical information on lateral design equations, see *AF&PA's Technical Report 12: General Dowel Equations for Calculating Lateral Connection Values* (137).

C11.3.2 Dowel Bearing Strength

C11.3.2.1 The limiting wood stresses used in the yield limit equations are based on the load at which the load-deformation curve from a fastener embedment test intersects a line represented by the initial tangent modulus offset 5 percent of the fastener diameter (120). This nominal yield point is intermediate between the proportional limit and maximum loads for the material.

The effect of specific gravity on dowel bearing strength was established from 3/4" dowel embedment tests on Douglas fir, southern pine, spruce-pine-fir, Sitka spruce, red oak, yellow poplar, and aspen. Diameter effects were evaluated from tests of 1/4", 1/2", 3/4", 1", and 1-1/2" inch dowels in southern pine using bolt holes 1/16" larger than the dowel diameter. Diameter was found to be a significant variable only in perpendicular to grain loading. Bearing specimens were 1/2" or thicker such that width and number of growth rings did not influence results (158).

The specific gravity values given in NDS Table 11.3.2A for each specie or species group are those used to establish dowel bearing strength values, F_e, tabulated in NDS Table 11.3.2. These specific gravity values represent average values from in-grade lumber test programs or are based on information from ASTM D2555.

The equations provided in footnote 2 of NDS Table 11.3.2 were used to calculate tabulated values in NDS Table 11.3.2. These equations were derived from test data using methods described in ASTM D5764 (158, 18).

C11.3.2.2 Dowel bearing strengths for wood structural panels in NDS Table 11.3.2B are based on research conducted by APA – The Engineered Wood Association (25).

C11.3.2.3 Dowel bearing strengths for structural composite lumber are determined for each product using equivalency methods described in ASTM D5456 (16).

C11.3.3 Dowel Bearing Strength at an Angle to Grain

NDS Equation 11.3-11 (and Equation J-2 in NDS Appendix J) is used to calculate the dowel bearing strength for a main or side member loaded at an angle to grain. This equation is a form of the bearing angle to grain equation (NDS Equation J-1). The equation is entered with the parallel and perpendicular dowel bearing strengths for the member and the reference bolt design value is determined from the yield limit equations using $F_{e\theta}$ as the dowel bearing strength for the main or side member.

The reference design value obtained from the yield limit equations using dowel bearing strength at an angle to grain is similar to that obtained from using parallel to grain and perpendicular to grain Z values in NDS Equation J-3 to obtain a Z_θ design value for the connection (157). Determining a Z_θ design value using this latter approach can be used as an alternative to calculating $F_{e\theta}$ for use in each yield limit equation and allows the use of tabulated Z values from the Specification.

C11.3.4 Dowel Bearing Length

Sensitivity studies of the yield limit equations indicate that inclusion of a tapered tip length of up to two diameters (2D) in the dowel bearing length does not significantly impact the estimated fastener capacities when the fastener penetration exceeds 10 times the fastener diameter (10D). For fastener penetrations less than 10D, the tapered tip may influence the calculations and should not be included. For wood screws and nails, the length of the tapered tip is not generally standardized. However, tip lengths for diamond-point nails, such as common and box nails, range from approximately 1.3 to 2.0 nail diameters in length.

C11.3.5 Dowel Bending Yield Strength

The bending yield strength, F_{yb}, of fasteners such as nails (79), wood screws, lag screws, and bolts are given in NDS Appendix I. For A36 and stronger steels, F_{yb} equal to 45,000 psi is a conservative value and is equivalent to the bolt strength reported in the original bolt test research (146).

C11.3.6 Dowel Diameter

The reduced moment resistance in the threaded portion of dowel-type fasteners can be accounted for by use of root diameter, D_r, in calculation of reference lateral design values. Use of diameter, D, is permitted when the threaded portion of the fastener is sufficiently far away from the connection shear plane(s). For more information, see NDS Appendix I.5.

Reference lateral design values for reduced body diameter lag screw and rolled thread wood screw connections are based on root diameter, D_r, to account for the reduced diameter of these fasteners. These values, while conservative, can also be used for full-body diameter lag screws and cut thread wood screws. For bolted connections, reference lateral design values are based on diameter, D.

One alternate method of accounting for the moment and bearing resistance of the threaded portion of the fastener and moment acting along the length of the fastener is provided in AF&PA's *Technical Report 12 - General Dowel Equations for Calculating Lateral Connection Values* (137). A general set of equations permits use of different fastener diameters for bearing resistance and moment resistance in each member.

C11.3.7 Asymmetric Three Member Connections, Double Shear

Conservatively, the Specification requires the use of minimum side member bearing length and minimum dowel diameter in the calculation of design values for asymmetric three member connections. Inherent in this calculation is the assumption that the load to each side member is equivalent. Where other load distributions occur, more complex analysis may be needed.

C11.3.8 Multiple Shear Connections

The Specification requires evaluation of each individual shear plane using the yield limit equations of NDS 11.3.1 and then assigning the lowest value to the other shear planes. Interior members should be checked for the combined loading from the adjacent shear planes to ensure that sufficient bearing capacity exists (such as would exist in a double shear connection limited by Mode I_m).

C11.3.9 Load at an Angle to Fastener Axis

Two member connections in which the load acts at an angle to the axis of the fastener are checked using the component of the load acting at 90° to the axis and member thicknesses equal to the length of the fastener in each member measured at the centerline of the fastener (see NDS Figure 11E). Reference design values for connections in which the load acts at an angle to the fastener axis are based on the yield limit equations of NDS 11.3.1. The lowest value of Z obtained, using t_m and t_s equal to the length of fastener in each member, divided by the cosine of the angle of intersection of the two members is the maximum reference design value for the connection.

The adequacy of the bearing area under washers and plates to resist the component of force acting parallel to the fastener axis can be checked using adjusted compression design values perpendicular to grain, $F_{c\perp}'$.

C11.3.10 Drift Bolts and Drift Pins

Reference lateral design values for drift bolts or pins (181) are 75 percent of the reference design value for common bolts of the same diameter to compensate for the absence of head, nut, and washer. End distance, edge distance, and spacing requirements, and group action adjustments that are applicable to bolts, are also applicable to drift bolts and drift pins.

C11.4 Combined Lateral and Withdrawal Loads

C11.4.1 Lag Screws and Wood Screws

Results of lag screw tests indicated that loading at an angle to the fastener axis to induce lateral and withdrawal components did not reduce the maximum connection capacity. However, when joint resistance was evaluated at the design load level, an interaction of the load components was observed with larger diameter screws at load angles less than 45° (87). Analysis at design load level was performed due to the differences in design level to maximum capacity ratios for lateral and withdrawal. NDS Equation 11.4-1 can also be used to determine the reference design value of lag screws embedded at an angle to grain in the wood member and loaded in a direction normal to the wood member. For this condition, α, would be defined as the angle perpendicular to the fastener axis.

C11.4.2 Nails and Spikes

It is assumed that current adjustments for toe-nailed connections address the effects of combined lateral and withdrawal loading and do not require further modification.

Research on the effects of combined lateral and withdrawal loading on nailed connections (37) involved tests of Engelmann spruce, Douglas fir, and red oak single shear connections made with 8d common nails. Nail penetration depths of 6, 10, and 14 diameters into the main member and load angles of 0°, 90°, and six intermediate directions were investigated. Two tests were conducted at each load angle. The interaction equation found to best describe maximum connection load results for each species and penetration depth was of the form:

$$P = \frac{(1 + K \sin 2\alpha)(W'pZ')}{(W'p)\cos\alpha + (Z')\sin\alpha} \qquad \text{(C11.4.2-1)}$$

where:

  P = maximum load at angle to grain, α

  $W'p$ = maximum load at 90° (withdrawal load perpendicular to grain per inch of penetration in the main member times the penetration depth)

  Z' = maximum load at 0° (lateral load)

  α = angle between wood surface and direction of applied load, and

  K = factor based on least squares analysis of test data for each species-penetration group

The average value of K for the six species and penetration groups evaluated was 0.535, and ranged from 0.151 to 1.406. Average K values by species were 0.432, 0.864, and 0.309 for Douglas fir, Engelmann spruce, and red oak, respectively. When K is conservatively assumed to equal 0, Equation C11.4.2-1 reduces to NDS Equation 11.4-2 or, in another format the following:

$$\frac{R_W}{W'p} + \frac{R_Z}{Z'} \leq 1 \qquad \text{(C11.4.2-2)}$$

where:

  R_W = connection withdrawal force, and

  R_Z = connection lateral force.

C11.5 Adjustment of Reference Design Values

C11.5.1 Geometry Factor, C_Δ

C11.5.1.1 For fasteners with diameters less than 1/4", no reduction for geometry is specified.

C11.5.1.2 For fasteners with diameters equal to or greater than 1/4", the geometry factor provides a proportionate reduction of reference design values for less than full end distance or less than full spacing distance. The lowest geometry factor for any fastener applies to all other fasteners in that same connection, not just to the end fastener or a pair of fasteners in a row. It should be noted that further reductions may be necessary when checking stresses in members at connections (see NDS 10.1.2).

The requirement that fastener design values for multiple shear plane connections or asymmetric three member connections be based on the application of the lowest geometry factor for any shear plane to all fasteners in the joint assumes that the total joint capacity is proportional to the number of shear planes.

Edge Distance: Requirements in NDS Table 11.5.1A for parallel to grain loading of 1.5D or the greater of 1.5D or 1/2 the spacing between rows for ℓ/D greater than 6, and for loaded edge - perpendicular to grain loading of 4D are based on early research (146). The unloaded edge perpendicular to grain minimum of 1.5D is a good practice recommendation.

NDS Section 11.5.1 does not provide specific guidance on edge distance requirements for loads applied at angles other than 0° and 90°, nor does it provide specific geometry factors for reduced edge distances.

The ratio of the fastener length in side member to fastener diameter, ℓ/D, in NDS Table 11.5.1A is based on the total thickness of both wood side members when connections of three or more wood members are involved. For connections involving metal main or side members, only the ℓ/D ratio for the wood members are considered for determination of edge distance requirements in this section. Metal parts must still be designed per NDS 10.2.3.

Avoidance of heavy or medium suspended loads below the neutral axis of a beam was added as a result of several reported field problems involving structural glued laminated timber beams subject to a line of concentrated loads applied through bolted hangers or ledger strips attached in the tension zone or at the bottom edge of the beam. Concentrated loads less than 100 pounds and spaced more than 24" apart may be considered a light load condition.

For perpendicular to grain connections, the member is required to be checked for shear in accordance with NDS 3.4.3.3 using a reduced depth, d_e, equivalent to the beam depth, d, less the distance from the unloaded edge of the beam to the center of the nearest fastener.

End Distance: Requirements in NDS 11.5.1.2(a) and NDS Table 11.5.1B for parallel to grain loading are based on early recommendations (146). For tension loads (fasteners bearing toward the member end), the minimum end distances of 7D for softwoods and 5D for hardwoods for C_Δ = 1.0 were established by test. For compression loads (fasteners bearing away from the member end), the minimum end distance of 4D for C_Δ = 1.0 was based on the minimum spacing of fasteners in a row for C_Δ = 1.0 (146). End distances for angle to grain tension loadings may be linearly interpolated from those for perpendicular to grain and tension parallel to grain design values.

The provisions for use of reduced end distances for connections when proportionate reductions ($0.5 \leq C_\Delta \leq 1.0$) are made in design values are supported by early research (184, 181, 146) which showed a linear relationship between end distance and joint proportional limit strength. A subsequent study showed that a minimum end distance of only $5D$ was sufficient to develop the full proportional limit load of Douglas fir joints made with metal side plates and loaded in tension parallel to grain (119). Other research further substantiates the adequacy of the end distance requirements for connections loaded in both compression and tension parallel to grain (102, 110). End distances less than 50 percent of those required for $C_\Delta = 1.0$ are not allowed.

Shear Area: Requirements in NDS 11.5.1(b) are for members loaded at an angle to the fastener axis. End distance requirements are expressed in terms of equivalent shear areas. Shear area for such a joint is defined as the triangular area in the thickness plane of the member which is enclosed between the tip of the member and the centerline of the fastener (NDS Figure 11E). This shear area for the angled member is compared to the shear area of a joint in which both members are loaded perpendicular to the fastener axis (members parallel to each other) and which meet end distance requirements. The equivalent shear area for the parallel member joint is the product of the required end distance and the length of the fastener in the member.

As with end distance requirements for parallel member connections, reduced shear areas less than 50 percent of those required for $C_\Delta = 1.0$ are not allowed. It is recommended as good practice that the distance between the fastener axis and the inside juncture of the angled side member and the main member (see NDS Figure 11E) be at least $1.5D$.

Spacing Requirements for Fasteners in a Row: For fasteners in a row, the spacing requirements contained in NDS 11.5.1(c) and NDS Table 11.5.1C are assumed to be sufficient to cover the effects of non-uniform distribution of shear stresses through the thickness of the member (concentrated at the edges) that occur as the fastener bends (146). Reduced spacings less than 75 percent of those required for $C_\Delta = 1.0$ are not allowed.

If the direction of loading is perpendicular to grain, the minimum spacing for $C_\Delta = 1.0$ is based on the attached member. If the attached member is steel, then steel spacing controls from the appropriate steel standards (125). If the attached member is a wood member loaded parallel to grain, then parallel to grain spacing controls. If the attached member is wood loaded perpendicular to grain, then $4D$

should be adequate. Evaluating the wood members for shear per NDS 3.4.3.3 would also be advisable.

Spacing Requirements Between Rows: For perpendicular to grain loading, NDS Table 11.5.1D provisions are based on early research (146). These requirements relate the tendency of the fasteners to bend and cause non-uniform bearing stresses and the resistance of the wood between rows to resist splitting. It is for this reason that staggering of fasteners loaded perpendicular to grain is desirable (see NDS 11.6.1). In computing the ℓ/D ratio for determining the appropriate minimum spacing between rows for perpendicular to grain loading, the ratio for side members is based on the sum of the bearing length in each side member where three or more wood member joints are involved.

For parallel to grain loading, NDS Table 11.5.1D permits rows of fasteners to be spaced 1.5D; however, additional spacing may be required when installing bolts and lag screws to accommodate larger head and washer dimensions and clearance requirements for wrench sockets. Note that the steel industry recommends a minimum center-to-center spacing between holes of 2.67D, with a preferred distance of 3D (125).

For parallel or perpendicular to grain loading, limiting the maximum distance between outer rows of fasteners on the same splice plate to 5" was introduced to avoid splitting that could occur in members at connections as a result of restraint of shrinkage associated with drying in service.

The limitation on row spacing applies to metal as well as wood side plates, to members loaded perpendicular as well as parallel to grain, and to three or more member connections occurring at truss panel points.

C11.5.2 End Grain Factor, C_{eg}

C11.5.2.1 Reducing reference withdrawal design values for lag screws 25 percent when the screw is inserted in the end grain (radial-tangential plane) of the main member rather than the side grain (radial-longitudinal or tangential-longitudinal plane) is based on lag screw joint tests (100).

Early tests of wood screws in withdrawal from end grain surfaces of oak, southern pine, maple, and cypress gave somewhat erratic results relative to those for withdrawal from side grain (43). These irregular results were attributed to the tendency of the screw to split the wood in the end grain configuration. Average ratios of end grain withdrawal resistance to side grain withdrawal resistance ranged from 52 to 108 percent (43). Because of this variability, structural loading of wood screws in withdrawal from end grain has been prohibited. Where splitting is avoided, use of an end grain to side grain withdrawal design value ratio of 75 percent has been suggested (184, 183).

Reduction of withdrawal design values up to 50 percent have been reported for nails driven in end grain surfaces (radial-tangential plane) as compared to side grain (radial-longitudinal or tangential-longitudinal planes) surfaces (184, 118). When coupled with the effects of seasoning in service after fabrication, such reductions are considered too great for reliable design. It is considered to be on this basis that loading of nails and spikes in withdrawal from end grain has been prohibited.

C11.5.2.2 The use of a 0.67 adjustment factor on reference lateral design values for lag screws, wood screws, nails, or spikes driven in the end grain is based on early research on joints made with softwood species (181, 184).

C11.5.3 Diaphragm Factor, C_{di}

Diaphragms are large, flat structural units acting like a deep relatively thin beam or girder. Horizontal wood diaphragms consist of floor or roof decks acting as webs and lumber, structural glued laminated timber members, SCL, or I-joists acting as the flanges. Such assemblies distribute horizontal forces acting on the flanges to vertical resisting elements (103). Shear walls consisting of wall sheathing materials attached to top and bottom plates and vertical framing members also are diaphragms. Such shear walls or vertical diaphragms act to transfer loads from horizontal diaphragms down to the supporting foundation. The diaphragm factor, C_{di}, applies to both horizontal and vertical diaphragms (144, 145).

C11.5.4 Toe-Nail Factor, C_{tn}

C11.5.4.1 The 0.67 adjustment of reference withdrawal design values for toe-nailing is based on the results of joint tests comparing slant driving and straight driving (184) and of typical toe-nailed and end nailed joints used in frame wall construction (118) where the attached member is pulled directly away from the main member. It is applicable to joints fabricated at all levels of seasoning. This includes multiple nail joints fabricated of unseasoned wood and then loaded after seasoning (184, 183, 118). Toe-nailing with cross slant driving can produce stronger joints than end or face nailing. For example, a stud to plate joint made of four 8d toe-nails was reported to be stronger than the same joint made with two 16d end nails (181, 118). Where toe-nailed connections are resisting withdrawal, the depth of penetration of the nail in the member holding the point may be taken as the actual length of nail in the member as shown in Figure C11.5.4-1.

Figure C11.5.4-1 Effective Penetration and Side Member Thickness for Toe-Nails Subject to Lateral Loads

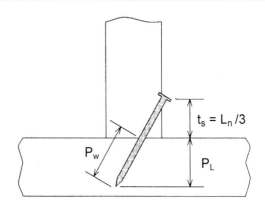

C11.5.4.2 The toe-nail factor of 0.83 is an adjustment based on the intermediate condition between the full lateral design value for side-grain connections and the full lateral design value for end grain conditions where $C_{eg} = 0.67$. Where toe-nailed connections are resisting lateral loads, the bearing length, L_m, of the nail in the member holding the point may be taken as the vertically projected length of nail in the member (see Figure C11.5.4-1) calculated as:

$$L_m = L_n cos30° - L_n/3 \qquad (C11.5.4-1)$$

where:

L_n = length of nail, in.

For purposes of establishing the single shear reference lateral design value applicable to a toe-nailed connection, the side member bearing length, L_s, of the nail (see Figure C11.5.4-1) shall be taken as:

$$L_s = L_n/3 \qquad (C11.5.4-2)$$

Equation C11.5.4-2 only applies to nails driven at an angle of approximately 30° to the face of the member being attached and 1/3 the nail length from the end of that member.

C11.6 Multiple Fasteners

C11.6.1 Symmetrically Staggered Fasteners

See C11.5.1.2 Spacing Requirements Between Rows.

C11.6.2 Fasteners Loaded at an Angle to Grain

General provisions for the placement and spacing of fasteners to cover all of the directions of loading and any number of members in a connection are beyond the scope of the Specification. For this reason, the gravity axis of all members must pass through the center of fastener resistance to maintain uniform stress in main members and uniform distribution of load to all fasteners. If it is not possible to achieve intersection of member gravity axes with the center of resistance of the fastener group, the designer has the responsibility to fully evaluate and account for the effects of the resultant eccentric loading on both the load-carrying capacity of the members and the capacity of the connection (see C10.1.3).

C11.6.3 Local Stresses in Connections

See C10.1.2.

COMMENTARY: DOWEL-TYPE FASTENERS

C12 SPLIT RING AND SHEAR PLATE CONNECTORS

C12.1 General

Background

Split ring and shear plate connectors act like dowels or keys in distributing loads from one member to another in a joint (184). The large diameters of the rings or plates, relative to the diameters of bolts, and the relatively shallow depth of the connectors in the members provide for increased bearing areas without penalizing reductions in net section areas. As a result, these connectors can develop significantly higher design values than those obtainable from bolts alone.

Split ring connectors are installed in precut grooves made with a special power-driven drill and cutting tool. They are used in wood-to-wood joints where high lateral joint loads are involved; such as in bowstring trusses, arches, and bridges. The bolt or lag screw passing through the center of the ring holds the faces of the joint members in contact.

Similar to split rings, shear plates are installed in precut grooves but are flush to the surface when fully seated. Two shear plates are the equivalent of one split ring, with the load being transferred from one plate to the other in the joint through shear in the bolt or lag screw. Shear plates are primarily used in wood-to-steel connections; such as steel gusset plate joints or column-foundation connections where the metal replaces one of the plates, and in demountable wood-to-wood connections, such as stadium bleachers (142).

The design provisions for split ring and shear plate connectors in the Specification are based on early research (104, 117).

C12.1.1 Terminology

A connector unit is expressed in terms of the metal parts required for a single shear plane. For a split ring connection, one ring is used in matching grooves in the members adjacent to one plane. For shear plate connections, two matching shear plates, one in appropriate grooves in each member, are used in wood-to-wood joints. In a wood-to-metal joint, the steel strap or plate replaces one of the shear plates. In all three cases, the bolt or lag screw tying the joint together is considered loaded in single shear. Where more than one connector unit is on the same bolt, as in the case of a three member joint where the main

member has connectors on the same bolt on both faces, an adjusted single shear design value for each shear plane is provided in the design value tables (see NDS Tables 12.2A and 12.2B).

C12.1.2 Quality of Split Ring and Shear Plate Connectors

C12.1.2.1 The split ring is wedge shaped (beveled toward the edges) to facilitate installation and assure a tight fit when fully seated. The diameter of the inside groove for the split ring is 2 percent larger than the inside diameter of the ring, thus requiring the ring to be sprung slightly when inserted. This provides for any subsequent shrinkage of the members and for simultaneous bearing of the inner surface of the connector against the inner core of wood created by the grooving operation and bearing of the outer surface of the connector on the opposite side against the outside wall of the groove (117, 142). The position of the tongue-slot joint in the ring relative to the direction of loading is not significant (117).

The two small perforations in the central portion of pressed steel shear plates serve to facilitate temporary attachment of the connector to the joint member when off-site fabrication is employed and in the erection and dismantling of temporary structures in the field. The perforations do not affect plate load-carrying performance.

C12.1.2.2 Design values in NDS Tables 12.2A and 12.2B correspond to the dimensions for split rings and shear plates, respectively, in NDS Appendix K. In addition to connector diameter, the depth of the connector in the member and its thickness affect joint load-carrying capacity. Only those split rings that have equivalent or larger inside diameter, metal depth, and metal thickness than those given in NDS Appendix K qualify for the connector design values provided in NDS Table 12.2A. Similarly, only those shear plates that have equivalent or larger plate diameter, plate depth, and plate thickness than those given in NDS Appendix K qualify for the connector design values provided in NDS Table 12.2B.

The projected areas given in NDS Appendix K for split rings are calculated as the sum of the inside groove diameter and twice the groove width times the groove depth. The projected areas for shear plates given in NDS

Appendix K are based on the groove diameter times the groove depth for the nominal shear plate dimensions shown. Tabulated projected areas for split ring and shear plate connectors given in NDS Appendix K are to be used in checking localized wood stresses in accordance with NDS 10.1.2 and NDS 12.3.7.3.

C12.1.2.3 Bolts used with split rings or shear plates are required to meet the quality provisions of NDS 11.1.2 for full body diameter bolts to prevent use of undersized fasteners that do not provide full bearing with the connectors.

C12.1.2.4 Lag screws used with split rings or shear plates are required to meet the quality provisions of NDS 11.1.3 for full body diameter lag screws to prevent use of undersized fasteners that do not provide full bearing with the connectors.

C12.1.3 Fabrication and Assembly

C12.1.3.1 Cutterheads should be designed specifically for the dimensions provided by the particular connector manufacturer.

C12.1.3.3 Washers may be used in shear plate connections involving steel straps and plates when use of a longer bolt or lag screw is necessary to avoid bearing of the threaded portion of the bolt or screw on the strap or plate.

C12.2 Reference Design Values

C12.2.1 Reference Design Values

Early connector tests of joints made with Douglas fir, southern pine, white oak, and other representative species showed that joint load-carrying capacity was directly related to the specific gravity of the wood members (184, 181, 104, 117).

Reference design values in NDS Tables 12.2A and 12.2B represent maximum joint test loads reduced by a factor of 3.6 that includes adjustments for variability and load duration (184, 181, 117). These reference design values, applicable to normal loading conditions, are considered to be less than 70 percent of proportional limit test loads (181, 117). Reference design values apply only to those joint designs which meet the minimum thickness requirements in NDS Tables 12.2A or 12.2B and the end distance, edge distance, and spacing requirements corresponding to $C_\Delta = 1.0$ in NDS Table 12.3. Net thickness requirements refer to the actual thickness of the member before grooving.

C12.1.3.4 Reference design values for split ring and shear plate connectors apply to joints in which the members are in contact, are fabricated of wood having a moisture content of 15 percent or lower to a depth of at least 3/4" from the surface, and will remain dry in service. Effects of normal variations in moisture content that occur in dry conditions of service are accounted for in the reference values.

When connectors are installed in unseasoned or partially seasoned wood intended for use in dry conditions of service, reference design values are to be adjusted in accordance with the factors in NDS 10.3.3. Such joints will need to be tightened as the members season in service by periodically turning down the nuts on the bolts until service equilibrium moisture content is reached.

It is good practice to exclude visible face knots within a distance of 1/2 the connector diameter along the grain from the edge of the connector unit (181, 117). Where visible knots are included within a 1/2 connector diameter distance of the critical section, the net section based on the projected area of the connector unit and bolt or screw should be further reduced for the cross-sectional area of such included knots (see NDS 3.1.2.3).

C12.2.1.1 Reference design values for split ring connections in NDS Table 12.2A and for shear plate connections in NDS Table 12.2B are given in terms of the number of faces a member has with a connector on the same bolt and on the thickness of that member. The lowest reference design value for the two members being joined is the reference design value for the shear plane.

C12.2.1.2 The 2,900 pound limit for the 2-5/8" shear plate is the maximum reference bearing load for a pressed steel plate without a reinforcing hub about the bolt hole. The 4,400 and 6,000 pound limit for the 4" plates used with 3/4" and 7/8" bolts, respectively, are the maximum reference shear design values for A307 bolts of these diameters. The 4" plates have integral re-enforcing hubs about the central bolt hole. The limiting values specified in footnote 2 of NDS Table 12.2B are based on metal strength; therefore, these metal parts should be designed per NDS 10.2.3. The strength of metal parts should not be adjusted by factors given in NDS 10.3.1 (e.g., ASD Load Duration Factor, C_D).

C12.2.2 Thickness of Wood Members

C12.2.2.1 The minimum member thicknesses required for use of the split ring and shear plate connector values in NDS Tables 12.2A and 12.2B, respectively, have been established from the results of joint tests (117).

C12.2.2.2 The provision for use of linear interpolation between minimum thicknesses and those required from maximum design values is based on the original connector research (117).

C12.2.3 Penetration Depth Factor, C_d

Adjustments for reduced lag screw penetration depths are permitted to be interpolated between the values for $C_d = 1.0$ and $C_d = 0.75$ using the corresponding penetrations, respectively, for each species group.

C12.2.4 Metal Side Plate Factor, C_{st}

Increases for metal side plates used with 4" shear plate connectors are based on original connector research involving claw plates (117). The increased values for 4" shear plates loaded parallel to grain are still limited by footnote 2 of NDS Table 12.2B.

C12.2.5 Load at Angle to Grain

Use of the standard bearing angle to grain equation (NDS Equation 12.2-1 and NDS Appendix J) to determine reference design values for split ring and shear plate connectors located in a shear plane that is loaded at an angle to grain between 0° and 90° are based on claw plate connector research (117). In this same study, tests of split ring connectors showed the relationship between maximum design value and grain angle could be described by a linear relationship without appreciable error. For consistency with the provisions for other fastener types, the standard angle to grain equation is conservatively used in the Specification to adjust both split ring and shear plate connector reference design values for grain angle.

C12.2.6 Split Ring and Shear Plate Connectors in End Grain

Design of connectors in end grain surfaces are frequently encountered in practice, such as those at the peak of A-frames or similar arches. Reference design values for split ring and shear plate connectors in end grain surfaces are keyed to use of a reference design value for connectors in square-cut end surfaces equal to 60 percent of the reference design value for connectors in side grain surfaces loaded perpendicular to grain.

The use of $0.60\ Q'$ as the reference design value for a square-cut end surface was originally based on experience with connector design with structural glued laminated timber (140). Available data from a comprehensive study of the capacity of shear plates in sloping grain end surfaces in Douglas fir (80) generally confirm the use of the 0.60 ratio. This ratio is slightly more conservative than the 0.67 value assumed for square-cut end surface design values in Canada (32, 75).

For split ring and shear plate connectors used in sloping end grain surfaces, the thickness of the member is taken as the distance between the edge of the connector and the nearest point on the outside edge of the member located on a line parallel to the bolt or lag screw axis. Where the end grain surface is square cut, the thickness of the member may be taken as the length of the lag screw in the member.

C12.3 Placement of Split Ring and Shear Plate Connectors

C12.3.1 Terminology

Edge and end distances and spacings for split ring and shear plate connectors are referenced to the center not the edge of the connectors.

C12.3.2 Geometry Factor, C_Δ

The geometry factor adjusts reference design values for use of end distances, edge distances, and/or spacings which are less than those required for $C_\Delta = 1.0$. The smallest geometry factor for any split ring or shear plate connector in a joint is to be applied to all connectors in that joint regardless of their alignment relative to one another.

C12.3.3 Edge Distance

C12.3.3.1 Connector edge distance requirements and related geometry factors in NDS Table 12.3 are based on the original connector research (117).

C12.3.3.2 The edge distance for the loaded edge establishes the geometry factor for edge distance that must be applied.

C12.3.4 End Distance

C12.3.4.1 The end distance requirements in NDS Table 12.3 are based on the original connector research (117). These requirements vary depending upon whether the member is being loaded in tension or compression, with the latter also differing depending upon whether loading is parallel or perpendicular to grain.

C12.3.4.2 Linear interpolation between tabulated end distances for parallel and perpendicular to grain loading is permitted to determine end distance requirements for members loaded at angles to grain between 0° and 90°.

C12.3.5 Spacing

C12.3.5.1 Spacing requirements in NDS Table 12.3 are based on the original connector research (117, 142) with the following two exceptions:

- The factor for the perpendicular loading and spacing case was dropped from 0.83 to 0.75 for purposes of uniformity.
- The geometry factor for minimum allowed spacings was reduced from 0.75 to 0.50 as part of an effort to simplify adjustment of connector design values for end distances and longitudinal spacing (181).

The original connector research indicated that the load-carrying capacity of a joint made with two or more connectors aligned parallel to grain and loaded perpendicular to grain was less than the sum of the maximum design values for the same connectors acting singly (181, 117). Staggering or offsetting of connectors so that they do not act along the same line along the grain of the transverse loaded member was found to give somewhat higher design values (181). When such offsetting is used, the line connecting the centers of two or more connectors located in the same contact face, the connector axis, φ, may not be oriented parallel or perpendicular to the grain of the member or to the direction of load, θ. Spacings intermediate to those given in NDS Table 12.3 for reduced and full reference design values are applicable to such cases. Because the variables involved are not linearly related, a graphical method has been developed for determining spacing requirements for designs for these cases where the connector axis is at an angle to the grain of the member (140, 142). This graphical method is based on numerical procedures (see C12.3.5.2).

Linear interpolation to establish geometry factors for spacings are permitted.

C12.3.5.2 The graphical method for determining minimum spacing requirements for members loaded at an angle to grain (140, 142) is based on numerical procedures. These procedures, which combine the effects of both variable connector axis angle, φ, and variable angle to grain loading, θ, are given below.

Minimum spacing, R, required for full reference design value for any connector axis angle, φ, between 0° and 90° and for any angle of load to grain, θ, between 0° and 90° is determined from the equation:

$$R = \frac{A\,B}{\sqrt{A^2\,sin^2\,\varphi\ +\ B^2\,cos^2\,\varphi}} \qquad (C12.3\text{-}1)$$

where:

A and B are spacing values selected from Table C12.3-1 for the applicable connector type and size and angle of load to grain.

The value of R determined from Equation C12.3-1 is the required spacing for $C_\Delta = 1.0$. The value of C from Table C12.3-1 is the minimum allowed spacing which is associated with $C_\Delta = 0.50$. For a load angle of 0°, values of A and B are the spacings from NDS Table 12.3 for the parallel spacing-parallel loading case. For a load angle of 90°, the values of A and B are the spacings from NDS Table 12.3 for the perpendicular spacing-perpendicular loading case.

For angles of load to grain, θ, intermediate to those tabulated, values of A and B may be obtained by linear interpolation. For actual spacing, S, between R and C, the geometry factor, $C_{\Delta s}$, is determined by linear interpolation or:

$$C_{\Delta s} = 0.50\ +\ \frac{(S - C)(1.0 - 0.50)}{(R - C)} \qquad (C12.3\text{-}2)$$

C12.3.6 Split Ring and Shear Plate Connectors in End Grain

C12.3.6.1 Procedures for establishing minimum and full reference design value spacing and edge and end distances for connectors in end grain surfaces follow the same logic as that employed to establish reference design values for such configurations in NDS 12.2.6.

C12.3.6.2 Shear capacity of members supported by connectors in end grain surfaces should be checked using provisions of NDS 3.4.3.3. Where the slope of the surface cut, α, is other than 90°, the component of the vertical force on the connector shear plane that is normal to the outside or uncut edge of the member should be taken as the shear force, V. The effective depth of the member, d_e, should be taken as the component of the distance from the loaded edge of the member to the unloaded edge of the connector that is normal to the outside or uncut edge of the member.

Table C12.3-1 Connector Spacing Values

Connector type and size	Angle of load to grain θ	A in.	B in.	C (min. for $C_\Delta = 0.5$) in.
2-1/2 in. split ring or 2-5/8 in. shear plate	0°	6-3/4	3-1/2	3-1/2
	15°	6	3-3/4	3-1/2
	30°	5-1/8	3-7/8	3-1/2
	45°	4-1/4	4-1/8	3-1/2
	60° to 90°	3-1/2	4-1/4	3-1/2
4 in. split ring or 4 in. shear plate	0°	9	5	5
	15°	8	5-1/4	5
	30°	7	5-1/2	5
	45°	6	5-3/4	5
	60° to 90°	5	6	5

C12.3.7 Multiple Split Ring or Shear Plate Connectors

C12.3.7.1 The group action factor, C_g, applies only to a row of two or more connectors which are in the same shear plane, are aligned in the direction of load, and are on separate bolts or lag screws (see C10.3.6). The factor need not be applied to connections involving two or more connector units on two or more contact faces concentric to the same bolt axis.

C12.3.7.2 When two sizes of split ring grooves are cut concentrically on the same wood surface and rings are installed in both grooves, the total load on the joint is limited to the reference design value for the larger ring only.

C12.3.7.3 Localized wood stresses should be checked in accordance with NDS 10.1.2.

C13 TIMBER RIVETS

C13.1 General

Timber rivets, also known as glulam rivets, were originally developed in Canada more than 35 years ago to connect pre-drilled steel plates to structural glued laminated timber (41). Typical applications include tension splices, beam hangers, and moment splices. The rivets have flattened-oval shanks with tapered heads that, when driven, wedge tightly into holes in the steel plate (see NDS Appendix M). The resulting head fixity adds to the strength and stiffness of the connection. The number of rivet rows in each plate and the number of rivets per row can both range from 2 to 20 (see NDS Figure 13A and NDS Tables 13.2.1 and 13.2.2).

The Specification presently limits use of timber rivets to attachment of steel side plates to structural glued laminated timber.

C13.1.1 Quality of Rivets and Steel Side Plates

Provisions of the Specification are applicable only to timber rivets that are hot-dipped galvanized. Rivets are made with fixed shank cross section and head dimensions (NDS Appendix M) and vary only by length.

Steel plates used in timber rivet connections must be a minimum of 1/8" thick and, when used in wet service conditions, must be hot-dipped galvanized. Strength reductions apply for steel plates less than 1/4" thick (see NDS Table 13.2.3). Due to rivet and plate hole dimensions and tolerances, fabrication of joints with plates greater than 1/4" is not practical and is generally avoided. Also, the reduced penetration of the rivet into the wood associated with greater plate thickness can limit connection capacity by reducing the area of wood available to resist the tension and shear loads being applied around the rivet group.

C13.1.2 Fabrication and Assembly

C13.1.2.1 Rivets, whose shank dimensions are nominally 1/4" by 1/8", must be driven with the wider dimension oriented parallel to the grain of the wood member. This orientation provides maximum connection capacity for both parallel and perpendicular to the grain loading and minimizes any splitting that may occur (41). Further, rivets are not driven flush with the plate but only to the point where the tapered heads wedge tightly into the predrilled holes in the plate. It is assumed that approximately 1/8"

of the rivet head will protrude from the face of the plate after driving (see NDS Appendix M).

To minimize splitting in rivet groups involving more than two rows and more than two rivets per row, rivets are driven around the perimeter first and then in successive inner rectangles toward the center.

C13.1.2.2 The limit on maximum penetration of rivets of 70 percent of wood member thickness is intended to prevent through splitting of the piece.

C13.1.2.3 Connections in which rivets driven through plates on both sides of a member penetrate beyond the midpoint of the member are not generally used. Where such overlap of rivets does occur, the length of overlap is limited to 20 percent of the member thickness (see NDS 13.1.2.2) and the rivets on both sides are required to be spaced (see NDS 13.3.1) as though they were all driven from one side. The capacity of the connection is then determined as if all rivets were driven from one side and with spacings parallel, s_p, and perpendicular, s_q, to grain (see NDS Figure 13A) determined as the distances between adjacent rivets (one from each side but assumed on one side) at their points. Under these provisions, NDS Equations 13.2-1 and 13.2-2 and NDS Tables 13.2.1A through 13.2.1F and 13.2.2A and 13.2.2B are entered with twice the number of rows and twice the number of rivets per row as those actually driven from one of the sides. Also, NDS Tables 13.2.1A through 13.2.1F are entered with the member dimension of a connection with only one plate, which as footnoted in these tables, is twice the thickness of the wood member.

The procedure for determining the capacity of plates on two sides with rivets overlapping is based on the derivation of the design methodology and supporting data for single plate connections.

C13.2 Reference Design Values

C13.2.1 Parallel to Grain Loading

Design equations for timber rivets are based on Canadian research (24, 47, 45, 48, 69). The ultimate load capacity of such connections are limited by rivet bending and localized crushing of wood at the rivets or by the tension or shear strength of the wood at the perimeter of the rivet group (45). As load is applied to the connection, end rivets carry a larger portion of the load than rivets in the center. As yielding occurs, the load is redistributed to the less-loaded fasteners, until at maximum connection load, all of the individual rivets are considered to have reached their ultimate bearing capacity (45). This mode of failure will occur as long as the tension and shear strengths of the wood around the group of rivets is sufficient to resist the total applied load. However, if shear failure of the wood on the side and bottom of the rivet group occurs, followed by tension failure at the interior end of the group perimeter, the block of wood into which the rivets have been driven can be pulled out of the member before the maximum rivet bending load has been reached (45). Thus timber rivet design loads are based on the lower of the maximum rivet bending load and the maximum load based on wood strength.

The constant and exponent in NDS Equation 13.2-1 are based on tests of single rivets in Douglas fir at penetrations of 1", 2", and 3" (47). The rivet capacity obtained from the equation represents average ultimate test values reduced by a factor of 3.36, the same factor used for test values limited by wood capacity and represents a 1.6 reduction for variability and 2.1 factor for load duration and factor of safety (45). NDS Equation 13.2-1 also includes an additional adjustment of 0.88 to account for specifying use of rivet of lower hardness and associated lower ultimate tensile and yield strength than the rivet used in the original research (48, 41). The change in rivet specification was made to avoid the possibility of hydrogen embrittlement occurring in service conditions involving high temperature and high humidity (48).

Because of the complexity of the equations used to check wood capacity in timber rivet connections loaded parallel to grain, only tabular values for a range of rivet penetrations, spacings, and rivet group sizes are given in the Specification (NDS Tables 13.2.1A through 13.2.1F). The loads in these tables are the lesser of the reference wood tension capacity or the reference wood shear capacity as determined from the equations developed in the original research and verified by tests of full-size connections representing a range of rivet group sizes and spacings in Douglas fir structural glued laminated timbers (45).

The maximum normal (tension) stress is checked assuming an area equal to the rivet penetration times the width of the rivet group. The induced stress on this area is calculated as a function of coefficients which are derived from equations involving the variables of rivets per row, number of rows, spacing between rivets, spacing between rows, and the ratio of member thickness to rivet penetration (45). The lower the ratio, the larger the load component resisted by the normal stress and the lower the load component resisted by shear stress. It is this effect that is being accounted for by entering NDS Tables 13.2.1A through 13.2.1F with a wood member dimension for a single plate connection which is twice the member thickness of a connection with plates on both sides.

In the original research involving evaluation of rivet connections made with Douglas fir members, an average ultimate tension stress parallel to grain of 5600 psi was found in connections whose ultimate load was either a result of rivet bending or wood shear failure (45). For determination of reference connection capacity limited by normal stress, this tension ultimate was reduced to 1600 psi to account for variability (1.6) and load duration and factor of safety (approximately 2.1).

The maximum shear stress in the rivet connection is checked assuming an area equal to twice the rivet penetration times the length of the rivet group. The load on this area is calculated as a function of coefficients which are based on different equations but involving the same variables as those used to determine normal stress plus end distance. These equations account for shear resistance on the bottom of the rivet group acting on the plane at the rivet tips as well as the lateral shear on the sides by proportioning the total shear loads carried by the bottom and side surfaces (45).

Rather than use shear stress values based on the ASTM D143 block shear specimen, the reference shear stress used in the shear checking equation for rivet connections was developed using a Weibull weakest link model in which strength is inversely related to volume. Based on experimental data, it was determined that the shear strength of a unit volume of Douglas fir under uniform shear at 0.5 survival probability was 2526 psi (45). Employing this value in the equation developed in the original research for maximum lateral shear stress and reducing the equation constants by a factor of 3.36 (1.6 variability and 2.1 load duration and factor of safety) gives a reference shear stress for evaluating shear loads in rivet connections of 743 psi. As verification of the shear checking equation, a mean ratio of estimated to observed ultimate loads of 1.03 was obtained for eight rivet connection configurations in Douglas fir that exhibited wood shear failure. Test connections involved configurations containing 25, 50, 100, and 150 rivets and rivet spacings of 1/2", 1", and 1-1/2" (45).

It is to be noted that calculated P_r values and P_w values tabulated in NDS Tables 13.2.1A through 13.2.1F apply to connections made with 1/4" side plates and to one plate with associated rivets. For connections with thinner side plates, the adjustments in NDS Table 13.2.3 apply. Where connections involve plates on two sides of the wood member, the limiting P_r or applicable tabular P_w value is doubled to determine the reference capacity of the connection.

Because of the species test results and property values used to develop the rivet bending and wood capacity equations, use of reference design values based on the provisions of NDS 13.2.2 should be limited to Douglas fir-Larch and southern pine structural glued laminated timber.

C13.2.2 Perpendicular to Grain Loading

As with parallel to grain loading, design loads for timber rivet connections in which the loads act perpendicular to the grain of the wood member are based on the lower of the maximum rivet bending load and the maximum load based on wood strength. However, strength in tension perpendicular to grain is the controlling wood property rather than tension parallel and shear strength properties. The mode of wood failure in the perpendicular load case is a separation along the grain just above the first line of rivets nearest the unloaded edge, as contrasted to the pull out of the block of wood containing the rivet group that occurs in the parallel load case (45).

NDS Equation 13.2-2 is the same as that for the parallel to grain loading case (NDS Equation 13.2-1) except for the value of the constant, 160 compared to 280. The ratio of the two values (0.57) represents the ratio of the average ultimate lateral load-carrying capacities of single rivet joints in Douglas fir structural glued laminated test specimens loaded perpendicular to grain and parallel to grain (47, 69).

The wood capacity of rivet connections loaded perpendicular to the grain is a function of penetration, number and configuration of rivets, rivet spacings, and unloaded edge distance (45). Checking equations assume the connection load acts on an area equal to the width of the rivet group times the rivet penetration. However, the distribution of stress is not uniform over this area, but is a maximum at the surface of the member and decreases sharply along the penetration depth and on either side of the center of the rivet group (24). This non-uniform distribution is accounted for in the basic design equations.

Based on tests that showed tension perpendicular to grain strength decreases with increase in cross-sectional area and/or length, a Weibull brittle fracture model was used to establish a reference wood stress for checking wood capacity in rivet connections loaded perpendicular to grain. Using results from tests of blocks cut from Douglas fir structural glued laminated timber beams and ranging from 16 to 3600 in.^{3} in volume, a tension perpendicular to grain strength for unit volume under uniform stress at a 95 percent survival probability of 267 psi was established (24). Reducing this value by a factor of 2.1 for load duration and factor of safety gives a reference tension perpendicular to grain stress of 127 psi. This unit value is adjusted in the checking equations for volume through introduction of a variable based on the distance between the unloaded edge of the member and the first line of rivets in the connection.

In lieu of presenting the complex equations required to determine wood capacity for perpendicular to grain loading, a simplified equation (NDS Equation 13.2-3) is given in the Specification enabling such capacity to be calculated for any rivet penetration and plate thickness using loads and factors from NDS Tables 13.2.2A and 13.2.2B that account for the effects of a range of rivet configurations, spacings, and unloaded edge distances. The unit load values given in NDS Table 13.2.2A include an adjustment factor to account for stress distribution effects in connections with two side plates; thus the load values in this table are conservative for a single plate application. It is to be noted that NDS Equations 13.2-2 and 13.2-3 provide reference design values for connections with one side plate. Reference design values obtained from either equation are doubled for connections having two side plates.

Because of the species test results and property values used to develop the rivet bending and wood capacity equations, use of reference design values based on the provisions of NDS 13.2.2 should be limited to Douglas fir-Larch and southern pine structural glued laminated timber.

C13.2.3 Metal Side Plate Factor, C_{st}

Supporting experimental data for timber rivet design equations involved tests of connections made with 1/4" thick steel side plates (45, 69). Use of thinner plates reduces the amount of fixity of the rivet head which in turn reduces rivet bending capacity.

Reference design values determined in accordance with NDS 13.2.1 and 13.2.2 assume 1/4" side plates are used. For connections made with 3/16" and 1/8" plates, reference design values based on rivet capacity (P_r and Q_r) are adjusted by the side plate factors of 0.90 and 0.80 given in NDS Table 13.2.3.

C13.2.4 Load at Angle to Grain

The equation for calculating reference design values for timber rivet connections loaded at angles to grain other than 0° and 90° is the same form as the bearing angle to grain equation (see NDS Appendix J).

C13.2.5 Timber Rivets in End Grain

The 50 percent reduction for timber rivets used in end grain is based on Canadian design practice (41). It can be compared with the end grain adjustment factor of 0.67 for nails and spikes (see C11.5.2).

C13.2.6 Design of Metal Parts

Timber rivet connections can carry relatively high loads. It is the responsibility of the designer to assure the metal side plates on such connections are of adequate strength to carry the total load being transferred.

C13.3 Placement of Timber Rivets

C13.3.1 Spacing Between Rivets

See C13.3.2.

C13.3.2 End and Edge Distance

Effects of rivet spacing and edge and end distances have been evaluated using the basic rivet design equations (45). For parallel to grain loading and with other variables constant, wider rivet spacings are associated with the rivet bending failure mode while closer spacings induce wood shear failures. Similarly, with other factors constant, longer end distances allow rivet bending to control while shorter end distances cause wood shear capacity to control.

Minimum spacings and minimum end and edge distance requirements given in NDS 13.3 and NDS Table 13.3.2 minimize the occurrence of premature wood failure in favor of more ductile rivet yielding based on Canadian design standards (41).

C14 SHEAR WALLS AND DIAPHRAGMS

C14.1 General

Shear walls and diaphragms are assemblies that are designed to transfer in-plane lateral forces. Any sheathed assembly provides some level of resistance to in-plane forces. In structural applications, properly designed and constructed sheathed wall, floor, and roof assemblies can be used to resist high lateral loads from such events as hurricanes and earthquakes. Specific design of shear walls and diaphragms are covered in a separate specification entitled *Special Design Provisions for Wind and Seismic (SDPWS)* (124).

C15 SPECIAL LOADING CONDITIONS

C15.1 General

C15.1.1 Lateral Distribution of a Concentrated Load for Moment

The lateral distribution of concentrated loads is particularly important to obtain efficient design of bending members in structures such as bridges and warehouse or industrial buildings where heavy wheel loads are involved. Easily applied methods for determining the maximum moment and maximum shear in bending members subject to concentrated wheel loads are given in NDS 15.1. These methods, which are based on the thickness of the flooring or decking involved (2" to 6" thick) and the spacing of the beams or stringers, have long been used in timber bridge design (129). The procedures have been verified through test and shown to be generally conservative, particularly when the portion of the load distributed to adjacent members is 40 percent or less (42).

The lateral distribution factors for moment in NDS Table 15.1.1 are keyed to the stiffness of the flooring or decking through use of nominal thickness and spacing of beams. These factors are based on recommendations of the American Association of State Highway and Transportation Officials (129). For cases where the factor exceeds 1.0 (S/denominator > 1.0), the load is assumed to be fully on the beam. Where the concentrated load is applied to the deck between the beams, the load is distributed to the adjacent beams assuming the deck acts as a simply supported beam. For cases where the factor is less than or equal to 1.0 and the concentrated load is applied to the deck between the beams, provisions of NDS 15.1.1 can be conservatively used or a more rigorous method of analysis should be considered.

The 2" plank floor refers to one made of pieces of lumber laid edge to edge with the wide faces bearing on the supporting beams or stringers. The 4" and 6" laminated floors refer to those made of pieces of lumber laid face to face with the narrow edges bearing on the supporting beams or stringers, with each piece being nailed to the preceding piece (129). Nails typically penetrate into two adjacent pieces, are staggered, and are alternated on the top and bottom edges (42). Flooring is typically attached to stringers by toe-nailed connections.

The lateral distribution factors apply to bridges designed for one traffic lane and to interior beams and stringers only. The computed factor gives the fraction of the wheel load (both front and rear of tractor or trailer axles on one side) positioned to give maximum bending moment at mid-span of the beam or stringer closest to the wheel load (129, 42).

The live load bending moment for outside beams or stringers is calculated using a load equal to the reaction of the wheel load assuming the flooring or decking between the outside and adjacent stringer is acting as a simply supported beam (129).

Lateral distribution factors determined in accordance with NDS Table 15.1.1 can be used for any type of fixed or moving concentrated load. The lateral distribution factors determined from the table have been verified by field tests on five timber bridges ranging from 15 to 46 feet in span and by laboratory tests on three full-size bridge deck and stringer assemblies 16 to 28 feet in span (42). These tests indicate the factors are somewhat conservative, particularly at ratios greater than 0.60.

For bridges of two or more traffic lanes, the American Association of State Highway and Transportation Officials (129) provides other lateral distribution factors.

Generally all designs involving multiple parallel bending members that are loaded through transverse elements such as flooring, decking, or sheathing are capable of some lateral distribution of a concentrated load on one member to adjacent members on either side. The repetitive member factor (see NDS 4.3.9, 7.3.6, 8.3.7) partially accounts for such load redistribution.

C15.1.2 Lateral Distribution of a Concentrated Load for Shear

The lateral distribution factors for shear relate the lateral distribution of concentrated load at the center of the beam or stringer span as determined under NDS 15.1.1, or by other means, to the distribution of load at the quarter points of the span. The quarter points are considered to be near the points of maximum shear in the stringers for timber bridge design.

The tabulated values of the percentage of a concentrated load on the center beam at the quarter point of the span and the percentage of the same load on the center beam at midspan is closely described by the following relation:

$$P_{1/4} = -1.807 + 1.405 \log (P_m) \qquad \text{(C15.1-1)}$$

where:

$P_{1/4}$ = percentage of load at 1/4 point of center beam

P_m = percentage of load at mid-span of center beam

= S/denominator from NDS Table 15.1.1 or other basis

Values of $P_{1/4}$ from NDS Table 15.1.2 are used to determine the actual shear stress from the wheel or other concentrated load being considered. Field and laboratory tests of full-size timber bridges verify the appropriateness of the NDS Table 15.1.2 values and indicate they are conservative at S/denominator ratios above 0.50 (42).

C15.2 Spaced Columns

C15.2.1 General

Spaced columns refer to two or more individual members oriented with their longitudinal axis parallel, separated at the ends and in the middle portion of their length by blocking, and joined at the ends by split ring or shear plate connectors capable of developing required shear resistance (181). The end-fixity developed by the connectors and end blocks increases the buckling resistance of the individual members in the direction perpendicular to the wide faces when loaded in compression parallel to grain (parallel to the d_1 dimension in NDS Figure 15A).

C15.2.1.1 In the design of spaced columns, the adjusted compression stress for an individual member is determined in accordance with the provisions of NDS 15.2 and other applicable provisions of the Specification. The actual compression stress parallel to grain, f_c, on the members of the spaced column is not to exceed the adjusted compression design value parallel to grain, F_c', for these members based on all provisions of NDS 3.6 and 3.7 except as modified or extended by the provisions of NDS 15.2. The net section requirements of NDS 3.6.3 are to be applied to the members of spaced columns.

C15.2.1.2 The advantage of a spaced column is the increase in the critical buckling design value for compression members obtained by the partial end-fixity of the individual members. This increase in capacity, 2-1/2 or 3 times the value for a solid column with the same slenderness ratio, applies only to buckling in the direction perpendicular to the wide face of the members (buckling limited by the ℓ_1/d_1 ratio). If there was no slip in the end connections and full fixity of the ends were provided by the end block fastenings, the buckling stress would be four times that of a solid column because of the 50 percent reduction in effective column length (141).

The increase in the critical buckling stress associated with the ℓ_1/d_1 slenderness ratio obtained through the use of spaced column design may make capacity in the direction parallel to the wide face of the members (buckling associated with the ℓ_2/d_2 ratio) the limiting case. The adjusted compression design value parallel to grain in this direction is not affected by spacing the individual members and, therefore, must be checked in accordance with NDS 3.7.

C15.2.2 Spacer and End Block Provisions

C15.2.2.1 Where more than one spacer block is used, the distance ℓ_3 (see NDS Figure 15A) is the distance from the center of one spacer block to the centroid of the connectors in the nearest end block.

C15.2.2.2 Spacer blocks located within the middle 1/10 of the column length are not required to be joined to the compression members by split ring or shear plate connectors. Such blocks should be fastened to assure the compression members maintain their spacing under load (181). A web member joined by connectors to two truss chords making up a spaced truss chord (spaced column) may be considered a spacer block.

Where it is not feasible to use a single middle spacer block, two or more spacer blocks joined to compression members by split ring or shear plate connectors may be required to meet the ℓ_3/d_1 ratio limit of 40 (see NDS 15.2.3.2). Connectors used in such spacer blocks must meet the same requirements as those applicable to end blocks and the distance between two adjacent spacer blocks is not to exceed 1/2 the distance between the centroids of connectors in the end blocks. Connectors are required for spacer blocks not located in the middle of the column length to provide the shear resistance necessary to assure the two members act as a unit under load.

C15.2.2.3 Spaced columns are used as compression chords in bowstring and other large span trusses (141). In this case, the web members of the truss serve as the end blocks. The distance between panel points, which are laterally supported, is taken as the length of such columns. Spaced-column web members may be designed using the procedures of NDS 15.2 if the joints at both ends of the web member are laterally supported.

C15.2.2.4 The thickness of end and spacer blocks is required to be equal to or larger than the thickness of the compression members and meet the minimum requirements for split ring or shear plate connections in NDS Chapter 12 (181). The length of end blocks and spacer blocks located at other than mid-length of the column should be sufficient to meet the end distance requirements for split ring or shear plate connectors given in NDS Chapter 12. In this regard, the load on the connectors in the end blocks shall be considered applied in either direction parallel to the longitudinal axes of the compression members.

C15.2.2.5 Connectors used in spaced columns are designed to restrain differential displacement between the individual compression members. Since the forces causing differential movement decrease as the ℓ/d of the individual members decrease, connector design value requirements vary with slenderness ratio (181).

The equations for end spacer block constants in NDS 15.2.2.5 are based on K_S of zero when $\ell_1/d_1 \leq 11$ and a K_S equal to 1/4 of the clear wood compression design value parallel to grain for the species group when ℓ_1/d_1 is $\geq$ 60 (181). The equations give K_S values for intermediate slenderness ratios based on linear interpolation between these limits.

The limiting K_S values of 468, 399, 330, and 261 for species groups A, B, C, and D (defined in NDS Table 12A), respectively, represent 1/4 the normal load, unseasoned clear wood compression design value parallel to grain applicable to representative species in each group in 1955 (181). The representative species were dense Douglas fir and dense southern pine for Group A, Douglas fir and southern pine for Group B, western hemlock for Group C, and white firs-balsam fir for Group D.

The connector or connectors on each face of each end spacer block should be able to carry a load equal to the cross-sectional area of one of the individual compression members (without reduction for cuts made to receive connectors) times the end spacer block constant, K_S.

C15.2.3 Column Stability Factor, C$_P$

C15.2.3.1 Effective column length for spaced columns is determined in accordance with NDS Figure 15A and adjusted by any applicable buckling length coefficient, K_e, greater than one as specified in NDS Appendix G. It is to be noted that ℓ_1 is the distance between points of lateral support restraining movement perpendicular to the wide faces of the individual members, and ℓ_2 is the distance between points of lateral support restraining movement parallel to the wide faces of the individual members. ℓ_1 and ℓ_2 are not necessarily equal.

C15.2.3.2 The slenderness ratio, ℓ_1/d_1, limit of 80 for the individual members is a conservative good practice recommendation recognizing that the individual members are continuous at the bracing locations. The limit of 50 on the slenderness ratio ℓ_2/d_2 is the limit applied to solid columns (see NDS 3.7.1.4). The limit of 40 on the ℓ_3/d_1 ratio also is a conservative good practice recommendation to assure the length between end and spacer blocks in a spaced column is not a controlling factor in the column design.

C15.2.3.3 The column stability factor for an individual member in a spaced column is calculated using the slenderness ratio ℓ_1/d_1 and the same equation as that applicable to solid columns (see NDS 3.7.1.5) except that the critical buckling design value for compression, F_{cE}, is modified by the spaced column fixity coefficient, K_x.

The actual compression stress parallel to grain, F_c, calculated by dividing the total load on the spaced column by the sum of the cross-sectional areas of the individual members, is checked against the product, F_c', of the column stability factor, C_P, the reference compression design value parallel to grain, F_c, and all other applicable adjustment factors (see NDS 2.3). If connectors are required to join spacer (interior) blocks to individual members, and such blocks are in a part of the column that is most subject to potential buckling, f_c is to be calculated using the reduced or net section area remaining at the connector location (see NDS 3.1.2) when comparing with the C_P adjusted compression design value parallel to grain, F_c'.

In spaced column designs, the actual compression stress parallel to grain, f_c, based on the net section area of the individual members at the end blocks is checked against the product of the reference compression design value parallel to grain and all applicable adjustment factors except the column stability factor (see NDS 3.6.3).

C15.2.3.4 Use of the lesser adjusted compression design value parallel to grain, F_c', for a spaced column having members of different species or grades for all members is conservative. Where the design involves the use of compression members of different thicknesses, the F_c' value for the thinnest member is to be applied to all other members.

C15.2.3.5 The actual compression stress parallel to grain, f_c, in spaced columns also is to be checked in all cases against the adjusted compression design value parallel to grain, F_c', based on the slenderness ratio ℓ_2/d_2 and a C_P factor calculated in accordance with the provisions of NDS 3.7 without use of the spaced column fixity coefficient, K_x. Use of connectors to join individual compression members through end blocks is assumed to only increase the load-carrying capacity of spaced columns in a direction perpendicular to the wide face of the members. When the ratio of the width to thickness of the individual compression members is less than the square root of the spaced column fixity coefficient, K_x, the adjusted compression stress parallel to grain, F_c', based on the slenderness ratio ℓ_2/d_2 may control.

C15.2.3.6 See C3.7.1.6.

C15.2.3.7 Design provisions for spaced beams joined by end blocks and connectors are not included in the Specification. The beam-column equations of NDS 3.9 therefore apply only to those spaced columns that are subject to loads on the narrow edges of the members that cause bending in a plane parallel to their wide face.

C15.3 Built-Up Columns

As with spaced columns, built-up columns obtain their efficiency by increasing the buckling resistance of the individual laminations. The smaller the amount of slip occurring between laminations under compressive load, the greater the relative capacity of that column compared to a solid column of the same slenderness ratio made with the same quality of material. Based on tests of columns of various lengths (114, 116), the capacity of two equivalent column types can be expressed as a percentage of the strength of a solid column made with material of the same grade and species. For mechanically connected built-up columns, efficiencies ranged from a value of 82 percent at an ℓ/d ratio of 6, decreasing to a low of 65 percent at an ℓ/d of 18, and then increasing to 82 percent at an ℓ/d of 26.

The NDS design provisions for built-up columns made with various types of mechanical fasteners are based on more recent modeling and testing (82, 83). This model can be used to determine the strength of any built-up column on the basis of the slip between members of the column in both the elastic and inelastic ranges. The theoretical formulas were verified through extensive testing including 400 column tests and evaluation of the load-slip properties of 250 different types of connections. The formulas are entered with fastener load-slip values based on beam-on-elastic-foundation principles (71).

C15.3.1 General

The provisions of NDS 15.3 apply only to multi-ply columns in which the laminations are of the same width and are continuous along the length. The limitations on number of laminations are based on the range of columns that were tested (83) that met the connection requirements of NDS 15.3.3 and 15.3.4. The minimum lamination thickness requirement assures use of lumber for which reference design values are available in the Specification.

C15.3.2 Column Stability Factor, C_P

Provisions in NDS 15.3.2 are the same as those applicable to solid columns in NDS 3.7.1 except for the addition of the column stability coefficients, K_f, in NDS Equation 15.3-1.

When nailed in accordance with the provisions of NDS 15.3.3, the capacity of built-up columns has been shown to be more than 60 percent of that of an equivalent solid column at all ℓ/d ratios (82). Efficiencies are higher for columns in the shorter ($\ell/d < 15$) and longer ($\ell/d > 30$) slenderness ratio ranges than those for columns in the intermediate range.

The efficiency of bolted built-up columns conforming to the connection requirements of NDS 15.3.4 is more than 75 percent for all ℓ/d ratios (82). As with nailed columns, efficiencies of short and long bolted built-up columns are higher than those for intermediate ones. The greater efficiency of bolted compared to nailed columns is reflective of the higher load-slip moduli obtainable with bolted connections.

In accordance with NDS 3.7.1.3, NDS Equation 15.3-1 is entered with a value of F_{cE} based on the larger of ℓ_{e1}/d_1 or ℓ_{e2}/d_2, where d_2 is the dimension of the built-up member across the weak axis of the individual laminations (sum of the thicknesses of individual laminations). Research (82) has shown that buckling about the weak axis of the individual laminations is a function of the amount of slip and load transfer that occurs at fasteners between laminations.

When the controlling slenderness ratio is the strong axis of the individual laminations, ℓ_{e1}/d_1, then $K_f = 1.0$. It is also necessary to compare C_p based on ℓ_{e1}/d_1 and $K_f = 1.0$ with C_p based on ℓ_{e2}/d_2 and $K_f = 0.6$ or 0.75 to determine the adjusted compression design value parallel to grain, F_c'.

Due to the conservatism of using a single factor for all ℓ_{e2}/d_2 ratios, F_c' values for individual laminations designed as solid columns can be greater than F_c' values for built-up columns for relatively small ℓ_{e2}/d_2 ratios. In these cases, the column capacity should not be limited to the built-up column capacities.

C15.3.3 Nailed Built-Up Columns

C15.3.3.1 Nailing requirements in NDS 15.3.3.1(a), (b), and (g) and the maximum spacing requirements of (d) and (e) are based on the conditions for which the column stability coefficient, K_f, of 60 percent was established (82). The maximum spacing between nails in a row of six times the thickness of the thinnest lamination minimizes the potential for buckling of the individual laminations between connection points. End, edge, and minimum spacing requirements are good practice recommendations for preventing splitting of members (32) and for assuring fasteners are well distributed across and along the face of the laminations.

The requirement for adjacent nails to be driven from opposite sides of the column applies to adjacent nails aligned both along the grain of the laminations and across their width.

In the nailing requirements of NDS 15.3.3.1, a nail row refers to those nails aligned parallel to the grain of the laminations and in the direction of the column length. Where only one longitudinal row of nails is required, such nails are required to be staggered along either side of the center line of the row. Adjacent offset nails in such a con-figuration should be driven from opposite faces.

Where three rows of nails are required by spacing and edge distance requirements, nails in adjacent rows are to be staggered and adjacent nails beginning with the first in each row driven from opposite sides as if nails were aligned across the face of the laminations.

C15.3.4 Bolted Built-Up Columns

C15.3.4.1 Maximum spacing limits for bolts and rows, and number of row requirements in NDS 15.3.4.1(d), (e), and (g), respectively, are based on conditions for which the bolted built-up column efficiency factor, K_f, was established (82). Maximum end distance limits in (c) are good practice recommendations (32) to assure end bolts are placed close to the ends of the column where interlaminar shear forces are largest. Minimum end distance, spacing between adjacent bolts in a row, spacing between rows, and edge distance in (c), (d), (e), and (f) correspond to provisions governing bolted joints in NDS 11.5.

As with nailed columns, a bolt row refers to those bolts aligned parallel to the grain of the laminations and in the direction of the column length. The maximum spacing of bolts in a row of six times the lamination thickness minimizes the potential for buckling of individual laminations between connection points.

C15.4 Wood Columns with Side Loads and Eccentricity

C15.4.1 General Equations

Equations for wood columns are based on theoretical analyses (186). The equations in NDS 15.4.1 for combined bending and eccentric axial compression loads are an expansion of the interaction equation given in NDS 3.9.2 to the general case of any combination of side loads, end loads, and eccentric end loads (189).

For the case of a bending load on the narrow face and an eccentric axial load producing a moment in the same direction as the bending load, the general interaction equation in NDS 15.4-1 reduces to:

$$\left(\frac{f_c}{F_c'}\right)^2 +$$

$$\frac{f_{b1} + f_c(6e_1/d_1)[1 + 0.234(f_c/F_{cE1})]}{F_{b1}'[1-(f_c/F_{cE1})]} \leq 1.0 \quad (C15.4\text{-}1)$$

or

$$\left(\frac{f_c}{F_c'}\right)^2 +$$

$$\frac{f_{b1} + f_c(6e_1/d_1)[1.234 - 0.234C_{m1}]}{C_{m1}F_{b1}'} \leq 1.0 \quad (C15.4\text{-}2)$$

where:

e_1 = eccentricity

C_{m1} = moment magnification factor = $1 - f_c / F_{cE1}$

C15.4.2 Columns with Side Brackets

The procedure for calculating the portion of an axial load applied through a bracket that is assumed to act as a side load at mid-height of the column is based on early recommendations (184). The application of a side load, P_s, acting at mid-span of a simply supported beam is assumed to produce a maximum moment ($P_s\ell/4$) equal to 3/4 of the moment produced by the eccentric load on the bracket, Pa, times the ratio of the bracket height (ℓ_p) to the column length (ℓ).

When the bracket is at the top of the column, results obtained by entering NDS Equation 15.4-1 (or NDS Equation 3.9-3) with a concentric axial load and the calculated side load, P_s, will give a 25 percent lower combined stress index than that obtained from the eccentric axial end load formula, NDS Equation 15.4-2. This difference is a result of the latter being based on the assumption of eccentric loads on both ends of the column (constant moment along the length of the column) whereas the procedure in NDS 15.4.2 assumes the moment due to the bracket load decreases linearly from the point of application to zero at the column base.

C16 FIRE DESIGN OF WOOD MEMBERS

C16.1 General

The design provisions in the Specification are intended for use in allowable stress design (ASD). For load and resistance factor design (LRFD) there are currently no standardized loads for use in an accidental fire loading condition.

Introduction to Fire Design

The model building codes in the US cover virtually every safety-related topic related to the construction of buildings, and fire-related issues comprise a surprisingly large portion of the model codes. Designing for fire safety is a complex and multi-faceted issue. The following information provides an overview of the subject.

To provide fire safety in any structure, many approaches are considered. This involves a combination of (1) preventing fire occurrence by reducing potential ignition sources, (2) controlling fire growth, and (3) providing protection to life and property. All need systematic attention to provide a high degree of economical fire safety. The building design professional can control fire growth within the structure by generating plans that include features such as protecting occupants, confining fire in compartment areas, and incorporating fire suppression and smoke or heat venting devices at critical locations.

Controlling construction features to facilitate rapid egress, protection of occupants in given areas, and preventing fire growth or spread are regulated by codes as a function of building occupancy. If the design professional rationally blends protection solutions for these items with the potential use of a fire-suppression system (sprinklers, for example), economical fire protection can be achieved.

Although attention could be given to all protection techniques available to the building design professional, this discussion is limited to the provisions that limit fire growth and limit spread of fire to neighboring compartments or buildings.

Fire-Rated Assemblies

The previous section explained that some occupancies require the use of fire-rated assemblies or members to prevent collapse or fire spread from one compartment of a building to another or from one building to another.

Members and assemblies are rated for their ability either to continue to carry design loads during fire exposure or to prevent the spread of fire through them. Such ratings are arrived at either by calculation or experiment for both members and assemblies. The standard fire exposure is defined in ASTM E119. A 1-hour fire-resistance rating for wall, floor, and floor-ceiling assemblies incorporating nominal 2" structural lumber can be accomplished through the use of fire-resistive membranes such as gypsum wallboard. However, fastening of these surface materials is critical for assembly performance and is carefully specified. For some wood assemblies, 2-hour ratings have been achieved.

Experimental ratings are available for several generic assemblies. Ratings for proprietary assemblies are typically supplied by the producers. Typically rated floor-ceiling assemblies for various products are provided in the product chapters of the *ASD/LRFD Manual for Engineered Wood Construction*. AF&PA's *DCA No. 3 - Fire Rated Wood Floor and Wall Assemblies,* available at http://www.awc.org, also provides information on code recognized 1- and 2-hour fire rated wood-frame floor and wall assemblies.

Analytically Rated

In lieu of experimentally rating the fire endurance of members and assemblies, major building codes will accept engineering calculations of the expected fire endurance, based upon engineering principles and material properties. This applies to the rating of previously untested members or assemblies, or in cases where it is desired to substitute one material or component for another. Although calculation procedures may be conservative, they have the advantage of quickly rating an assembly or member and allowing interpolation or some extrapolation of expected performance. Additional details regarding the analytical approach are provided in AF&PA's *DCA No. 4 - Component Additive Method (CAM) for Calculating and Demonstrating Assembly Fire Endurance*, available at http://www.awc.org.

C

Beams and Columns

Heavy timber construction has traditionally been recognized to provide a fire-resistant building. This is primarily due to the large size of the members, the connection details, and the lack of concealed spaces. Such a construction type has often satisfied the fire-resistive requirement in all building codes by simple prescription. Although heavy timber construction has not been "rated" in the United States, Canada has assigned it a 45-minute fire-endurance rating.

Using calculations, glulam timber columns and beams can be designed for desired fire-endurance ratings. Additional details regarding the analytical approach are provided in *NDS* Chapter 16 and AF&PA's *DCA No. 2 - Design of Fire-Resistive Exposed Wood Members*, available at http://www.awc.org.

Fireblocking and Draftstopping

In all construction types, no greater emphasis can be placed on the control of construction to reduce the fire growth hazard than the emplacement of fire and draft stops in concealed spaces. The spread of fire and smoke through these concealed openings within large rooms or between rooms is a continuous cause of major life and property loss. As a result, most building codes enforce detailing of fireblocking and draftstopping within building plans. Fireblocking considered acceptable are (1) 2" nominal lumber, (2) two thicknesses of 1" nominal lumber, and (3) two thicknesses of 3/4" plywood, with staggered joints.

Draftstopping does not require fire resistance of fireblocking. Therefore, draftstopping material is not required to be as thick. Typical draftstop materials and their minimum thicknesses are (1) 1/2" gypsum wallboard and (2) 3/8" plywood. Building codes consider an area between draftstops of 1,000 square feet as reasonable. Concealed spaces consisting of open-web floor truss components in protected floor-ceiling assemblies are an important location to draftstop parallel to the component. Areas of 500 square feet in single-family dwellings and 1,000 square feet in other buildings are recommended, and areas between family compartments are absolutely necessary. Critical draftstop locations are in the concealed spaces in floor-ceiling assemblies and in attics of multi-family dwellings when separation walls do not extend to the roof sheathing above.

Other important locations to fireblock in wood-frame construction are in the following concealed spaces:

1. Stud walls and partitions at ceiling and floor levels.
2. Intersections between concealed horizontal and vertical spaces such as soffits.
3. Top and bottom of stairs between stair stringers.
4. Openings around vents, pipes, ducts, chimneys (and fireplaces at ceiling and floor levels) with noncombustible fire stops.

Flame Spread

Regulation of materials used on interior building surfaces (and sometimes exterior surfaces) of other than one- and two-family structures is provided to minimize the danger of rapid flame spread. ASTM E84 gives the method used to obtain the flame-spread property for regulatory purposes of paneling materials. Materials are classified as having a flame spread of more or less than that of red oak, which has an assigned flame spread of 100. A noncombustible inorganic reinforced cement board has an assigned flame spread of zero. A list of accredited flame-spread ratings for various commercial woods and wood products is given in AF&PA's *DCA No. 1 - Flame Spread Performance of Wood Products*, available at http://www.awc.org.

Fire Retardant Treatments

It is possible to make wood highly resistant to the spread of fire by pressure impregnating it with an approved chemical formulation. Wood will char if exposed to fire or fire temperatures, even if it is treated with a fire retardant solution, but the rate of its destruction and the transmission of heat can be retarded by chemicals. However, the most significant contribution of chemicals is reducing the spread of fire. Wood that has absorbed adequate amounts of a fire retardant solution will not support combustion or contribute fuel and will cease to burn as soon as the source of ignition is removed.

Two general methods of improving resistance of wood to fire are (1) impregnation with an effective chemical and (2) coating the surface with a layer of intumescent paint. The first method is more effective. For interiors or locations protected from weather, impregnation treatments can be considered permanent and have considerable value in preventing ignition. These surface applications offer the principal means of increasing fire retardant properties of existing structures. However, these coatings may require periodic renewal if their effectiveness is to be maintained. In the past, the only effective chemicals were water soluble, making fire retardant treatments unadaptable to weather exposure. Impregnated fire retardants that are resistant to both high humidity and exterior exposures are becoming increasingly available on the market for treated lumber and plywood products. See product-specific recommendations regarding proper procedures for preservative treatment of that product.

C16.2 Design Procedures for Exposed Wood Members

The mechanics-based design procedures in the Specification for exposed wood members are based on research described in AF&PA's *Technical Report 10: Calculating the Fire Resistance of Exposed Wood Members* (136). The design procedure calculates the capacity of exposed wood members using basic wood engineering mechanics. Actual mechanical and physical properties of the wood are used and member capacity is directly calculated for a given period of time. Section properties are computed assuming an effective char rate, β_{eff}, at a given time, t. Reductions of strength and stiffness of wood directly adjacent to the char layer are addressed by accelerating the char rate 20 percent. Average member strength properties are approximated from existing accepted procedures used to calculate design properties. Finally, wood members are designed using accepted engineering procedures found in NDS for allowable stress design.

C16.2.1 Char Rate

To estimate the reduced cross-sectional dimensions, the location of the char base must be determined as a function of time on the basis of empirical charring rate data. The char layer can be assumed to have zero strength and stiffness. The physical shape of the remaining section and its load-carrying capacity should be adjusted to account for rounding at the corners, and for loss of strength and stiffness in the heated zone. In design there are various documented approaches to account for these results:

- additional reduction of the remaining section;
- uniform reduction of the maximum strength and stiffness; or
- more detailed analysis with subdivision of the remaining section into several zones at different temperatures.

Extensive char rate data is available for one-dimensional wood slabs. Data is also available for two-dimensional timbers, but most of this data is limited to larger cross sections. Evaluation of linear char rate models using one-dimensional char rate data suggests that charring of wood is slightly nonlinear, and estimates using linear models tend to underestimate char depth for short time periods (< 60 minutes) and overestimate char depth for longer time periods (> 60 minutes). To account for char rate nonlinearity, a nonlinear, one-dimensional char rate model based on the results of 40 one-dimensional wood slab charring tests of various species was developed (154). This non-linear model addressed accelerated charring which occurs early in fire exposure by applying a power factor to the char depth, x_{char}, to adjust for char rate non-linearity:

$$t = m(x_{char})^{1.23}$$

(C16.2-1)

where:

t = exposure time (min)

m = char slope (min/in.$^{1.23}$)

x_{char} = char depth (in.)

However, application of this model is limited since the char slope (min/in.$^{1.23}$), m, is species-specific and limited data exists for different wood species fit to the model. In addition, the model is limited to one-dimensional slabs.

To develop a two-dimensional, nonlinear char rate model, one-dimensional non-linear char rate model was modified to enable values for the slope factor, m, to be estimated using nominal char rate values (in./hr), β_n. The nominal char rate values, β_n, are calculated using measured char depth at approximately 1 hour. Substituting and solving for the char depth, x_{char}, in terms of time, t:

$$x_{char} = \beta_n t^{0.813}$$

(C16.2-2)

To account for rounding at the corners and reduction of strength and stiffness of the heated zone, the nominal char rate value, β_n, is increased 20 percent in NDS Equation 16.2-1.

Section properties can be calculated using standard equations for area, section modulus, and moment of inertia using reduced cross-sectional dimensions. The dimensions are reduced by $\beta_{eff}t$ for each surface exposed to fire. Cross-sectional properties for a member exposed on all four sides are:

Table C16.2-1 Cross-Sectional Properties for Four-Sided Exposure

Cross-sectional Property	Four-Sided Example
Area of the cross section, in.^{2}	$A(t) = (B - 2\beta_{eff}\, t)(D - 2\beta_{eff}\, t)$
Section Modulus in the major-axis direction, in.^{3}	$S(t) = (B - 2\beta_{eff}\, t)(D - 2\beta_{eff}\, t)^2/6$
Section Modulus in the minor-axis direction, in.^{3}	$S(t) = (B - 2\beta_{eff}\, t)^2(D - 2\beta_{eff}\, t)/6$
Moment of Inertia in the major-axis direction, in.^{4}	$I(t) = (D_{min} - 2\beta_{eff}\, t)(D_{max} - 2\beta_{eff}\, t)^3/12$
Moment of Inertia in the minor-axis direction, in.^{4}	$I(t) = (D_{min} - 2\beta_{eff}\, t)^3(D_{max} - 2\beta_{eff}\, t)/12$

Other exposures can be calculated using this method.

C16.2.2 Member Strength

Generally, average unheated member strength can be approximated from tests or by using design stresses derived from actual member strength data. To approximate an average member strength using a reference design value, the reference design value can be multiplied by an adjustment factor, K, to adjust from a 5 percent exclusion value allowable design value to an average ultimate value. The adjustment factor, K, has two components, the inverse of the applicable design value adjustment factor, $1/k$, and the inverse of the variability adjustment factor, c. To develop general design procedures for solid-sawn lumber, structural glued laminated timber, and structural composite lumber, the following design value adjustment factors and estimates of COV were used to conservatively develop an allowable design stress to average ultimate strength adjustment factor, K:

Table C16.2-2 Allowable Design Stress to Average Ultimate Strength Adjustment Factors

	F	1/k	c	Assumed COV	K
Bending Strength	F_b	2.1 [1]	$1 - 1.645\, COV_b$	0.16 [2]	2.85
Tensile Strength	F_t	2.1 [1]	$1 - 1.645\, COV_t$	0.16 [2]	2.85
Compression Strength	F_c	1.9 [1]	$1 - 1.645\, COV_c$	0.16 [2]	2.58
Buckling Strength	E_{05}	1.66 [3]	$1 - 1.645\, COV_E$	0.11 [3]	2.03

1. Taken from Table 10 of ASTM D245 *Standard Practice for Establishing Structural Grades and Related Allowable Properties for Visually Graded Lumber.*
2. Taken from Table 4-6 of *1999 Wood Handbook.*
3. Taken from NDS Appendices D and H.

C16.2.3 Design of Members

The induced stress can not exceed the average member capacity of a wood member exposed to fire for a given time, t. The average member capacity can be estimated using cross-sectional properties reduced for fire exposure and average ultimate strength properties derived from reference design values.

C16.2.4 Special Provisions for Structural Glued Laminated Timber Beams

The outer laminations of structural glued laminated timber bending members in Table 5A of the NDS Supplement are typically higher strength laminations. When the beam is exposed to fire, these laminations are the first to be charred. In order to maintain the ultimate capacity of the beam when these laminations are completely charred, core laminations should be replaced with the higher strength laminations in the beam layup. For unbalanced beams, only the core laminations adjacent to the tension side lamination need to be replaced. For balanced beams, the core laminations adjacent to the outer laminations on both sides need to be replaced.

16.2.5 Provisions for Timber Decks

Sides of individual timber decking members are shielded from full fire exposure by adjacent members collectively acting as a joint. Partial exposure can occur as members shrink and joints between members open. The degree of exposure is a function of the view angle of the radiant flame and the ability of hot volatile gases to pass through the joints. When the joint is completely open, such as can occur with butt-jointed timber decking, hot gases will carry into the joint and the sides of the decking members will char. This charring can be conservatively approximated assuming the sides of a member along the joint char at the effective char rate. When the joint is open but covered by sheathing, as with butt-jointed timber decking covered with wood structural panels, passage of hot gases is limited, and tests have shown that charring can be approximated assuming a partial exposure char rate along the joint equal to 1/3 of the effective char rate. For joints which are not open, as with tongue-and-groove timber decking, tests have shown that charring of the sides of members is negligible and can be ignored.

REFERENCES

1. Alpin, E. N., Factors Affecting the Stiffness and Strength of Metal Plate Connector Joints, Information Report OP-X-57, Ottawa, Ontario, Department of Environment, Canadian Forestry Service, Eastern Forest Products Laboratory, 1973.

2. ANSI/AITC Standard A190.1-2002, Structural Glued Laminated Timber, American Institute of Timber Construction, Centennial, CO, 2002.

3. ASCE Standard 7-02, Minimum Design Loads for Buildings and Other Structures, American Society of Civil Engineers, Reston, VA, 2003.

4. ASTM Standard D 2915-03, Standard Practice for Evaluating Allowable Properties for Grades of Structural Lumber, ASTM, West Conshohocken, PA, 2003.

5. ASTM Standard D 143-94 (2000), Standard Methods of Testing Small Clear Specimens of Timber, ASTM, West Conshohocken, PA, 2000.

6. ASTM Standard D 1760-01, Pressure Treatment of Timber Products, ASTM, West Conshohocken, PA, 2001.

7. ASTM Standard D 1990-00e1 (2002), Establishing Allowable Properties for Visually Graded Dimension Lumber from In-Grade Tests of Full-Size Specimens, ASTM, West Conshohocken, PA, 2002.

8. ASTM Standard D 245-00e1 (2002), Establishing Structural Grades and Related Allowable Properties for Visually Graded Lumber, ASTM, West Conshohocken, PA, 2002.

9. ASTM Standard D 2555-98e1, Establishing Clear Wood Strength Values, ASTM, West Conshohocken, PA, 1998.

10. ASTM Standard D 25-91, Round Timber Piles, ASTM, West Conshohocken, PA, 1991.

11. ASTM Standard D 2899-95, Establishing Design Stresses for Round Timber Piles, ASTM, West Conshohocken, PA, 1995.

12. ASTM Standard D 3200-74 (2000), Establishing Recommended Design Stresses for Round Timber Construction Poles, ASTM, West Conshohocken, PA, 2000.

13. ASTM Standard D 3737-03, Establishing Stresses for Structural Glued Laminated Timber (Glulam), ASTM, West Conshohocken, PA, 2003.

14. ASTM Standard D 4761-05, Standard Test Methods for Mechanical Properties of Lumber and Wood-Based Structural Material, ASTM, West Conshohocken, PA, 2005.

15. ASTM Standard D 5055-04, Establishing and Monitoring Structural Capacities of Prefabricated Wood I-Joists, ASTM, West Conshohocken, PA, 2004.

16. ASTM Standard D 5456-03, Evaluation of Structural Composite Lumber Products, ASTM, West Conshohocken, PA, 2003.

17. ASTM Standard D 5457-04, Standard Specification for Computing the Reference Resistance of Wood-Based Materials and Structural Connections for Load and Resistance Factor Design, ASTM, West Conshohocken, PA, 2004.

18. ASTM Standard D 5764-97a(2002), Standard Test Method for Evaluating Dowel-Bearing Strength of Wood and Wood-Based Products, ASTM, West Conshohocken, PA, 2002.

19. ASTM Standard D 6555-03, Standard Guide for Evaluating System Effects in Repetitive-Member Wood Assemblies, ASTM, West Conshohocken, PA, 2003.

20. Auune, P. and M. Patton-Mallory, Lateral Load-Bearing Capacity of Nailed Joints Based on the Yield Theory: Experimental Verification, Research Paper FPL 470, Madison, WI, U.S. Department of Agriculture, Forest Service, Forest Products Laboratory, 1986.

21. Auune, P. and M. Patton-Mallory, Lateral Load-Bearing Capacity of Nailed Joints Based on the Yield Theory: Theoretical Development, Research Paper FPL 469, Madison, WI, U.S. Department of Agriculture, Forest Service, Forest Products Laboratory, 1986.

22. AWPA Book of Standards, American Wood-Preservers' Association, Selma, AL, 2003.

23. Barrett, J. D., R. O. Foschi, and S. P. Fox, Perpendicular to Grain Strength of Douglas fir, Ottawa, Ontario, Canadian Journal of Civil Engineering, Vol. 2, No. 1: 50-57, 1975.

24. Barrett, J. D., Effect of Size on Tension Perpendicular to Grain Strength of Douglas fir, Wood and Fiber, 6(2): 126-143, 1974.

25. Bearing Strength of OSB to be used for the EYM Design Method, APA – The Engineered Wood Association, Tacoma, WA, 1996.

26. Bendsten, B. A. and W. L. Galligan, Mean and Tolerance Limit Stresses and Stress Modeling for Compression Perpendicular to Grain in Hardwood and Softwood Species, Research Paper FPL 337, Madison, WI, U.S. Department of Agriculture, Forest Service, Forest Products Laboratory, 1979.

27. Bendsten, B. A. and W. L. Galligan, Modeling the Stress-Compression Relationships in Wood in Compression Perpendicular to Grain, Madison, WI, Forest Products Research Society (Forest Products Society), Forest Products Journal, Vol. 29, No. 2: 42-48, 1979.

28. Bonnicksen, L. W. and S. K. Suddarth, Structural Reliability Analysis of Wood Load-Sharing System, Paper No. 82, Philadelphia, PA, ASTM, Fifth Pacific Area National Meeting, 1965.

29. Borkenhagen, E. H. and H. J. Kuelling, Clinching of Nails in Container Construction, Report No. R1777, Madison, WI, U.S. Department of Agriculture, Forest Service, Forest Products Laboratory, 1948.

30. Buchanan, A. H., Strength Model and Design Methods for Bending and Axial Load Interaction in Timber Members, Thesis, Vancouver, British Columbia, University of British Columbia, Department of Civil Engineering, 1984.

31. Call, R. D. and R. Bjorhawde, Wood Connections with Heavy Bolts and Steel Plates, New York, NY, American Society of Civil Engineers, Journal of Structural Engineering, Vol. 116, No. 11, 1990.

32. Canadian Standards Association, Engineering Design in Wood (Working Stress Design), CAN/CSA-086-M89, Rexdale, Ontario, Canadian Standards Association, 1989.

33. Cline, M. and A. L. Heim, Tests of Structural Timbers, Bulletin 108, Washington, DC, U.S. Department of Agriculture, Forest Service, 1912.

34. Clouser, W. S., Creep of Small Wood Beams Under Constant Bending Load, Report No. 2150, Madison, WI, U.S. Department of Agriculture, Forest Service, Forest Products Laboratory, 1959.

35. Cramer, C. O., Load Distribution in Multiple-Bolt Tension Joints, New York, NY, Proceedings of the American Society of Civil Engineers, Journal of the Structural Division, Vol. 94, No. ST5: 1101-1117, 1968.

36. Criswell, M. E., New Design Equations for Tapered Columns, Portland, OR, Wood Products Information Center, Wood Design Focus, Components, Vol. 2, No. 3: 4-7, 1991.

37. DeBonis, A. L. and J. Bodig, Nailed Wood Joints Under Combined Loading, Springer-Verlag, Wood Science and Technology, Vol. 9: 129-144, 1975.

38. Design/Construction Guide — Diaphragms and Shear Walls, Form L350, APA — The Engineered Wood Association, Tacoma, WA, 2001.

39. Doyle, D. V., Performance of Joints with Light Bolts in Laminated Douglas fir, Research Paper FPL 10, Madison, WI, U.S. Department of Agriculture, Forest Service, Forest Products Laboratory, 1964.

40. Doyle, D. V. and J. A. Scholten, Performance of Bolted Joints in Douglas fir, Research Paper FPL 2, Madison, WI, U.S. Department of Agriculture, Forest Service, Forest Products Laboratory, 1963.

41. Engineering Design in Wood (Limit States Design) CAN/CSA-088.1-M89, Rexdale, Ontario, Canadian Standards Association, 1989.

42. Erickson, E. C. O. and K. M. Romstad, Distribution of Wheel Loads on Timber Bridges, Research Paper FPL 44, Madison, WI, U.S. Department of Agriculture, Forest Service, Forest Products Laboratory, 1965.

43. Fairchild, I. J., Holding Power of Wood Screws, Technologic Papers of the Bureau of Standards No. 319, Washington, DC, Department of Commerce, Bureau of Standards, 1926.

44. Forest Products Laboratory, Communication of August 13, 1935 to National Lumber Manufacturers Association, Madison, WI, U.S. Department of Agriculture, Forest Service, Forest Products Laboratory, 1935.

45. Foschi, R. O. and J. Longworth, Analysis and Design of Griplam Nailed Connections, New York, NY, American Society of Civil Engineers, Journal of the Structural Division, Vol. 101, No. Stp12: 2536-2555, 1974.

46. Foschi, R. O. and S. P. Fox, Radial Stresses in Curved Timber Beams, New York, NY, Proceedings of the American Society of Civil Engineers, Journal of the Structural Division, Vol. 96, No. ST10: 1997-2008, 1970.

47. Foschi, R. O., Load-Slip Characteristics of Nails, Madison, WI, Forest Products Research Society (Forest Products Society), Wood Science, Vol. 9, No. 1: 69-76, 1974.

48. Fox, S. P., Connection Capacity of New Griplam Nails, Ottawa, Ontario, Canadian Journal of Civil Engineering, Vol. 6, No. 1: 59-64, 1979.

49. Freas, A. D. and M. L. Selbo, Fabrication and Design of Glued Laminated Wood Structural Members, Technical Bulletin No. 1069, Washington, DC, U.S. Department of Agriculture, Forest Service, 1954.

50. General Observations on the Nailing of Wood, Technical Note 243, Madison, WI, U.S. Department of Agriculture, Forest Service, Forest Products Laboratory, 1940.

51. Gerhards, C. C., Effect of Moisture Content and Temperature on the Mechanical Properties of Wood: An Analysis of Immediate Effects, Madison, WI, Society of Wood Science and Technology, Wood and Fiber, Vol. 14, No. 1: 4-36, 1982.

52. Gerhards, C. C., Time-Dependent Bending Deflections of Douglas fir 2 by 4's, Madison, WI, Forest Products Research Society (Forest Products Society), Forest Products Journal, Vol. 35, No. 4: 18-26, 1985.

53. Goodman, J. R. and J. Bodig, Contribution of Plywood Sheathing to Buckling Stiffness of Residential Roof Truss Chord Members, Report and Supplemental Report to National Forest Products Association, Fort Collins, CO, Colorado State University, Department of Civil Engineering, 1977.

54. Goodman, J. R. and J. Bodig, Orthotropic Strength of Wood in Compression, Madison, WI, Forest Products Research Society (Forest Products Society), Wood Science, Vol. 4, No. 2: 83-94, 1971.

55. Goodman, J. R. and M. E. Criswell, Contribution of Plywood Sheathing to Buckling Stiffness of Residential Roof Truss Chord Members, Supplemental Report to National Forest Products Association, Fort Collins, CO, Colorado State University, Department of Civil Engineering, 1980.

56. Gopu, V. K. A., J. R. Goodman, M. D. Vanderbilt, E. G. Thompson, and J. Bodig, Behavior and Design of Double-Tapered Pitched and Curved Glulam Beams, Structural Research Report No. 16, Fort Collins, CO, Colorado State University, Civil Engineering Department, 1976.

57. Grenoble, H. S., Bearing Strength of Bolts in Wood, Project I-228-7, Madison, WI, U.S. Department of Agriculture, Forest Service, Forest Products Laboratory, 1923.

58. Gurfinkel, G., Wood Engineering, New Orleans, LA, Southern Forest Products Association, 1973.

59. Hankinson, R. L., Investigation of Crushing Strength of Spruce at Varying Angles of Grain, Material Section Paper No. 130, McCook Field, NE, United States Army Engineering Division, U.S. Air Service Information Circular, Vol. III, No. 257, 1921.

60. Hooley, R. F. and B. Madsen, Lateral Stability of Glued Laminated Beams, New York, NY, Proceedings of the American Society of Civil Engineers, Journal of the Structural Division, Vol. 90, ST3: 201-218, 1964.

61. Hooley, R. F. and R. H. Duval, Lateral Buckling of Simply Supported Glued Laminated Beams, Report to Laminated Timber Institute of Canada, Vancouver, British Columbia, University of British Columbia, Department of Civil Engineering, 1972.

62. Hoyle, R. J., Jr., M. C. Griffith, and R.Y. Itani, Primary Creep in Douglas fir Beams of Commercial Size and Quality, Madison, WI, Society of Wood Science and Technology, Wood and Fiber Science, Vol. 17, No. 3: 300-314, 1985.

63. Hunt, G. M. and G. A. Garratt, Wood Preservation, 2nd ed. New York, NY, McGraw Hill, 1953.

64. Hyer, O. C., Study of Temperature in Wood Parts of Homes Throughout the United States, Research Note FPL-012, Madison, WI, U.S. Department of Agriculture, Forest Service, Forest Products Laboratory, 1963.

65. In-Grade Testing Program Technical Committee, In-Grade Testing of Structural Lumber, Proceedings 47363, Madison, WI, Forest Products Research Society (Forest Products Society), 1989.

66. Isyumov, N., Load Distribution in Multiple Shear-Plate Joints in Timber, Departmental Publication No. 1203, Ottawa, ON Canada, Department of Forestry and Rural Development, Forestry Branch, 1967.

67. Johansen, K. W., Theory of Timber Connections, Zurich, Switzerland, Publications of International Association for Bridge and Structural Engineering, Vol. 9: 249-262, 1949.

68. Johns, K. C. and A. H. Buchanan, Strength of Timber Members in Combined Bending and Axial Loading, Boras, Sweden, International Union of Forest Research Organizations, Proceedings IUFRO Wood Engineering Group S5.02, 343-368, 1982.

69. Karacabeyli, E. and H. Fraser, Short-Term Strength of Glulam Rivet Connections Made with Spruce and Douglas fir Glulam and Douglas fir Solid Timber, Ottawa, Ontario, Canadian Journal of Civil Engineering, Vol. 17, 166-172, 1990.

70. Kolberk, A. and M. Birnbaum, Transverse Strength of Screws in Wood, Ithaca, NY, Cornell University, The Cornell Civil Engineer, Vol. 22, No. 2: 31-41, 1913.

71. Kuenzi, E. W. Theoretical Design of a Nailed or Bolted Joint, Report No. D1951, Madison, WI, U.S. Department of Agriculture, Forest Service, Forest Products Laboratory, 1955.

72. Kunesh, R. H. and J. W. Johnson, Strength of Multiple-Bolt Joints: Influence of Spacing and Other Variables, Report T-24, Corvallis, OR, Oregon State University, School of Forestry, Forest Research Laboratory, 1968.

73. Lam, F. and P. I. Morris, Effect of Double-Density Incising on Bending Strength of Lumber, Madison, WI, Forest Products Research Society (Forest Products Society), Forest Products Journal, Vol. 41, No. 9: 43-47, 1991.

74. Lam, F. and P. I. Morris, Effect of Double-Density Incising on Bending Strength of Lumber, Madison, WI, Forest Products Research Society (Forest Products Society), Forest Products Journal, Vol. 41, No. 9: 43-47, 1991.

75. Laminated Timber Institute of Canada, Timber Design Manual, Ottawa, Ontario, Laminated Timber Institute of Canada, 1980.

76. Lane, W. W., A Study of the Effects of Lag Screw Spacing on the Strength of Timber Joints, Building Research Laboratory Report No. BR 4-1, Columbus, OH, Ohio State University, Engineering Experiment Station, 1963.

77. Lantos, G., Load Distribution in a Row of Fasteners Subjected to Lateral Load, Madison, WI, Forest Products Research Society (Forest Products Society), Wood Science, Vol. 1, No. 3: 129-136, 1969.

78. Larsen, H. J., The Yield of Bolted and Nailed Joints, South Africa, International Union of Forest Research Organizations, Proceedings of Division 5 Conference, 646-654, 1973.

79. Loferski, J. R. and T. E. McLain, Static and Impact Flexural Properties of Common Wire Nails, Philadelphia, PA, ASTM, Journal of Testing and Evaluation, Vol. 19, No. 4: 297-304, 1991.

80. Longworth, J., Behavior of Shear Plate Connections in Sloping Grain Surfaces, Madison, WI, Forest Products Research Society (Forest Products Society), Forest Products Journal, Vol. 17, No. 7: 49-63, 1967.

81. Malhotra, S. K., A Rational Approach to the Design of Solid Timber Columns, Study No. 7, Applications of Solid Mechanics, Waterloo, Ontario, University of Waterloo, 1972.

82. Malhotra, S. K. and A. P. Sukumar, A Simplified Procedure for Built-Up Wood Compression Members, St, John's, Newfoundland, Annual Conference, Canadian Society for Civil Engineering, June 1-18, 1989.

83. Malhotra, S. K. and D. B. Van Dyer, Rational Approach to the Design of Built-Up Timber Columns, Madison, WI, Forest Products Research Society (Forest Products Society), Wood Science, Vol. 9, No. 4: 174-186, 1977.

84. Markwardt, L. J. and T. R. C. Wilson, Strength and Related Properties of Woods Grown in the United States, Technical Bulletin No. 479, Washington, DC, U.S. Department of Agriculture, Forest Service, 1935.

85. McLain, T. E., Influence of Metal Side Plates on the Strength of Bolted Wood Joints, Blacksburg, VA, Virginia Polytechnic Institute and State University, Department of Forest Products, 1981.

86. McLain, T. E., Strength of Lag Screw Connections, Blacksburg, VA, Virginia Polytechnic Institute and State University, Department of Wood Science and Forest Products, 1991.

87. McLain, T. E. and J. D. Carroll, Combined Load Capacity of Threaded Fastener-Wood Connections, New York, NY, American Society of Civil Engineers, Journal of Structural Engineering, Vol. 116, No. 9: 2419-2432, 1990.

88. McLain, T. E. and S. Thangjithan, Bolted Wood-Joint Yield Model, New York, NY, American Society of Civil Engineers, Journal of Structural Engineering, Vol. 109, No. 8: 1820-1835, 1983.

89. McLain, T. E., P. Pellicane, L. Soltis, T. L. Wilkinson and J. Zahn, Comparison of EYM-Predicted Yield Loads and Current ASD Loads for Nails, Bolts and Screws, Washington, DC, National Forest Products Association, 1990.

90. Moody, R. C., R. H. Falk, and T. G. Williamson, Strength of Glulam Beams – Volume Effects, Tokyo, Japan, Proceedings of the 1990 International Timber Engineering Conference, Vol. 1: 176-182, 1990.

91. Murphy, J. F., Strength and Stiffness Reduction of Large Notched Beams, New York, NY, American Society of Civil Engineers, Journal of Structural Engineering, Vol. 112, No. 9: 1989-1999, 1986.

92. Murphy, J. F., Using Fracture Mechanics to Predict Fracture in Notched Wood Beams, Vancouver, British Columbia, Forintek Canada Corporation, Western Forest Products Laboratory, Proceedings of the First International Conference on Wood Fracture, 1978.

93. Murphy, J. F., B. R. Ellingwood, and E. M. Hendrickson, Damage Accumulation in Wood Structural Members Under Stochastic Live Loads, Madison, WI, Society of Wood Science and Technology, Wood and Fiber Science, Vol. 19, No. 4: 453-463, 1987.

94. Nail Holding Power of American Woods, Technical Note 236, Washington, DC, U.S. Department of Agriculture, Forest Service, Forest Products Laboratory, 1931.

95. Nail-Withdrawal Resistance of American Woods, Research Note FPL-093, Madison, WI, U.S. Department of Agriculture, Forest Service, Forest Products Laboratory, 1965.

96. National Design Specification for Stress-Grade Lumber and its Fastenings, Washington, DC, National Lumber Manufacturers Association (American Forest & Paper Association), 1944.

97. Neubauer, L. W., Full-Size Stud Tests Confirm Superior Strength of Square-End Wood Columns, Annual Meeting Paper No. 70-408, St. Joseph, MI, American Society of Agricultural Engineers, 1970.

98. Newlin, J. A. and G. W. Trayer, Form Factors of Beams Subjected to Transverse Loading Only, Report No. 1310, Madison, WI, U.S. Department of Agriculture, Forest Service, Forest Products Laboratory, 1941, (Also Report 181 of the National Advisory Committee for Aeronautics, 1924).

99. Newlin, J. A. and G. W. Trayer, Stresses in Wood Members Subjected to Combined Column and Beam Action, National Advisory Committee for Aeronautics Report 188 (Forest Products Laboratory Report No. 1311), Madison, WI, U.S. Department of Agriculture, Forest Service, Forest Products Laboratory, 1924.

100. Newlin, J. A. and J. M. Gahagan, Lag-Screw Joints: Their Behavior and Design, Technical Bulletin No. 597, Washington, DC, U.S. Department of Agriculture, Forest Service, Forest Products Laboratory, 1938.

101. Parker, J. E., A Study of the Strength of Short and Intermediate Wood Columns by Experimental and Analytical Methods, Research Note FPL-028, Madison, WI, U.S. Department of Agriculture, Forest Service, Forest Products Laboratory, 1964.

102. Patton-Mallory, M., End Distance Effects Comparing Tensile and Compression Loads on Bolted Wood Connections, Seattle, WA, Proceedings of the 1988 International Conference on Timber Engineering, Vol. 2: 313-324, 1988.

103. Perkins, N. S., Plywood: Properties, Design and Construction, Tacoma, WA, Douglas fir Plywood Association (APA – The Engineered Wood Association), 1962.

104. Perkins, N. S., P. Landsem, and G. W. Trayer, Modern Connectors in Timber Construction, Washington, DC, U.S. Department of Commerce, National Committee on Wood Utilization and U.S. Department of Agriculture, Forest Service, Forest Products Laboratory, 1933.

105. Perrin, P. W., Review of Incising and its Effects on Strength and Preservative Treatment of Wood, Madison, WI, Forest Products Research Society (Forest Products Society), Forest Products Journal, Vol. 28, No. 9: 27-33, 1978.

106. Plywood Design Specification and Supplements, Form Y510, APA – The Engineered Wood Association, Tacoma, WA, 1997.

107. Polensek, A. and G. H. Atherton, Compression-Bending Strength and Stiffness of Walls Made with Utility Grade Studs, Madison, WI, Forest Products Research Society (Forest Products Society), Forest Products Journal, Vol. 26, No. 11: 17-25, 1976.

108. Popov, E. P., Mechanics of Materials, Englewood Cliffs, NJ, Prentice-Hall, 1976.

109. Radcliffe, B. F. and A. Sliker, Effect of Variables on Performance of Trussed Rafters, Research Report 21, East Lansing, MI, Michigan State University, Agricultural Experiment Station, 1964.

110. Rahman, M. V., Y. J. Chiang, and R. E. Rowlands, Stress and Failure Analysis of Double-Bolted Joints in Douglas- Fir and Sitka Spruce, Madison, WI, Society of Wood Science and Technology, Wood and Fiber Science, Vol. 23, No. 4: 567-589, 1991.

111. Rosowsky, D. and B. Ellingwood, Reliability of Wood Systems Subjected to Stochastic Loads, Madison, WI, Society of Wood Science and Technology, Wood and Fiber Science, Vol. 24, No. 1: 47-59, 1992.

112. Schniewind, A. and D. E. Lyon, Further Experiments on Creep-Rupture Life Under Cyclic Environmental Conditions, Madison, WI, Society of Wood Science and Technology, Wood and Fiber, Vol. 4, No. 4: 334-341, 1973.

113. Schniewind, A. P. and D. E. Lyon, A Fracture Mechanics Approach to the Tensile Strength Perpendicular to Grain of Dimension Lumber, New York, NY, Springer-Verlag, Wood Science and Technology, Vol. 7: 45-49, 1973.

114. Scholten, J. A., Built-Up Wood Columns Conserve Lumber, New York, NY, Engineering News Record, Vol. 107, No. 9, 1931.

115. Scholten, J. A., Rounding Notches Makes Stronger Joist, Chicago, IL, Pacific Logging Congress, American Lumberman, Vol. 46, 1935.

116. Scholten, J. A., Tests of Built-Up Wood Columns, Project L-273-1J4, Madison, WI, U.S. Department of Agriculture, Forest Service, Forest Products Laboratory, 1931.

117. Scholten, J. A., Timber-Connector Joints, Their Strength and Design, Technical Bulletin No. 865, Washington, DC, U.S. Department of Agriculture, Forest Service, Forest Products Laboratory, 1944.

118. Scholten, J. A. and E. G. Molander, Strength of Nailed Joints in Frame Walls, Madison, WI, U.S. Department of Agriculture, Forest Service, Forest Products Laboratory, 1950.

119. Snodgrass, J. D. and W. W. Gleaves, Effect of End-Distance on Strength of Single-Bolt Joints, Corvallis, OR, Oregon State University, Oregon Forest Research Center, 1960.

120. Soltis, L. A., European Yield Model for Wood Connections, New York, NY, American Society of Civil Engineers, Proceedings of Structures Congress 1991, Indianapolis, Indiana, 60-63, 1991.

121. Soltis, L. A. and T. L. Wilkinson, Bolted Connection Design, General Research Report FPL-GRT-54, Madison, WI, U.S. Department of Agriculture, Forest Service, Forest Products Laboratory, 1987.

122. Soltis, L. A. and T. L. Wilkinson, Timber Bolted Connection Design, New York, NY, American Society of Civil Engineers, Proceedings of Structural Congress 1987, Orlando, Florida, 205-220, 1987.

123. Soltis, L. A., W. Nelson, and J. L. Hills, Creep of Structural Lumber, New York, NY, American Society of Mechanical Engineers, Proceedings of 3rd Joint ASCE/ASME Mechanics Conference, San Diego, 216-221, 1989.

124. Special Design Provisions for Wind and Seismic (SDPWS-05), American Forest & Paper Association, Washington, DC, 2005.

125. Specification for Structural Steel Buildings – Allowable Stress Design and Plastic Design, American Institute of Steel Construction (AISC), Chicago, IL, 1989.

126. Specification for the Design of Cold-Formed Steel Structural Members, American Iron and Steel Institute (AISI), Washington, DC, 1996.

127. Stamm, A. J., Wood and cellulose science, New York, NY, Ronald Press, 1964.

128. Standard Appearance Grades for Structural Glued Laminated Timber, AITC 110-2001, American Institute of Timber Construction, Centennial, CO, 2001.

129. Standard Specifications for Highway Bridges, American Association of State Highway and Transportation Officials (AASHTO), Washington, DC, 1987.

130. Standard Specifications for Structural Glued Laminated Timber of Hardwood Species, AITC 119-96, American Institute of Timber Construction, Centennial, CO, 1996.

131. Standard Specifications for Structural Glued Laminated Timber of Softwood Species, AITC 117-2004, American Institute of Timber Construction, Centennial, CO, 2004.

132. Stieda, C. K. A., Stress Concentrations in Notched Timber Beams, Contribution No. P-49, Vancouver, British Columbia, Department of Forestry of Canada, Vancouver Laboratory, Forest Products Research Branch, 1964.

133. Structural Glued Laminated Timber, Commercial Standard CS 253-63, U.S. Department of Commerce, National Bureau of Standards, Washington, DC, 1963.

134. Structural Glued Laminated Timber, Voluntary Product Standard PS 56-73, U.S. Department of Commerce, National Bureau of Standards, Washington, DC, 1973.

135. Suddarth, S. K., Test Performance of 1-1/2 Inch Bolts in Glulam – Row Effects and Effect of Subsequent Drying, Portland, OR, Wood Products Information Center, Wood Design Focus, Components, Vol. 1, No.1, 1990.

136. Technical Report 10 – Calculating the Fire Resistance of Exposed Wood Members, American Forest & Paper Association, Washington, DC, 2003.

137. Technical Report 12 – General Dowel Equations for Calculating Lateral Connection Values, American Forest & Paper Association, Washington, DC, 1999.

138. Technical Report 14 – Designing for Lateral-Torsional Stability in Wood Members, American Forest & Paper Association, Washington DC, 2003.

139. Tiemann, H. D., Some Results of Dead Load Bending Tests by Means of a Recording Deflectometer, Philadelphia, PA, Proceedings of the American Society for Testing Materials, Vol. 9: 534-548, 1909.

140. Timber Construction Manual, American Institute of Timber Construction, John Wiley & Sons, 2004.

141. Timber Engineering Company, Design Manual for TECO Timber-Connector Construction, Washington, DC, National Lumber Manufacturers Association (American Forest & Paper Association), Timber Engineering Company, 1955.

142. Timber Engineering Company, Timber Design and Construction Handbook, New York, NY, F.W, Dodge, 1956.

143. Tissell, J. R., Horizontal Plywood Diaphragm Tests, Laboratory Report No. 106, Tacoma, WA, American Plywood Association (APA – The Engineered Wood Association), 1967.

144. Tissell, J. R., Plywood Diaphragms, Research Report 138, Tacoma, WA, American Plywood Association (APA – The Engineered Wood Association), 1990.

145. Tissell, J. R., Structural Panel Shear Walls, Research Report 154, Tacoma, WA, American Plywood Association (APA – The Engineered Wood Association), 1990.

146. Trayer, G. W., The Bearing Strength of Wood Under Bolts, Technical Bulletin No. 332, Washington, DC, U.S. Department of Agriculture, Forest Service, Forest Products Laboratory, 1932.

147. Trayer, G. W. and H. W. March, Elastic Instability of Members Having Sections Common in Aircraft Construction, Report No. 382, Washington, DC, National Advisory Committee for Aeronautics, 1931.

148. Truss Plate Institute, Commentary and Recommendations for Bracing Wood Trusses, BWT-76, Madison, WI, Truss Plate Institute, 1976.

149. Vanderbilt, M. D., J. R. Goodman, and J. Bodig, A Rational Analysis and Design Procedure for Wood Joist Floor Systems, Final Report to the National Science Foundation for Grant GK-30853, Fort Collins, CO, Colorado State University, Department of Civil Engineering, 1974.

150. Voluntary Product Standard (PS 1-95), Construction and Industrial Plywood, United States Department of Commerce, National Institute of Standards and Technology, Gaithersburg, MD, 1995.

151. Voluntary Product Standard (PS 2-04), Performance Standard for Wood-Based Structural-Use Panels, United States Department of Commerce, National Institute of Standards and Technology, Gaithersburg, MD, 2004.

152. Voluntary Product Standard (PS 20-99), American Softwood Lumber Standard, United States Department of Commerce, National Institute of Standards and Technology, Gaithersburg, MD, 1999.

153. War Production Board, National Emergency Specifications for the Design, Fabrication and Erection of Stress Grade Lumber and its Fastenings for Buildings, Directive No. 29, Washington, DC, War Production Board, Conservation Division, 1943.

154. White, R. H., Charring Rates of Different Wood Species, PhD Thesis, University of Wisconsin, Madison, WI, 1988.

155. Wilkinson, T. L., Analyses of Nailed Joints with Dissimilar Members, New York, NY, American Society of Civil Engineers, Journal of the Structural Division, Vol. 98, No. ST9: 2005-2013, 1972.

156. Wilkinson, T. L., Assessment of Modification Factors for a Row of Bolts in Timber Connections, Research Paper FPL 376, Madison, WI, U.S. Department of Agriculture, Forest Service, Forest Products Laboratory, 1980.

157. Wilkinson, T. L., Bolted Connection Allowable Loads Based on the European Yield Model, Madison, WI, U.S. Department of Agriculture, Forest Service, Forest Products Laboratory, 1991.

158. Wilkinson, T. L., Dowel Bearing Strength, Research Paper FPL-RP-505, Madison, WI, U.S. Department of Agriculture, Forest Service, Forest Products Laboratory, 1991.

159. Wilkinson, T. L., Elastic Bearing Constants for Sheathing Materials, Research Paper FPL 192, Madison, WI, U.S. Department of Agriculture, Forest Service, Forest Products Laboratory, 1974.

160. Wilkinson, T. L., Formulas for Working Stresses for Timber Piles, Madison, WI, U.S. Department of Agriculture, Forest Service, Forest Products Laboratory, 1969.

161. Wilkinson, T. L., Strength Evaluation of Round Timber Piles, Research Paper FPL 101, Madison, WI, U.S. Department of Agriculture, Forest Service, Forest Products Laboratory, 1968.

162. Wilkinson, T. L., Strength of Bolted Wood Joints with Various Ratios of Member Thickness, Research Paper FPL 314, Madison, WI, U.S. Department of Agriculture, Forest Service, Forest Products Laboratory, 1978.

163. Wilkinson, T. L. and T. R. Laatsch, Lateral and Withdrawal Resistance of Tapping Screws in Three Densities of Wood, Madison, WI, Forest Products Research Society (Forest Products Society), Forest Products Journal, Vol. 20, No. 7: 35-41, 1971.

164. Williamson, T. G. and B. Hill, Waiver of Metal Hanger Torsional Restraint Requirements, Communication to ICBO Evaluation Service, Vancouver, WA, American Institute of Timber Construction, (November), 1989.

165. Williamson, T. G., R. Gregg, and H. Brooks, Wood Design: A Commentary on the Performance of Deep and Narrow Re-Sawn Glulam Purlins, Los Angles, CA, Structural Engineers Association of Southern California, (June), 1990.

166. Wilson, T. R. C., Glued Laminated Wooden Arch, Technical Bulletin No. 691, Washington, DC, U.S. Department of Agriculture, Forest Service, 1939.

167. Wilson, T. R. C., Guide to the Grading of Structural Timbers and the Determination of Working Stresses, U.S. Department of Agriculture Miscellaneous Publication 185, Washington, DC, U.S. Department of Agriculture, 1934.

168. Winandy, J. E., ACA and CCA Preservative Treatment and Redrying Effects on Bending Properties of Douglas fir, Stevensville, MD, American Wood-Preservers' Association Proceedings, Vol. 85: 106-118, 1989.

169. Winandy, J. E., CCA Preservative Treatment and Redrying Effects on the Bending Properties of 2 by 4 Southern Pine, Madison, WI, Forest Products Research Society (Forest Products Society), Forest Products Journal, Vol. 39, No. 9: 14-21, 1989.

170. Winandy, J. E., Effects of Treatment and Redrying on Mechanical Properties of Wood, Madison, WI, Forest Products Research Society (Forest Products Society), Proceedings 47358 of Conference on Wood Protection Techniques and the Use of Treated Wood in Construction, 54-62, 1988.

171. Winandy, J. E. and H. M. Barnes, Influence of Initial Kiln-Drying Temperature on CCA-Treatment Effects on Strength, Stevensville, MD, American Wood-Preservers' Association Proceedings, Vol. 87, 1991.

172. Winandy, J. E. and R. S. Boone, The Effects of CCA Preservative Treatment and Redrying on the Bending Properties of 2 x 6 Southern Pine Lumber, Madison, WI, Society of Wood Science and Technology, Wood and Fiber Science, Vol. 20, No. 3: 350-364, 1988.

173. Winandy, J. E., Influence of Time-to-Failure on Strength of CCA-Treated Lumber, Madison, WI, Forest Products Research Society (Forest Products Society), Forest Products Journal, Vol. 45, No. 2: 82-85, 1995.

174. Winandy, J. E., J. J. Morell, and S. T. Lebow, Review of Effects of Incising on Treatability and Strength, Madison, WI, Forest Products Society Conference, Savannah, GA, Wood Preservation: In the '90s and Beyond, 1994.

175. Winandy, J. E., R. S. Boone, and B. A. Bendsten, Interaction of CCA Preservative Treatment and Redrying: Effect on the Mechanical Properties of Southern Pine, Madison, WI, Forest Products Research Society (Forest Products Society), Forest Products Journal, Vol. 35, No. 10: 62-68, 1985.

176. Wolfe, R. W., Allowable Stresses for the Upside-Down Timber Industry, Madison, WI, U.S. Department of Agriculture, Forest Service, Forest Products Laboratory, 1989.

177. Wolfe, R. W., Performance of Light-Frame Redundant Assemblies, Tokyo, Japan, Proceedings of the 1990 International Timber Engineering Conference, Vol. 1: 124-131, 1990.

178. Wolfe, R. W., Research Dealing with Effects of Bearing Length on Compression Perpendicular to the Grain, Madison, WI, U.S. Department of Agriculture, Forest Service, Forest Products Laboratory, 1983.

179. Wolfe, R. W. and T. LaBissoniere, Structural Performance of Light-Frame Roof Assemblies, II, Conventional Truss Assemblies, Research Paper FPL-RP-499, Madison, WI, U.S. Department of Agriculture, Forest Service, Forest Products Laboratory, 1991.

180. Wood Construction Data 1 (WCD 1) Details for Conventional Wood Frame Construction, Washington, DC, American Forest & Paper Association, 2001.

181. Wood Handbook, Agriculture Handbook No. 72, Washington, DC, U.S. Department of Agriculture, Forest Service, Forest Products Laboratory, 1955.

182. Wood Handbook, Agriculture Handbook No. 72, Washington, DC, U.S. Department of Agriculture, Forest Service, Forest Products Laboratory, 1974.

183. Wood Handbook, Agriculture Handbook No. 72, Washington, DC, U.S. Department of Agriculture, Forest Service, Forest Products Laboratory, 1987.

184. Wood Handbook, Washington, DC, U.S. Department of Agriculture, Forest Service, Forest Products Laboratory, 1935.

185. Wood, L. W., Behavior of Wood Under Continued Loading, New York, NY, Engineering News Record, Vol. 139, No. 24: 108-111, 1947.

186. Wood, L. W., Formulas for Columns with Side Loads and Eccentricity, Report No. R1782, Madison, WI, U.S. Department of Agriculture, Forest Service, Forest Products Laboratory, 1950.

187. Zahn, J. J., Combined-Load Stability Criterion for Wood Beam-Columns, New York, NY, American Society of Civil Engineers, Journal of Structural Engineering, Vol. 114, No. 11: 2612-2618, 1986.

188. Zahn, J. J., Design Equation for Multiple-Fastener Wood Connections, Madison, WI, U.S. Department of Agriculture, Forest Service, Forest Products Laboratory, 1991.

189. Zahn, J. J., Design of Wood Members Under Combined Load, New York, NY, American Society of Civil Engineers, Journal of Structural Engineering, Vol. 112, No. 9: 2109-2126, 1986.

190. Zahn, J. J., Interaction of Crushing and Buckling in Wood Columns and Beams, Madison, WI, U.S. Department of Agriculture, Forest Service, Forest Products Laboratory, 1990.

191. Zahn, J. J., Progress Report to NFPA on Column Research at FPL, Madison, WI, U.S. Department of Agriculture, Forest Service, Forest Products Laboratory, 1989.

192. Zahn, J. J., Proposed Design Formula for Wood Beam Columns, Paper No. 87-4002, Baltimore, MD, Proceedings of American Society of Agricultural Engineers, 1987.

193. Zahn, J. J., Strength of Lumber Under Combined Bending and Compression, Research Paper FPL 391, Madison, WI, U.S. Department of Agriculture, Forest Service, Forest Products Laboratory, 1982.

194. Zahn, J. J., Strength of Multiple-Member Structures, Research Paper FPL 139, Madison, WI, U.S. Department of Agriculture, Forest Service, Forest Products Laboratory, 1970.

195. Wilkinson, T. L., Moisture Cycling of Trussed Rafter Joints, Research Paper FPL 67, Madison, WI, U.S. Department of Agriculture, Forest Service, Forest Products Laboratory, 1966.

2005 EDITION

S U P P L E M E N T

N D S®

NATIONAL DESIGN SPECIFICATION®

DESIGN VALUES FOR WOOD CONSTRUCTION

American
Forest &
Paper
Association

American Wood Council

2005 Edition

S U P P L E M E N T

N D S®

NATIONAL DESIGN SPECIFICATION®

DESIGN VALUES FOR
WOOD CONSTRUCTION

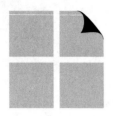

Introduction

This Supplement is an integral part of the *National Design Specification® (NDS®) for Wood Construction*, 2005 Edition. It provides reference design values for structural sawn lumber and structural glued laminated timber.

Lumber

The reference design values for lumber in this Supplement are obtained from grading rules published by seven agencies: National Lumber Grades Authority (a Canadian agency), Northeastern Lumber Manufacturers Association, Northern Softwood Lumber Bureau, Redwood Inspection Service, Southern Pine Inspection Bureau, West Coast Lumber Inspection Bureau, and Western Wood Products Association. The grading rules promulgated by these agencies, including the reference design values therein, have been approved by the Board of Review of the American Lumber Standards Committee and certified for conformance with U.S. Department of Commerce Voluntary Product Standard PS 20-99 (American Softwood Lumber Standard).

Reference design values for most species and grades of visually graded dimension lumber are based on the provisions of ASTM Standard D 1990-00$^{\varepsilon1}$ (Establishing Allowable Properties for Visually Graded Dimension Lumber from In-Grade Tests of Full-Size Specimens). Reference design values for visually graded timbers, decking, and some species and grades of dimension lumber are based on the provisions of ASTM Standard D 245-00$^{\varepsilon1}$ (Establishing Structural Grades and Related Allowable Properties for Visually Graded Lumber). The methods in ASTM Standard D 245-00$^{\varepsilon1}$ involve adjusting the strength properties of small clear specimens of wood, as given in ASTM Standard D 2555-98 (Establishing Clear Wood Strength Values), for the effects of knots, slope of grain, splits, checks, size, duration of load, moisture content, and other influencing factors, to obtain reference design values applicable to normal conditions of service. Lumber structures designed on the basis of working stresses derived from ASTM Standard D 245 procedures and standard design criteria have a long history of satisfactory performance.

Reference design values for machine stress rated (MSR) lumber and machine evaluated lumber (MEL) are based on nondestructive testing of individual pieces. Certain visual grade requirements also apply to such lumber. The stress rating system used for MSR and MEL lumber is regularly checked by the responsible grading agency for conformance to established certification and quality control procedures.

For additional information on development and applicability of lumber reference design values, the grading rules published by the individual agencies and the referenced ASTM Standards should be consulted.

Structural Glued Laminated Timber

Reference design values in this Supplement for structural glued laminated timber are developed and published by the American Institute of Timber Construction (AITC) and APA–The Engineered Wood Association (APA) in accordance with principles originally established by the U.S. Forest Products Laboratory in the early 1950s. These principles involve adjusting strength properties of clear straight grained lumber to account for knots, slope of grain, density, size of member, number of laminations, and other factors unique to laminated timber.

Specific methods used to establish reference design values have been periodically revised and improved to reflect the results of tests of large structural glued laminated timber members conducted by the U.S. Forest Products Laboratory and other accredited testing agencies. The performance history of structures made with structural glued laminated timber conforming to AITC specifications and manufactured in accordance with American National Standard ANSI/AITC A190.1-2002 (Structural Glued Laminated Timber) has demonstrated the validity of the methods used to establish structural glued laminated timber reference design values.

Conditions of Use

Reference design values presented in this Supplement are for normal load duration under dry conditions of service. Because the strength of wood varies with conditions under which it is used, these reference design values should only be applied in conjunction with appropriate design and service recommendations from the *NDS*. Additionally, the reference design values in this Supplement apply only to material identified by the grade mark of, or certificate of inspection issued by, a grading or inspection bureau or agency recognized as being competent.

TABLE OF CONTENTS

LIST OF TABLES

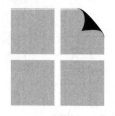

SAWN LUMBER GRADING AGENCIES

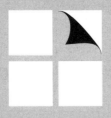

AMERICAN FOREST & PAPER ASSOCIATION

1.1 List of Sawn Lumber Grading Agencies

Following is a list of agencies certified by the American Lumber Standard Committee Board of Review (as of 2004) for inspection and grading of untreated lumber under the rules indicated. For the most up-to-date list of certified agencies contact:

American Lumber Standard Committee
P.O. Box 210
Germantown, Maryland 20875-0210
www.alsc.org

Rules Writing Agencies

Rules for which grading is authorized

Northeastern Lumber Manufacturers Association (NELMA) .... NELMA, NLGA, NSLB, SPIB, WCLIB, WWPA
   272 Tuttle Road, P.O. Box 87A, Cumberland Center, Maine 04021
Northern Softwood Lumber Bureau (NSLB) .... NLGA, NSLB, WCLIB, WWPA
   272 Tuttle Road, P.O. Box 87A, Cumberland Center, Maine 04021
Redwood Inspection Service (RIS) .... RIS, WCLIB, WWPA
   405 Enfrente Drive, Suite 200, Novato, California 94949
Southern Pine Inspection Bureau (SPIB) .... NELMA, NLGA, NSLB, SPIB, WCLIB, WWPA
   4709 Scenic Highway, Pensacola, Florida 32504
West Coast Lumber Inspection Bureau (WCLIB) .... NLGA, RIS, SPIB, WCLIB, WWPA
   6980 SW Varnes Road, P.O. Box 23145, Tigard, Oregon 97223
Western Wood Products Association (WWPA) .... NLGA, RIS, SPIB, WCLIB, WWPA
   522 SW Fifth Avenue, Suite 500, Portland, Oregon 97204
National Lumber Grades Authority (NLGA)
   960 Quayside Dr., New Westminster, BC, Canada V3M 6G2

Non-Rules Writing Agencies

Pacific Lumber Inspection Bureau, Inc. .... RIS, WCLIB, WWPA, NLGA
Renewable Resource Associates, Inc. .... NELMA, NLGA, NSLB, SPIB, WCLIB, WWPA
Stafford Inspection and Consulting, LLC .... SPIB
Timber Products Inspection .... NELMA, NLGA, NSLB, RIS, SPIB, WCLIB, WWPA

Alberta Forest Products Association .... NLGA
Canadian Lumbermen's Association .... NELMA, NLGA
Canadian Mill Services Association .... NLGA, WWPA
Canadian Softwood Inspection Agency, Inc. .... NLGA, WCLIB, WWPA
Central Forest Products Association .... NELMA, NLGA
Council of Forest Industries .... NLGA, WWPA
Macdonald Inspection .... NLGA, WCLIB, WWPA
Maritime Lumber Bureau .... NELMA, NLGA
Newfoundland and Labrador Lumber Producers Association .... NLGA
Ontario Lumber Manufacturers Association .... NELMA, NLGA
Pacific Lumber Inspection Bureau .... NLGA, RIS, WCLIB, WWPA
Quebec Forest Industry Council .... NELMA, NLGA

2

SPECIES COMBINATIONS

2.1 List of Sawn Lumber Species Combinations

Species or Species Combination	Species That May Be Included in Combination	Grading Rules Agencies	Design Values Provided in Tables
Alaska Cedar		WCLIB	4A
Alaska Hemlock		WWPA	4A
Alaska Spruce	Alaska Sitka Spruce Alaska White Spruce	WWPA	4A
Alaska Yellow Cedar		WCLIB, WWPA	4A
Aspen	Big Tooth Aspen Quaking Aspen	NELMA NSLB WWPA	4A
Baldcypress		SPIB	4A, 4D
Balsam Fir		NELMA NSLB	4D, 4E
Beech-Birch-Hickory	American Beech Bitternut Hickory Mockernut Hickory Nutmeg Hickory Pecan Hickory Pignut Hickory Shagbark Hickory Shellbark Hickory Sweet Birch Water Hickory Yellow Birch	NELMA	4A, 4D
Coast Sitka Spruce		NLGA	4D, 4E
Coast Species	Amabilis Fir Coast Sitka Spruce Douglas Fir Western Hemlock Western Larch	NLGA	4E
Cottonwood		NSLB	4A
Douglas Fir-Larch	Douglas Fir Western Larch	WCLIB WWPA	4A, 4C, 4D, 4E
Douglas Fir-Larch (North)	Douglas Fir Western Larch	NLGA	4A, 4C, 4D, 4E
Douglas Fir-South		WWPA	4A, 4C, 4D, 4E
Eastern Hemlock		NELMA NSLB	4D
Eastern Hemlock-Balsam Fir	Balsam Fir Eastern Hemlock Tamarack	NELMA	4A
Eastern Hemlock-Tamarack	Eastern Hemlock Tamarack	NELMA NSLB	4A, 4D, 4E
Eastern Hemlock-Tamarack (North)	Eastern Hemlock Tamarack	NLGA	4D, 4E

Species or Species Combination	Species That May Be Included in Combination	Grading Rules Agencies	Design Values Provided in Tables
Eastern Softwoods	Balsam Fir Black Spruce Eastern Hemlock Eastern White Pine Jack Pine Norway (Red) Pine Pitch Pine Red Spruce Tamarack White Spruce	NELMA NSLB	4A
Eastern Spruce	Black Spruce Red Spruce White Spruce	NELMA NSLB	4D, 4E
Eastern White Pine		NELMA NSLB	4A, 4D, 4E
Eastern White Pine (North)		NLGA	4E
Hem-Fir	California Red Fir Grand Fir Noble Fir Pacific Silver Fir Western Hemlock White Fir	WCLIB WWPA	4A, 4C, 4D, 4E
Hem-Fir (North)	Amabilis Fir Western Hemlock	NLGA	4A, 4C, 4D, 4E
Mixed Maple	Black Maple Red Maple Silver Maple Sugar Maple	NELMA	4A, 4D
Mixed Oak	All Oak Species graded under NELMA rules	NELMA	4A, 4D
Mixed Southern Pine	Any species in the Southern Pine species combination, plus either or both of the following: Pond Pine Virginia Pine	SPIB	4B, 4C, 4D
Mountain Hemlock		WWPA, WCLIB	4D
Northern Pine	Jack Pine Norway (Red) Pine Pitch Pine	NELMA NSLB	4D, 4E
Northern Red Oak	Black Oak Northern Red Oak Pin Oak Scarlet Oak	NELMA	4A, 4D
Northern Species	Any species graded under NLGA rules except Red Alder, White Birch, and Norway Spruce	NLGA	4A, 4C, 4E
Northern White Cedar		NELMA	4A, 4D, 4E
Ponderosa Pine		NLGA	4D, 4E

SPECIES COMBINATIONS

Species or Species Combination	Species That May Be Included in Combination	Grading Rules Agencies	Design Values Provided in Tables
Red Maple		NELMA	4A, 4D
Red Oak	Black Oak Cherrybark Oak Laurel Oak Northern Red Oak Pin Oak Scarlet Oak Southern Red Oak Water Oak Willow Oak	NELMA	4A, 4D
Red Pine		NLGA	4D, 4E
Redwood		RIS	4A, 4D, 4E
Sitka Spruce		WWPA, WCLIB	4D, 4E
Southern Pine	Loblolly Pine Longleaf Pine Shortleaf Pine Slash Pine	SPIB	4B, 4C, 4D, 4E
Spruce-Pine-Fir	Alpine Fir Balsam Fir Black Spruce Engelmann Spruce Jack Pine Lodgepole Pine Red Spruce White Spruce	NLGA	4A, 4C, 4D, 4E
Spruce-Pine-Fir (South)	Balsam Fir Black Spruce Engelmann Spruce Jack Pine Lodgepole Pine Norway (Red) Pine Red Spruce Sitka Spruce White Spruce	NELMA NSLB WCLIB WWPA	4A, 4C, 4D, 4E
Western Cedars	Alaska Cedar Incense Cedar Port Orford Cedar Western Red Cedar	WCLIB WWPA	4A, 4C, 4D, 4E
Western Cedars (North)	Pacific Coast Yellow Cedar Western Red Cedar	NLGA	4D, 4E
Western Hemlock		WWPA, WCLIB	4D, 4E
Western Hemlock (North)		NLGA	4D, 4E
Western White Pine		NLGA	4D, 4E

Species or Species Combination	Species That May Be Included in Combination	Grading Rules Agencies	Design Values Provided in Tables

Western Woods	Any species in the Douglas Fir-Larch, Douglas Fir-South, Hem-Fir, and Spruce-Pine-Fir (South) species combinations, plus any or all of the following:
	    Alpine Fir
	    Idaho White Pine
	    Mountain Hemlock
	    Ponderosa Pine
	    Sugar Pine
		WCLIB
		WWPA
			4A, 4C, 4D, 4E

White Oak	Bur Oak Chestnut Oak Live Oak Overcup Oak Post Oak Swamp Chestnut Oak Swamp White Oak White Oak	NELMA	4A, 4D
Yellow Poplar		NSLB	4A

SPECIES COMBINATIONS

2

2.2 List of Non-North American Sawn Lumber Species Combinations

Species or Species Combination	Species That May Be Included in Combination	Grading Rules Agency	Design Values Provided in Tables
Austrian Spruce - Austria & The Czech Republic		WCLIB	4F
Douglas Fir/European Larch - Austria, The Czech Republic, & Bavaria	Douglas Fir European Larch	WCLIB	4F
Montane Pine - South Africa		WCLIB	4F
Norway Spruce - Estonia & Lithuania		WCLIB	4F
Norway Spruce - Finland		WCLIB	4F
Norway Spruce - Germany, NE France, & Switzerland		WCLIB	4F
Norway Spruce - Romania & the Ukraine		WCLIB	4F
Norway Spruce - Sweden		WCLIB	4F
Scots Pine - Austria, The Czech Republic, Romania, & the Ukraine		WCLIB	4F
Scots Pine - Estonia & Lithuania		WCLIB	4F
Scots Pine - Finland		WCLIB	4F
Scots Pine - Germany*		WCLIB	4F
Scots Pine - Sweden		WCLIB	4F
Silver Fir (Abies alba) - Germany, NE France, & Switzerland		WCLIB	4F
Southern Pine - Misiones Argentina		SPIB	4F
Southern Pine - Misiones Argentina, Free of Heart Center and Medium Grade Density		SPIB	4F

* Does not include states of Baden-Wurttemburg and Saarland.

2.3 List of Structural Glued Laminated Timber Species Combinations

Species or Species Group	Symbol	Species That May Be Included in Group	Design Values Provided in Tables
Alaska Cedar	AC	Alaska Cedar	5A, 5B
Douglas Fir-Larch	DF	Douglas Fir, Western Larch	5A, 5B
Hem-Fir	HF	California Red Fir Grand Fir Noble Fir Pacific Silver Fir Western Hemlock White Fir	5A, 5B
Softwood Species	SW	Alpine Fir Balsam Fir Black Spruce Douglas Fir Douglas Fir South Engelmann Spruce Idaho White Pine Jack Pine Lodgepole Pine Mountain Hemlock Ponderosa Pine Red Spruce Sugar Pine Western Larch Western Red Cedar White Spruce	5A, 5B
Southern Pine	SP	Loblolly Pine Longleaf Pine Shortleaf Pine Slash Pine	5A, 5B

Species or Species Group	Symbol	Species That May Be Included in Group	Design Values Provided in Tables
Group A Hardwoods	A	Ash, White Beech, American Birch, Sweet Birch, Yellow Hickory, Bitternut Hickory, Mockernut Hickory, Nutmeg Hickory, Pecan Hickory, Pignut Hickory, Shagbark Hickory, Shellbark Hickory, Water Oak, Northern Red Oak, White	5C, 5D

Group B Hardwoods	B	Elm, Rock
		Maple, Black
		Maple, Red
		Mixed Oak:
		    Black
		    Bur
		    Cherrybark
		    Chestnut
		    Laurel
		    Live
		    Northern Red
		    Overcup
		    Pin
		    Post
		    Scarlet
		    Southern Red
		    Swamp Chestnut
		    Swamp White
		    Water
		    White
		Sweetgum
			5C, 5D

Group C Hardwoods	C	Ash, Black Elm, American Tupulo, Water Yellow Poplar	5C, 5D

Group D Hardwoods	D	Aspen, Bigtooth
		Aspen, Quaking
		Cottonwood, Eastern
		Mixed Maple:
		    Black
		    Red
		    Silver
		    Sugar
			5C, 5D

SECTION PROPERTIES

3

3.1 Section Properties of Sawn Lumber and Structural Glued Laminated Timber

3.1.1 Standard Sizes of Sawn Lumber

Details regarding the dressed sizes of various species of lumber in the grading rules of the agencies which formulate and maintain such rules. The dressed sizes in Table 1A conform to the sizes set forth in U.S. Department of Commerce Voluntary Product Standard PS 20-99 (American Softwood Lumber Standard). While these sizes are generally available on a commercial basis, it is good practice to consult the local lumber dealer to determine what sizes are on hand or can be readily secured.

Dry lumber is defined as lumber which has been seasoned to a moisture content of 19% or less. Green lumber is defined as lumber having a moisture content in excess of 19%.

3.1.2 Properties of Standard Dressed Sizes

Certain mathematical expressions of the properties or elements of sections are used in design calculations for various member shapes and loading conditions. The section properties for selected standard sizes of boards, dimension lumber, and timbers are given in Table 1B. Section properties for selected standard sizes of structural glued laminated timber are given in Table 1C and 1D.

3.1.3 Definitions

NEUTRAL AXIS, in the cross section of a beam, is the line on which there is neither tension nor compression stress.

Figure 1A Dimensions for Rectangular Cross Section

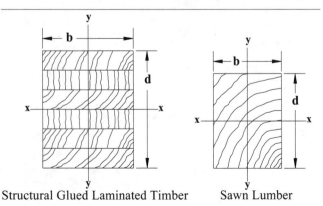

Structural Glued Laminated Timber   Sawn Lumber

MOMENT OF INERTIA, I, of the cross section of a beam is the sum of the products of each of its elementary areas multiplied by the square of their distance from the neutral axis of the section.

SECTION MODULUS, S, is the moment of inertia divided by the distance from the neutral axis to the extreme fiber of the section.

CROSS SECTION is a section taken through the member perpendicular to its longitudinal axis.

The following symbols and formulas apply to rectangular beam cross sections:

$X\text{-}X$ = neutral axis for edgewise bending (load applied to narrow face)

$Y\text{-}Y$ = neutral axis for flatwise bending (load applied to wide face)

b = breadth of rectangular bending member, in.

d = depth of rectangular bending member, in.

$A = bd$ = area of cross section, in.^{2}

c = distance from neutral axis to extreme fiber of cross section, in.

$I_x = bd^3/12$ = moment of inertia about the X-X axis, in.^{4}

$I_y = db^3/12$ = moment of inertia about the Y-Y axis, in.^{4}

$r_x = \sqrt{I_x/A} = d/\sqrt{12}$ = radius of gyration about the X-X axis, in.

$r_y = \sqrt{I_y/A} = b/\sqrt{12}$ = radius of gyration about the Y-Y axis, in.

$S_x = I_x/c = bd^2/6$ = section modulus about the X-X axis, in.^{3}

$S_y = I_y/c = db^2/6$ = section modulus about the Y-Y axis, in.^{3}

The following formula shall be used to determine the density in lb./ft.^{3} of wood:

$$\text{density} = 62.4\left[\frac{G}{1+G(0.009)(\text{m.c.})}\right]\left[1+\frac{\text{m.c.}}{100}\right]$$

where:

G = specific gravity of wood (see NDS Table 11.3.2A)

m.c. = moisture content of wood, %

Table 1A   Nominal and Minimum Dressed Sizes of Sawn Lumber

Item	Thickness (in.)			Face Widths (in.)		
	Nominal	Minimum dressed		Nominal	Minimum dressed	
		Dry	Green		Dry	Green
Boards	3/4	5/8	11/16	2	1-1/2	1-9/16
	1	3/4	25/32	3	2-1/2	2-9/16
	1-1/4	1	1-1/32	4	3-1/2	3-9/16
	1-1/2	1-1/4	1-9/32	5	4-1/2	4-5/8
				6	5-1/2	5-5/8
				7	6-1/2	6-5/8
				8	7-1/4	7-1/2
				9	8-1/4	8-1/2
				10	9-1/4	9-1/2
				11	10-1/4	10-1/2
				12	11-1/4	11-1/2
				14	13-1/4	13-1/2
				16	15-1/4	15-1/2
Dimension Lumber	2	1-1/2	1-9/16	2	1-1/2	1-9/16
	2-1/2	2	2-1/16	3	2-1/2	2-9/16
	3	2-1/2	2-9/16	4	3-1/2	3-9/16
	3-1/2	3	3-1/16	5	4-1/2	4-5/8
	4	3-1/2	3-9/16	6	5-1/2	5-5/8
	4-1/2	4	4-1/16	8	7-1/4	7-1/2
				10	9-1/4	9-1/2
				12	11-1/4	11-1/2
				14	13-1/4	13-1/2
				16	15-1/4	15-1/2
Timbers	5 & thicker	—	1/2 off	5 & wider	—	1/2 off

Table 1B Section Properties of Standard Dressed (S4S) Sawn Lumber

Nominal Size b × d	Standard Dressed Size (S4S) b × d inches × inches	Area of Section A in.²	X-X Axis Section Modulus S_{xx} in.³	X-X Axis Moment of Inertia I_{xx} in.⁴	Y-Y Axis Section Modulus S_{yy} in.³	Y-Y Axis Moment of Inertia I_{yy} in.⁴	Approximate weight in pounds per linear foot (lb./ft.) of piece when density of wood equals: 25 lb./ft.³	30 lb./ft.³	35 lb./ft.³	40 lb./ft.³	45 lb./ft.³	50 lb./ft.³
1 × 3	3/4 × 2-1/2	1.875	0.781	0.977	0.234	0.088	0.326	0.391	0.456	0.521	0.586	0.651
1 × 4	3/4 × 3-1/2	2.625	1.531	2.680	0.328	0.123	0.456	0.547	0.638	0.729	0.820	0.911
1 × 6	3/4 × 5-1/2	4.125	3.781	10.40	0.516	0.193	0.716	0.859	1.003	1.146	1.289	1.432
1 × 8	3/4 × 7-1/4	5.438	6.570	23.82	0.680	0.255	0.944	1.133	1.322	1.510	1.699	1.888
1 × 10	3/4 × 9-1/4	6.938	10.70	49.47	0.867	0.325	1.204	1.445	1.686	1.927	2.168	2.409
1 × 12	3/4 × 11-1/4	8.438	15.82	88.99	1.055	0.396	1.465	1.758	2.051	2.344	2.637	2.930
2 × 3	1-1/2 × 2-1/2	3.750	1.563	1.953	0.938	0.703	0.651	0.781	0.911	1.042	1.172	1.302
2 × 4	1-1/2 × 3-1/2	5.250	3.063	5.359	1.313	0.984	0.911	1.094	1.276	1.458	1.641	1.823
2 × 5	1-1/2 × 4-1/2	6.750	5.063	11.39	1.688	1.266	1.172	1.406	1.641	1.875	2.109	2.344
2 × 6	1-1/2 × 5-1/2	8.250	7.563	20.80	2.063	1.547	1.432	1.719	2.005	2.292	2.578	2.865
2 × 8	1-1/2 × 7-1/4	10.88	13.14	47.63	2.719	2.039	1.888	2.266	2.643	3.021	3.398	3.776
2 × 10	1-1/2 × 9-1/4	13.88	21.39	98.93	3.469	2.602	2.409	2.891	3.372	3.854	4.336	4.818
2 × 12	1-1/2 × 11-1/4	16.88	31.64	178.0	4.219	3.164	2.930	3.516	4.102	4.688	5.273	5.859
2 × 14	1-1/2 × 13-1/4	19.88	43.89	290.8	4.969	3.727	3.451	4.141	4.831	5.521	6.211	6.901
3 × 4	2-1/2 × 3-1/2	8.750	5.104	8.932	3.646	4.557	1.519	1.823	2.127	2.431	2.734	3.038
3 × 5	2-1/2 × 4-1/2	11.25	8.438	18.98	4.688	5.859	1.953	2.344	2.734	3.125	3.516	3.906
3 × 6	2-1/2 × 5-1/2	13.75	12.60	34.66	5.729	7.161	2.387	2.865	3.342	3.819	4.297	4.774
3 × 8	2-1/2 × 7-1/4	18.13	21.90	79.39	7.552	9.440	3.147	3.776	4.405	5.035	5.664	6.293
3 × 10	2-1/2 × 9-1/4	23.13	35.65	164.9	9.635	12.04	4.015	4.818	5.621	6.424	7.227	8.030
3 × 12	2-1/2 × 11-1/4	28.13	52.73	296.6	11.72	14.65	4.883	5.859	6.836	7.813	8.789	9.766
3 × 14	2-1/2 × 13-1/4	33.13	73.15	484.6	13.80	17.25	5.751	6.901	8.051	9.201	10.35	11.50
3 × 16	2-1/2 × 15-1/4	38.13	96.90	738.9	15.89	19.86	6.619	7.943	9.266	10.59	11.91	13.24
4 × 4	3-1/2 × 3-1/2	12.25	7.146	12.51	7.146	12.51	2.127	2.552	2.977	3.403	3.828	4.253
4 × 5	3-1/2 × 4-1/2	15.75	11.81	26.58	9.188	16.08	2.734	3.281	3.828	4.375	4.922	5.469
4 × 6	3-1/2 × 5-1/2	19.25	17.65	48.53	11.23	19.65	3.342	4.010	4.679	5.347	6.016	6.684
4 × 8	3-1/2 × 7-1/4	25.38	30.66	111.1	14.80	25.90	4.405	5.286	6.168	7.049	7.930	8.811
4 × 10	3-1/2 × 9-1/4	32.38	49.91	230.8	18.89	33.05	5.621	6.745	7.869	8.993	10.12	11.24
4 × 12	3-1/2 × 11-1/4	39.38	73.83	415.3	22.97	40.20	6.836	8.203	9.570	10.94	12.30	13.67
4 × 14	3-1/2 × 13-1/4	46.38	102.4	678.5	27.05	47.34	8.051	9.661	11.27	12.88	14.49	16.10
4 × 16	3-1/2 × 15-1/4	53.38	135.7	1034	31.14	54.49	9.266	11.12	12.97	14.83	16.68	18.53
5 × 5	4-1/2 × 4-1/2	20.25	15.19	34.17	15.19	34.17	3.516	4.219	4.922	5.625	6.328	7.031
6 × 6	5-1/2 × 5-1/2	30.25	27.73	76.26	27.73	76.26	5.252	6.302	7.352	8.403	9.453	10.50
6 × 8	5-1/2 × 7-1/2	41.25	51.56	193.4	37.81	104.0	7.161	8.594	10.03	11.46	12.89	14.32
6 × 10	5-1/2 × 9-1/2	52.25	82.73	393.0	47.90	131.7	9.071	10.89	12.70	14.51	16.33	18.14
6 × 12	5-1/2 × 11-1/2	63.25	121.2	697.1	57.98	159.4	10.98	13.18	15.37	17.57	19.77	21.96
6 × 14	5-1/2 × 13-1/2	74.25	167.1	1128	68.06	187.2	12.89	15.47	18.05	20.63	23.20	25.78
6 × 16	5-1/2 × 15-1/2	85.25	220.2	1707	78.15	214.9	14.80	17.76	20.72	23.68	26.64	29.60
6 × 18	5-1/2 × 17-1/2	96.25	280.7	2456	88.23	242.6	16.71	20.05	23.39	26.74	30.08	33.42
6 × 20	5-1/2 × 19-1/2	107.3	348.6	3398	98.31	270.4	18.62	22.34	26.07	29.79	33.52	37.24
6 × 22	5-1/2 × 21-1/2	118.3	423.7	4555	108.4	298.1	20.53	24.64	28.74	32.85	36.95	41.06
6 × 24	5-1/2 × 23-1/2	129.3	506.2	5948	118.5	325.8	22.44	26.93	31.41	35.90	40.39	44.88
8 × 8	7-1/2 × 7-1/2	56.25	70.31	263.7	70.31	263.7	9.766	11.72	13.67	15.63	17.58	19.53
8 × 10	7-1/2 × 9-1/2	71.25	112.8	535.9	89.06	334.0	12.37	14.84	17.32	19.79	22.27	24.74
8 × 12	7-1/2 × 11-1/2	86.25	165.3	950.5	107.8	404.3	14.97	17.97	20.96	23.96	26.95	29.95
8 × 14	7-1/2 × 13-1/2	101.3	227.8	1538	126.6	474.6	17.58	21.09	24.61	28.13	31.64	35.16
8 × 16	7-1/2 × 15-1/2	116.3	300.3	2327	145.3	544.9	20.18	24.22	28.26	32.29	36.33	40.36
8 × 18	7-1/2 × 17-1/2	131.3	382.8	3350	164.1	615.2	22.79	27.34	31.90	36.46	41.02	45.57
8 × 20	7-1/2 × 19-1/2	146.3	475.3	4634	182.8	685.5	25.39	30.47	35.55	40.63	45.70	50.78
8 × 22	7-1/2 × 21-1/2	161.3	577.8	6211	201.6	755.9	27.99	33.59	39.19	44.79	50.39	55.99
8 × 24	7-1/2 × 23-1/2	176.3	690.3	8111	220.3	826.2	30.60	36.72	42.84	48.96	55.08	61.20
10 × 10	9-1/2 × 9-1/2	90.25	142.9	678.8	142.9	678.8	15.67	18.80	21.94	25.07	28.20	31.34
10 × 12	9-1/2 × 11-1/2	109.3	209.4	1204	173.0	821.7	18.97	22.76	26.55	30.35	34.14	37.93
10 × 14	9-1/2 × 13-1/2	128.3	288.6	1948	203.1	964.5	22.27	26.72	31.17	35.63	40.08	44.53
10 × 16	9-1/2 × 15-1/2	147.3	380.4	2948	233.1	1107	25.56	30.68	35.79	40.90	46.02	51.13
10 × 18	9-1/2 × 17-1/2	166.3	484.9	4243	263.2	1250	28.86	34.64	40.41	46.18	51.95	57.73
10 × 20	9-1/2 × 19-1/2	185.3	602.1	5870	293.3	1393	32.16	38.59	45.03	51.46	57.89	64.32
10 × 22	9-1/2 × 21-1/2	204.3	731.9	7868	323.4	1536	35.46	42.55	49.64	56.74	63.83	70.92
10 × 24	9-1/2 × 23-1/2	223.3	874.4	10270	353.5	1679	38.76	46.51	54.26	62.01	69.77	77.52

Nominal Size b × d	Standard Dressed Size (S4S) b × d inches × inches	Area of Section A in.²	X-X Axis Section Modulus S_x in.³	X-X Axis Moment of Inertia I_x in.⁴	Y-Y Axis Section Modulus S_y in.³	Y-Y Axis Moment of Inertia I_y in.⁴	Approximate weight in pounds per linear foot (lb./ft.) of piece when density of wood equals: 25 lb./ft.³	30 lb./ft.³	35 lb./ft.³	40 lb./ft.³	45 lb./ft.³	50 lb./ft.³
12 × 12	11-1/2 × 11-1/2	132.3	253.5	1458	253.5	1458	22.96	27.55	32.14	36.74	41.33	45.92
12 × 14	11-1/2 × 13-1/2	155.3	349.3	2358	297.6	1711	26.95	32.34	37.73	43.13	48.52	53.91
12 × 16	11-1/2 × 15-1/2	178.3	460.5	3569	341.6	1964	30.95	37.14	43.32	49.51	55.70	61.89
12 × 18	11-1/2 × 17-1/2	201.3	587.0	5136	385.7	2218	34.94	41.93	48.91	55.90	62.89	69.88
12 × 20	11-1/2 × 19-1/2	224.3	728.8	7106	429.8	2471	38.93	46.72	54.51	62.29	70.08	77.86
12 × 22	11-1/2 × 21-1/2	247.3	886.0	9524	473.9	2725	42.93	51.51	60.10	68.68	77.27	85.85
12 × 24	11-1/2 × 23-1/2	270.3	1058	12440	518.0	2978	46.92	56.30	65.69	75.07	84.45	93.84
14 × 14	13-1/2 × 13-1/2	182.3	410.1	2768	410.1	2768	31.64	37.97	44.30	50.63	56.95	63.28
14 × 16	13-1/2 × 15-1/2	209.3	540.6	4189	470.8	3178	36.33	43.59	50.86	58.13	65.39	72.66
14 × 18	13-1/2 × 17-1/2	236.3	689.1	6029	531.6	3588	41.02	49.22	57.42	65.63	73.83	82.03
14 × 20	13-1/2 × 19-1/2	263.3	855.6	8342	592.3	3998	45.70	54.84	63.98	73.13	82.27	91.41
14 × 22	13-1/2 × 21-1/2	290.3	1040	11180	653.1	4408	50.39	60.47	70.55	80.63	90.70	100.8
14 × 24	13-1/2 × 23-1/2	317.3	1243	14600	713.8	4818	55.08	66.09	77.11	88.13	99.14	110.2
16 × 16	15-1/2 × 15-1/2	240.3	620.6	4810	620.6	4810	41.71	50.05	58.39	66.74	75.08	83.42
16 × 18	15-1/2 × 17-1/2	271.3	791.1	6923	700.7	5431	47.09	56.51	65.93	75.35	84.77	94.18
16 × 20	15-1/2 × 19-1/2	302.3	982.3	9578	780.8	6051	52.47	62.97	73.46	83.96	94.45	104.9
16 × 22	15-1/2 × 21-1/2	333.3	1194	12840	860.9	6672	57.86	69.43	81.00	92.57	104.1	115.7
16 × 24	15-1/2 × 23-1/2	364.3	1427	16760	941.0	7293	63.24	75.89	88.53	101.2	113.8	126.5
18 × 18	17-1/2 × 17-1/2	306.3	893.2	7816	893.2	7816	53.17	63.80	74.44	85.07	95.70	106.3
18 × 20	17-1/2 × 19-1/2	341.3	1109	10810	995.3	8709	59.24	71.09	82.94	94.79	106.6	118.5
18 × 22	17-1/2 × 21-1/2	376.3	1348	14490	1097	9602	65.32	78.39	91.45	104.5	117.6	130.6
18 × 24	17-1/2 × 23-1/2	411.3	1611	18930	1199	10500	71.40	85.68	99.96	114.2	128.5	142.8
20 × 20	19-1/2 × 19-1/2	380.3	1236	12050	1236	12050	66.02	79.22	92.42	105.6	118.8	132.0
20 × 22	19-1/2 × 21-1/2	419.3	1502	16150	1363	13280	72.79	87.34	101.9	116.5	131.0	145.6
20 × 24	19-1/2 × 23-1/2	458.3	1795	21090	1489	14520	79.56	95.47	111.4	127.3	143.2	159.1
22 × 22	21-1/2 × 21-1/2	462.3	1656	17810	1656	17810	80.25	96.30	112.4	128.4	144.5	160.5
22 × 24	21-1/2 × 23-1/2	505.3	1979	23250	1810	19460	87.72	105.3	122.8	140.3	157.9	175.4
24 × 24	23-1/2 × 23-1/2	552.3	2163	25420	2163	25420	95.88	115.1	134.2	153.4	172.6	191.8

3

SECTION PROPERTIES

Table 1C Section Properties of *Western Species* Structural Glued Laminated Timber

Depth d (in.)	Area A (in.²)	X-X Axis I_x (in.⁴)	X-X Axis S_x (in.³)	X-X Axis r_x (in.)	Y-Y Axis I_y (in.⁴)	Y-Y Axis S_y (in.³)
		2-1/2 in. Width			**(r_y = 0.722 in.)**	
6	15.00	45.00	15.00	1.732	7.813	6.250
7-1/2	18.75	87.89	23.44	2.165	9.766	7.813
9	22.50	151.9	33.75	2.598	11.72	9.375
10-1/2	26.25	241.2	45.94	3.031	13.67	10.94
12	30.00	360.0	60.00	3.464	15.63	12.50
13-1/2	33.75	512.6	75.94	3.897	17.58	14.06
15	37.50	703.1	93.75	4.330	19.53	15.63
16-1/2	41.25	935.9	113.4	4.763	21.48	17.19
18	45.00	1215	135.0	5.196	23.44	18.75
19-1/2	48.75	1545	158.4	5.629	25.39	20.31
21	52.50	1929	183.8	6.062	27.34	21.88
		3-1/8 in. Width			**(r_y = 0.902 in.)**	
6	18.75	56.25	18.75	1.732	15.26	9.766
7-1/2	23.44	109.9	29.30	2.165	19.07	12.21
9	28.13	189.8	42.19	2.598	22.89	14.65
10-1/2	32.81	301.5	57.42	3.031	26.70	17.09
12	37.50	450.0	75.00	3.464	30.52	19.53
13-1/2	42.19	640.7	94.92	3.897	34.33	21.97
15	46.88	878.9	117.2	4.330	38.15	24.41
16-1/2	51.56	1170	141.8	4.763	41.96	26.86
18	56.25	1519	168.8	5.196	45.78	29.30
19-1/2	60.94	1931	198.0	5.629	49.59	31.74
21	65.63	2412	229.7	6.062	53.41	34.18
22-1/2	70.31	2966	263.7	6.495	57.22	36.62
24	75.00	3600	300.0	6.928	61.04	39.06
		3-1/2 in. Width			**(r_y = 1.010 in.)**	
6	21.00	63.00	21.00	1.732	21.44	12.25
7-1/2	26.25	123.0	32.81	2.165	26.80	15.31
9	31.50	212.6	47.25	2.598	32.16	18.38
10-1/2	36.75	337.6	64.31	3.031	37.52	21.44
12	42.00	504.0	84.00	3.464	42.88	24.50
13-1/2	47.25	717.6	106.3	3.897	48.23	27.56
15	52.50	984.4	131.3	4.330	53.59	30.63
16-1/2	57.75	1310	158.8	4.763	58.95	33.69
18	63.00	1701	189.0	5.196	64.31	36.75
19-1/2	68.25	2163	221.8	5.629	69.67	39.81
21	73.50	2701	257.3	6.062	75.03	42.88
22-1/2	78.75	3322	295.3	6.495	80.39	45.94
24	84.00	4032	336.0	6.928	85.75	49.00

Table 1C Section Properties of *Western Species* Structural Glued Laminated Timber (Cont.)

Depth d (in.)	Area A (in.^{2})	X-X Axis			Y-Y Axis	
		I_x (in.^{4})	S_x (in.^{3})	r_x (in.)	I_y (in.^{4})	S_y (in.^{3})
5-1/8 in. Width					**($r_y = 1.479$ in.)**	
6	30.75	92.25	30.75	1.732	67.31	26.27
7-1/2	38.44	180.2	48.05	2.165	84.13	32.83
9	46.13	311.3	69.19	2.598	101.0	39.40
10-1/2	53.81	494.4	94.17	3.031	117.8	45.96
12	61.50	738.0	123.0	3.464	134.6	52.53
13-1/2	69.19	1051	155.7	3.897	151.4	59.10
15	76.88	1441	192.2	4.330	168.3	65.66
16-1/2	84.56	1919	232.5	4.763	185.1	72.23
18	92.25	2491	276.8	5.196	201.9	78.80
19-1/2	99.94	3167	324.8	5.629	218.7	85.36
21	107.6	3955	376.7	6.062	235.6	91.93
22-1/2	115.3	4865	432.4	6.495	252.4	98.50
24	123.0	5904	492.0	6.928	269.2	105.1
25-1/2	130.7	7082	555.4	7.361	286.0	111.6
27	138.4	8406	622.7	7.794	302.9	118.2
28-1/2	146.1	9887	693.8	8.227	319.7	124.8
30	153.8	11530	768.8	8.660	336.5	131.3
31-1/2	161.4	13350	847.5	9.093	353.4	137.9
33	169.1	15350	930.2	9.526	370.2	144.5
34-1/2	176.8	17540	1017	9.959	387.0	151.0
36	184.5	19930	1107	10.39	403.8	157.6
5-1/2 in. Width					**($r_y = 1.588$ in.)**	
6	33.00	99.00	33.00	1.732	83.19	30.25
7-1/2	41.25	193.4	51.56	2.165	104.0	37.81
9	49.50	334.1	74.25	2.598	124.8	45.38
10-1/2	57.75	530.6	101.1	3.031	145.6	52.94
12	66.00	792.0	132.0	3.464	166.4	60.50
13-1/2	74.25	1128	167.1	3.897	187.2	68.06
15	82.50	1547	206.3	4.330	208.0	75.63
16-1/2	90.75	2059	249.6	4.763	228.8	83.19
18	99.00	2673	297.0	5.196	249.6	90.75
19-1/2	107.3	3398	348.6	5.629	270.4	98.31
21	115.5	4245	404.3	6.062	291.2	105.9
22-1/2	123.8	5221	464.1	6.495	312.0	113.4
24	132.0	6336	528.0	6.928	332.8	121.0
25-1/2	140.3	7600	596.1	7.361	353.5	128.6
27	148.5	9021	668.3	7.794	374.3	136.1
28-1/2	156.8	10610	744.6	8.227	395.1	143.7
30	165.0	12380	825.0	8.660	415.9	151.3
31-1/2	173.3	14330	909.6	9.093	436.7	158.8
33	181.5	16470	998.3	9.526	457.5	166.4
34-1/2	189.8	18820	1091	9.959	478.3	173.9
36	198.0	21380	1188	10.39	499.1	181.5

3

SECTION PROPERTIES

Table 1C   Section Properties of *Western Species* Structural Glued Laminated Timber (Cont.)

Depth	Area	X-X Axis			Y-Y Axis	
d (in.)	A (in.^{2})	I_x (in.^{4})	S_x (in.^{3})	r_x (in.)	I_y (in.^{4})	S_y (in.^{3})
		6-3/4 in. Width			(r_y = 1.949 in.)	
7-1/2	50.63	237.3	63.28	2.165	192.2	56.95
9	60.75	410.1	91.13	2.598	230.7	68.34
10-1/2	70.88	651.2	124.0	3.031	269.1	79.73
12	81.00	972.0	162.0	3.464	307.5	91.13
13-1/2	91.13	1384	205.0	3.897	346.0	102.5
15	101.3	1898	253.1	4.330	384.4	113.9
16-1/2	111.4	2527	306.3	4.763	422.9	125.3
18	121.5	3281	364.5	5.196	461.3	136.7
19-1/2	131.6	4171	427.8	5.629	499.8	148.1
21	141.8	5209	496.1	6.062	538.2	159.5
22-1/2	151.9	6407	569.5	6.495	576.7	170.9
24	162.0	7776	648.0	6.928	615.1	182.3
25-1/2	172.1	9327	731.5	7.361	653.5	193.6
27	182.3	11070	820.1	7.794	692.0	205.0
28-1/2	192.4	13020	913.8	8.227	730.4	216.4
30	202.5	15190	1013	8.660	768.9	227.8
31-1/2	212.6	17580	1116	9.093	807.3	239.2
33	222.8	20210	1225	9.526	845.8	250.6
34-1/2	232.9	23100	1339	9.959	884.2	262.0
36	243.0	26240	1458	10.39	922.6	273.4
37-1/2	253.1	29660	1582	10.83	961.1	284.8
39	263.3	33370	1711	11.26	999.5	296.2
40-1/2	273.4	37370	1845	11.69	1038	307.5
42	283.5	41670	1985	12.12	1076	318.9
43-1/2	293.6	46300	2129	12.56	1115	330.3
45	303.8	51260	2278	12.99	1153	341.7
46-1/2	313.9	56560	2433	13.42	1192	353.1
48	324.0	62210	2592	13.86	1230	364.5
49-1/2	334.1	68220	2757	14.29	1269	375.9
51	344.3	74620	2926	14.72	1307	387.3
52-1/2	354.4	81400	3101	15.16	1346	398.7
54	364.5	88570	3281	15.59	1384	410.1
55-1/2	374.6	96160	3465	16.02	1422	421.5
57	384.8	104200	3655	16.45	1461	432.8
58-1/2	394.9	112600	3850	16.89	1499	444.2
60	405.0	121500	4050	17.32	1538	455.6

Depth	Area	X-X Axis			Y-Y Axis	
d (in.)	A (in.^{2})	I_x (in.^{4})	S_x (in.^{3})	r_x (in.)	I_y (in.^{4})	S_y (in.^{3})
		8-3/4 in. Width			**(r_y = 2.526 in.)**	
9	78.75	531.6	118.1	2.598	502.4	114.8
10-1/2	91.88	844.1	160.8	3.031	586.2	134.0
12	105.0	1260	210.0	3.464	669.9	153.1
13-1/2	118.1	1794	265.8	3.897	753.7	172.3
15	131.3	2461	328.1	4.330	837.4	191.4
16-1/2	144.4	3276	397.0	4.763	921.1	210.5
18	157.5	4253	472.5	5.196	1005	229.7
19-1/2	170.6	5407	554.5	5.629	1089	248.8
21	183.8	6753	643.1	6.062	1172	268.0
22-1/2	196.9	8306	738.3	6.495	1256	287.1
24	210.0	10080	840.0	6.928	1340	306.3
25-1/2	223.1	12090	948.3	7.361	1424	325.4
27	236.3	14350	1063	7.794	1507	344.5
28-1/2	249.4	16880	1185	8.227	1591	363.7
30	262.5	19690	1313	8.660	1675	382.8
31-1/2	275.6	22790	1447	9.093	1759	402.0
33	288.8	26200	1588	9.526	1842	421.1
34-1/2	301.9	29940	1736	9.959	1926	440.2
36	315.0	34020	1890	10.39	2010	459.4
37-1/2	328.1	38450	2051	10.83	2094	478.5
39	341.3	43250	2218	11.26	2177	497.7
40-1/2	354.4	48440	2392	11.69	2261	516.8
42	367.5	54020	2573	12.12	2345	535.9
43-1/2	380.6	60020	2760	12.56	2428	555.1
45	393.8	66450	2953	12.99	2512	574.2
46-1/2	406.9	73310	3153	13.42	2596	593.4
48	420.0	80640	3360	13.86	2680	612.5
49-1/2	433.1	88440	3573	14.29	2763	631.6
51	446.3	96720	3793	14.72	2847	650.8
52-1/2	459.4	105500	4020	15.16	2931	669.9
54	472.5	114800	4253	15.59	3015	689.1
55-1/2	485.6	124700	4492	16.02	3098	708.2
57	498.8	135000	4738	16.45	3182	727.3
58-1/2	511.9	146000	4991	16.89	3266	746.5
60	525.0	157500	5250	17.32	3350	765.6

3

SECTION PROPERTIES

Table 1C Section Properties of *Western Species* Structural Glued Laminated Timber (Cont.)

Depth d (in.)	Area A (in.²)	X-X Axis			Y-Y Axis	
		I_x (in.⁴)	S_x (in.³)	r_x (in.)	I_y (in.⁴)	S_y (in.³)
		10-3/4 in. Width			**(r_y = 3.103 in.)**	
12	129.0	1548	258.0	3.464	1242	231.1
13-1/2	145.1	2204	326.5	3.897	1398	260.0
15	161.3	3023	403.1	4.330	1553	288.9
16-1/2	177.4	4024	487.8	4.763	1708	317.8
18	193.5	5225	580.5	5.196	1863	346.7
19-1/2	209.6	6642	681.3	5.629	2019	375.6
21	225.8	8296	790.1	6.062	2174	404.5
22-1/2	241.9	10200	907.0	6.495	2329	433.4
24	258.0	12380	1032	6.928	2485	462.3
25-1/2	274.1	14850	1165	7.361	2640	491.1
27	290.3	17630	1306	7.794	2795	520.0
28-1/2	306.4	20740	1455	8.227	2950	548.9
30	322.5	24190	1613	8.660	3106	577.8
31-1/2	338.6	28000	1778	9.093	3261	606.7
33	354.8	32190	1951	9.526	3416	635.6
34-1/2	370.9	36790	2133	9.959	3572	664.5
36	387.0	41800	2322	10.39	3727	693.4
37-1/2	403.1	47240	2520	10.83	3882	722.3
39	419.3	53140	2725	11.26	4037	751.2
40-1/2	435.4	59510	2939	11.69	4193	780.0
42	451.5	66370	3161	12.12	4348	808.9
43-1/2	467.6	73740	3390	12.56	4503	837.8
45	483.8	81630	3628	12.99	4659	866.7
46-1/2	499.9	90070	3874	13.42	4814	895.6
48	516.0	99070	4128	13.86	4969	924.5
49-1/2	532.1	108700	4390	14.29	5124	953.4
51	548.3	118800	4660	14.72	5280	982.3
52-1/2	564.4	129600	4938	15.16	5435	1011
54	580.5	141100	5225	15.59	5590	1040
55-1/2	596.6	153100	5519	16.02	5746	1069
57	612.8	165900	5821	16.45	5901	1098
58-1/2	628.9	179300	6132	16.89	6056	1127
60	645.0	193500	6450	17.32	6211	1156

Table 1C Section Properties of *Western Species* Structural Glued Laminated Timber (Cont.)

Depth	Area	X-X Axis			Y-Y Axis	
d (in.)	A (in.^{2})	I_x (in.^{4})	S_x (in.^{3})	r_x (in.)	I_y (in.^{4})	S_y (in.^{3})
		12-1/4 in. Width			(r_y = 3.536 in.)	
13-1/2	165.4	2512	372.1	3.897	2068	337.6
15	183.8	3445	459.4	4.330	2298	375.2
16-1/2	202.1	4586	555.8	4.763	2528	412.7
18	220.5	5954	661.5	5.196	2757	450.2
19-1/2	238.9	7569	776.3	5.629	2987	487.7
21	257.3	9454	900.4	6.062	3217	525.2
22-1/2	275.6	11630	1034	6.495	3447	562.7
24	294.0	14110	1176	6.928	3677	600.3
25-1/2	312.4	16930	1328	7.361	3906	637.8
27	330.8	20090	1488	7.794	4136	675.3
28-1/2	349.1	23630	1658	8.227	4366	712.8
30	367.5	27560	1838	8.660	4596	750.3
31-1/2	385.9	31910	2026	9.093	4825	787.8
33	404.3	36690	2223	9.526	5055	825.3
34-1/2	422.6	41920	2430	9.959	5285	862.9
36	441.0	47630	2646	10.39	5515	900.4
37-1/2	459.4	53830	2871	10.83	5745	937.9
39	477.8	60550	3105	11.26	5974	975.4
40-1/2	496.1	67810	3349	11.69	6204	1013
42	514.5	75630	3602	12.12	6434	1050
43-1/2	532.9	84030	3863	12.56	6664	1088
45	551.3	93020	4134	12.99	6893	1125
46-1/2	569.6	102600	4415	13.42	7123	1163
48	588.0	112900	4704	13.86	7353	1201
49-1/2	606.4	123800	5003	14.29	7583	1238
51	624.8	135400	5310	14.72	7813	1276
52-1/2	643.1	147700	5627	15.16	8042	1313
54	661.5	160700	5954	15.59	8272	1351
55-1/2	679.9	174500	6289	16.02	8502	1388
57	698.3	189100	6633	16.45	8732	1426
58-1/2	716.6	204400	6987	16.89	8962	1463
60	735.0	220500	7350	17.32	9191	1501

3

SECTION PROPERTIES

Table 1D   Section Properties of *Southern Pine* Structural Glued Laminated Timber

Depth	Area	X-X Axis				Y-Y Axis	
d (in.)	A (in.^{2})	I_x (in.^{4})	S_x (in.^{3})	r_x (in.)	I_y (in.^{4})	S_y (in.^{3})	
2-1/2 in. Width					$(r_y = 0.722$ in.$)$		
5-1/2	13.75	34.66	12.60	1.588	7.161	5.729
6-7/8	17.19	67.70	19.69	1.985	8.952	7.161
8-1/4	20.63	117.0	28.36	2.382	10.74	8.594
9-5/8	24.06	185.8	38.60	2.778	12.53	10.03
11	27.50	277.3	50.42	3.175	14.32	11.46
12-3/8	30.94	394.8	63.81	3.572	16.11	12.89
13-3/4	34.38	541.6	78.78	3.969	17.90	14.32
15-1/8	37.81	720.9	95.32	4.366	19.69	15.76
16-1/2	41.25	935.9	113.4	4.763	21.48	17.19
17-7/8	44.69	1190	133.1	5.160	23.27	18.62
19-1/4	48.13	1486	154.4	5.557	25.07	20.05
20-5/8	51.56	1828	177.2	5.954	26.86	21.48
22	55.00	2218	201.7	6.351	28.65	22.92
23-3/8	58.44	2661	227.7	6.748	30.44	24.35
3 in. Width					$(r_y = 0.866$ in.$)$		
5-1/2	16.50	41.59	15.13	1.588	12.38	8.250
6-7/8	20.63	81.24	23.63	1.985	15.47	10.31
8-1/4	24.75	140.4	34.03	2.382	18.56	12.38
9-5/8	28.88	222.9	46.32	2.778	21.66	14.44
11	33.00	332.8	60.50	3.175	24.75	16.50
12-3/8	37.13	473.8	76.57	3.572	27.84	18.56
13-3/4	41.25	649.9	94.53	3.969	30.94	20.63
15-1/8	45.38	865.0	114.4	4.366	34.03	22.69
16-1/2	49.50	1123	136.1	4.763	37.13	24.75
17-7/8	53.63	1428	159.8	5.160	40.22	26.81
19-1/4	57.75	1783	185.3	5.557	43.31	28.88
20-5/8	61.88	2193	212.7	5.954	46.41	30.94
22	66.00	2662	242.0	6.351	49.50	33.00
23-3/8	70.13	3193	273.2	6.748	52.59	35.06
3-1/8 in. Width					$(r_y = 0.902$ in.$)$		
5-1/2	17.19	43.33	15.76	1.588	13.99	8.952
6-7/8	21.48	84.62	24.62	1.985	17.48	11.19
8-1/4	25.78	146.2	35.45	2.382	20.98	13.43
9-5/8	30.08	232.2	48.25	2.778	24.48	15.67
11	34.38	346.6	63.02	3.175	27.97	17.90
12-3/8	38.67	493.5	79.76	3.572	31.47	20.14
13-3/4	42.97	677.0	98.47	3.969	34.97	22.38
15-1/8	47.27	901.1	119.1	4.366	38.46	24.62
16-1/2	51.56	1170	141.8	4.763	41.96	26.86
17-7/8	55.86	1487	166.4	5.160	45.46	29.09
19-1/4	60.16	1858	193.0	5.557	48.96	31.33
20-5/8	64.45	2285	221.6	5.954	52.45	33.57
22	68.75	2773	252.1	6.351	55.95	35.81
23-3/8	73.05	3326	284.6	6.748	59.45	38.05

Depth	Area	X-X Axis			Y-Y Axis	
d (in.)	A (in.^{2})	I_x (in.^{4})	S_x (in.^{3})	r_x (in.)	I_y (in.^{4})	S_y (in.^{3})
3-1/2 in. Width					**(r_y = 1.010 in.)**	
5-1/2	19.25	48.53	17.65	1.588	19.65	11.23
6-7/8	24.06	94.78	27.57	1.985	24.56	14.04
8-1/4	28.88	163.8	39.70	2.382	29.48	16.84
9-5/8	33.69	260.1	54.04	2.778	34.39	19.65
11	38.50	388.2	70.58	3.175	39.30	22.46
12-3/8	43.31	552.7	89.33	3.572	44.21	25.27
13-3/4	48.13	758.2	110.3	3.969	49.13	28.07
15-1/8	52.94	1009	133.4	4.366	54.04	30.88
16-1/2	57.75	1310	158.8	4.763	58.95	33.69
17-7/8	62.56	1666	186.4	5.160	63.87	36.49
19-1/4	67.38	2081	216.2	5.557	68.78	39.30
20-5/8	72.19	2559	248.1	5.954	73.69	42.11
22	77.00	3106	282.3	6.351	78.60	44.92
23-3/8	81.81	3725	318.7	6.748	83.52	47.72
5 in. Width					**(r_y = 1.443 in.)**	
6-7/8	34.38	135.4	39.39	1.985	71.61	28.65
8-1/4	41.25	234.0	56.72	2.382	85.94	34.38
9-5/8	48.13	371.5	77.20	2.778	100.3	40.10
11	55.00	554.6	100.8	3.175	114.6	45.83
12-3/8	61.88	789.6	127.6	3.572	128.9	51.56
13-3/4	68.75	1083	157.6	3.969	143.2	57.29
15-1/8	75.63	1442	190.6	4.366	157.6	63.02
16-1/2	82.50	1872	226.9	4.763	171.9	68.75
17-7/8	89.38	2380	266.3	5.160	186.2	74.48
19-1/4	96.25	2972	308.8	5.557	200.5	80.21
20-5/8	103.1	3656	354.5	5.954	214.8	85.94
22	110.0	4437	403.3	6.351	229.2	91.67
23-3/8	116.9	5322	455.3	6.748	243.5	97.40
24-3/4	123.8	6317	510.5	7.145	257.8	103.1
26-1/8	130.6	7429	568.8	7.542	272.1	108.9
27-1/2	137.5	8665	630.2	7.939	286.5	114.6
28-7/8	144.4	10030	694.8	8.335	300.8	120.3
30-1/4	151.3	11530	762.6	8.732	315.1	126.0
31-5/8	158.1	13180	833.5	9.129	329.4	131.8
33	165.0	14970	907.5	9.526	343.8	137.5
34-3/8	171.9	16920	984.7	9.923	358.1	143.2
35-3/4	178.8	19040	1065	10.32	372.4	149.0

3

SECTION PROPERTIES

Table 1D   Section Properties of *Southern Pine* Structural Glued Laminated Timber (Cont.)

Depth d (in.)	Area A (in.^{2})	X-X Axis			Y-Y Axis	
		I_x (in.^{4})	S_x (in.^{3})	r_x (in.)	I_y (in.^{4})	S_y (in.^{3})
5-1/8 in. Width					**(r_y = 1.479 in.)**	
6-7/8	35.23	138.8	40.37	1.985	77.12	30.10
8-1/4	42.28	239.8	58.14	2.382	92.55	36.12
9-5/8	49.33	380.8	79.13	2.778	108.0	42.13
11	56.38	568.4	103.4	3.175	123.4	48.15
12-3/8	63.42	809.4	130.8	3.572	138.8	54.17
13-3/4	70.47	1110	161.5	3.969	154.2	60.19
15-1/8	77.52	1478	195.4	4.366	169.7	66.21
16-1/2	84.56	1919	232.5	4.763	185.1	72.23
17-7/8	91.61	2439	272.9	5.160	200.5	78.25
19-1/4	98.66	3047	316.5	5.557	215.9	84.27
20-5/8	105.7	3747	363.4	5.954	231.4	90.29
22	112.8	4548	413.4	6.351	246.8	96.31
23-3/8	119.8	5455	466.7	6.748	262.2	102.3
24-3/4	126.8	6475	523.2	7.145	277.6	108.3
26-1/8	133.9	7615	583.0	7.542	293.1	114.4
27-1/2	140.9	8882	646	7.939	308.5	120.4
28-7/8	148.0	10280	712.2	8.335	323.9	126.4
30-1/4	155.0	11820	781.6	8.732	339.3	132.4
31-5/8	162.1	13510	854.3	9.129	354.8	138.4
33	169.1	15350	930.2	9.526	370.2	144.5
34-3/8	176.2	17350	1009	9.923	385.6	150.5
35-3/4	183.2	19510	1092	10.32	401.0	156.5
5-1/2 in. Width					**(r_y = 1.588 in.)**	
6-7/8	37.81	148.9	43.33	1.985	95.32	34.66
8-1/4	45.38	257.4	62.39	2.382	114.4	41.59
9-5/8	52.94	408.7	84.92	2.778	133.4	48.53
11	60.50	610.0	110.9	3.175	152.5	55.46
12-3/8	68.06	868.6	140.4	3.572	171.6	62.39
13-3/4	75.63	1191	173.3	3.969	190.6	69.32
15-1/8	83.19	1586	209.7	4.366	209.7	76.26
16-1/2	90.75	2059	249.6	4.763	228.8	83.19
17-7/8	98.31	2618	292.9	5.160	247.8	90.12
19-1/4	105.9	3269	339.7	5.557	266.9	97.05
20-5/8	113.4	4021	389.9	5.954	286.0	104.0
22	121.0	4880	443.7	6.351	305.0	110.9
23-3/8	128.6	5854	500.9	6.748	324.1	117.8
24-3/4	136.1	6949	561.5	7.145	343.1	124.8
26-1/8	143.7	8172	625.6	7.542	362.2	131.7
27-1/2	151.3	9532	693.2	7.939	381.3	138.6
28-7/8	158.8	11030	764.3	8.335	400.3	145.6
30-1/4	166.4	12690	838.8	8.732	419.4	152.5
31-5/8	173.9	14500	916.8	9.129	438.5	159.4
33	181.5	16470	998.3	9.526	457.5	166.4
34-3/8	189.1	18620	1083	9.923	476.6	173.3
35-3/4	196.6	20940	1172	10.32	495.7	180.2

Table 1D Section Properties of *Southern Pine* Structural Glued Laminated Timber (Cont.)

Depth	Area	X-X Axis			Y-Y Axis	
d (in.)	A (in.^{2})	I_x (in.^{4})	S_x (in.^{3})	r_x (in.)	I_y (in.^{4})	S_y (in.^{3})
6-3/4 in. Width					**(r_y = 1.949 in.)**	
6-7/8	46.41	182.8	53.17	1.985	176.2	52.21
8-1/4	55.69	315.9	76.57	2.382	211.4	62.65
9-5/8	64.97	501.6	104.2	2.778	246.7	73.09
11	74.25	748.7	136.1	3.175	281.9	83.53
12-3/8	83.53	1066	172.3	3.572	317.2	93.97
13-3/4	92.81	1462	212.7	3.969	352.4	104.4
15-1/8	102.1	1946	257.4	4.366	387.6	114.9
16-1/2	111.4	2527	306.3	4.763	422.9	125.3
17-7/8	120.7	3213	359.5	5.160	458.1	135.7
19-1/4	129.9	4012	416.9	5.557	493.4	146.2
20-5/8	139.2	4935	478.6	5.954	528.6	156.6
22	148.5	5990	544.5	6.351	563.8	167.1
23-3/8	157.8	7184	614.7	6.748	599.1	177.5
24-3/4	167.1	8528	689.1	7.145	634.3	187.9
26-1/8	176.3	10030	767.8	7.542	669.6	198.4
27-1/2	185.6	11700	850.8	7.939	704.8	208.8
28-7/8	194.9	13540	938.0	8.335	740.0	219.3
30-1/4	204.2	15570	1029	8.732	775.3	229.7
31-5/8	213.5	17790	1125	9.129	810.5	240.2
33	222.8	20210	1225	9.526	845.8	250.6
34-3/8	232.0	22850	1329	9.923	881.0	261.0
35-3/4	241.3	25700	1438	10.32	916.2	271.5
37-1/8	250.6	28780	1551	10.72	951.5	281.9
38-1/2	259.9	32100	1668	11.11	986.7	292.4
39-7/8	269.2	35660	1789	11.51	1022	302.8
41-1/4	278.4	39480	1914	11.91	1057	313.2
42-5/8	287.7	43560	2044	12.30	1092	323.7
44	297.0	47920	2178	12.70	1128	334.1
45-3/8	306.3	52550	2316	13.10	1163	344.6
46-3/4	315.6	57470	2459	13.50	1198	355.0
48-1/8	324.8	62700	2606	13.89	1233	365.4
49-1/2	334.1	68220	2757	14.29	1269	375.9
50-7/8	343.4	74070	2912	14.69	1304	386.3
52-1/4	352.7	80240	3071	15.08	1339	396.8
53-5/8	362.0	86740	3235	15.48	1374	407.2
55	371.3	93590	3403	15.88	1410	417.7
56-3/8	380.5	100800	3575	16.27	1445	428.1
57-3/4	389.8	108300	3752	16.67	1480	438.5
59-1/8	399.1	116300	3933	17.07	1515	449.0
60-1/2	408.4	124600	4118	17.46	1551	459.4

Table 1D Section Properties of *Southern Pine* Structural Glued Laminated Timber (Cont.)

Depth	Area	X-X Axis			Y-Y Axis	
d (in.)	A (in.^{2})	I_x (in.^{4})	S_x (in.^{3})	r_x (in.)	I_y (in.^{4})	S_y (in.^{3})
		8-1/2 in. Width			**(r_y = 2.454 in.)**	
9-5/8	81.81	631.6	131.2	2.778	492.6	115.9
11	93.50	942.8	171.4	3.175	562.9	132.5
12-3/8	105.2	1342	216.9	3.572	633.3	149.0
13-3/4	116.9	1841	267.8	3.969	703.7	165.6
15-1/8	128.6	2451	324.1	4.366	774.1	182.1
16-1/2	140.3	3182	385.7	4.763	844.4	198.7
17-7/8	151.9	4046	452.6	5.160	914.8	215.2
19-1/4	163.6	5053	525.0	5.557	985.2	231.8
20-5/8	175.3	6215	602.6	5.954	1056	248.4
22	187.0	7542	685.7	6.351	1126	264.9
23-3/8	198.7	9047	774.1	6.748	1196	281.5
24-3/4	210.4	10740	867.8	7.145	1267	298.0
26-1/8	222.1	12630	966.9	7.542	1337	314.6
27-1/2	233.8	14730	1071	7.939	1407	331.1
28-7/8	245.4	17050	1181	8.335	1478	347.7
30-1/4	257.1	19610	1296	8.732	1548	364.3
31-5/8	268.8	22400	1417	9.129	1618	380.8
33	280.5	25460	1543	9.526	1689	397.4
34-3/8	292.2	28770	1674	9.923	1759	413.9
35-3/4	303.9	32360	1811	10.32	1830	430.5
37-1/8	315.6	36240	1953	10.72	1900	447.0
38-1/2	327.3	40420	2100	11.11	1970	463.6
39-7/8	338.9	44910	2253	11.51	2041	480.2
41-1/4	350.6	49720	2411	11.91	2111	496.7
42-5/8	362.3	54860	2574	12.30	2181	513.3
44	374.0	60340	2743	12.70	2252	529.8
45-3/8	385.7	66170	2917	13.10	2322	546.4
46-3/4	397.4	72370	3096	13.50	2393	562.9
48-1/8	409.1	78950	3281	13.89	2463	579.5
49-1/2	420.8	85910	3471	14.29	2533	596.1
50-7/8	432.4	93270	3667	14.69	2604	612.6
52-1/4	444.1	101000	3868	15.08	2674	629.2
53-5/8	455.8	109200	4074	15.48	2744	645.7
55	467.5	117800	4285	15.88	2815	662.3
56-3/8	479.2	126900	4502	16.27	2885	678.8
57-3/4	490.9	136400	4725	16.67	2955	695.4
59-1/8	502.6	146400	4952	17.07	3026	712.0
60-1/2	514.3	156900	5185	17.46	3096	728.5

Depth	Area	X-X Axis				Y-Y Axis	
d (in.)	A (in.^{2})	I_x (in.^{4})	S_x (in.^{3})	r_x (in.)		I_y (in.^{4})	S_y (in.^{3})
10-1/2 in. Width						**(r_y = 3.031 in.)**	
11	115.5	1165	211.8	3.175		1061	202.1
12-3/8	129.9	1658	268.0	3.572		1194	227.4
13-3/4	144.4	2275	330.9	3.969		1326	252.7
15-1/8	158.8	3028	400.3	4.366		1459	277.9
16-1/2	173.3	3931	476.4	4.763		1592	303.2
17-7/8	187.7	4997	559.2	5.160		1724	328.5
19-1/4	202.1	6242	648.5	5.557		1857	353.7
20-5/8	216.6	7677	744.4	5.954		1990	379.0
22	231.0	9317	847.0	6.351		2122	404.3
23-3/8	245.4	11180	956.2	6.748		2255	429.5
24-3/4	259.9	13270	1072	7.145		2388	454.8
26-1/8	274.3	15600	1194	7.542		2520	480.0
27-1/2	288.8	18200	1323	7.939		2653	505.3
28-7/8	303.2	21070	1459	8.335		2786	530.6
30-1/4	317.6	24220	1601	8.732		2918	555.8
31-5/8	332.1	27680	1750	9.129		3051	581.1
33	346.5	31440	1906	9.526		3183	606.4
34-3/8	360.9	35540	2068	9.923		3316	631.6
35-3/4	375.4	39980	2237	10.32		3449	656.9
37-1/8	389.8	44770	2412	10.72		3581	682.2
38-1/2	404.3	49930	2594	11.11		3714	707.4
39-7/8	418.7	55480	2783	11.51		3847	732.7
41-1/4	433.1	61420	2978	11.91		3979	758.0
42-5/8	447.6	67760	3180	12.30		4112	783.2
44	462.0	74540	3388	12.70		4245	808.5
45-3/8	476.4	81740	3603	13.10		4377	833.8
46-3/4	490.9	89400	3825	13.50		4510	859.0
48-1/8	505.3	97530	4053	13.89		4643	884.3
49-1/2	519.8	106100	4288	14.29		4775	909.6
50-7/8	534.2	115200	4529	14.69		4908	934.8
52-1/4	548.6	124800	4778	15.08		5040	960.1
53-5/8	563.1	134900	5032	15.48		5173	985.4
55	577.5	145600	5294	15.88		5306	1011
56-3/8	591.9	156800	5562	16.27		5438	1036
57-3/4	606.4	168500	5836	16.67		5571	1061
59-1/8	620.8	180900	6118	17.07		5704	1086
60-1/2	635.3	193800	6405	17.46		5836	1112

3

SECTION PROPERTIES

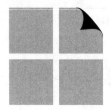

REFERENCE DESIGN VALUES

4

Table 4A Adjustment Factors

Repetitive Member Factor, C_r

Bending design values, F_b, for dimension lumber 2" to 4" thick shall be multiplied by the repetitive member factor, $C_r = 1.15$, when such members are used as joists, truss chords, rafters, studs, planks, decking, or similar members which are in contact or spaced not more than 24" on center, are not less than 3 in number and are joined by floor, roof, or other load distributing elements adequate to support the design load.

Wet Service Factor, C_M

When dimension lumber is used where moisture content will exceed 19% for an extended time period, design values shall be multiplied by the appropriate wet service factors from the following table:

Wet Service Factors, C_M

F_b	F_t	F_v	$F_{c\perp}$	F_c	E and E_{min}
0.85*	1.0	0.97	0.67	0.8**	0.9

* when $(F_b)(C_F) \leq 1{,}150$ psi, $C_M = 1.0$
** when $(F_c)(C_F) \leq 750$ psi, $C_M = 1.0$

Flat Use Factor, C_{fu}

Bending design values adjusted by size factors are based on edgewise use (load applied to narrow face). When dimension lumber is used flatwise (load applied to wide face), the bending design value, F_b, shall also be multiplied by the following flat use factors:

Flat Use Factors, C_{fu}

Width (depth)	Thickness (breadth)	
	2" & 3"	4"
2" & 3"	1.0	—
4"	1.1	1.0
5"	1.1	1.05
6"	1.15	1.05
8"	1.15	1.05
10" & wider	1.2	1.1

NOTE

To facilitate the use of Table 4A, shading has been employed to distinguish design values based on a 4" nominal width (Construction, Standard, and Utility grades) or a 6" nominal width (Stud grade) from design values based on a 12" nominal width (Select Structural, No.1 & Btr, No.1, No.2, and No.3 grades).

Size Factor, C_F

Tabulated bending, tension, and compression parallel to grain design values for dimension lumber 2" to 4" thick shall be multiplied by the following size factors:

Size Factors, C_F

Grades	Width (depth)	F_b		F_t	F_c
		Thickness (breadth)			
		2" & 3"	4"		
Select Structural, No.1 & Btr, No.1, No.2, No.3	2", 3", & 4"	1.5	1.5	1.5	1.15
	5"	1.4	1.4	1.4	1.1
	6"	1.3	1.3	1.3	1.1
	8"	1.2	1.3	1.2	1.05
	10"	1.1	1.2	1.1	1.0
	12"	1.0	1.1	1.0	1.0
	14" & wider	0.9	1.0	0.9	0.9
Stud	2", 3", & 4"	1.1	1.1	1.1	1.05
	5" & 6"	1.0	1.0	1.0	1.0
	8" & wider	Use No.3 Grade tabulated design values and size factors			
Construction, Standard	2", 3", & 4"	1.0	1.0	1.0	1.0
Utility	4"	1.0	1.0	1.0	1.0
	2" & 3"	0.4	—	0.4	0.6

Table 4A Reference Design Values for Visually Graded Dimension Lumber (2" - 4" thick)[1,2,3]

(All species except Southern Pine — see Table 4B) (Tabulated design values are for normal load duration and dry service conditions. See NDS 4.3 for a comprehensive description of design value adjustment factors.)

USE WITH TABLE 4A ADJUSTMENT FACTORS

Species and commercial grade	Size classification	Design values in pounds per square inch (psi)							Grading Rules Agency
		Bending F_b	Tension parallel to grain F_t	Shear parallel to grain F_v	Compression perpendicular to grain $F_{c\perp}$	Compression parallel to grain F_c	Modulus of Elasticity E	E_{min}	
ALASKA CEDAR									
Select Structural		1,150	625	165	525	1,000	1,400,000	510,000	
No.1		975	525	165	525	900	1,300,000	470,000	
No.2	2" & wider	800	425	165	525	750	1,200,000	440,000	
No.3		450	250	165	525	425	1,100,000	400,000	WCLIB
Stud	2" & wider	625	350	165	525	475	1,100,000	400,000	
Construction		900	500	165	525	950	1,200,000	440,000	
Standard	2" - 4" wide	500	275	165	525	775	1,100,000	400,000	
Utility		250	125	165	525	500	1,000,000	370,000	
ALASKA HEMLOCK									
Select Structural		1,300	825	185	440	1,200	1,700,000	620,000	
No.1		900	550	185	440	1,100	1,600,000	580,000	
No.2	2" & wider	825	475	185	440	1,050	1,500,000	550,000	
No.3		475	275	185	440	600	1,400,000	510,000	WWPA
Stud	2" & wider	650	375	185	440	650	1,400,000	510,000	
Construction		950	550	185	440	1,250	1,400,000	510,000	
Standard	2" - 4" wide	525	300	185	440	1,050	1,300,000	470,000	
Utility		250	150	185	440	700	1,200,000	440,000	
ALASKA SPRUCE									
Select Structural		1,400	900	160	330	1,200	1,600,000	580,000	
No.1		950	600	160	330	1,100	1,500,000	550,000	
No.2	2" & wider	875	500	160	330	1,050	1,400,000	510,000	
No.3		500	300	160	330	600	1,300,000	470,000	WWPA
Stud	2" & wider	675	400	160	330	675	1,300,000	470,000	
Construction		1,000	575	160	330	1,250	1,300,000	470,000	
Standard	2" - 4" wide	550	325	160	330	1,050	1,200,000	440,000	
Utility		275	150	160	330	700	1,100,000	400,000	
ALASKA YELLOW CEDAR									
Select Structural		1,350	800	225	510	1,200	1,500,000	550,000	
No.1		900	525	225	510	1,050	1,400,000	510,000	
No.2	2" & wider	800	450	225	510	1,000	1,300,000	470,000	
No.3		475	250	225	510	575	1,200,000	440,000	WCLIB
Stud	2" & wider	625	350	225	510	625	1,200,000	440,000	WWPA
Construction		925	500	225	510	1,250	1,300,000	470,000	
Standard	2" - 4" wide	500	275	225	510	1,050	1,100,000	400,000	
Utility		250	125	225	510	675	1,100,000	400,000	
ASPEN									
Select Structural		875	500	120	265	725	1,100,000	400,000	
No.1		625	375	120	265	600	1,100,000	400,000	
No.2	2" & wider	600	350	120	265	450	1,000,000	370,000	
No.3		350	200	120	265	275	900,000	330,000	NELMA
Stud	2" & wider	475	275	120	265	300	900,000	330,000	NSLB
Construction		700	400	120	265	625	900,000	330,000	WWPA
Standard	2" - 4" wide	375	225	120	265	475	900,000	330,000	
Utility		175	100	120	265	300	800,000	290,000	
BALDCYPRESS									
Select Structural		1,200	650	160	615	1,200	1,400,000	510,000	
No.1		1,000	550	160	615	1,050	1,400,000	510,000	
No.2	2" & wider	825	450	160	615	900	1,300,000	470,000	
No.3		475	250	160	615	525	1,200,000	440,000	SPIB
Stud	2" & wider	650	350	160	615	575	1,200,000	440,000	
Construction		925	500	160	615	1,100	1,200,000	440,000	
Standard	2" - 4" wide	525	275	160	615	925	1,100,000	400,000	
Utility		250	125	160	615	600	1,000,000	370,000	

Table 4A (Cont.) Reference Design Values for Visually Graded Dimension Lumber (2" - 4" thick)[1,2,3]

(All species except Southern Pine — see Table 4B) (Tabulated design values are for normal load duration and dry service conditions. See NDS 4.3 for a comprehensive description of design value adjustment factors.)

USE WITH TABLE 4A ADJUSTMENT FACTORS

Species and commercial grade	Size classification	Design values in pounds per square inch (psi)							Grading Rules Agency
		Bending F_b	Tension parallel to grain F_t	Shear parallel to grain F_v	Compression perpendicular to grain $F_{c\perp}$	Compression parallel to grain F_c	Modulus of Elasticity		
							E	E_{min}	
BEECH-BIRCH-HICKORY									
Select Structural		1,450	850	195	715	1,200	1,700,000	620,000	
No.1		1,050	600	195	715	950	1,600,000	580,000	
No.2	2" & wider	1,000	600	195	715	750	1,500,000	550,000	
No.3		575	350	195	715	425	1,300,000	470,000	NELMA
Stud	2" & wider	775	450	195	715	475	1,300,000	470,000	
Construction		1,150	675	195	715	1,000	1,400,000	510,000	
Standard	2" - 4" wide	650	375	195	715	775	1,300,000	470,000	
Utility		300	175	195	715	500	1,200,000	440,000	
COTTONWOOD									
Select Structural		875	525	125	320	775	1,200,000	440,000	
No.1		625	375	125	320	625	1,200,000	440,000	
No.2	2" & wider	625	350	125	320	475	1,100,000	400,000	
No.3		350	200	125	320	275	1,000,000	370,000	NSLB
Stud	2" & wider	475	275	125	320	300	1,000,000	370,000	
Construction		700	400	125	320	650	1,000,000	370,000	
Standard	2" - 4" wide	400	225	125	320	500	900,000	330,000	
Utility		175	100	125	320	325	900,000	330,000	
DOUGLAS FIR-LARCH									
Select Structural		1,500	1,000	180	625	1,700	1,900,000	690,000	
No.1 & Btr		1,200	800	180	625	1,550	1,800,000	660,000	
No.1	2" & wider	1,000	675	180	625	1,500	1,700,000	620,000	
No.2		900	575	180	625	1,350	1,600,000	580,000	WCLIB
No.3		525	325	180	625	775	1,400,000	510,000	WWPA
Stud	2" & wider	700	450	180	625	850	1,400,000	510,000	
Construction		1,000	650	180	625	1,650	1,500,000	550,000	
Standard	2" - 4" wide	575	375	180	625	1,400	1,400,000	510,000	
Utility		275	175	180	625	900	1,300,000	470,000	
DOUGLAS FIR-LARCH (NORTH)									
Select Structural		1,350	825	180	625	1,900	1,900,000	690,000	
No.1 & Btr		1,150	750	180	625	1,800	1,800,000	660,000	
No.1/No.2	2" & wider	850	500	180	625	1,400	1,600,000	580,000	
No.3		475	300	180	625	825	1,400,000	510,000	NLGA
Stud	2" & wider	650	400	180	625	900	1,400,000	510,000	
Construction		950	575	180	625	1,800	1,500,000	550,000	
Standard	2" - 4" wide	525	325	180	625	1,450	1,400,000	510,000	
Utility		250	150	180	625	950	1,300,000	470,000	
DOUGLAS FIR-SOUTH									
Select Structural		1,350	900	180	520	1,600	1,400,000	510,000	
No.1		925	600	180	520	1,450	1,300,000	470,000	
No.2	2" & wider	850	525	180	520	1,350	1,200,000	440,000	
No.3		500	300	180	520	775	1,100,000	400,000	WWPA
Stud	2" & wider	675	425	180	520	850	1,100,000	400,000	
Construction		975	600	180	520	1,650	1,200,000	440,000	
Standard	2" - 4" wide	550	350	180	520	1,400	1,100,000	400,000	
Utility		250	150	180	520	900	1,000,000	370,000	
EASTERN HEMLOCK-BALSAM FIR									
Select Structural		1,250	575	140	335	1,200	1,200,000	440,000	
No.1		775	350	140	335	1,000	1,100,000	400,000	
No.2	2" & wider	575	275	140	335	825	1,100,000	400,000	
No.3		350	150	140	335	475	900,000	330,000	NELMA
Stud	2" & wider	450	200	140	335	525	900,000	330,000	NSLB
Construction		675	300	140	335	1,050	1,000,000	370,000	
Standard	2" - 4" wide	375	175	140	335	850	900,000	330,000	
Utility		175	75	140	335	550	800,000	290,000	

Table 4A (Cont.) Reference Design Values for Visually Graded Dimension Lumber (2" – 4" thick)[1,2,3]

(All species except Southern Pine — see Table 4B) (Tabulated design values are for normal load duration and dry service conditions. See NDS 4.3 for a comprehensive description of design value adjustment factors.)

USE WITH TABLE 4A ADJUSTMENT FACTORS

Species and commercial grade	Size classification	Bending F_b	Tension parallel to grain F_t	Shear parallel to grain F_v	Compression perpendicular to grain $F_{c\perp}$	Compression parallel to grain F_c	Modulus of Elasticity E	E_{min}	Grading Rules Agency
EASTERN HEMLOCK-TAMARACK									
Select Structural		1,250	575	170	555	1,200	1,200,000	440,000	
No.1		775	350	170	555	1,000	1,100,000	400,000	
No.2	2" & wider	575	275	170	555	825	1,100,000	400,000	
No.3		350	150	170	555	475	900,000	330,000	NELMA
Stud	2" & wider	450	200	170	555	525	900,000	330,000	NSLB
Construction		675	300	170	555	1,050	1,000,000	370,000	
Standard	2" - 4" wide	375	175	170	555	850	900,000	330,000	
Utility		175	75	170	555	550	800,000	290,000	
EASTERN SOFTWOODS									
Select Structural		1,250	575	140	335	1,200	1,200,000	440,000	
No.1		775	350	140	335	1,000	1,100,000	400,000	
No.2	2" & wider	575	275	140	335	825	1,100,000	400,000	
No.3		350	150	140	335	475	900,000	330,000	NELMA
Stud	2" & wider	450	200	140	335	525	900,000	330,000	NSLB
Construction		675	300	140	335	1,050	1,000,000	370,000	
Standard	2" - 4" wide	375	175	140	335	850	900,000	330,000	
Utility		175	75	140	335	550	800,000	290,000	
EASTERN WHITE PINE									
Select Structural		1,250	575	135	350	1,200	1,200,000	440,000	
No.1		775	350	135	350	1,000	1,100,000	400,000	
No.2	2" & wider	575	275	135	350	825	1,100,000	400,000	
No.3		350	150	135	350	475	900,000	330,000	NELMA
Stud	2" & wider	450	200	135	350	525	900,000	330,000	NSLB
Construction		675	300	135	350	1,050	1,000,000	370,000	
Standard	2" - 4" wide	375	175	135	350	850	900,000	330,000	
Utility		175	75	135	350	550	800,000	290,000	
HEM-FIR									
Select Structural		1,400	925	150	405	1,500	1,600,000	580,000	
No.1 & Btr		1,100	725	150	405	1,350	1,500,000	550,000	
No.1	2" & wider	975	625	150	405	1,350	1,500,000	550,000	
No.2		850	525	150	405	1,300	1,300,000	470,000	
No.3		500	300	150	405	725	1,200,000	440,000	WCLIB
Stud	2" & wider	675	400	150	405	800	1,200,000	440,000	WWPA
Construction		975	600	150	405	1,550	1,300,000	470,000	
Standard	2" - 4" wide	550	325	150	405	1,300	1,200,000	440,000	
Utility		250	150	150	405	850	1,100,000	400,000	
HEM-FIR (NORTH)									
Select Structural		1,300	775	145	405	1,700	1,700,000	620,000	
No.1 & Btr	2" & wider	1,200	725	145	405	1,550	1,700,000	620,000	
No.1/No.2		1,000	575	145	405	1,450	1,600,000	580,000	
No.3		575	325	145	405	850	1,400,000	510,000	
Stud	2" & wider	775	450	145	405	925	1,400,000	510,000	NLGA
Construction		1,150	650	145	405	1,750	1,500,000	550,000	
Standard	2" - 4" wide	650	350	145	405	1,500	1,400,000	510,000	
Utility		300	175	145	405	975	1,300,000	470,000	
MIXED MAPLE									
Select Structural		1,000	600	195	620	875	1,300,000	470,000	
No.1		725	425	195	620	700	1,200,000	440,000	
No.2	2" & wider	700	425	195	620	550	1,100,000	400,000	
No.3		400	250	195	620	325	1,000,000	370,000	
Stud	2" & wider	550	325	195	620	350	1,000,000	370,000	NELMA
Construction		800	475	195	620	725	1,100,000	400,000	
Standard	2" - 4" wide	450	275	195	620	575	1,000,000	370,000	
Utility		225	125	195	620	375	900,000	330,000	

(All species except Southern Pine — see Table 4B) (Tabulated design values are for normal load duration and dry service conditions. See NDS 4.3 for a comprehensive description of design value adjustment factors.)

USE WITH TABLE 4A ADJUSTMENT FACTORS

Species and commercial grade	Size classification	Design values in pounds per square inch (psi)							Grading Rules Agency
		Bending F_b	Tension parallel to grain F_t	Shear parallel to grain F_v	Compression perpendicular to grain $F_{c\perp}$	Compression parallel to grain F_c	Modulus of Elasticity E	E_{min}	
MIXED OAK									
Select Structural		1,150	675	170	800	1,000	1,100,000	400,000	
No.1		825	500	170	800	825	1,000,000	370,000	
No.2	2" & wider	800	475	170	800	625	900,000	330,000	
No.3		475	275	170	800	375	800,000	290,000	NELMA
Stud	2" & wider	625	375	170	800	400	800,000	290,000	
Construction		925	550	170	800	850	900,000	330,000	
Standard	2" - 4" wide	525	300	170	800	650	800,000	290,000	
Utility		250	150	170	800	425	800,000	290,000	
NORTHERN RED OAK									
Select Structural		1,400	800	220	885	1,150	1,400,000	510,000	
No.1		1,000	575	220	885	925	1,400,000	510,000	
No.2	2" & wider	975	575	220	885	725	1,300,000	470,000	
No.3		550	325	220	885	425	1,200,000	440,000	NELMA
Stud	2" & wider	750	450	220	885	450	1,200,000	440,000	
Construction		1,100	650	220	885	975	1,200,000	440,000	
Standard	2" - 4" wide	625	350	220	885	750	1,100,000	400,000	
Utility		300	175	220	885	500	1,000,000	370,000	
NORTHERN SPECIES									
Select Structural		975	425	110	350	1,100	1,100,000	400,000	
No.1/No.2	2" & wider	625	275	110	350	850	1,100,000	400,000	
No.3		350	150	110	350	500	1,000,000	370,000	
Stud	2" & wider	475	225	110	350	550	1,000,000	370,000	NLGA
Construction		700	325	110	350	1,050	1,000,000	370,000	
Standard	2" - 4" wide	400	175	110	350	875	900,000	330,000	
Utility		175	75	110	350	575	900,000	330,000	
NORTHERN WHITE CEDAR									
Select Structural		775	450	120	370	750	800,000	290,000	
No.1		575	325	120	370	600	700,000	260,000	
No.2	2" & wider	550	325	120	370	475	700,000	260,000	
No.3		325	175	120	370	275	600,000	220,000	NELMA
Stud	2" & wider	425	250	120	370	300	600,000	220,000	
Construction		625	375	120	370	625	700,000	260,000	
Standard	2" - 4" wide	350	200	120	370	475	600,000	220,000	
Utility		175	100	120	370	325	600,000	220,000	
RED MAPLE									
Select Structural		1,300	750	210	615	1,100	1,700,000	620,000	
No.1		925	550	210	615	900	1,600,000	580,000	
No.2	2" & wider	900	525	210	615	700	1,500,000	550,000	
No.3		525	300	210	615	400	1,300,000	470,000	NELMA
Stud	2" & wider	700	425	210	615	450	1,300,000	470,000	
Construction		1,050	600	210	615	925	1,400,000	510,000	
Standard	2" - 4" wide	575	325	210	615	725	1,300,000	470,000	
Utility		275	150	210	615	475	1,200,000	440,000	
RED OAK									
Select Structural		1,150	675	170	820	1,000	1,400,000	510,000	
No.1		825	500	170	820	825	1,300,000	470,000	
No.2	2" & wider	800	475	170	820	625	1,200,000	440,000	
No.3		475	275	170	820	375	1,100,000	400,000	NELMA
Stud	2" & wider	625	375	170	820	400	1,100,000	400,000	
Construction		925	550	170	820	850	1,200,000	440,000	
Standard	2" - 4" wide	525	300	170	820	650	1,100,000	400,000	
Utility		250	150	170	820	425	1,000,000	370,000	

Table 4A (Cont.)   Reference Design Values for Visually Graded Dimension Lumber (2" - 4" thick)[1,2,3]

(All species except Southern Pine — see Table 4B) (Tabulated design values are for normal load duration and dry service conditions. See NDS 4.3 for a comprehensive description of design value adjustment factors.)

USE WITH TABLE 4A ADJUSTMENT FACTORS

Species and commercial grade	Size classification	Design values in pounds per square inch (psi)							Grading Rules Agency
		Bending F_b	Tension parallel to grain F_t	Shear parallel to grain F_v	Compression perpendicular to grain $F_{c\perp}$	Compression parallel to grain F_c	Modulus of Elasticity		
							E	E_{min}	
REDWOOD									
Clear Structural		1,750	1,000	160	650	1,850	1,400,000	510,000	
Select Structural		1,350	800	160	650	1,500	1,400,000	510,000	
Select Structural, open grain		1,100	625	160	425	1,100	1,100,000	400,000	
No.1		975	575	160	650	1,200	1,300,000	470,000	
No.1, open grain	2" & wider	775	450	160	425	900	1,100,000	400,000	
No.2		925	525	160	650	950	1,200,000	440,000	
No.2, open grain		725	425	160	425	700	1,000,000	370,000	RIS
No.3		525	300	160	650	550	1,100,000	400,000	
No.3, open grain		425	250	160	425	400	900,000	330,000	
Stud	2" & wider	575	325	160	425	450	900,000	330,000	
Construction		825	475	160	425	925	900,000	330,000	
Standard	2" - 4" wide	450	275	160	425	725	900,000	330,000	
Utility		225	125	160	425	475	800,000	290,000	
SPRUCE-PINE-FIR									
Select Structural		1,250	700	135	425	1,400	1,500,000	550,000	
No.1/No.2	2" & wider	875	450	135	425	1,150	1,400,000	510,000	
No.3		500	250	135	425	650	1,200,000	440,000	
Stud	2" & wider	675	350	135	425	725	1,200,000	440,000	NLGA
Construction		1,000	500	135	425	1,400	1,300,000	470,000	
Standard	2" - 4" wide	550	275	135	425	1,150	1,200,000	440,000	
Utility		275	125	135	425	750	1,100,000	400,000	
SPRUCE-PINE-FIR (SOUTH)									
Select Structural		1,300	575	135	335	1,200	1,300,000	470,000	
No.1		875	400	135	335	1,050	1,200,000	440,000	
No.2	2" & wider	775	350	135	335	1,000	1,100,000	400,000	NELMA
No.3		450	200	135	335	575	1,000,000	370,000	NSLB
Stud	2" & wider	600	275	135	335	625	1,000,000	370,000	WCLIB
Construction		875	400	135	335	1,200	1,000,000	370,000	WWPA
Standard	2" - 4" wide	500	225	135	335	1,000	900,000	330,000	
Utility		225	100	135	335	675	900,000	330,000	
WESTERN CEDARS									
Select Structural		1,000	600	155	425	1,000	1,100,000	400,000	
No.1		725	425	155	425	825	1,000,000	370,000	
No.2	2" & wider	700	425	155	425	650	1,000,000	370,000	
No.3		400	250	155	425	375	900,000	330,000	
Stud	2" & wider	550	325	155	425	400	900,000	330,000	WCLIB
Construction		800	475	155	425	850	900,000	330,000	WWPA
Standard	2" - 4" wide	450	275	155	425	650	800,000	290,000	
Utility		225	125	155	425	425	800,000	290,000	
WESTERN WOODS									
Select Structural		900	400	135	335	1,050	1,200,000	440,000	
No.1		675	300	135	335	950	1,100,000	400,000	
No.2	2" & wider	675	300	135	335	900	1,000,000	370,000	
No.3		375	175	135	335	525	900,000	330,000	WCLIB
Stud	2" & wider	525	225	135	335	575	900,000	330,000	WWPA
Construction		775	350	135	335	1,100	1,000,000	370,000	
Standard	2" - 4" wide	425	200	135	335	925	900,000	330,000	
Utility		200	100	135	335	600	800,000	290,000	

4

REFERENCE DESIGN VALUES

(All species except Southern Pine — see Table 4B) (Tabulated design values are for normal load duration and dry service conditions. See NDS 4.3 for a comprehensive description of design value adjustment factors.)

USE WITH TABLE 4A ADJUSTMENT FACTORS

Species and commercial grade	Size classification	Bending F_b	Tension parallel to grain F_t	Shear parallel to grain F_v	Compression perpendicular to grain $F_{c\perp}$	Compression parallel to grain F_c	Modulus of Elasticity E	E_{min}	Grading Rules Agency
WHITE OAK									
Select Structural		1,200	700	220	800	1,100	1,100,000	400,000	
No.1		875	500	220	800	900	1,000,000	370,000	
No.2	2" & wider	850	500	220	800	700	900,000	330,000	
No.3		475	275	220	800	400	800,000	290,000	NELMA
Stud	2" & wider	650	375	220	800	450	800,000	290,000	
Construction		950	550	220	800	925	900,000	330,000	
Standard	2" - 4" wide	525	325	220	800	725	800,000	290,000	
Utility		250	150	220	800	475	800,000	290,000	
YELLOW POPLAR									
Select Structural		1,000	575	145	420	900	1,500,000	550,000	
No.1		725	425	145	420	725	1,400,000	510,000	
No.2	2" & wider	700	400	145	420	575	1,300,000	470,000	
No.3		400	225	145	420	325	1,200,000	440,000	NSLB
Stud	2" & wider	550	325	145	420	350	1,200,000	440,000	
Construction		800	475	145	420	750	1,300,000	470,000	
Standard	2" - 4" wide	450	250	145	420	575	1,100,000	400,000	
Utility		200	125	145	420	375	1,100,000	400,000	

1. **LUMBER DIMENSIONS.** Tabulated design values are applicable to lumber that will be used under dry conditions such as in most covered structures. For 2" to 4" thick lumber the DRY dressed sizes shall be used (see Table 1A) regardless of the moisture content at the time of manufacture or use. In calculating design values, the natural gain in strength and stiffness that occurs as lumber dries has been taken into consideration as well as the reduction in size that occurs when unseasoned lumber shrinks. The gain in load carrying capacity due to increased strength and stiffness resulting from drying more than offsets the design effect of size reductions due to shrinkage.

2. **STRESS-RATED BOARDS.** Stress-rated boards of nominal 1", 1-¼" and 1-½" thickness, 2" and wider, of most species, are permitted to use the design values shown for Select Structural, No.1 & Btr, No.1, No.2, No.3, Stud, Construction, Standard, Utility, and Clear Structural grades as shown in the 2" to 4" thick categories herein, when graded in accordance with the stress-rated board provisions in the applicable grading rules. Information on stress-rated board grades applicable to the various species is available from the respective grading rules agencies. Information on additional design values may also be available from the respective grading rules agencies.

3. When individual species or species groups are combined, the design values to be used for the combination shall be the lowest design values for each individual species or species group for each design property.

Size Factor, C_F

Appropriate size adjustment factors have already been incorporated in the tabulated design values for most thicknesses of Southern Pine and Mixed Southern Pine dimension lumber. For dimension lumber 4" thick, 8" and wider (all grades except Dense Structural 86, Dense Structural 72, and Dense Structural 65), tabulated bending design values, F_b, shall be permitted to be multiplied by the size factor, $C_F = 1.1$. For dimension lumber wider than 12" (all grades except Dense Structural 86, Dense Structural 72, and Dense Structural 65), tabulated bending, tension and compression parallel to grain design values for 12" wide lumber shall be multiplied by the size factor, $C_F = 0.9$. When the depth, d, of Dense Structural 86, Dense Structural 72, or Dense Structural 65 dimension lumber exceeds 12", the tabulated bending design value, F_b, shall be multiplied by the following size factor:

$$C_F = (12/d)^{1/9}$$

Repetitive Member Factor, C_r

Bending design values, F_b, for dimension lumber 2" to 4" thick shall be multiplied by the repetitive member factor, $C_r = 1.15$, when such members are used as joists, truss chords, rafters, studs, planks, decking, or similar members which are in contact or spaced not more than 24" on center, are not less than 3 in number and are joined by floor, roof, or other load distributing elements adequate to support the design load.

Flat Use Factor, C_{fu}

Bending design values adjusted by size factors are based on edgewise use (load applied to narrow face). When dimension lumber is used flatwise (load applied to wide face), the bending design value, F_b, shall also be multiplied by the following flat use factors:

Flat Use Factors, C_{fu}

Width (depth)	Thickness (breadth)	
	2" & 3"	4"
2" & 3"	1.0	—
4"	1.1	1.0
5"	1.1	1.05
6"	1.15	1.05
8"	1.15	1.05
10" & wider	1.2	1.1

Wet Service Factor, C_M

When dimension lumber is used where moisture content will exceed 19% for an extended time period, design values shall be multiplied by the appropriate wet service factors from the following table (for surfaced dry Dense Structural 86, Dense Structural 72, and Dense Structural 65 use tabulated surfaced green design values for wet service conditions without further adjustment):

Wet Service Factors, C_M

F_b	F_t	F_v	$F_{c\perp}$	F_c	E and E_{min}
0.85*	1.0	0.97	0.67	0.8**	0.9

* when $(F_b)(C_F) \leq 1,150$ psi, $C_M = 1.0$
** when $(F_c) \leq 750$ psi, $C_M = 1.0$

Table 4B Reference Design Values for Visually Graded Southern Pine Dimension Lumber (2" – 4" thick)[1,2,3,4,5]

(Tabulated design values are for normal load duration and dry service conditions, unless specified otherwise. See NDS 4.3 for a comprehensive description of design value adjustment factors.)

USE WITH TABLE 4B ADJUSTMENT FACTORS

Species and commercial grade	Size classification	Design values in pounds per square inch (psi)							Grading Rules Agency
		Bending F_b	Tension parallel to grain F_t	Shear parallel to grain F_v	Compression perpendicular to grain $F_{c\perp}$	Compression parallel to grain F_c	Modulus of Elasticity E	E_{min}	
SOUTHERN PINE									
Dense Select Structural		3,050	1,650	175	660	2,250	1,900,000	690,000	
Select Structural		2,850	1,600	175	565	2,100	1,800,000	660,000	
Non-Dense Select Structural		2,650	1,350	175	480	1,950	1,700,000	620,000	
No.1 Dense		2,000	1,100	175	660	2,000	1,800,000	660,000	
No.1	2" - 4" wide	1,850	1,050	175	565	1,850	1,700,000	620,000	
No.1 Non-Dense		1,700	900	175	480	1,700	1,600,000	580,000	
No.2 Dense		1,700	875	175	660	1,850	1,700,000	620,000	
No.2		1,500	825	175	565	1,650	1,600,000	580,000	
No.2 Non-Dense		1,350	775	175	480	1,600	1,400,000	510,000	
No.3 and Stud		850	475	175	565	975	1,400,000	510,000	
Construction		1,100	625	175	565	1,800	1,500,000	550,000	
Standard	4" wide	625	350	175	565	1,500	1,300,000	470,000	
Utility		300	175	175	565	975	1,300,000	470,000	
Dense Select Structural		2,700	1,500	175	660	2,150	1,900,000	690,000	
Select Structural		2,550	1,400	175	565	2,000	1,800,000	660,000	
Non-Dense Select Structural		2,350	1,200	175	480	1,850	1,700,000	620,000	
No.1 Dense		1,750	950	175	660	1,900	1,800,000	660,000	
No.1	5" - 6" wide	1,650	900	175	565	1,750	1,700,000	620,000	
No.1 Non-Dense		1,500	800	175	480	1,600	1,600,000	580,000	
No.2 Dense		1,450	775	175	660	1,750	1,700,000	620,000	
No.2		1,250	725	175	565	1,600	1,600,000	580,000	
No.2 Non-Dense		1,150	675	175	480	1,500	1,400,000	510,000	
No.3 and Stud		750	425	175	565	925	1,400,000	510,000	
Dense Select Structural		2,450	1,350	175	660	2,050	1,900,000	690,000	
Select Structural		2,300	1,300	175	565	1,900	1,800,000	660,000	
Non-Dense Select Structural		2,100	1,100	175	480	1,750	1,700,000	620,000	SPIB
No.1 Dense		1,650	875	175	660	1,800	1,800,000	660,000	
No.1	8" wide	1,500	825	175	565	1,650	1,700,000	620,000	
No.1 Non-Dense		1,350	725	175	480	1,550	1,600,000	580,000	
No.2 Dense		1,400	675	175	660	1,700	1,700,000	620,000	
No.2		1,200	650	175	565	1,550	1,600,000	580,000	
No.2 Non-Dense		1,100	600	175	480	1,450	1,400,000	510,000	
No.3 and Stud		700	400	175	565	875	1,400,000	510,000	
Dense Select Structural		2,150	1,200	175	660	2,000	1,900,000	690,000	
Select Structural		2,050	1,100	175	565	1,850	1,800,000	660,000	
Non-Dense Select Structural		1,850	950	175	480	1,750	1,700,000	620,000	
No.1 Dense		1,450	775	175	660	1,750	1,800,000	660,000	
No.1	10" wide	1,300	725	175	565	1,600	1,700,000	620,000	
No.1 Non-Dense		1,200	650	175	480	1,500	1,600,000	580,000	
No.2 Dense		1,200	625	175	660	1,650	1,700,000	620,000	
No.2		1,050	575	175	565	1,500	1,600,000	580,000	
No.2 Non-Dense		950	550	175	480	1,400	1,400,000	510,000	
No.3 and Stud		600	325	175	565	850	1,400,000	510,000	
Dense Select Structural		2,050	1,100	175	660	1,950	1,900,000	690,000	
Select Structural		1,900	1,050	175	565	1,800	1,800,000	660,000	
Non-Dense Select Structural		1,750	900	175	480	1,700	1,700,000	620,000	
No.1 Dense		1,350	725	175	660	1,700	1,800,000	660,000	
No.1	12" wide	1,250	675	175	565	1,600	1,700,000	620,000	
No.1 Non-Dense		1,150	600	175	480	1,500	1,600,000	580,000	
No.2 Dense		1,150	575	175	660	1,600	1,700,000	620,000	
No.2		975	550	175	565	1,450	1,600,000	580,000	
No.2 Non-Dense		900	525	175	480	1,350	1,400,000	510,000	
No.3 and Stud		575	325	175	565	825	1,400,000	510,000	

(Tabulated design values are for normal load duration and dry service conditions, unless specified otherwise. See NDS 4.3 for a comprehensive description of design value adjustment factors.)

USE WITH TABLE 4B ADJUSTMENT FACTORS

Species and commercial grade	Size classification	Bending F_b	Tension parallel to grain F_t	Shear parallel to grain F_v	Compression perpendicular to grain $F_{c\perp}$	Compression parallel to grain F_c	Modulus of Elasticity E	E_{min}	Grading Rules Agency
SOUTHERN PINE		**(Surfaced Dry - Used in dry service conditions - 19% or less moisture content)**							
Dense Structural 86		2,600	1,750	175	660	2,000	1,800,000	660,000	
Dense Structural 72	2" & wider	2,200	1,450	175	660	1,650	1,800,000	660,000	SPIB
Dense Structural 65		2,000	1,300	175	660	1,500	1,800,000	660,000	
SOUTHERN PINE		**(Surfaced Green - Used in any service condition)**							
Dense Structural 86		2,100	1,400	165	440	1,300	1,600,000	580,000	
Dense Structural 72	2-1/2" & wider	1,750	1,200	165	440	1,100	1,600,000	580,000	SPIB
Dense Structural 65	2-1/2"-4" thick	1,600	1,050	165	440	1,000	1,600,000	580,000	
MIXED SOUTHERN PINE									
Select Structural		2,050	1,200	175	565	1,800	1,600,000	580,000	
No.1	2" - 4" wide	1,450	875	175	565	1,650	1,500,000	550,000	
No.2		1,300	775	175	565	1,650	1,400,000	510,000	
No.3 and Stud		750	450	175	565	950	1,200,000	440,000	
Construction		1,000	600	175	565	1,700	1,300,000	470,000	
Standard	4" wide	550	325	175	565	1,450	1,200,000	440,000	
Utility		275	150	175	565	950	1,100,000	400,000	
Select Structural		1,850	1,100	175	565	1,700	1,600,000	580,000	
No.1	5" - 6" wide	1,300	750	175	565	1,550	1,500,000	550,000	
No.2		1,150	675	175	565	1,550	1,400,000	510,000	
No.3 and Stud		675	400	175	565	875	1,200,000	440,000	SPIB
Select Structural		1,750	1,000	175	565	1,600	1,600,000	580,000	
No.1	8" wide	1,200	700	175	565	1,450	1,500,000	550,000	
No.2		1,050	625	175	565	1,450	1,400,000	510,000	
No.3 and Stud		625	375	175	565	850	1,200,000	440,000	
Select Structural		1,500	875	175	565	1,600	1,600,000	580,000	
No.1	10" wide	1,050	600	175	565	1,450	1,500,000	550,000	
No.2		925	550	175	565	1,450	1,400,000	510,000	
No.3 and Stud		525	325	175	565	825	1,200,000	440,000	
Select Structural		1,400	825	175	565	1,550	1,600,000	580,000	
No.1	12" wide	975	575	175	565	1,400	1,500,000	550,000	
No.2		875	525	175	565	1,400	1,400,000	510,000	
No.3 and Stud		500	300	175	565	800	1,200,000	440,000	

1. **LUMBER DIMENSIONS.** Tabulated design values are applicable to lumber that will be used under dry conditions such as in most covered structures. For 2" to 4" thick lumber the DRY dressed sizes shall be used (see Table 1A) regardless of the moisture content at the time of manufacture or use. In calculating design values, the natural gain in strength and stiffness that occurs as lumber dries has been taken into consideration as well as the reduction in size that occurs when unseasoned lumber shrinks. The gain in load carrying capacity due to increased strength and stiffness resulting from drying more than offsets the design effect of size reductions due to shrinkage.

2. **STRESS-RATED BOARDS.** Information for various grades of Southern Pine stress-rated boards of nominal 1", 1-¼", and 1-½" thickness, 2" and wider is available from the Southern Pine Inspection Bureau (SPIB) in the *Standard Grading Rules for Southern Pine Lumber*.

3. **SPRUCE PINE.** To obtain recommended design values for Spruce Pine graded to SPIB rules, multiply the appropriate design values for Mixed Southern Pine by the corresponding conversion factor shown below and round to the nearest 100,000 psi for E; to the nearest 10,000 psi for E_{min}; to the next lower multiple of 5 psi for F_v and $F_{c\perp}$; to the next lower multiple of 50 psi for F_b, F_t, and F_c if 1,000 psi or greater, 25 psi otherwise.

CONVERSION FACTORS FOR DETERMINING DESIGN VALUES FOR SPRUCE PINE

	Bending F_b	Tension parallel to grain F_t	Shear parallel to grain F_v	Compression perpendicular to grain $F_{c\perp}$	Compression parallel to grain F_c	Modulus of Elasticity E and E_{min}
Conversion Factor	0.78	0.78	0.98	0.73	0.78	0.82

4. **SIZE FACTOR.** For sizes wider than 12", use size factors for F_b, F_t, and F_c specified for the 12" width. Use 100% of the F_v, $F_{c\perp}$, E, and E_{min} specified for the 12" width.

5. When individual species or species groups are combined, the design values to be used for the combination shall be the lowest design values for each individual species or species group for each design property.

Flat Use Factor, C_{fu}

Bending design values adjusted by size factors are based on edgewise use (load applied to narrow face). When dimension lumber is used flatwise (load applied to wide face), the bending design value, F_b, shall also be multiplied by the following flat use factors:

Flat Use Factors, C_{fu}

Width (depth)	Thickness (breadth)
	2"
2" & 3"	1.0
4"	1.1
5"	1.1
6"	1.15
8"	1.15
10" & wider	1.2

Repetitive Member Factor, C_r

Bending design values, F_b, for dimension lumber 2" to 4" thick shall be multiplied by the repetitive member factor, $C_r = 1.15$, when such members are used as joists, truss chords, rafters, studs, planks, decking, or similar members which are in contact or spaced not more than 24" on center, are not less than 3 in number and are joined by floor, roof, or other load distributing elements adequate to support the design load.

Wet Service Factor, C_M

When dimension lumber is used where moisture content will exceed 19% for an extended time period, design values shall be multiplied by the appropriate wet service factors from the following table:

Wet Service Factors, C_M

F_b	F_t	F_v	$F_{c\perp}$	F_c	E and E_{min}
0.85*	1.0	0.97	0.67	0.8**	0.9

* when $F_b \leq 1,150$ psi, $C_M = 1.0$
** when $F_c \leq 750$ psi, $C_M = 1.0$

Table 4C   Reference Design Values for Mechanically Graded Dimension Lumber[1,2,3]

(Tabulated design values are for normal load duration and dry service conditions, unless specified otherwise. See NDS 4.3 for a comprehensive description of design value adjustment factors.)

USE WITH TABLE 4C ADJUSTMENT FACTORS

Species and commercial grade	Size classification	Design values in pounds per square inch (psi)					Grading Rules Agency
		Bending F_b	Tension parallel to grain F_t	Compression parallel to grain F_c	Modulus of Elasticity E	E_{min}	
MACHINE STRESS RATED (MSR) LUMBER							
900f-1.0E		900	350	1,050	1,000,000	510,000	WCLIB, WWPA, NELMA, NSLB
1200f-1.2E		1,200	600	1,400	1,200,000	610,000	NLGA, WCLIB, WWPA, NELMA, NSLB
1250f-1.4E		1,250	800	1,475	1,400,000	710,000	WCLIB, WWPA
1350f-1.3E		1,350	750	1,600	1,300,000	660,000	NLGA, WCLIB, WWPA, NELMA, NSLB
1400f-1.2E		1,400	800	1,600	1,200,000	610,000	NLGA, WWPA
1450f-1.3E		1,450	800	1,625	1,300,000	660,000	NLGA, WCLIB, WWPA, NELMA, NSLB
1450f-1.5E		1,450	875	1,625	1,500,000	760,000	WCLIB, WWPA
1500f-1.4E		1,500	900	1,650	1,400,000	710,000	NLGA, WCLIB, WWPA, NELMA, NSLB
1600f-1.4E		1,600	950	1,675	1,400,000	710,000	NLGA, WWPA
1650f-1.3E		1,650	1,020	1,700	1,300,000	660,000	NLGA, WWPA
1650f-1.5E		1,650	1,020	1,700	1,500,000	760,000	NLGA, SPIB, WCLIB, WWPA, NELMA, NSLB
1650f-1.6E-1075f_t		1,650	1,075	1,700	1,600,000	810,000	WCLIB, WWPA
1650f-1.6E		1,650	1,175	1,700	1,600,000	810,000	WCLIB, WWPA
1650f-1.8E		1,650	1,020	1,750	1,800,000	910,000	WCLIB, WWPA
1700f-1.6E	2" and less in thickness	1,700	1,175	1,725	1,600,000	810,000	WCLIB, WWPA
1750f-2.0E		1,750	1,125	1,725	2,000,000	1,020,000	WCLIB, WWPA
1800f-1.5E		1,800	1,300	1,750	1,500,000	760,000	NLGA, WWPA
1800f-1.6E	2" and wider	1,800	1,175	1,750	1,600,000	810,000	NLGA, SPIB, WCLIB, WWPA, NELMA, NSLB
1800f-1.8E		1,800	1,200	1,750	1,800,000	910,000	WCLIB, WWPA
1950f-1.5E		1,950	1,375	1,800	1,500,000	760,000	SPIB, WWPA
1950f-1.7E		1,950	1,375	1,800	1,700,000	860,000	NLGA, SPIB, WCLIB, WWPA, NELMA, NSLB
2000f-1.6E		2,000	1,300	1,825	1,600,000	810,000	NLGA, WWPA
2100f-1.8E		2,100	1,575	1,875	1,800,000	910,000	NLGA, SPIB, WCLIB, WWPA, NELMA, NSLB
2250f-1.7E		2,250	1,750	1,925	1,700,000	860,000	NLGA, WWPA
2250f-1.8E		2,250	1,750	1,925	1,800,000	910,000	NLGA, WCLIB, WWPA
2250f-1.9E		2,250	1,750	1,925	1,900,000	970,000	NLGA, SPIB, WCLIB, WWPA, NELMA, NSLB
2250f-2.0E-1600f_t		2,250	1,600	1,925	2,000,000	1,020,000	WCLIB, WWPA
2250f-2.0E		2,250	1,750	1,925	2,000,000	1,020,000	WCLIB, WWPA
2400f-1.8E		2,400	1,925	1,975	1,800,000	910,000	NLGA, WWPA
2400f-2.0E		2,400	1,925	1,975	2,000,000	1,020,000	NLGA, SPIB, WCLIB, WWPA, NELMA, NSLB
2500f-2.2E		2,500	1,750	2,000	2,200,000	1,120,000	WCLIB, WWPA
2500f-2.2E-1925f_t		2,500	1,925	2,000	2,200,000	1,120,000	WCLIB, WWPA
2550f-2.1E		2,550	2,050	2,025	2,100,000	1,070,000	NLGA, SPIB, WCLIB, WWPA, NELMA, NSLB
2700f-2.0E		2,700	1,800	2,100	2,000,000	1,020,000	WCLIB, WWPA
2700f-2.2E		2,700	2,150	2,100	2,200,000	1,120,000	NLGA, SPIB, WCLIB, WWPA, NELMA, NSLB
2850f-2.3E		2,850	2,300	2,150	2,300,000	1,170,000	NLGA, SPIB, WCLIB, WWPA, NELMA, NSLB
3000f-2.4E		3,000	2,400	2,200	2,400,000	1,220,000	NLGA, SPIB

AMERICAN FOREST & PAPER ASSOCIATION

Table 4C (Cont.) **Reference Design Values for Mechanically Graded Dimension Lumber**[1,2,3]

(Tabulated design values are for normal load duration and dry service conditions, unless specified otherwise. See NDS 4.3 for a comprehensive description of design value adjustment factors.)

USE WITH TABLE 4C ADJUSTMENT FACTORS

Species and commercial grade	Size classification	Design values in pounds per square inch (psi)					Grading Rules Agency
		Bending F_b	Tension parallel to grain F_t	Compression parallel to grain F_c	Modulus of Elasticity E	E_{min}	
MACHINE EVALUATED LUMBER (MEL)							
M-5		900	500	1,050	1,100,000	510,000	SPIB
M-6		1,100	600	1,300	1,000,000	470,000	SPIB
M-7		1,200	650	1,400	1,100,000	510,000	SPIB
M-8		1,300	700	1,500	1,300,000	610,000	SPIB
M-9		1,400	800	1,600	1,400,000	650,000	SPIB
M-10		1,400	800	1,600	1,200,000	560,000	NLGA, SPIB
M-11		1,550	850	1,675	1,500,000	700,000	NLGA, SPIB
M-12		1,600	850	1,675	1,600,000	750,000	NLGA, SPIB
M-13		1,600	950	1,675	1,400,000	650,000	NLGA, SPIB
M-14		1,800	1,000	1,750	1,700,000	790,000	NLGA, SPIB
M-15		1,800	1,100	1,750	1,500,000	700,000	NLGA, SPIB
M-16	2" and less in thickness	1,800	1,300	1,750	1,500,000	700,000	SPIB
M-17[4]		1,950	1,300	2,050	1,700,000	790,000	SPIB
M-18		2,000	1,200	1,825	1,800,000	840,000	NLGA, SPIB
M-19	2" and wider	2,000	1,300	1,825	1,600,000	750,000	NLGA, SPIB
M-20[4]		2,000	1,600	2,100	1,900,000	890,000	SPIB
M-21		2,300	1,400	1,950	1,900,000	890,000	NLGA, SPIB
M-22		2,350	1,500	1,950	1,700,000	790,000	NLGA, SPIB
M-23		2,400	1,900	1,975	1,800,000	840,000	NLGA, SPIB
M-24		2,700	1,800	2,100	1,900,000	890,000	NLGA, SPIB
M-25		2,750	2,000	2,100	2,200,000	1,030,000	NLGA, SPIB
M-26		2,800	1,800	2,150	2,000,000	930,000	NLGA, SPIB
M-27[4]		3,000	2,000	2,400	2,100,000	980,000	SPIB
M-28		2,200	1,600	1,900	1,700,000	790,000	SPIB
M-29		1,550	850	1,650	1,700,000	790,000	SPIB
M-30		2,050	1,050	1,850	1,700,000	790,000	SPIB
M-31		2,850	1,600	2,150	1,900,000	890,000	SPIB

Table 4C Footnotes

1. **LUMBER DIMENSIONS.** Tabulated design values are applicable to lumber that will be used under dry conditions such as in most covered structures. For 2" to 4" thick lumber the DRY dressed sizes shall be used (see Table 1A) regardless of the moisture content at the time of manufacture or use. In calculating design values, the natural gain in strength and stiffness that occurs as lumber dries has been taken into consideration as well as the reduction in size that occurs when unseasoned lumber shrinks. The gain in load carrying capacity due to increased strength and stiffness resulting from drying more than offsets the design effect of size reductions due to shrinkage.

2. **SPECIFIC GRAVITY, G, SHEAR PARALLEL TO GRAIN, F_v, AND COMPRESSION PERPENDICULAR TO GRAIN, $F_{c\perp}$.** Values for specific gravity, G, shear parallel to grain, F_v, and compression perpendicular to grain, $F_{c\perp}$, are provided below for MSR and MEL lumber. For species or species groups not shown below, the G, F_v, and $F_{c\perp}$ values for visually graded lumber may be used. Higher G values may be claimed when (a) specifically assigned by the rules writing agency or (b) when qualified by test, quality controlled for G and provided for on the grade stamp. When a different G value is provided on the grade stamp, higher F_v and $F_{c\perp}$ design values may be calculated in accordance with the grading rule requirements.

Species	Modulus of Elasticity E (x10⁶), psi	Design Values			Grading Rules Agency
		Specific Gravity G	Shear Parallel to Grain F_v, psi	Compression Perpendicular to Grain $F_{c\perp}$, psi	
Douglas Fir-Larch	1.0 and higher	0.50	180	625	WCLIB, WWPA
	2.0	0.51	180	670	WCLIB, WWPA
	2.1	0.52	180	690	
	2.2	0.53	180	715	
	2.3	0.54	185	735	
	2.4	0.55	185	760	
Douglas Fir-Larch (N)	1.2 to 1.9	0.49	180	625	
	2.0 to 2.2	0.53	180	715	NLGA
	2.3 and higher	0.57	190	715	NLGA
Douglas Fir-South	1.0 and higher	0.46	180	520	WWPA
Englemann Spruce-Lodgepole Pine	1.0 and higher	0.38	135	335	WWPA
	1.5 and higher	0.46	160	555	WWPA
Hem-Fir	1.0 and higher	0.43	150	405	WCLIB, WWPA
	1.6	0.44	155	510	
	1.7	0.45	160	535	
	1.8	0.46	160	555	
	1.9	0.47	165	580	WCLIB, WWPA
	2.0	0.48	170	600	
	2.1	0.49	170	625	
	2.2	0.50	175	645	
	2.3	0.51	190	670	
	2.4	0.52	190	690	
Hem-Fir (N)	1.0 and higher	0.46	145	405	NLGA
Southern Pine	1.0 and higher	0.55	175	565	SPIB
	1.8 and higher	0.57	190	805	SPIB
Spruce-Pine-Fir	1.2 and higher	0.42	135	425	NLGA
	1.8 to 1.9	0.46	160	525	NLGA
	2.0 and higher	0.50	170	615	NLGA
Spruce-Pine-Fir (South)	1.0 and higher	0.36	135	335	NELMA, NSLB, WCLIB, WWPA
	1.2 to 1.9	0.42	150	465	NELMA, NSLB
	1.2 to 1.7	0.42	150	465	WWPA
	1.8 to 1.9	0.46	160	555	
	2.0 and higher	0.50	175	645	NELMA, NSLB, WWPA
Western Cedars	1.0 and higher	0.36	155	425	WCLIB, WWPA
Western Woods	1.0 and higher	0.36	135	335	WCLIB, WWPA

3. **MODULUS OF ELASTICITY, E, AND TENSION PARALLEL TO GRAIN, F_t.** For any given bending design value, F_b, the modulus of elasticity, E, and tension parallel to grain, F_t, design value may vary depending upon species, timber source, or other variables. The "E" and "F_t" values included in the "F_b-E" grade designations in Table 4C are those usually associated with each "F_b" level. Grade stamps may show higher or lower values if machine rating indicates the assignment is appropriate. Where the "E" or "F_t" values shown on a grade stamp differ from Table 4C values associated with the "F_b" on the grade stamp, the values on the stamp shall be used in design, and the "F_c" value associated with the "F_b" value in Table 4C shall be used.

4. **COMPRESSION PARALLEL TO GRAIN, F_c.** This grade requires "F_c" qualification and quality control.

Table 4D Adjustment Factors

Size Factor, C_F

When the depth, d, of a beam, stringer, post, or timber exceeds 12", the tabulated bending design value, F_b, shall be multiplied by the following size factor:

$$C_F = (12/d)^{1/9}$$

When beams and stringers are subjected to loads applied to the wide face, tabulated design values shall be multiplied by the following size factors:

Size Factors, C_F

Grade	F_b	E and E_{min}	Other Properties
Select Structural	0.86	1.00	1.00
No.1	0.74	0.90	1.00
No.2	1.00	1.00	1.00

Wet Service Factor, C_M

When timbers are used where moisture content will exceed 19% for an extended time period, design values shall be multiplied by the appropriate wet service factors from the following table (for Southern Pine and Mixed Southern Pine use tabulated design values without further adjustment):

Wet Service Factors, C_M

F_b	F_t	F_v	$F_{c\perp}$	F_c	E and E_{min}
1.00	1.00	1.00	0.67	0.91	1.00

Table 4D   Reference Design Values for Visually Graded Timbers (5" x 5" and larger)[1,3]

(Tabulated design values are for normal load duration and dry service conditions, unless specified otherwise. See NDS 4.3 for a comprehensive description of design value adjustment factors.)

USE WITH TABLE 4D ADJUSTMENT FACTORS

Species and commercial grade	Size classification	Design values in pounds per square inch (psi)							Grading Rules Agency
		Bending F_b	Tension parallel to grain F_t	Shear parallel to grain F_v	Compression perpendicular to grain $F_{c\perp}$	Compression parallel to grain F_c	Modulus of Elasticity		
							E	E_{min}	
ALASKA CEDAR									
Select Structural	Beams and Stringers	1,400	675	155	525	925	1,200,000	440,000	
No.1		1,150	475	155	525	775	1,200,000	440,000	
No.2		750	300	155	525	500	1,000,000	370,000	WCLIB
Select Structural	Posts and Timbers	1,300	700	155	525	975	1,200,000	440,000	
No.1		1,050	575	155	525	850	1,200,000	440,000	
No.2		625	350	155	525	600	1,000,000	370,000	
BALDCYPRESS									
Select Structural	5"x5" and Larger	1,150	750	200	615	1,050	1,300,000	470,000	
No.1		1,000	675	200	615	925	1,300,000	470,000	SPIB
No.2		625	425	175	615	600	1,000,000	370,000	
BALSAM FIR									
Select Structural	Beams and Stringers	1,350	900	125	305	950	1,400,000	510,000	
No.1		1,100	750	125	305	800	1,400,000	510,000	
No.2		725	350	125	305	500	1,100,000	400,000	NELMA
Select Structural	Posts and Timbers	1,250	825	125	305	1,000	1,400,000	510,000	NSLB
No.1		1,000	675	125	305	875	1,400,000	510,000	
No.2		575	375	125	305	400	1,100,000	400,000	
BEECH-BIRCH-HICKORY									
Select Structural	Beams and Stringers	1,650	975	180	715	975	1,500,000	550,000	
No.1		1,400	700	180	715	825	1,500,000	550,000	
No.2		900	450	180	715	525	1,200,000	440,000	NELMA
Select Structural	Posts and Timbers	1,550	1,050	180	715	1,050	1,500,000	550,000	
No.1		1,250	850	180	715	900	1,500,000	550,000	
No.2		725	475	180	715	425	1,200,000	440,000	
COAST SITKA SPRUCE									
Select Structural	Beams and Stringers	1,150	675	115	455	775	1,500,000	550,000	
No.1		950	475	115	455	650	1,500,000	550,000	
No.2		625	325	115	455	425	1,200,000	440,000	NLGA
Select Structural	Posts and Timbers	1,100	725	115	455	825	1,500,000	550,000	
No.1		875	575	115	455	725	1,500,000	550,000	
No .2		525	350	115	455	500	1,200,000	440,000	
DOUGLAS FIR-LARCH									
Dense Select Structural		1,900	1,100	170	730	1,300	1,700,000	620,000	
Select Structural	Beams and Stringers	1,600	950	170	625	1,100	1,600,000	580,000	
Dense No.1		1,550	775	170	730	1,100	1,700,000	620,000	
No.1		1,350	675	170	625	925	1,600,000	580,000	
No.2		875	425	170	625	600	1,300,000	470,000	WCLIB
Dense Select Structural		1,750	1,150	170	730	1,350	1,700,000	620,000	
Select Structural	Posts and Timbers	1,500	1,000	170	625	1,150	1,600,000	580,000	
Dense No.1		1,400	950	170	730	1,200	1,700,000	620,000	
No.1		1,200	825	170	625	1,000	1,600,000	580,000	
No.2		750	475	170	625	700	1,300,000	470,000	
Dense Select Structural		1,900	1,100	170	730	1,300	1,700,000	620,000	
Select Structural	Beams and Stringers	1,600	950	170	625	1,100	1,600,000	580,000	
Dense No.1		1,550	775	170	730	1,100	1,700,000	620,000	
No.1		1,350	675	170	625	925	1,600,000	580,000	
No.2 Dense		1,000	500	170	730	700	1,400,000	510,000	
No.2		875	425	170	625	600	1,300,000	470,000	WWPA
Dense Select Structural		1,750	1,150	170	730	1,350	1,700,000	620,000	
Select Structural	Posts and Timbers	1,500	1,000	170	625	1,150	1,600,000	580,000	
Dense No.1		1,400	950	170	730	1,200	1,700,000	620,000	
No.1		1,200	825	170	625	1,000	1,600,000	580,000	
No.2 Dense		850	550	170	730	825	1,400,000	510,000	
No.2		750	475	170	625	700	1,300,000	470,000	

Table 4D (Cont.) Reference Design Values for Visually Graded Timbers (5" x 5" and larger)[1,3]

(Tabulated design values are for normal load duration and dry service conditions, unless specified otherwise. See NDS 4.3 for a comprehensive description of design value adjustment factors.)

USE WITH TABLE 4D ADJUSTMENT FACTORS

Species and commercial grade	Size classification	Bending F_b	Tension parallel to grain F_t	Shear parallel to grain F_v	Compression perpendicular to grain $F_{c\perp}$	Compression parallel to grain F_c	Modulus of Elasticity E	E_{min}	Grading Rules Agency
DOUGLAS FIR-LARCH (NORTH)									
Select Structural	Beams and	1,600	950	170	625	1,100	1,600,000	580,000	
No.1	Stringers	1,300	675	170	625	925	1,600,000	580,000	
No.2		875	425	170	625	600	1,300,000	470,000	NLGA
Select Structural	Posts and	1,500	1,000	170	625	1,150	1,600,000	580,000	
No.1	Timbers	1,200	825	170	625	1,000	1,600,000	580,000	
No.2		725	475	170	625	700	1,300,000	470,000	
DOUGLAS FIR-SOUTH									
Select Structural	Beams and	1,550	900	165	520	1,000	1,200,000	440,000	
No.1	Stringers	1,300	625	165	520	850	1,200,000	440,000	
No.2		825	425	165	520	550	1,000,000	370,000	WWPA
Select Structural	Posts and	1,450	950	165	520	1,050	1,200,000	440,000	
No.1	Timbers	1,150	775	165	520	925	1,200,000	440,000	
No.2		675	450	165	520	650	1,000,000	370,000	
EASTERN HEMLOCK									
Select Structural	Beams and	1,350	925	155	550	950	1,200,000	440,000	
No.1	Stringers	1,150	775	155	550	800	1,200,000	440,000	
No.2		750	375	155	550	550	900,000	330,000	NELMA
Select Structural	Posts and	1,250	850	155	550	1,000	1,200,000	440,000	NSLB
No.1	Timbers	1,050	700	155	500	875	1,200,000	440,000	
No.2		600	400	155	550	400	900,000	330,000	
EASTERN HEMLOCK-TAMARACK									
Select Structural	Beams and	1,400	925	155	555	950	1,200,000	440,000	
No.1	Stringers	1,150	775	155	555	800	1,200,000	440,000	
No.2		750	375	155	555	500	900,000	330,000	NELMA
Select Structural	Posts and	1,300	875	155	555	1,000	1,200,000	440,000	NSLB
No.1	Timbers	1,050	700	155	555	875	1,200,000	440,000	
No.2		600	400	155	555	400	900,000	330,000	
EASTERN HEMLOCK-TAMARACK (N)									
Select Structural	Beams and	1,450	850	165	555	950	1,300,000	470,000	
No.1	Stringers	1,200	600	165	555	800	1,300,000	470,000	
No.2		775	400	165	555	500	1,100,000	400,000	NLGA
Select Structural	Posts and	1,350	900	165	555	1,000	1,300,000	470,000	
No.1	Timbers	1,100	725	165	555	875	1,300,000	470,000	
No.2		650	425	165	555	600	1,100,000	400,000	
EASTERN SPRUCE									
Select Structural	Beams and	1,050	725	135	390	750	1,400,000	510,000	
No.1	Stringers	900	600	135	390	625	1,400,000	510,000	
No.2		575	275	135	390	375	1,000,000	370,000	NELMA
Select Structural	Posts and	1,000	675	135	390	775	1,400,000	510,000	NSLB
No.1	Timbers	800	550	135	390	675	1,400,000	510,000	
No.2		450	300	135	390	300	1,000,000	370,000	
EASTERN WHITE PINE									
Select Structural	Beams and	1,050	700	125	350	675	1,100,000	400,000	
No.1	Stringers	875	600	125	350	575	1,100,000	400,000	
No.2		575	275	125	350	400	900,000	330,000	NELMA
Select Structural	Posts and	975	650	125	350	725	1,100,000	400,000	NSLB
No.1	Timbers	800	525	125	350	625	1,100,000	400,000	
No.2		450	300	125	350	325	900,000	330,000	

(Tabulated design values are for normal load duration and dry service conditions, unless specified otherwise. See NDS 4.3 for a comprehensive description of design value adjustment factors.)

USE WITH TABLE 4D ADJUSTMENT FACTORS

Species and commercial grade	Size classification	Bending F_b	Tension parallel to grain F_t	Shear parallel to grain F_v	Compression perpendicular to grain $F_{c\perp}$	Compression parallel to grain F_c	Modulus of Elasticity E	E_{min}	Grading Rules Agency
HEM-FIR									
Select Structural	Beams and	1,300	750	140	405	925	1,300,000	470,000	
No.1	Stringers	1,050	525	140	405	750	1,300,000	470,000	
No.2		675	350	140	405	500	1,100,000	400,000	WCLIB
Select Structural	Posts and	1,200	800	140	405	975	1,300,000	470,000	WWPA
No.1	Timbers	975	650	140	405	850	1,300,000	470,000	
No.2		575	375	140	405	575	1,100,000	400,000	
HEM-FIR (NORTH)									
Select Structural	Beams and	1,250	725	135	405	900	1,300,000	470,000	
No.1	Stringers	1,000	500	135	405	750	1,300,000	470,000	
No.2		675	325	135	405	475	1,100,000	400,000	NLGA
Select Structural	Posts and	1,150	775	135	405	950	1,300,000	470,000	
No.1	Timbers	925	625	135	405	850	1,300,000	470,000	
No.2		550	375	135	405	575	1,100,000	400,000	
MIXED MAPLE									
Select Structural	Beams and	1,150	700	180	620	725	1,100,000	400,000	
No.1	Stringers	975	500	180	620	600	1,100,000	400,000	
No.2		625	325	180	620	375	900,000	330,000	NELMA
Select Structural	Posts and	1,100	725	180	620	750	1,100,000	400,000	
No.1	Timbers	875	600	180	620	650	1,100,000	400,000	
No.2		500	350	180	620	300	900,000	330,000	
MIXED OAK									
Select Structural	Beams and	1,350	800	155	800	825	1,000,000	370,000	
No.1	Stringers	1,150	550	155	800	700	1,000,000	370,000	
No.2		725	375	155	800	450	800,000	290,000	NELMA
Select Structural	Posts and	1,250	850	155	800	875	1,000,000	370,000	
No.1	Timbers	1,000	675	155	800	775	1,000,000	370,000	
No.2		575	400	155	800	350	800,000	290,000	
MIXED SOUTHERN PINE[2]		**(Wet Service Conditions)**							
Select Structural	5"x5" and	1,500	1,000	165	375	900	1,300,000	470,000	
No.1	Larger	1,350	900	165	375	800	1,300,000	470,000	SPIB
No.2		850	550	165	375	525	1,000,000	370,000	
MOUNTAIN HEMLOCK									
Select Structural	Beams and	1,350	775	170	570	875	1,100,000	400,000	
No.1	Stringers	1,100	550	170	570	725	1,100,000	400,000	
No.2		725	375	170	570	475	900,000	330,000	WCLIB
Select Structural	Posts and	1,250	825	170	570	925	1,100,000	400,000	WWPA
No.1	Timbers	1,000	675	170	570	800	1,100,000	400,000	
No.2		625	400	170	570	550	900,000	330,000	
NORTHERN PINE									
Select Structural	Beams and	1,250	850	135	435	850	1,300,000	470,000	
No.1	Stringers	1,050	700	135	435	725	1,300,000	470,000	
No.2		675	350	135	435	450	1,000,000	370,000	NELMA
Select Structural	Posts and	1,150	800	135	435	900	1,300,000	470,000	NSLB
No.1	Timbers	950	650	135	435	800	1,300,000	470,000	
No.2		550	375	135	435	375	1,000,000	370,000	
NORTHERN RED OAK									
Select Structural	Beams and	1,600	950	205	885	950	1,300,000	470,000	
No.1	Stringers	1,350	675	205	885	800	1,300,000	470,000	
No.2		875	425	205	885	500	1,000,000	370,000	NELMA
Select Structural	Posts and	1,500	1,000	205	885	1,000	1,300,000	470,000	
No.1	Timbers	1,200	800	205	885	875	1,300,000	470,000	
No.2		700	475	205	885	400	1,000,000	370,000	

(Tabulated design values are for normal load duration and dry service conditions, unless specified otherwise. See NDS 4.3 for a comprehensive description of design value adjustment factors.)

USE WITH TABLE 4D ADJUSTMENT FACTORS

Species and commercial grade	Size classification	Bending F_b	Tension parallel to grain F_t	Shear parallel to grain F_v	Compression perpendicular to grain $F_{c\perp}$	Compression parallel to grain F_c	Modulus of Elasticity E	Modulus of Elasticity E_{min}	Grading Rules Agency
NORTHERN WHITE CEDAR									
Select Structural	Beams and Stringers	900	600	115	370	600	700,000	260,000	
No.1	Stringers	750	500	115	370	500	700,000	260,000	NELMA
No.2		500	250	115	370	325	600,000	220,000	
Select Structural	Posts and Timbers	850	575	115	370	650	700,000	260,000	
No.1		675	450	115	370	550	700,000	260,000	
No.2		400	250	115	370	250	600,000	220,000	
PONDEROSA PINE									
Select Structural	Beams and Stringers	1,100	725	130	535	750	1,100,000	400,000	
No.1		925	500	130	535	625	1,100,000	400,000	NLGA
No.2		600	300	130	535	400	900,000	330,000	
Select Structural	Posts and Timbers	1,000	675	130	535	800	1,100,000	400,000	
No.1		825	550	130	535	700	1,100,000	400,000	
No.2		475	325	130	535	325	900,000	330,000	
RED MAPLE									
Select Structural	Beams and Stringers	1,500	875	195	615	900	1,500,000	550,000	
No.1		1,250	625	195	615	750	1,500,000	550,000	NELMA
No.2		800	400	195	615	475	1,200,000	440,000	
Select Structural	Posts and Timbers	1,400	925	195	615	950	1,500,000	550,000	
No.1		1,150	750	195	615	825	1,500,000	550,000	
No.2		650	425	195	615	375	1,200,000	440,000	
RED OAK									
Select Structural	Beams and Stringers	1,350	800	155	820	825	1,200,000	440,000	
No.1		1,150	550	155	820	700	1,200,000	440,000	NELMA
No.2		725	375	155	820	450	1,000,000	370,000	
Select Structural	Posts and Timbers	1,250	850	155	820	875	1,200,000	440,000	
No.1		1,000	675	155	820	775	1,200,000	440,000	
No.2		575	400	155	820	350	1,000,000	370,000	
RED PINE									
Select Structural	Beams and Stringers	1,050	625	130	440	725	1,100,000	400,000	
No.1		875	450	130	440	600	1,100,000	400,000	NLGA
No.2		575	300	130	440	375	900,000	330,000	
Select Structural	Posts and Timbers	1,000	675	130	440	775	1,100,000	400,000	
No.1		800	550	130	440	675	1,100,000	400,000	
No.2		475	325	130	440	475	900,000	330,000	
REDWOOD									
Clear Structural	5" x 5" and Larger	1,850	1,250	145	650	1,650	1,300,000	470,000	
Select Structural		1,400	950	145	650	1,200	1,300,000	470,000	
Select Structural OG		1,100	750	145	420	900	1,000,000	370,000	
No.1		1,200	800	145	650	1,050	1,300,000	470,000	RIS
No.1 OG		950	650	145	420	800	1,000,000	370,000	
No.2		1,000	525	145	650	900	1,100,000	400,000	
No.2 OG		750	400	145	420	650	900,000	330,000	
SITKA SPRUCE									
Select Structural	Beams and Stringers	1,200	675	140	435	825	1,300,000	470,000	
No.1		1,000	500	140	435	675	1,300,000	470,000	WCLIB
No.2		650	325	140	435	450	1,000,000	370,000	
Select Structural	Posts and Timbers	1,150	750	140	435	875	1,300,000	470,000	
No.1		925	600	140	435	750	1,300,000	470,000	
No.2		550	350	140	435	525	1,000,000	370,000	
Select Structural	Beams and Stringers	1,200	675	140	435	825	1,300,000	470,000	
No.1		1,000	500	140	435	675	1,300,000	470,000	WWPA
No.2		650	325	140	435	450	1,100,000	400,000	
Select Structural	Posts and Timbers	1,150	750	140	435	875	1,300,000	470,000	
No.1		925	600	140	435	750	1,300,000	470,000	
No.2		550	350	140	435	525	1,100,000	400,000	

(Tabulated design values are for normal load duration and dry service conditions, unless specified otherwise. See NDS 4.3 for a comprehensive description of design value adjustment factors.)

USE WITH TABLE 4D ADJUSTMENT FACTORS

Species and commercial grade	Size classification	Design values in pounds per square inch (psi)							Grading Rules Agency
		Bending F_b	Tension parallel to grain F_t	Shear parallel to grain F_v	Compression perpendicular to grain $F_{c\perp}$	Compression parallel to grain F_c	Modulus of Elasticity E	E_{min}	
SOUTHERN PINE		**(Wet Service Conditions)**							
Dense Select Structural	5" x 5" and Larger	1,750	1,200	165	440	1,100	1,600,000	580,000	
Select Structural		1,500	1,000	165	375	950	1,500,000	550,000	
No.1 Dense		1,550	1,050	165	440	975	1,600,000	580,000	
No.1		1,350	900	165	375	825	1,500,000	550,000	
No.2 Dense		975	650	165	440	625	1,300,000	470,000	SPIB
No.2		850	550	165	375	525	1,200,000	440,000	
Dense Select Structural 86		2,100	1,400	165	440	1,300	1,600,000	580,000	
Dense Select Structural 72		1,750	1,200	165	440	1,100	1,600,000	580,000	
Dense Select Structural 65		1,600	1,050	165	440	1,000	1,600,000	580,000	
SPRUCE-PINE-FIR									
Select Structural	Beams and Stringers	1,100	650	125	425	775	1,300,000	470,000	
No.1		900	450	125	425	625	1,300,000	470,000	
No.2		600	300	125	425	425	1,000,000	370,000	NLGA
Select Structural	Posts and Timbers	1,050	700	125	425	800	1,300,000	470,000	
No.1		850	550	125	425	700	1,300,000	470,000	
No.2		500	325	125	425	500	1,000,000	370,000	
SPRUCE-PINE-FIR (SOUTH)									
Select Structural	Beams and Stringers	1,050	625	125	335	675	1,200,000	440,000	
No.1		900	450	125	335	550	1,200,000	440,000	NELMA
No.2		575	300	125	335	375	1,000,000	370,000	NSLB
Select Structural	Posts and Timbers	1,000	675	125	335	700	1,200,000	440,000	WWPA
No.1		800	550	125	335	625	1,200,000	440,000	WCLIB
No.2		475	325	125	335	425	1,000,000	370,000	
WESTERN CEDARS									
Select Structural	Beams and Stringers	1,150	675	140	425	875	1,000,000	370,000	
No.1		975	475	140	425	725	1,000,000	370,000	
No.2		625	325	140	425	475	800,000	290,000	WCLIB
Select Structural	Posts and Timbers	1,100	725	140	425	925	1,000,000	370,000	WWPA
No.1		875	600	140	425	800	1,000,000	370,000	
No.2		550	350	140	425	550	800,000	290,000	
WESTERN CEDARS (NORTH)									
Select Structural	Beams and Stringers	1,150	675	130	425	850	1,000,000	370,000	
No.1		925	475	130	425	700	1,000,000	370,000	
No.2		625	300	130	425	450	800,000	290,000	NLGA
Select Structural	Posts and Timbers	1,050	700	130	425	900	1,000,000	370,000	
No.1		875	575	130	425	800	1,000,000	370,000	
No.2		500	350	130	425	550	800,000	290,000	
WESTERN HEMLOCK									
Select Structural	Beams and Stringers	1,400	825	170	410	1,000	1,400,000	510,000	
No.1		1,150	575	170	410	850	1,400,000	510,000	
No.2		750	375	170	410	550	1,100,000	400,000	WCLIB
Select Structural	Posts and Timbers	1,300	875	170	410	1,100	1,400,000	510,000	WWPA
No.1		1,050	700	170	410	950	1,400,000	510,000	
No.2		650	425	170	410	650	1,100,000	400,000	
WESTERN HEMLOCK (NORTH)									
Select Structural	Beams and Stringers	1,400	825	135	410	1,000	1,400,000	510,000	
No.1		1,150	575	135	410	850	1,400,000	510,000	
No.2		750	375	135	410	550	1,100,000	400,000	NLGA
Select Structural	Posts and Timbers	1,300	875	135	410	1,100	1,400,000	510,000	
No.1		1,050	700	135	410	950	1,400,000	510,000	
No.2		650	425	135	410	650	1,100,000	400,000	

4

REFERENCE DESIGN VALUES

Table 4D (Cont.) Reference Design Values for Visually Graded Timbers (5" x 5" and larger)[1,3]

(Tabulated design values are for normal load duration and dry service conditions, unless specified otherwise. See NDS 4.3 for a comprehensive description of design value adjustment factors.)

USE WITH TABLE 4D ADJUSTMENT FACTORS

| Species and commercial grade | Size classification | Design values in pounds per square inch (psi) | | | | | | | Grading Rules Agency |
| | | Bending F_b | Tension parallel to grain F_t | Shear parallel to grain F_v | Compression perpendicular to grain $F_{c\perp}$ | Compression parallel to grain F_c | Modulus of Elasticity | | |
							E	E_{min}	
WESTERN WHITE PINE									
Select Structural	Beams and Stringers	1,050	600	120	375	775	1,300,000	470,000	
No.1		850	425	120	375	625	1,300,000	470,000	
No.2		550	275	120	375	400	1,000,000	370,000	NLGA
Select Structural	Posts and Timbers	975	650	120	375	800	1,300,000	470,000	
No.1		775	525	120	375	700	1,300,000	470,000	
No.2		450	300	120	375	500	1,000,000	370,000	
WESTERN WOODS									
Select Structural	Beams and Stringers	1,050	625	125	345	750	1,100,000	400,000	
No.1		900	450	125	345	625	1,100,000	400,000	
No.2		575	300	125	345	425	900,000	330,000	WCLIB
Select Structural	Posts and Timbers	1,000	675	125	345	800	1,100,000	400,000	WWPA
No.1		800	525	125	345	700	1,100,000	400,000	
No.2		475	325	125	345	475	900,000	330,000	
WHITE OAK									
Select Structural	Beams and Stringers	1,400	825	205	800	900	1,000,000	370,000	
No.1		1,200	575	205	800	775	1,000,000	370,000	
No.2		750	375	205	800	475	800,000	290,000	NELMA
Select Structural	Posts and Timbers	1,300	875	205	800	950	1,000,000	370,000	
No.1		1,050	700	205	800	825	1,000,000	370,000	
No.2		600	400	205	800	400	800,000	290,000	

Footnotes to Table 4D

1. LUMBER DIMENSIONS. Tabulated design values are applicable to lumber that will be used under dry conditions such as in most covered structures. For 5" and thicker lumber, the GREEN dressed sizes shall be permitted to be used (see Table 1A) because design values have been adjusted to compensate for any loss in size by shrinkage which may occur.

2. SPRUCE PINE. To obtain recommended design values for Spruce Pine graded to Southern Pine Inspection Bureau (SPIB) rules, multiply the appropriate design values for Mixed Southern Pine by the corresponding conversion factor shown below and round to the nearest 100,000 psi for E; to the nearest 10,000 psi for E_{min}; to the next lower multiple of 5 psi for F_v and $F_{c\perp}$; to the next lower multiple of 50 psi for F_b, F_t, and F_c if 1,000 psi or greater, 25 psi otherwise.

CONVERSION FACTORS FOR DETERMINING DESIGN VALUES FOR SPRUCE PINE

	Bending F_b	Tension parallel to grain F_t	Shear parallel to grain F_v	Compression perpendicular to grain $F_{c\perp}$	Compression parallel to grain F_c	Modulus of Elasticity E and E_{min}
Conversion Factor	0.78	0.78	0.98	0.73	0.78	0.82

3. When individual species or species groups are combined, the design values to be used for the combination shall be the lowest design values for each individual species or species group for each design property.

Size Factor, C_F

Bending design values for all species of decking except Redwood are based on 4" thick decking. When 2" thick or 3" thick decking is used, the bending design values, F_b, for all species except Redwood shall be multiplied by the following size factors:

Size Factors, C_F

Thickness	C_F
2"	1.10
3"	1.04

Repetitive Member Factor, C_r

Tabulated bending design values for repetitive member uses, $(F_b)(C_r)$, for decking have already been multiplied by the repetitive member factor, C_r.

Flat Use Factor, C_{fu}

Tabulated bending design values, F_b, for decking have already been adjusted for flatwise usage (load applied to wide face).

Wet Service Factor, C_M

When decking is used where moisture content will exceed 19% for an extended time period, design values shall be multiplied by the appropriate wet service factors from the following table (for surfaced dry Southern Pine decking use tabulated surfaced green design values for wet service conditions without further adjustment):

Wet Service Factors, C_M

F_b	$F_{c\perp}$	E and E_{min}
0.85*	0.67	0.9

* when $(F_b)(C_F) \leq 1,150$ psi, $C_M = 1.0$

REFERENCE DESIGN VALUES

4

Table 4E   Reference Design Values for Visually Graded Decking[1,2]

(Tabulated design values are for normal load duration and dry service conditions, unless specified otherwise. See NDS 4.3 for a comprehensive description of design value adjustment factors.)

USE WITH TABLE 4E ADJUSTMENT FACTORS

Species and commercial grade	Size classification	Bending Single Member F_b	Bending Repetitive Member $(F_b)(C_r)$	Compression perpendicular to grain $F_{c\perp}$	Modulus of Elasticity E	Modulus of Elasticity E_{min}	Grading Rules Agency
BALSAM FIR							
Select	2" - 4" thick	—	1,650	—	1,500,000	550,000	NELMA
Commercial	4" - 12" wide	—	1,400	—	1,300,000	470,000	
COAST SITKA SPRUCE							
Select	2" - 4" thick	1,250	1,450	455	1,700,000	620,000	NLGA
Commercial	4" & wider	1,050	1,200	455	1,500,000	550,000	
COAST SPECIES							
Select	2" - 4" thick	1,250	1,450	370	1,500,000	550,000	NLGA
Commercial	4" & wider	1,050	1,200	370	1,400,000	510,000	
DOUGLAS FIR-LARCH							
Select Dex	2" - 4" thick	1,750	2,000	625	1,800,000	660,000	WCLIB
Commercial Dex	6" - 8" wide	1,450	1,650	625	1,700,000	620,000	
Selected	2" - 4" thick	1,750	2,000	625	1,800,000	660,000	WWPA
Commercial	4" & wider	1,450	1,650	625	1,700,000	620,000	
DOUGLAS FIR-LARCH (NORTH)							
Select	2" - 4" thick	1,750	2,000	625	1,800,000	660,000	NLGA
Commercial	4" & wider	1,450	1,650	625	1,700,000	620,000	
DOUGLAS FIR-SOUTH							
Selected	2" - 4" thick	1,650	1,900	520	1,400,000	510,000	WWPA
Commercial	4" & wider	1,400	1,600	520	1,300,000	470,000	
EASTERN HEMLOCK-TAMARACK							
Select	2" - 4" thick	—	1,700	—	1,300,000	470,000	NELMA
Commercial	4" - 12" wide	—	1,450	—	1,100,000	400,000	
EASTERN HEMLOCK-TAMARACK (NORTH)							
Select	2" - 4" thick	1,500	1,700	555	1,300,000	470,000	NLGA
Commercial	4" & wider	1,250	1,450	555	1,100,000	400,000	
EASTERN SPRUCE							
Select	2" - 4" thick	—	1,300	—	1,500,000	550,000	NELMA
Commercial	4" - 12" wide	—	1,100	—	1,400,000	510,000	
EASTERN WHITE PINE							
Select	2" - 4" thick	—	1,300	—	1,200,000	440,000	NELMA
Commercial	4" - 12"wide	—	1,100	—	1,100,000	400,000	
EASTERN WHITE PINE (NORTH)							
Select	2" - 4" thick	900	1,050	350	1,200,000	440,000	NLGA
Commercial	4" & wider	775	875	350	1,100,000	400,000	
HEM-FIR							
Select Dex	2" - 4" thick	1,400	1,600	405	1,500,000	550,000	WCLIB
Commercial Dex	6" - 8" wide	1,150	1,350	405	1,400,000	510,000	
Selected	2" - 4" thick	1,400	1,600	405	1,500,000	550,000	WWPA
Commercial	4" & wider	1,150	1,350	405	1,400,000	510,000	
HEM-FIR (NORTH)							
Select	2" - 4" thick	1,350	1,500	405	1,500,000	550,000	NLGA
Commercial	4" & wider	1,100	1,300	405	1,400,000	510,000	
NORTHERN PINE							
Select	2" - 4" thick	—	1,550	—	1,400,000	510,000	NELMA
Commercial	4" - 12" wide	—	1,300	—	1,300,000	470,000	
NORTHERN SPECIES							
Select	2" - 4" thick	900	1,050	350	1,100,000	400,000	NLGA
Commercial	4" & wider	775	875	350	1,000,000	370,000	

Table 4E (Cont.) Reference Design Values for Visually Graded Decking[1,2]

(Tabulated design values are for normal load duration and dry service conditions, unless specified otherwise. See NDS 4.3 for a comprehensive description of design value adjustment factors.)

USE WITH TABLE 4E ADJUSTMENT FACTORS

Species and commercial grade	Size classification	Bending Single Member F_b	Bending Repetitive Member $(F_b)(C_r)$	Compression perpendicular to grain $F_{c\perp}$	Modulus of Elasticity E	Modulus of Elasticity E_{min}	Grading Rules Agency
NORTHERN WHITE CEDAR							
Select	2" - 4" thick	—	1,100	—	800,000	290,000	NELMA
Commercial	4" - 12" wide	—	950	—	700,000	260,000	
PONDEROSA PINE							
Select	2" - 4" thick	1,200	1,450	535	1,300,000	470,000	NLGA
Commercial	4" & wider	1,000	1,250	535	1,100,000	400,000	
RED PINE							
Select	2" - 4" thick	1,150	1,350	440	1,300,000	470,000	NLGA
Commercial	4" & wider	975	1,100	440	1,200,000	440,000	
REDWOOD							
Select, Close grain	2" thick	1,850	2,150	—	1,400,000	510,000	
Select		1,450	1,700	—	1,100,000	400,000	
Commercial	6" & wider	1,200	1,350	—	1,000,000	370,000	
Deck Heart and	2" thick 4" wide	400	450	420	900,000	330,000	RIS
Deck Common	2" thick 6" wide	700	800	420	900,000	330,000	
SITKA SPRUCE							
Select Dex	2" - 4" thick	1,300	1,500	435	1,500,000	550,000	WCLIB
Commercial Dex	6" - 8" wide	1,100	1,250	435	1,300,000	470,000	
SOUTHERN PINE	(Surfaced dry – Used in dry service conditions — 19% or less moisture content)						
Dense Standard		2,000	2,300	660	1,800,000	660,000	
Dense Select	2" - 4" thick	1,650	1,900	660	1,600,000	580,000	
Select		1,400	1,650	565	1,600,000	580,000	SPIB
Dense Commercial	2" & wider	1,650	1,900	660	1,600,000	580,000	
Commercial		1,400	1,650	565	1,600,000	580,000	
SOUTHERN PINE	(Surfaced Green – Used in any service condition)						
Dense Standard		1,600	1,800	440	1,600,000	580,000	
Dense Select	2-1/2" - 4" thick	1,350	1,500	440	1,400,000	510,000	
Select		1,150	1,300	375	1,400,000	510,000	SPIB
Dense Commercial	2" & wider	1,350	1,500	440	1,400,000	510,000	
Commercial		1,150	1,300	375	1,400,000	510,000	
SPRUCE-PINE-FIR							
Select	2" - 4" thick	1,200	1,400	425	1,500,000	550,000	NLGA
Commercial	4" & wider	1,000	1,150	425	1,300,000	470,000	
SPRUCE-PINE-FIR (SOUTH)							
Selected	2" - 4" thick	1,150	1,350	335	1,400,000	510,000	NELMA
Commercial	4" & wider	950	1,100	335	1,200,000	440,000	WWPA
WESTERN CEDARS							
Select Dex	2" - 4" thick	1,250	1,450	425	1,100,000	400,000	WCLIB
Commercial Dex	6" - 8" wide	1,050	1,200	425	1,000,000	370,000	
Selected	2" - 4" thick	1,250	1,450	425	1,100,000	400,000	WWPA
Commercial	4" & wider	1,050	1,200	425	1,000,000	370,000	
WESTERN CEDARS (NORTH)							
Select	2" - 4" thick	1,200	1,400	425	1,100,000	400,000	NLGA
Commercial	4" & wider	1,050	1,200	425	1,000,000	370,000	
WESTERN HEMLOCK							
Select Dex	2" - 4" thick	1,500	1,750	410	1,600,000	580,000	WCLIB
Commercial Dex	6" & wider	1,300	1,450	410	1,400,000	510,000	

(Tabulated design values are for normal load duration and dry service conditions, unless specified otherwise. See NDS 4.3 for a comprehensive description of design value adjustment factors.)

USE WITH TABLE 4E ADJUSTMENT FACTORS

Species and commercial grade	Size classification	Design values in pounds per square inch (psi)					Grading Rules Agency
		Bending		Compression perpendicular to grain $F_{c\perp}$	Modulus of Elasticity		
		Single Member F_b	Repetitive Member $(F_b)(C_r)$		E	E_{min}	
WESTERN HEMLOCK (NORTH)							
Select	2" - 4" thick	1,500	1,750	410	1,600,000	580,000	NLGA
Commercial	4" & wider	1,300	1,450	410	1,400,000	510,000	
WESTERN WHITE PINE							
Select	2" - 4" thick	1,100	1,300	375	1,400,000	510,000	NLGA
Commercial	4" & wider	925	1,050	375	1,300,000	470,000	
WESTERN WOODS							
Selected	2" - 4" thick	1,150	1,300	335	1,200,000	440,000	WWPA
Commercial	4" & wider	950	1,100	335	1,100,000	400,000	

1. **LUMBER DIMENSIONS.** Tabulated design values are applicable to lumber that will be used under dry conditions such as in most covered structures. For 2" to 4" thick lumber the DRY dressed sizes shall be used (see Table 1A) regardless of the moisture content at the time of manufacture or use. In calculating design values, the natural gain in strength and stiffness that occurs as lumber dries has been taken into consideration as well as the reduction in size that occurs when unseasoned lumber shrinks. The gain in load carrying capacity due to increased strength and stiffness resulting from drying more than offsets the design effect of size reductions due to shrinkage.

2. When individual species or species groups are combined, the design values to be used for the combination shall be the lowest design values for each individual species or species group for each design property.

Table 4F Adjustment Factors

Repetitive Member Factor, C_r

Bending design values, F_b, for dimension lumber 2" to 4" thick shall be multiplied by the repetitive member factor, $C_r = 1.15$, when such members are used as joists, truss chords, rafters, studs, planks, decking, or similar members which are in contact or spaced not more than 24" on center, are not less than 3 in number, and are joined by floor, roof, or other load distributing elements adequate to support the design load.

Wet Service Factor, C_M

When dimension lumber is used where moisture content will exceed 19% for an extended time period, design values shall be multiplied by the appropriate wet service factors from the following table:

Wet Service Factors, C_M

F_b	F_t	F_v	$F_{c\perp}$	F_c	E and E_{min}
0.85*	1.0	0.97	0.67	0.8**	0.9

* when $(F_b)(C_F) \leq 1,150$ psi, $C_M = 1.0$
** when $(F_c)(C_F) \leq 750$ psi, $C_M = 1.0$

Flat Use Factor, C_{fu}

Bending design values adjusted by size factors are based on edgewise use (load applied to narrow face). When dimension lumber is used flatwise (load applied to wide face), the bending design value, F_b, shall also be multiplied by the following flat use factors:

Flat Use Factors, C_{fu}

Width (depth)	Thickness (breadth)	
	2" & 3"	4"
2" & 3"	1.0	—
4"	1.1	1.0
5"	1.1	1.05
6"	1.15	1.05
8"	1.15	1.05
10" & wider	1.2	1.1

NOTE

To facilitate the use of Table 4F, shading has been employed to distinguish design values based on a 4" nominal width (Construction, Standard, and Utility grades) or a 6" nominal width (Stud grade) from design values based on a 12" nominal width (Select Structural, No.1 & Btr, No.1, No.2, and No.3 grades).

Size Factor, C_F

Tabulated bending, tension, and compression parallel to grain design values for dimension lumber 2" to 4" thick shall be multiplied by the following size factors:

Size Factors, C_F

Grades	Width (depth)	F_b		F_t	F_c
		Thickness (breadth)			
		2" & 3"	4"		
Select Structural, No.1 & Btr, No.1, No.2, No.3	2", 3", & 4"	1.5	1.5	1.5	1.15
	5"	1.4	1.4	1.4	1.1
	6"	1.3	1.3	1.3	1.1
	8"	1.2	1.3	1.2	1.05
	10"	1.1	1.2	1.1	1.0
	12"	1.0	1.1	1.0	1.0
	14" & wider	0.9	1.0	0.9	0.9
Stud	2", 3", & 4"	1.1	1.1	1.1	1.05
	5" & 6"	1.0	1.0	1.0	1.0
	8" & wider	Use No.3 Grade tabulated design values and size factors			
Construction, Standard	2", 3", & 4"	1.0	1.0	1.0	1.0
Utility	4"	1.0	1.0	1.0	1.0
	2" & 3"	0.4	—	0.4	0.6

4

REFERENCE DESIGN VALUES

Table 4F　Reference Design Values for Non-North American Visually Graded Dimension Lumber (2" - 4" thick)[1,3,4]

(Tabulated design values are for normal load duration and dry service conditions. See NDS 4.3 for a comprehensive description of design value adjustment factors.)

USE WITH TABLE 4F ADJUSTMENT FACTORS

Species and commercial grade	Size classification	Design values in pounds per square inch (psi)							Grading Rules Agency
		Bending F_b	Tension parallel to grain F_t	Shear parallel to grain F_v	Compression perpendicular to grain $F_{c\perp}$	Compression parallel to grain F_c	Modulus of Elasticity		
							E	E_{min}	
AUSTRIAN SPRUCE - Austria & The Czech Republic									
Select Structural		1,500	675	175	260	1,250	1,700,000	620,000	
No.1		1,000	450	175	260	1,100	1,600,000	580,000	
No.2	2" & wider	925	400	175	260	1,050	1,500,000	550,000	
No.3		525	225	175	260	625	1,300,000	470,000	WCLIB
Stud	2" & wider	725	325	175	260	675	1,300,000	470,000	
Construction		1,050	475	175	260	1,300	1,400,000	510,000	
Standard	2" - 4" wide	575	250	175	260	1,100	1,300,000	470,000	
Utility		275	125	175	260	725	1,200,000	440,000	
DOUGLAS FIR/EUROPEAN LARCH - Austria, The Czech Republic, & Bavaria[2]									
Select Structural		1,900	850	195	440	1,400	1,800,000	660,000	
No.1		1,400	625	195	440	1,250	1,700,000	620,000	
No.2	2" & wider	1,350	600	195	440	1,250	1,600,000	580,000	
No.3		775	350	195	440	700	1,400,000	510,000	WCLIB
Stud	2" & wider	800	350	195	440	700	1,400,000	510,000	
Construction		1,000	450	195	440	1,250	1,500,000	550,000	
Standard	2" - 4" wide	575	250	195	440	1,100	1,300,000	470,000	
Utility		275	125	195	440	700	1,300,000	470,000	
MONTANE PINE - South Africa									
Select Structural		975	425	135	325	1,100	1,300,000	470,000	
No.1		650	300	135	325	950	1,100,000	400,000	
No.2	2" & wider	600	275	135	325	850	1,000,000	370,000	
No.3		350	150	135	325	475	900,000	330,000	WCLIB
Stud	2" & wider	475	200	135	325	525	900,000	330,000	
Construction		675	300	135	325	1,050	900,000	330,000	
Standard	2" - 4" wide	375	175	135	325	875	800,000	290,000	
Utility		175	75	135	325	575	800,000	290,000	
NORWAY SPRUCE - Estonia & Lithuania									
Select Structural		1,200	550	150	430	1,200	1,500,000	550,000	
No.1		800	375	150	430	1,050	1,400,000	510,000	
No.2	2" & wider	700	300	150	430	925	1,200,000	440,000	
No.3		400	175	150	430	525	1,100,000	400,000	WCLIB
Stud	2" & wider	550	250	150	430	575	1,100,000	400,000	
Construction		800	350	150	430	1,150	1,100,000	400,000	
Standard	2" - 4" wide	450	200	150	430	950	1,000,000	370,000	
Utility		200	100	150	430	625	1,000,000	370,000	
NORWAY SPRUCE - Finland									
Select Structural		1,350	600	125	220	1,200	1,500,000	550,000	
No.1		825	375	125	220	1,000	1,400,000	510,000	
No.2	2" & wider	625	275	125	220	875	1,200,000	440,000	
No.3		375	175	125	220	500	1,100,000	400,000	WCLIB
Stud	2" & wider	575	250	125	220	600	1,100,000	400,000	
Construction		725	325	125	220	1,100	1,100,000	400,000	
Standard	2" - 4" wide	400	175	125	220	900	1,000,000	370,000	
Utility		200	75	125	220	600	1,000,000	370,000	
NORWAY SPRUCE - Germany, NE France, & Switzerland									
Select Structural		1,200	550	170	355	1,200	1,600,000	580,000	
No.1		825	375	170	355	1,050	1,400,000	510,000	
No.2	2" & wider	725	325	170	355	950	1,200,000	440,000	
No.3		425	200	170	355	550	1,100,000	400,000	WCLIB
Stud	2" & wider	575	250	170	355	600	1,100,000	400,000	
Construction		825	375	170	355	1,200	1,100,000	400,000	
Standard	2" - 4" wide	475	200	170	355	975	1,000,000	370,000	
Utility		225	100	170	355	650	900,000	330,000	

Table 4F (Cont.) Reference Design Values for Non-North American Visually Graded Dimension Lumber (2" - 4" thick)[1,3,4]

(Tabulated design values are for normal load duration and dry service conditions. See NDS 4.3 for a comprehensive description of design value adjustment factors.)

USE WITH TABLE 4F ADJUSTMENT FACTORS

| Species and commercial grade | Size classification | Design values in pounds per square inch (psi) | | | | | Modulus of Elasticity | | Grading Rules Agency |
		Bending F_b	Tension parallel to grain F_t	Shear parallel to grain F_v	Compression perpendicular to grain $F_{c\perp}$	Compression parallel to grain F_c	E	E_{min}	
NORWAY SPRUCE - Romania & the Ukraine									
Select Structural		1,250	575	100	275	1,200	1,500,000	550,000	
No.1		850	375	100	275	1,050	1,400,000	510,000	
No.2	2" & wider	725	325	100	275	950	1,200,000	440,000	
No.3		425	200	100	275	550	1,100,000	400,000	WCLIB
Stud	2" & wider	575	250	100	275	600	1,100,000	400,000	
Construction		850	375	100	275	1,200	1,100,000	400,000	
Standard	2" - 4" wide	475	200	100	275	1,000	1,000,000	370,000	
Utility		225	100	100	275	650	1,000,000	370,000	
NORWAY SPRUCE - Sweden									
Select Structural		1,250	550	170	285	1,200	1,600,000	580,000	
No.1		825	375	170	285	1,050	1,400,000	510,000	
No.2	2" & wider	675	300	170	285	925	1,200,000	440,000	
No.3		400	175	170	285	525	1,100,000	400,000	WCLIB
Stud	2" & wider	550	250	170	285	575	1,100,000	400,000	
Construction		775	350	170	285	1,150	1,200,000	440,000	
Standard	2" - 4" wide	425	200	170	285	950	1,100,000	400,000	
Utility		200	100	170	285	625	1,000,000	370,000	
SCOTS PINE - Austria, The Czech Republic, Romania, & the Ukraine									
Select Structural		1,300	600	135	270	1,200	1,700,000	620,000	
No.1		900	400	135	270	1,050	1,600,000	580,000	
No.2	2" & wider	775	350	135	270	1,000	1,400,000	510,000	
No.3		450	200	135	270	575	1,300,000	470,000	WCLIB
Stud	2" & wider	600	275	135	270	625	1,300,000	470,000	
Construction		875	400	135	270	1,200	1,300,000	470,000	
Standard	2" - 4" wide	500	225	135	270	1,000	1,200,000	440,000	
Utility		225	100	135	270	675	1,100,000	400,000	
SCOTS PINE - Estonia & Lithuania									
Select Structural		1,100	500	130	430	1,150	1,500,000	550,000	
No.1		750	350	130	430	1,000	1,300,000	470,000	
No.2	2" & wider	650	300	130	430	900	1,100,000	400,000	
No.3		375	175	130	430	525	1,000,000	370,000	WCLIB
Stud	2" & wider	525	225	130	430	575	1,000,000	370,000	
Construction		750	325	130	430	1,100	1,100,000	400,000	
Standard	2" - 4" wide	425	200	130	430	925	1,000,000	370,000	
Utility		200	100	130	430	600	900,000	330,000	
SCOTS PINE - Finland									
Select Structural		1,300	600	150	210	1,200	1,500,000	550,000	
No.1		950	425	150	210	1,100	1,400,000	510,000	
No.2	2" & wider	925	425	150	210	1,100	1,300,000	470,000	
No.3		525	250	150	210	625	1,200,000	440,000	WCLIB
Stud	2" & wider	725	325	150	210	675	1,200,000	440,000	
Construction		1,050	475	150	210	1,300	1,200,000	440,000	
Standard	2" - 4" wide	600	275	150	210	1,100	1,100,000	400,000	
Utility		275	125	150	210	725	1,000,000	370,000	
SCOTS PINE - Germany[5]									
Select Structural		1,200	550	160	395	1,200	1,600,000	580,000	
No.1		800	375	160	395	1,050	1,400,000	510,000	
No.2	2" & wider	700	325	160	395	950	1,100,000	400,000	
No.3		400	175	160	395	550	1,000,000	370,000	WCLIB
Stud	2" & wider	550	250	160	395	600	1,000,000	370,000	
Construction		800	375	160	395	1,150	1,100,000	400,000	
Standard	2" - 4" wide	450	200	160	395	975	1,000,000	370,000	
Utility		225	100	160	395	625	900,000	330,000	

Table 4F (Cont.) Reference Design Values for Non-North American Visually Graded Dimension Lumber (2" - 4" thick)[1,3,4]

(Tabulated design values are for normal load duration and dry service conditions. See NDS 4.3 for a comprehensive description of design value adjustment factors.)

USE WITH TABLE 4F ADJUSTMENT FACTORS

Species and commercial grade	Size classification	Design values in pounds per square inch (psi)							Grading Rules Agency
		Bending F_b	Tension parallel to grain F_t	Shear parallel to grain F_v	Compression perpendicular to grain $F_{c\perp}$	Compression parallel to grain F_c	Modulus of Elasticity		
							E	E_{min}	
SCOTS PINE - Sweden									
Select Structural		1,350	600	120	410	1,200	1,700,000	620,000	
No.1		825	375	120	410	1,000	1,500,000	550,000	
No.2	2" & wider	575	250	120	410	825	1,200,000	440,000	
No.3		325	150	120	410	475	1,100,000	400,000	WCLIB
Stud	2" & wider	450	200	120	410	525	1,100,000	400,000	
Construction		650	300	120	410	1,050	1,200,000	440,000	
Standard	2" - 4" wide	375	175	120	410	850	1,100,000	400,000	
Utility		175	75	120	410	550	1,000,000	370,000	
SILVER FIR (Abies alba) - Germany, NE France, & Switzerland									
Select Structural		950	425	125	400	1,100	1,500,000	550,000	
No.1		725	325	125	400	975	1,400,000	510,000	
No.2	2" & wider	725	325	125	400	950	1,300,000	470,000	
No.3		425	200	125	400	550	1,100,000	400,000	WCLIB
Stud	2" & wider	575	250	125	400	600	1,100,000	400,000	
Construction		825	375	125	400	1,150	1,200,000	440,000	
Standard	2" - 4" wide	475	200	125	400	975	1,100,000	400,000	
Utility		225	100	125	400	650	1,000,000	370,000	
SOUTHERN PINE - Misiones Argentina									
Select Structural		1,100	500	150	440	1,150	1,200,000	440,000	
No.1		775	350	150	440	1,000	1,100,000	400,000	
No.2	2" & wider	725	325	150	440	950	1,100,000	400,000	
No.3		425	200	150	440	550	900,000	330,000	SPIB
Stud	2" & wider	575	250	150	440	600	900,000	330,000	
Construction		825	375	150	440	1,150	1,000,000	370,000	
Standard	2" - 4" wide	475	200	150	440	975	900,000	330,000	
Utility		225	100	150	440	650	800,000	290,000	
SOUTHERN PINE - Misiones Argentina, Free of Heart Center and Medium Grain Density									
Select Structural		1,700	775	210	710	1,250	1,500,000	550,000	
No.1		1,150	525	210	710	1,150	1,500,000	550,000	
No.2	2" & wider	1,000	450	210	710	1,100	1,500,000	550,000	
No.3		575	250	210	710	650	1,400,000	510,000	SPIB
Stud	2" & wider	800	350	210	710	700	1,400,000	510,000	
Construction		1,150	525	210	710	1,350	1,400,000	510,000	
Standard	2" - 4" wide	650	300	210	710	1,150	1,300,000	470,000	
Utility		300	125	210	710	750	1,200,000	440,000	

1. **LUMBER DIMENSIONS.** Tabulated design values are applicable to lumber that will be used under dry conditions such as in most covered structures. For 2" to 4" thick lumber the DRY dressed sizes shall be used (see Table 1A) regardless of the moisture content at the time of manufacture or use. In calculating design values, the natural gain in strength and stiffness that occurs as lumber dries has been taken into consideration as well as the reduction in size that occurs when unseasoned lumber shrinks. The gain in the load carrying capacity due to increased strength and stiffness resulting from drying more than offsets the design effect of size reductions due to shrinkage.

2. Design values are applicable only for 2x4 dimensional lumber and shall not be multiplied by the size factor adjustment.

3. Specific Gravity, G, values for Non-North American Species are provided below in lieu of providing G values in NDS Table 11.3.2A

Species or Species Combination	Specific Gravity	Species or Species Combination	Specific Gravity
Austrian Spruce - Austria & The Czech Republic	0.43	Scots Pine - Austria, The Czech Republic, Romania, & the Ukraine	0.50
Douglas Fir/European Larch - Austria, The Czech Republic, & Bavaria	0.48	Scots Pine - Estonia & Lithuania	0.45
		Scots Pine - Finland	0.48
Montane Pine - South Africa	0.45	Scots Pine - Germany*	0.53
Norway Spruce - Estonia & Lithuania	0.43	Scots Pine - Sweden	0.47
Norway Spruce - Finland	0.42	Silver Fir (Abies alba) - Germany, NE France, & Switzerland	0.43
Norway Spruce - Germany, NE France, & Switzerland	0.42	Southern Pine - Misiones Argentina, Free of Heart Center and Medium Grain Density	0.5
Norway Spruce - Romania & the Ukraine	0.38		
Norway Spruce - Sweden	0.42	Southern Pine - Misiones Argentina	0.45

* See footnote 5.

4. When individual species or species groups are combined, the design values to be used for the combination shall be the lowest design values for each individual species or species group for each design property.

5. Does not include states of Baden-Wurttemburg and Saarland.

Volume Factor, C_V

Tabulated bending design values for loading perpendicular to wide faces of laminations, F_{bx}, for structural glued laminated bending members shall be multiplied by the following volume factor:

$$C_V = (21/L)^{1/x}(12/d)^{1/x}(5.125/b)^{1/x} \le 1.0$$

where:

L = length of bending member between points of zero moment, ft

d = depth of bending member, in.

b = width (breadth) of bending member, in. For multiple piece width, b = width of widest piece in the layup. Thus b ≤ 10.75".

x = 20 for Southern Pine

x = 10 for all other species

The volume factor shall not apply simultaneously with the beam stability factor (see 5.3.6). Therefore, the lesser of these adjustment factors shall apply.

Flat Use Factor, C_{fu}

Tabulated bending design values for loading parallel to wide faces of laminations, F_{by}, shall be multiplied by the following flat use factors when the member dimension parallel to wide faces of laminations is less than 12":

Flat Use Factors, C_{fu}

Member dimension parallel to wide faces of laminations	C_{fu}
10-3/4" or 10-1/2"	1.01
8-3/4" or 8-1/2"	1.04
6-3/4"	1.07
5-1/8" or 5"	1.10
3-1/8" or 3"	1.16
2-1/2"	1.19

Wet Service Factor, C_M

When structural glued laminated timber is used where moisture content will be 16% or greater, design values shall be multiplied by the appropriate wet service factors from the following table:

Wet Service Factors, C_M

F_b	F_t	F_v	$F_{c\perp}$	F_c	E and E_{min}
0.8	0.8	0.875	0.53	0.73	0.833

4

REFERENCE DESIGN VALUES

Table 5A Reference Design Values for Structural Glued Laminated Softwood Timber

(Members stressed primarily in bending) (Tabulated design values are for normal load duration and dry service conditions. See NDS 5.3 for a comprehensive description of design value adjustment factors.)

Use with Table 5A Adjustment Factors

Stress Class	Bending About X-X Axis — Loaded Perpendicular to Wide Faces of Laminations						Bending About Y-Y Axis — Loaded Parallel to Wide Faces of Laminations					Axially Loaded			Fasteners
	Extreme Fiber in Bending		Compression Perpendicular to Grain	Shear Parallel to Grain (Horizontal)	Modulus of Elasticity	Modulus of Elasticity for Beam and Column Stability	Extreme Fiber in Bending	Compression Perpendicular to Grain	Shear Parallel to Grain (Horizontal)	Modulus of Elasticity	Modulus of Elasticity for Beam and Column Stability	Tension Parallel to Grain	Compression Parallel to Grain	Modulus of Elasticity	Specific Gravity for Fastener Design
	Tension Zone Stressed in Tension (Positive Bending)	Compression Zone Stressed in Tension (Negative Bending)													
	F_{bx}^{+}	F_{bx}^{-} [1]	F_{cLx}	F_{vx} [4]	E_x	$E_{x\,min}$	F_{by}	F_{cLy}	F_{vy} [4][5]	E_y	$E_{y\,min}$	F_t	F_c	E_{axial}	G
	(psi)	(psi)	(psi)	(psi)	(10^6 psi)	(10^6 psi)	(psi)	(psi)	(psi)	(10^6 psi)	(10^6 psi)	(psi)	(psi)	(10^6 psi)	
16F-1.3E	1600	925	315	195	1.3	0.67	800	315	170	1.1	0.57	675	925	1.2	0.42
20F-1.5E	2000	1100	425	210 [6]	1.5	0.78	800	315	185	1.2	0.62	725	925	1.3	0.42
24F-1.7E	2400	1450	500	210 [6]	1.7	0.88	1050	315	185	1.3	0.67	775	1000	1.4	0.42
24F-1.8E	2400	1450 [2]	650	265 [3]	1.8	0.93	1450	560	230 [3]	1.6	0.83	1100	1600	1.7	0.50 [10]
26F-1.9E [7]	2600	1950	650	265 [3]	1.9	0.98	1600	560	230 [3]	1.6	0.83	1150	1600	1.7	0.50 [10]
28F-2.1E SP [7]	2800	2300	740	300	2.1 [9]	1.09 [9]	1600	650	260	1.7	0.88	1250	1750	1.7	0.55
30F-2.1E SP [7][8]	3000	2400	740	300	2.1 [9]	1.09 [9]	1750	650	260	1.7	0.88	1250	1750	1.7	0.55

1. For balanced layups, F_{bx}^{-} shall be equal to F_{bx}^{+} for the stress class. Designer shall specify when balanced layup is required.
2. Negative bending stress, F_{bx}^{-}, is permitted to be increased to 1,850 psi for Douglas Fir and to 1,950 psi for Southern Pine for specific combinations. Designer shall specify when these increased stresses are required.
3. For structural glued laminated timber of Southern Pine, the basic shear design values, F_{vx} and F_{vy}, are permitted to be increased to 300 psi and 260 psi, respectively.
4. The design value for shear, F_{vx} and F_{vy}, shall be decreased by multiplying by a factor of 0.72 for non-prismatic members, notched members, and for all members subject to impact or cyclic loading. The reduced design value shall be used for design of members at connections that transfer shear by mechanical fasteners (NDS 3.4.3.3). The reduced design value shall also be used for determination of design values for radial tension (NDS 5.2.2).
5. Design values are for timbers with laminations made from a single piece of lumber across the width or multiple pieces that have been edge bonded. For timbers manufactured from multiple piece laminations (across width) that are not edge bonded, value shall be multiplied by 0.4 for members with 5, 7, or 9 laminations or by 0.5 for all other members. This reduction shall be cumulative with the adjustment in footnote (4).
6. Certain Southern Pine combinations may contain lumber with wane. If lumber with wane is used, the design value for shear parallel to grain, F_{vx}, shall be multiplied by 0.67 if wane is allowed on both sides. If wane is limited to one side, F_{vx} shall be multiplied by 0.83. This reduction shall be cumulative with the adjustment in footnote (4).
7. 26F, 28F, and 30F beams are not produced by all manufacturers, therefore, availability may be limited. Contact supplier or manufacturer for details.
8. 30F combinations are restricted to a maximum 6" nominal width.
9. For 28F and 30F members with more than 15 laminations, $E_x = 2.0$ million psi and $E_{x\,min} = 1.04$ million psi.
10. For structural glued laminated timber of Southern Pine, specific gravity for fastener design is permitted to be increased to 0.55.

Design values in this table represent design values for groups of similar structural glued laminated timber combinations. Higher design values may be obtained by specifying a particular combination listed in Table 5A Expanded. Design values are for members with 4 or more laminations. For 2 and 3 lamination members, see Table 5B. Some stress classes are not available in all species. Contact structural glued laminated timber manufacturer for availability.

Table 5A Expanded – Reference Design Values for Structural Glued Laminated Softwood Timber Combinations[1]

(Members stressed primarily in bending) (Tabulated design values are for normal load duration and dry service conditions.) Table 5A Expanded is an expanded list of structural glued laminated timber combinations from AITC 117 and APA-EWS Y117 that meet the requirements of each stress class in the new structural glued laminated timber stress class system. Table 5A Expanded is provided to allow easy conversion from the old combination symbols system to the new stress class system.

Use with Table 5A Adjustment Factors

Combination Symbol	Species Outer/Core	Bending About X-X Axis (Loaded Perpendicular to Wide Faces of Laminations)							Bending About Y-Y Axis (Loaded Parallel to Wide Faces of Laminations)					Axially Loaded			Fasteners (Specific Gravity for Fastener Design)	
		Extreme Fiber in Bending F_{bx}^{+} (Tension Zone Stressed in Tension) (psi)	Extreme Fiber in Bending F_{bx}^{-} (Compression Zone Stressed in Tension) (psi)	Comp. Perp. to Grain Tension Face (psi)	Comp. Perp. to Grain Compression Face F_{cLx} (psi)	Shear Parallel to Grain (Horizontal) F_{vx} (3) (psi)	Modulus of Elasticity E_x (10⁶ psi)	M.O.E. for Beam and Column Stability $E_{x\,min}$ (10⁶ psi)	Extreme Fiber in Bending F_{by} (psi)	Comp. Perp. to Grain F_{cLy} (psi)	Shear Parallel to Grain (Horizontal) F_{vy} (4) (psi)	Modulus of Elasticity E_y (10⁶ psi)	M.O.E. for Beam and Column Stability $E_{y\,min}$ (10⁶ psi)	Tension Parallel to Grain F_t (psi)	Compression Parallel to Grain F_c (psi)	Modulus of Elasticity E_{axial} (10⁶ psi)	Top or Bottom Face	Side Face — G
16F-1.3E		**1600**	**925**	**315**		**195**	**1.3**	**0.67**	**800**	**315**	**170**	**1.1**	**0.57**	**675**	**925**	**1.2**	**0.42**	
16F-V6	DF/DF	1600	1600	560	560	265	1.5	0.78	1450	560	230	1.5	0.78	900	1550	1.6	0.5	0.5
16F-E2	HF/HF	1600	1050	375	375	215	1.3	0.67	1200	375	190	1.3	0.67	825	1200	1.4	0.43	0.43
16F-E3	DF/DF	1600	1200	560	560	215	1.6	0.83	1450	560	190	1.5	0.78	925	1600	1.6	0.5	0.5
16F-E6	DF/DF	1600	1600	560	560	265	1.6	0.83	1550	560	230	1.5	0.78	975	1600	1.6	0.5	0.5
16F-E7	HF/HF	1600	1600	375	375	215	1.4	0.73	1450	375	190	1.4	0.73	1000	1450	1.5	0.43	0.43
16F-V2	SP/SP	1600	1350	650	650	300	1.4	0.73	1450	650	260	1.4	0.73	975	1350	1.5	0.55	0.55
16F-V3	SP/SP	1600	1450	740	740	300	1.4	0.73	1450	650	260	1.4	0.73	925	1400	1.4	0.55	0.55
16F-V5	SP/SP	1600	1600	650	650	300	1.4	0.73	1750	650	260	1.4	0.73	1000	1500	1.5	0.55	0.55
16F-E1	SP/SP	1600	1250	650	650	300	1.6	0.83	1750	650	260	1.5	0.78	1050	1550	1.6	0.55	0.55
16F-E3	SP/SP	1600	1600	650	650	300	1.6	0.83	1750	650	260	1.5	0.78	1100	1600	1.6	0.55	0.55
20F-1.5E		**2000**	**1100**	**425**		**210**	**1.5**	**0.78**	**800**	**315**	**185**	**1.2**	**0.62**	**725**	**925**	**1.3**	**0.42**	
20F-V3	DF/DF	2000	1450	650	560	265	1.6	0.83	1450	560	230	1.5	0.78	975	1550	1.6	0.5	0.5
20F-V7	DF/DF	2000	2000	650	650	265	1.6	0.83	1450	560	230	1.6	0.83	1000	1550	1.6	0.5	0.5
20F-V9	HF/HF	2000	2000	500	500	215	1.5	0.78	1350	375	190	1.4	0.73	975	1400	1.5	0.43	0.43
20F-V12	AC/AC	2000	1400	560	560	265	1.5	0.78	1250	470	230	1.4	0.73	900	1500	1.4	0.46	0.46
20F-V13	AC/AC	2000	2000	560	560	265	1.5	0.78	1250	470	230	1.4	0.73	925	1550	1.5	0.46	0.46
20F-E2	HF/HF	2000	1400	500	500	215	1.6	0.83	1200	375	190	1.4	0.73	925	1350	1.5	0.43	0.43
20F-E3	DF/DF	2000	1200	560	560	265	1.7	0.88	1450	560	230	1.6	0.83	1000	1600	1.7	0.5	0.5
20F-E6	DF/DF	2000	2000	560	560	265	1.7	0.88	1550	560	230	1.6	0.83	1100	1650	1.7	0.5	0.5
20F-E7	HF/HF	2000	2000	500	500	215	1.6	0.83	1450	375	190	1.4	0.73	1050	1450	1.5	0.43	0.43
20F-V2	SP/SP	2000	1550	740	650	300	1.5	0.78	1450	650	260	1.4	0.73	975	1350	1.5	0.55	0.55
20F-V3	SP/SP	2000	1450	650	650	300	1.5	0.78	1750	650	260	1.4	0.73	1050	1400	1.5	0.55	0.55
20F-V5	SP/SP	2000	2000	740	740	300	1.6	0.83	1450	650	260	1.5	0.78	1050	1500	1.5	0.55	0.55
20F-E1	SP/SP	2000	1250	650	650	300	1.7	0.88	1750	650	260	1.6	0.78	1050	1550	1.6	0.55	0.55
20F-E3	SP/SP	2000	2000	650	650	300	1.7	0.88	1900	650	260	1.6	0.78	1150	1650	1.6	0.55	0.55
24F-1.7E		**2400**	**1450**	**500**		**210**	**1.7**	**0.88**	**1050**	**315**	**185**	**1.3**	**0.67**	**775**	**1000**	**1.4**	**0.42**	
24F-V5	DF/HF	2400	1600	650	650	215	1.7	0.88	1200	375	190	1.5	0.78	1150	1450	1.6	0.5	0.5
24F-V10	DF/HF	2400	2400	650	650	215	1.8	0.93	1450	375	190	1.5	0.78	1100	1550	1.6	0.5	0.5
24F-E11	HF/HF	2400	2400	500	500	215	1.8	0.93	1550	375	190	1.5	0.78	1150	1550	1.6	0.43	0.43
24F-E15	HF/HF	2400	1600	500	500	215	1.8	0.93	1200	375	190	1.5	0.78	975	1500	1.6	0.43	0.43
24F-V1	SP/SP	2400	1750	740	650	300	1.7	0.88	1450	650	260	1.5	0.78	1100	1550	1.6	0.55	0.55
24F-V4 (5)	SP/SP	2400	1450	740	650	210	1.7	0.88	1050	470	185	1.3	0.67	875	1000	1.5	0.55	0.43
24F-V5	SP/SP	2400	2400	740	740	300	1.7	0.88	1750	650	260	1.5	0.78	1150	1650	1.6	0.55	0.55

Table 5A Expanded – Reference Design Values for Structural Glued Laminated Softwood Timber Combinations[1] (Cont.)

(Members stressed primarily in bending) (Tabulated design values are for normal load duration and dry service conditions.) Table 5A Expanded is an expanded list of structural glued laminated timber combinations from AITC 117 and APA-EWS Y117 that meet the requirements of each stress class in the new structural glued laminated timber stress class system. Table 5A Expanded is provided to allow easy conversion from the old combination symbols system to the new stress class system.

Use with Table 5A Adjustment Factors

Combination Symbol	Species Outer/Core	Bending About X-X Axis (Loaded Perpendicular to Wide Faces of Laminations)							Bending About Y-Y Axis (Loaded Parallel to Wide Faces of Laminations)					Axially Loaded			Fasteners	
		Extreme Fiber in Bending		Compression Perpendicular to Grain		Shear Parallel to Grain (Horizontal)	Modulus of Elasticity	Modulus of Elasticity for Beam and Column Stability	Extreme Fiber in Bending	Compression Perpendicular to Grain	Shear Parallel to Grain (Horizontal)	Modulus of Elasticity	Modulus of Elasticity for Beam and Column Stability	Tension Parallel to Grain	Compression Parallel to Grain	Modulus of Elasticity	Specific Gravity for Fastener Design	
		Tension Zone Stressed in Tension [2]	Compression Zone Stressed in Tension	Tension Face	Compression Face												Top or Bottom Face	Side Face
		F_{bx}^{+} (psi)	F_{bx}^{-} (psi)	F_{cLx} (psi)	F_{cLx} (psi)	F_{vx} [3] (psi)	E_x (10⁶ psi)	$E_{x\,min}$ (10⁶ psi)	F_{by} (psi)	F_{cLy} (psi)	F_{vy} [3][4] (psi)	E_y (10⁶ psi)	$E_{y\,min}$ (10⁶ psi)	F_t (psi)	F_c (psi)	E_{axial} (10⁶ psi)	G	
24F-1.8E		2400	1450	650	650	265	1.8	0.93	1450	560	230	1.6	0.83	1100	1600	1.7	0.5	
24F-V4	DF/DF	2400	1850	650	650	265	1.8	0.93	1450	560	230	1.6	0.83	1100	1650	1.7	0.5	0.5
24F-V8	DF/DF	2400	2400	650	650	265	1.8	0.93	1450	560	230	1.6	0.83	1100	1650	1.7	0.5	0.5
24F-E4	DF/DF	2400	1450	650	650	265	1.8	0.88	1450	560	230	1.7	0.88	1100	1700	1.8	0.5	0.5
24F-E13	DF/DF	2400	2400	650	650	265	1.8	0.88	1750	560	230	1.7	0.88	1200	1700	1.8	0.5	0.5
24F-E18	DF/DF	2400	2400	650	650	265	1.9	0.98	1550	560	230	1.7	0.88	1100	1700	1.8	0.5	0.5
24F-V3	SP/SP	2400	1950	740	740	300	1.8	0.93	1750	650	260	1.6	0.83	1150	1650	1.7	0.55	0.55
24F-E1	SP/SP	2400	1450	740	650	300	1.8	0.93	1750	650	260	1.6	0.83	1100	1600	1.7	0.55	0.55
24F-E4	SP/SP	2400	2400	740	740	300	1.9	0.98	2200	650	260	1.7	0.88	1450	1850	1.8	0.55	0.55
26F-1.9E [6]		2600	1950	650	650	265	1.9	0.98	1600	560	230	1.6	0.83	1150	1600	1.7	0.5	
26F-V1	DF/DF	2600	1950	650	650	265	2.0	1.04	1750	560	230	1.8	0.93	1300	1850	1.9	0.5	0.5
26F-V2	DF/DF	2600	2600	650	650	265	2.0	1.04	1750	560	230	1.8	0.93	1300	1850	1.9	0.5	0.5
26F-V1	SP/SP	2600	1950	740	740	300	1.8	0.93	1900	650	260	1.6	0.83	1150	1600	1.7	0.55	0.55
26F-V2	SP/SP	2600	2100	740	740	300	1.9	0.98	2200	740	260	1.8	0.93	1250	1650	1.9	0.55	0.55
26F-V3	SP/SP	2600	2100	740	740	300	1.9	0.98	2100	650	260	1.8	0.93	1200	1600	1.9	0.55	0.55
26F-V4	SP/SP	2600	2600	740	740	300	1.9	0.98	2100	650	260	1.8	0.93	1200	1600	1.9	0.55	0.55
28F-2.1E [6]		2800	2300	740	740	300	2.1 [8]	1.09 [8]	1600	650	260	1.7	0.88	1250	1750	1.7	0.55	
28F-E1	SP/SP	2800	2300	740	740	300	2.1 [8]	1.09 [8]	1600	650	260	1.7	0.88	1300	1850	1.7	0.55	
28F-E2	SP/SP	2800	2800	740	740	300	2.1 [8]	1.09 [8]	2000	650	260	1.7	0.88	1300	1850	1.7	0.55	
30F-2.1E [6][7]		3000	2400	740	740	300	2.1 [8]	1.09 [8]	1750	650	260	1.7	0.88	1250	1750	1.7	0.55	
30F-E1	SP/SP	3000	2400	740	740	300	2.1 [8]	1.09 [8]	1750	650	260	1.7	0.88	1250	1750	1.7	0.55	
30F-E2	SP/SP	3000	3000	740	740	300	2.1 [8]	1.09 [8]	1750	650	260	1.7	0.88	1350	1750	1.7	0.55	

Footnotes to Expanded Table 5A

1. The combinations in this table are applicable to members consisting of 4 or more laminations and are intended primarily for members stressed in bending due to loads applied perpendicular to the wide faces of the laminations. However, design values are tabulated for loading both perpendicular and parallel to the wide faces of the laminations. For combinations and design values applicable to members loaded primarily axially or parallel to the wide faces of the laminations, see Table 5B. For members of 2 or 3 laminations, see Table 5B.

2. The tabulated design values in this column, for bending about the X-X axis (F_{bx}), require the use of special tension laminations. If these special tension laminations are omitted, value shall be multiplied by 0.75 for members greater than or equal to 15" in depth or by 0.85 for members less than 15" in depth.

3. The design value for shear, F_{vx} and F_{vy}, shall be decreased by multiplying by a factor of 0.72 for non-prismatic members, notched members, and for all members subject to impact or cyclic loading. The reduced design value shall be used for design of members at connections (NDS 3.4.3.3) that transfer shear by mechanical fasteners. The reduced design value shall also be used for detrmination of design values for radial tension (NDS 5.2.2).

4. Design values are for timbers with laminations made from a single piece of lumber across the width or multiple pieces that have been edge bonded. For timber manufactured from multiple piece laminations (across width) that are not edge-bonded, value shall be multiplied by 0.4 for members with 5, 7, or 9 laminations or by 0.5 for all other members. This reduction shall be cumulative with the adjustment in footnote (3).

5. This combination may contain lumber with wane. If lumber with wane is used, the design value for shear parallel to grain, F_{vx}, shall be multiplied by 0.67 if wane is allowed on both sides. If wane is limited to one side, F_{vx} shall be multiplied by 0.83. This reduction shall be cumulative with the adjustment in footnote (3).

6. 26F, 28F, and 30F beams are not produced by all manufacturers, therefore, availability may be limited. Contact supplier or manufacturer for details.

7. 30F combinations are restricted to a maximum 6" nominal width.

8. For 28F and 30F members with more than 15 laminations, E_x = 2.0 million psi and $E_{x\,min}$ = 1.04 million psi.

4

REFERENCE DESIGN VALUES

Volume Factor, C_V

Tabulated bending design values for loading perpendicular to wide faces of laminations, F_{bx}, for structural glued laminated bending members shall be multiplied by the following volume factor:

$$C_V = (21/L)^{1/x} (12/d)^{1/x} (5.125/b)^{1/x} \leq 1.0$$

where:

L = length of bending member between points of zero moment, ft

d = depth of bending member, in.

b = width (breadth) of bending member, in. For multiple piece width layups, b = width of widest piece in the layup. Thus $b \leq 10.75"$.

x = 20 for Southern Pine

x = 10 for all other species

The volume factor shall not apply simultaneously with the beam stability factor (see 5.3.6). Therefore, the lesser of these adjustment factors shall apply.

Wet Service Factor, C_M

When structural glued laminated timber is used where moisture content will be 16% or greater, design values shall be multiplied by the appropriate wet service factors from the following table:

Wet Service Factors, C_M

F_b	F_t	F_v	$F_{c\perp}$	F_c	E and E_{min}
0.8	0.8	0.875	0.53	0.73	0.833

Flat Use Factor, C_{fu}

Tabulated bending design values for loading parallel to wide faces of laminations, F_{by}, shall be multiplied by the following flat use factors when the member dimension parallel to wide faces of laminations is less than 12":

Flat Use Factors, C_{fu}

Member dimension parallel to wide faces of laminations	C_{fu}
10-3/4" or 10-1/2"	1.01
8-3/4" or 8-1/2"	1.04
6-3/4"	1.07
5-1/8" or 5"	1.10
3-1/8" or 3"	1.16
2-1/2"	1.19

Table 5B Reference Design Values for Structural Glued Laminated Softwood Timber

(Members stressed primarily in axial tension or compression)[1,2] (Tabulated design values are for normal load duration and dry service conditions. See NDS 5.3 for a comprehensive description of design value adjustment factors.)

Use with Table 5B Adjustment Factors

Identification Number	Species	Grade	Modulus of Elasticity E (10^6 psi)	Modulus of Elasticity for Beam and Column Stability E_{min} (10^6 psi)	Compression Perpendicular to Grain $F_{c⊥}$ (psi)	Tension Parallel to Grain 2 or More Laminations F_t (psi)	Compression Parallel to Grain 4 or More Laminations F_c (psi)	Compression Parallel to Grain 2 or 3 Laminations F_c (psi)	Bending 4 or More Laminations F_{by} (psi)	Bending 3 Laminations F_{by} (psi)	Bending 2 Laminations F_{by} (psi)	Shear Parallel to Grain[1,2,3] F_{vy} (psi)	Bending[4] 2 Laminations to 15 in. Deep[5] F_{bx} (psi)	Shear Parallel to Grain[3] F_{vx} (psi)
Visually Graded Western Species														
1	DF	L3	1.5	0.78	560	900	1550	1200	1450	1250	1000	230	1250	265
2	DF	L2	1.6	0.83	560	1250	1950	1600	1800	1600	1300	230	1700	265
3	DF	L2D	1.9	0.98	650	1450	2300	1850	2100	1850	1550	230	2000	265
4	DF	L1CL	1.9	0.98	590	1400	2100	1900	2200	2000	1650	230	1900	265
5	DF	L1D	2.0	1.04	650	1600	2400	2100	2400	2100	1800	230	2200	265
14	HF	L3	1.3	0.67	375	800	1100	975	1200	1050	850	190	1100	215
15	HF	L2	1.4	0.73	375	1050	1350	1300	1500	1350	1100	190	1450	215
16	HF	L1	1.6	0.83	375	1200	1500	1450	1750	1550	1300	190	1600	215
17	HF	L1D	1.7	0.88	500	1400	1750	1700	2000	1850	1550	190	1900	215
22[6]	SW	L3	1.0	0.52	315	525	850	675	800	700	550	170	725	195
69	AC	L3	1.2	0.62	470	725	1150	1100	1100	975	775	230	1000	265
70	AC	L2	1.3	0.67	470	975	1450	1450	1400	1250	1000	230	1350	265
71	AC	L1D	1.6	0.83	560	1250	1900	1900	1850	1650	1400	230	1700	265
72	AC	L1S	1.6	0.83	560	1250	1900	1900	1850	1650	1400	230	1900	265
E-Rated Western Species														
27	DF	1.9E2	1.8	0.93	560	900	1750	1200	1450	1250	1000	230	1250	265
28	DF	2.1E2	2.0	1.04	650	1100	2000	1400	1650	1450	1150	230	1500	265
29	DF	2.3E2	2.2	1.14	650	1250	2250	1550	1900	1650	1350	230	1700	265
30	DF	1.9E6	1.8	0.93	560	1550	2100	1700	2400	2400	2100	230	1800	265
31	DF	2.1E6	2.0	1.04	650	1800	2400	1950	2400	2400	2400	230	2100	265
32	DF	2.3E6	2.2	1.14	650	1800	2400	2200	2400	2400	2400	230	2400	265
62	DF	2.2E2	2.1	1.09	650	1150	1850	1500	1800	1550	1250	230	1800	265
63	DF	2.2E6	2.1	1.09	650	1950	2300	2000	2400	2400	2400	230	2200	265
33	HF	1.6E2	1.5	0.78	375	800	1050	950	1200	1050	850	190	1100	215
34	HF	1.9E2	1.8	0.93	500	900	1500	1200	1450	1250	1000	190	1300	215
35	HF	2.1E2	2.0	1.04	500	1100	1550	1400	1650	1450	1150	190	1850	215
36	HF	1.6E4	1.5	0.78	375	1200	1450	1350	2100	1900	1700	190	1400	215
37	HF	1.9E6	1.8	0.93	500	1550	1950	1700	2400	2400	2100	190	1800	215
38	HF	2.1E6	2.0	1.04	500	1800	2400	1950	2400	2400	2400	190	2100	215
39[6]	SW	1.6E2	1.5	0.78	315	800	1200	950	1200	1050	850	170	1100	195
40[6]	SW	1.9E2	1.8	0.93	315	900	1500	1200	1450	1250	1000	170	1250	195
41[6]	SW	2.1E2	2.0	1.04	315	1100	1750	1400	1650	1450	1150	170	1550	195
42[6]	SW	1.6E4	1.5	0.78	315	1200	1550	1350	2100	1900	1700	170	1400	195
43[6]	SW	1.9E6	1.8	0.93	315	1550	1950	1700	2400	2400	2100	170	1800	195
44[6]	SW	2.1E6	2.0	1.04	315	1800	2100	1950	2400	2400	2400	170	2100	195

Column groupings: **All Loading** (Modulus of Elasticity, Modulus of Elasticity for Beam and Column Stability, Compression Perpendicular to Grain); **Axially Loaded** (Tension Parallel to Grain, Compression Parallel to Grain); **Bending about Y-Y Axis** — Loaded Parallel to Wide Faces of Laminations (Bending, Shear Parallel to Grain); **Bending About X-X Axis** — Loaded Perpendicular to Wide Faces of Laminations (Bending, Shear Parallel to Grain).

Table 5B Reference Design Values for Structural Glued Laminated Softwood Timber (Cont.)

(Members stressed primarily in axial tension or compression)[1,2] (Tabulated design values are for normal load duration and dry service conditions. See NDS 5.3 for a comprehensive description of design value adjustment factors.)

Use with Table 5B Adjustment Factors

Identification Number	Species	Grade	All Loading E (10^6 psi)	All Loading E_{min} (10^6 psi)	Compression Perpendicular to Grain F_{cL} (psi)	Tension Parallel to Grain 2 or More Laminations F_t (psi)	Compression Parallel to Grain 4 or More Laminations F_c (psi)	Compression Parallel to Grain 2 or 3 Laminations F_c (psi)	Bending 4 or More Laminations F_{by} (psi)	Bending 3 Laminations F_{by} (psi)	Bending 2 Laminations F_{by} (psi)	Shear Parallel to Grain F_{vy} (psi)	Bending 2 Laminations to 15 in. Deep F_{bx} (psi)	Shear Parallel to Grain F_{vx} (psi)
Visually Graded Southern Pine														
47 1:10	SP	N2M14	1.4	0.73	650	1200	1900	1150	1750	1550	1300	260	1400	300
47 1:10	SP	N2M10	1.4	0.73	650	1150	1700	1150	1750	1550	1300	260	1400	300
47 1:8	SP	N2M	1.4	0.73	650	1000	1500	1150	1600	1550	1300	260	1350	300
48	SP	N2D14	1.7	0.88	740	1400	2200	1350	2000	1800	1500	260	1600	300
48 1:10	SP	N2D10	1.7	0.88	740	1350	2000	1350	2000	1800	1500	260	1600	300
48 1:8	SP	N2D	1.7	0.88	740	1150	1750	1350	1850	1800	1500	260	1600	300
49	SP	N1M16	1.7	0.88	650	1350	2100	1450	1950	1750	1500	260	1800	300
49 1:12	SP	N1M12	1.7	0.88	650	1300	1900	1450	1950	1750	1500	260	1750	300
49 1:10	SP	N1M	1.7	0.88	650	1150	1700	1450	1850	1750	1500	260	1550	300
50	SP	N1D14	1.9	0.98	740	1550	2300	1700	2300	2100	1750	260	2100	300
50 1:12	SP	N1D12	1.9	0.98	740	1550	2200	1700	2300	2100	1750	260	2100	300
50 1:10	SP	N1D	1.9	0.98	740	1350	2000	1700	2100	2100	1750	260	1800	300
E-Rated Southern Pine														
54	SP	2.1E2	2.0	1.04	740	1100	2300	1400	1650	1450	1150	260	1500	300
55	SP	2.3E2	2.2	1.14	740	1250	2400	1550	1900	1650	1350	260	1700	300
56	SP	1.9E6	1.8	0.93	650	1550	1850	1700	2400	2400	2100	260	1800	300
57	SP	2.1E6	2.0	1.04	740	1800	2300	1950	2400	2400	2400	260	2100	300
58	SP	2.3E6	2.2	1.14	740	1800	2400	2200	2400	2400	2400	260	2400	300

Column group headings: **All Loading**; **Axially Loaded**; **Bending about Y-Y Axis** (Loaded Parallel to Wide Faces of Laminations); **Bending About X-X Axis** (Loaded Perpendicular to Wide Faces of Laminations).

1. For members with 2 or 3 laminations, the shear design value for transverse loads parallel to the wide faces of the laminations, F_{vy}, shall be reduced by multiplying by a factor of 0.84 or 0.95, respectively.
2. The shear design value for transverse loads applied parallel to the wide faces of the laminations, F_{vy}, shall be multiplied by 0.4 for members with 5, 7, or 9 laminations manufactured from multiple piece laminations (across width) that are not edge bonded. The shear design value, F_{vy}, shall be multiplied by 0.5 for all other members manufactured from multiple piece laminations with unbonded edge joints. This reduction shall be cumulative with the adjustment in footnote (1) and (3).
3. The design value for shear, F_{vx} and F_{vy}, shall be decreased by multiplying by a factor of 0.72 for non-prismatic members, notched members, and for all members subject to impact or cyclic loading. The reduced design value shall be used for design of members at connections (NDS 3.4.3.3) that transfer shear by mechanical fasteners. The reduced design value shall also be used for determination of design values for radial tension (NDS 5.2.2).
4. Tabulated design values are for members without special tension laminations. If special tension laminations are used, the design value for bending, F_{bx}, shall be permitted to be increased by multiplying by 1.18. This factor shall not be applied cumulatively with the adjustment in footnote (5).
5. For members greater than 15" deep and without special tension laminations, the bending design value, F_{bx}, shall be reduced by multiplying by a factor of 0.88. This factor shall not be applied cumulatively with the adjustment in footnote (4).
6. When Western Cedars, Western Cedars (North), Western Woods, and Redwood (open grain) are used in combinations for Softwood Species (SW), the design value for E shall be reduced by 100,000 psi and E_{min} shall be reduced by 50,000 psi. When Coast Sitka Spruce, Coast Species, Western White Pine, and Eastern White Pine are used in combinations for Softwood Species (SW) tabulated design values for shear parallel to grain, F_{vx} and F_{vy}, shall be reduced by 10 psi, before applying any other adjustments.

Volume Factor, C_V

Tabulated bending design values for loading perpendicular to wide faces of laminations, F_{bx}, for structural glued laminated bending members shall be multiplied by the following volume factor:

$$C_V = (21/L)^{1/x} (12/d)^{1/x} (5.125/b)^{1/x} \leq 1.0$$

where:

L = length of bending member between points of zero moment, ft

d = depth of bending member, in.

b = width (breadth) of bending member, in. For multiple piece width layups, b = width of widest piece in the layup. Thus b ≤ 10.75".

x = 20 for Southern Pine

x = 10 for all other species

The volume factor shall not apply simultaneously with the beam stability factor (see 5.3.6). Therefore, the lesser of these adjustment factors shall apply.

Wet Service Factor, C_M

When structural glued laminated timber is used where moisture content will be 16% or greater, design values shall be multiplied by the appropriate wet service factors from the following table:

Wet Service Factors, C_M

F_b	F_t	F_v	$F_{c\perp}$	F_c	E and E_{min}
0.8	0.8	0.875	0.53	0.73	0.833

Flat Use Factor, C_{fu}

Tabulated bending design values for loading parallel to wide faces of laminations, F_{by}, shall be multiplied by the following flat use factors when the member dimension parallel to wide faces of laminations is less than 12":

Flat Use Factors, C_{fu}

Member dimension parallel to wide faces of laminations	C_{fu}
10-3/4" or 10-1/2"	1.01
8-3/4" or 8-1/2"	1.04
6-3/4"	1.07
5-1/8" or 5"	1.10
3-1/8" or 3"	1.16
2-1/2"	1.19

4

REFERENCE DESIGN VALUES

Table 5C   Reference Design Values for Structural Glued Laminated Hardwood Timber

(Members stressed primarily in bending)[1] (Tabulated design values are for normal load duration and dry service conditions. See NDS 5.3 for a comprehensive description of design value adjustment factors.)

Use with Table 5C Adjustment Factors

| Combination Symbol | Bending About X-X Axis (Loaded Perpendicular to Wide Faces of Laminations) | | | | | | Bending About Y-Y Axis (Loaded Parallel to Wide Faces of Laminations) | | | | | Axially Loaded | | | Fasteners[3] |
	Extreme Fiber in Bending — Tension Zone Stressed in Tension (Positive Bending) F_{bx}^{+} (psi)	Extreme Fiber in Bending — Compression Zone Stressed in Tension (Negative Bending) F_{bx}^{-} (psi)	Compression Perpendicular to Grain F_{cLx} (psi)	Shear Parallel to Grain (Horizontal) F_{vx} (psi)	Modulus of Elasticity E_x (10^6 psi)	Modulus of Elasticity for Beam and Column Stability $E_{x\,min}$ (10^6 psi)	Extreme Fiber in Bending F_{by} (psi)	Compression Perpendicular to Grain F_{cLy} (psi)	Shear Parallel to Grain (Horizontal) $F_{vy}^{(2)}$ (psi)	Modulus of Elasticity E_y (10^6 psi)	Modulus of Elasticity for Beam and Column Stability $E_{y\,min}$ (10^6 psi)	Tension Parallel to Grain F_t (psi)	Compression Parallel to Grain F_c (psi)	Modulus of Elasticity E_{axial} (10^6 psi)	Specific Gravity for Fastener Design G
Visually Graded Hardwoods															
12F-V1	1200	600	285	125	1.2	0.62	1050	285	110	1.0	0.52	600	800	1.0	0.39
12F-V2	1200	1200	285	125	1.2	0.62	1050	285	110	1.1	0.57	625	860	1.1	0.39
14F-V1	1400	700	405	155	1.3	0.67	1250	405	135	1.1	0.57	700	950	1.1	0.45
14F-V2	1400	700	590	180	1.3	0.67	1450	590	160	1.1	0.57	750	1200	1.1	0.53
14F-V3	1400	1400	405	155	1.3	0.67	1250	405	135	1.1	0.57	725	950	1.1	0.45
14F-V4	1400	1400	590	180	1.3	0.67	1450	590	160	1.1	0.57	775	1200	1.1	0.53
16F-V1	1600	800	590	180	1.4	0.73	1400	590	160	1.2	0.62	800	1200	1.2	0.53
16F-V2	1600	800	835	200	1.5	0.78	1700	835	175	1.3	0.67	875	1250	1.3	0.63
16F-V3	1600	1600	590	180	1.4	0.73	1400	590	160	1.2	0.62	850	1200	1.2	0.53
16F-V4	1600	1600	835	200	1.6	0.83	1700	835	175	1.3	0.67	900	1300	1.3	0.63
20F-V1	2000	1000	835	200	1.7	0.88	1700	835	175	1.4	0.73	975	1400	1.4	0.63
20F-V2	2000	2000	835	200	1.7	0.88	1700	835	175	1.4	0.73	1000	1400	1.4	0.63
E-Rated Hardwoods															
16F-E1	1600	800	440	125	1.4	0.73	1250	285	110	1.2	0.62	825	975	1.2	0.39
16F-E2	1600	1600	440	125	1.4	0.73	1400	285	110	1.2	0.62	900	1000	1.2	0.39
20F-E1	2000	1000	590	155	1.6	0.83	1350	405	135	1.3	0.67	950	1050	1.3	0.45
20F-E2	2000	2000	590	155	1.6	0.83	1600	405	135	1.3	0.67	1050	1100	1.3	0.45
24F-E1	2400	1200	770	180	1.8	0.93	1550	590	160	1.5	0.78	1050	1400	1.5	0.53
24F-E2	2400	2400	770	180	1.8	0.93	1650	590	160	1.5	0.78	1050	1400	1.5	0.53
24F-E3 YP	2400	1200	590	155	1.8	0.93	1450	405	135	1.5	0.78	975	1200	1.5	0.45
24F-E4 RM	2400	1200	895	220	1.8	0.93	1650	710	195	1.6	0.83	1050	1350	1.6	0.53
24F-E5 RO	2400	1200	1075	235	1.8	0.93	1700	900	205	1.5	0.78	1100	1450	1.5	0.63

1. Design values in this table were excerpted from AITC 119-96 *Standard Specifications for Structural Glued Laminated Timber of Hardwood Species.* Design values are applicable to members with 4 or more laminations. For 2 and 3 lamination members see Table 5D.
2. Design values are for timbers with laminations made from a single piece of lumber across the width or multiple pieces that have been edge bonded. For timbers manufactured from multiple piece laminations (across width) that are not edge bonded, value shall be multiplied by 0.4 for members with 5, 7, or 9 laminations or by 0.5 for all other members.
3. Fastener values are for groups of hardwood species permitted in each combination. If actual species is known, values for that species are permitted to be used.

Volume Factor, C_V

Tabulated bending design values for loading perpendicular to wide faces of laminations, F_{bx}, for structural glued laminated bending members shall be multiplied by the following volume factor:

$$C_V = (21/L)^{1/x} (12/d)^{1/x} (5.125/b)^{1/x} \leq 1.0$$

where:

> L = length of bending member between points of zero moment, ft
>
> d = depth of bending member, in.
>
> b = width (breadth) of bending member, in. For multiple piece width layups, b = width of widest piece in the layup. Thus $b \leq 10.75''$.
>
> x = 20 for Southern Pine
>
> x = 10 for all other species

The volume factor shall not apply simultaneously with the beam stability factor (see 5.3.6). Therefore, the lesser of these adjustment factors shall apply.

Wet Service Factor, C_M

When structural glued laminated timber is used where moisture content will be 16% or greater, design values shall be multiplied by the appropriate wet service factors from the following table:

Wet Service Factors, C_M

F_b	F_t	F_v	$F_{c\perp}$	F_c	E and E_{min}
0.8	0.8	0.875	0.53	0.73	0.833

Flat Use Factor, C_{fu}

Tabulated bending design values for loading parallel to wide faces of laminations, F_{by}, shall be multiplied by the following flat use factors when the member dimension parallel to wide faces of laminations is less than 12":

Flat Use Factors, C_{fu}

Member dimension parallel to wide faces of laminations	C_{fu}
10-3/4" or 10-1/2"	1.01
8-3/4" or 8-1/2"	1.04
6-3/4"	1.07
5-1/8" or 5"	1.10
3-1/8" or 3"	1.16
2-1/2"	1.19

4

REFERENCE DESIGN VALUES

Table 5D Reference Design Values for Structural Glued Laminated Hardwood Timber

(Members stressed primarily in axial tension or compression)[1,2] (Tabulated design values are for normal load duration and dry service conditions. See NDS 5.3 for a comprehensive description of design value adjustment factors.)

Use with Table 5D Adjustment Factors

Combination Symbol	Species Group	Grade	All Loading — Modulus of Elasticity E (10⁶ psi)	All Loading — Modulus of Elasticity for Beam and Column Stability E_{min} (10⁶ psi)	All Loading — Compression Perpendicular to Grain $F_{c\perp}$ (psi)	Axially Loaded — Tension Parallel to Grain 2 or More Laminations F_t (psi)	Axially Loaded — Compression Parallel to Grain 4 or More Laminations F_c (psi)	Axially Loaded — Compression Parallel to Grain 2 or 3 Laminations F_c (psi)	Bending about Y-Y Axis — Bending 4 or More Laminations F_{by} (psi)	Bending about Y-Y Axis — Bending 3 Laminations F_{by} (psi)	Bending about Y-Y Axis — Bending 2 Laminations F_{by} (psi)	Bending about Y-Y Axis — Shear Parallel 4 or More Laminations for members with multiple piece laminations[3] F_{vy} (psi)	Bending about Y-Y Axis — Shear Parallel 4 or More Laminations F_{vy} (psi)	Bending about Y-Y Axis — Shear Parallel 3 Laminations F_{vy} (psi)	Bending about Y-Y Axis — Shear Parallel 2 Laminations F_{vy} (psi)	Bending About X-X Axis — Bending 2 Laminations to 15 in. Deep[4] without Special Tension Lams F_{bx} (psi)	Bending About X-X Axis — Bending 4 or More Laminations with Special Tension Lams[5] F_{bx} (psi)	Bending About X-X Axis — Shear Parallel to Grain 2 or More Laminations F_{vx} (psi)
Visually Graded Hardwoods																		
H1	A	N3	1.3	0.67	835	425	900	900	1250	1100	875	90	175	165	150	925	1200	200
H2	A	N2	1.5	0.78	835	875	1300	1300	1700	1550	1300	90	175	165	150	1200	1500	200
H3	A	N1	1.7	0.88	835	1000	1450	1450	2000	1800	1550	90	175	165	150	1600	1800	200
H4	A	SS	1.7	0.88	835	1150	1600	1600	2000	1850	1600	90	175	165	150	1700	2000	200
H5	B	N3	1.2	0.62	590	350	800	800	1050	900	750	80	160	150	135	750	1000	180
H6	B	N2	1.3	0.67	590	750	1150	1150	1450	1300	1050	80	160	150	135	1000	1200	180
H7	B	N1	1.5	0.78	590	850	1300	1300	1650	1500	1300	80	160	150	135	1350	1600	180
H8	B	SS	1.5	0.78	590	950	1450	1450	1700	1550	1350	80	160	150	135	1400	1700	180
H9	C	N3	1.0	0.52	405	300	625	625	900	800	625	70	135	130	115	675	900	155
H10	C	N2	1.2	0.62	405	625	900	900	1200	1100	925	70	135	130	115	875	1100	155
H11	C	N1	1.3	0.67	405	725	1000	1000	1400	1300	1100	70	135	130	115	1150	1400	155
H12	C	SS	1.3	0.67	405	825	1100	1100	1450	1350	1150	70	135	130	115	1200	1500	155
H13	D	N3	0.9	0.47	285	250	575	575	775	675	550	55	110	105	95	575	775	125
H14	D	N2	1.1	0.57	285	550	825	825	1050	950	800	55	110	105	95	750	925	125
H15	D	N1	1.2	0.62	285	625	925	925	1200	1100	950	55	110	105	95	1000	1150	125
H16	D	SS	1.2	0.62	285	700	1050	1050	1250	1150	1000	55	110	105	95	1050	1300	125

Table 5D Reference Design Values for Structural Glued Laminated Hardwood Timber (Cont.)

(Members stressed primarily in axial tension or compression)[1,2] (Tabulated design values are for normal load duration and dry service conditions. See NDS 5.3 for a comprehensive description of design value adjustment factors.)

Use with Table 5D Adjustment Factors

Combination Symbol	Species Group	Grade	Modulus of Elasticity E (10^6 psi)	Modulus of Elasticity for Beam and Column Stability E_{min} (10^6 psi)	Compression Perpendicular to Grain $F_{c\perp}$ (psi)	Tension Parallel to Grain 2 or More Laminations F_t (psi)	Compression Parallel to Grain 4 or More Laminations F_c (psi)	Compression Parallel to Grain 2 or 3 Laminations F_c (psi)	Bending 4 or More Laminations F_{by} (psi)	Bending 3 Laminations F_{by} (psi)	Bending 2 Laminations F_{by} (psi)	Shear Parallel to Grain 4 or More Laminations for members with multiple piece laminations[3] F_{vy} (psi)	Shear Parallel to Grain 4 or More Laminations F_{vy} (psi)	Shear Parallel to Grain 3 Laminations F_{vy} (psi)	Shear Parallel to Grain 2 Laminations F_{vy} (psi)	Bending 2 Laminations to 15 in. Deep[4] without Special Tension Lams F_{bx} (psi)	Bending 4 or More Laminations with Special Tension Lams[5] F_{bx} (psi)	Shear Parallel to Grain 2 or More Laminations F_{vx} (psi)
E-Rated Hardwoods																		
H17	A	1.5E3	1.4	0.73	1015	1000	1500	1350	1850	1750	1550	90	175	165	150	1200	1450	200
H18	A	1.8E3	1.7	0.88	1015	1150	1950	1850	2100	2000	1750	90	175	165	150	1450	1850	200
H19	A	1.8E6	1.7	0.88	1015	1450	2000	1900	2300	2200	1950	90	175	165	150	1650	2000	200
H20	A	2.0E3	1.9	0.98	1015	1350	2600	2200	2400	2300	2100	90	175	165	150	1700	2200	200
H21	A	2.0E6	1.9	0.98	1015	1700	2430	2300	2400	2400	2300	90	175	165	150	2100	2600	200
H22	B	1.5E3	1.4	0.73	770	1000	1500	1350	1850	1750	1550	80	160	150	135	1200	1450	180
H23	B	1.8E3	1.7	0.88	770	1150	1950	1850	2100	2000	1750	80	160	150	135	1450	1850	180
H24	B	1.8E6	1.7	0.88	770	1450	2000	1900	2300	2200	1950	80	160	150	135	1650	2000	180
H25	B	2.0E3	1.9	0.98	770	1350	2300	2200	2400	2300	2100	80	160	150	135	1700	2200	180
H26	B	2.0E6	1.9	0.98	770	1700	2400	2300	2400	2400	2300	80	160	150	135	2100	2600	180
H27	C	1.5E3	1.4	0.73	590	1000	1500	1350	1850	1750	1550	70	135	130	115	1200	1450	155
H28	C	1.8E3	1.7	0.88	590	1150	1950	1850	2100	2000	1750	70	135	130	115	1450	1850	155
H29	C	1.8E6	1.7	0.88	590	1450	2000	1900	2300	2200	1950	70	135	130	115	1650	2000	155
H30	C	2.0E3	1.9	0.98	590	1350	2300	2200	2400	2300	2100	70	135	130	115	1700	2200	155
H31	C	2.0E6	1.9	0.98	590	1700	2400	2300	2400	2400	2300	70	135	130	115	2100	2600	155
H32	D	1.5E3	1.4	0.73	440	1000	1500	1350	1850	1750	1550	55	110	105	95	1200	1450	125
H33	D	1.5E6	1.4	0.73	440	1250	1500	1400	2000	1900	1700	55	110	105	95	1250	1600	125
H34	D	1.8E3	1.7	0.88	440	1150	1950	1850	2100	2000	1750	55	110	105	95	1450	1850	125
H35	D	1.8E6	1.7	0.88	440	1450	2000	1900	2300	2200	1950	55	110	105	95	1650	2000	125
H36	D	2.0E3	1.9	0.98	440	1350	2300	2200	2400	2300	2100	55	110	105	95	1700	2200	125
H37	D	2.0E6	1.9	0.98	440	1700	2400	2300	2400	2400	2300	55	110	105	95	2100	2600	125

1. Design values in this table are for combinations conforming to AITC 119-96 (*Standard Specifications for Structural Glued Laminated Timber of Hardwood Species*), by American Institute of Timber Construction, and manufactured in accordance with American National Standard ANSI/AITC A190.1-2002 (*Structural Glued Laminated Timber*).
2. The combinations in this table are intended primarily for members loaded axially or in bending with the loads acting parallel to the wide faces of the laminations (bending about Y-Y axis). Design values for bending due to loading applied perpendicular to the wide faces of the laminations (bending about X-X axis) are also included; however, the combinations in Table 5C are preferred for this condition of loading.
3. Values apply to members manufactured using multiple piece laminations with unbonded edge joints. For members with 5, 7, or 9 laminations, value shall be multiplied by 0.8.
4. For members greater than 15" deep, values shall be reduced by multiplying by a factor of 0.88.
5. These design values require the use of special tension laminations. If these design values are used, the designer shall specify the required design value as well as the combination symbol.

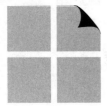

AMERICAN FOREST & PAPER ASSOCIATION
American Wood Council
Engineered and Traditional Wood Products

February 2007

2007 ERRATA/ADDENDUM
to the

2005 Edition of

the National Design Specification® (NDS®) for Wood Construction Supplement: Design Values for Wood Construction
(printed versions dated 04-05 2M, 09-05 2M, and 08-06 5M)

Page   **Revision**

4   In Table 2.1, revise the following:

Species or Species Combination	Species That May Be Included in Combination	Grading Rules Agencies	Design Values Provided in Tables
Coast Sitka Spruce	Coast Sitka Spruce	NLGA	4A, 4D, 4E
Yellow Cedar	Yellow Cedar	NLGA	4A

32   In Table 4A, add the following design values for Coast Sitka Spruce

Species and commercial grade	Size classification	Design values in pounds per square inch (psi)							Grading Rules Agency
		Bending F_b	Tension parallel to grain F_t	Shear parallel to grain F_v	Compression perpendicular to grain $F_{c\perp}$	Compression parallel to grain F_c	Modulus of Elasticity		
							E	E_{min}	
Coast Sitka Spruce[4]									
Select Structural	2" & wider	1300	950	125	455	1200	1,700,000	620,000	
No. 1 / No. 2		925	550	125	455	1100	1,500,000	550,000	
No. 3		525	325	125	455	625	1,400,000	510,000	
Stud	2" & wider	725	450	125	455	675	1,400,000	510,000	NLGA
Construction		1050	650	125	455	1300	1,400,000	510,000	
Standard	2"-4" wide	600	350	125	455	1100	1,300,000	470,000	
Utility		275	175	125	455	725	1,200,000	440,000	

34   In Table 4A, revise the following design values for Northern Species

Species and commercial grade	Size classification	Design values in pounds per square inch (psi)							Grading Rules Agency
		Bending F_b	Tension parallel to grain F_t	Shear parallel to grain F_v	Compression perpendicular to grain $F_{c\perp}$	Compression parallel to grain F_c	Modulus of Elasticity		
							E	E_{min}	
Northern Species									
Select Structural	2" & wider	~~1,000~~ 975	~~450~~ 425	110	350	1,100	1,100,000	400,000	
No. 1 / No. 2		~~600~~ 625	275	110	350	850	1,100,000	400,000	
No. 3		350	150	110	350	500	1,000,000	370,000	
Stud	2" & wider	475	225	110	350	550	1,000,000	370,000	NLGA
Construction		700	~~300~~ 325	110	350	1,050	1,000,000	370,000	
Standard	2"-4" wide	400	175	110	350	875	900,000	330,000	
Utility		175	75	110	350	575	900,000	330,000	

1111 Nineteenth Street, NW, Suite 800 - Washington, DC 20036 - 202 463-4713 - Fax: 202 463-2791 - www.awc.org
America's Forest & Paper People® - *Improving Tomorrow's Environment Today* ®

AMERICAN FOREST & PAPER ASSOCIATION

Page   Revision

36   In Table 4A, add the following design values for Yellow Cedar

Species and commercial grade	Size classification	Design values in pounds per square inch (psi)							Grading Rules Agency
		Bending F_b	Tension parallel to grain F_t	Shear parallel to grain F_v	Compression perpendicular to grain $F_{c\perp}$	Compression parallel to grain F_c	Modulus of Elasticity		
							E	E_{min}	
Yellow Cedar[4]									
Select Structural		1200	725	175	540	1200	1,600,000	580,000	
No. 1 / No. 2	2" & wider	800	475	175	540	1000	1,400,000	510,000	
No. 3		475	275	175	540	575	1,200,000	440,000	
Stud	2" & wider	625	375	175	540	650	1,200,000	440,000	NLGA
Construction		925	550	175	540	1200	1,300,000	470,000	
Standard	2"-4" wide	525	300	175	540	1050	1,200,000	440,000	
Utility		250	150	175	540	675	1,100,000	400,000	

36   In Table 4A, add the following footnote:

4. **SPECIFIC GRAVITY, G.** Specific gravity values are provided below for visually graded dimension lumber. Note that the value for Coast Sitka Spruce is applicable only for visually graded dimension lumber (2" – 4" thick). See NDS Table 11.3.2A for the specific gravity value applicable to Coast Sitka Spruce used as visually graded timber (5"x5" and larger) and visually graded decking.

Species	**Specific Gravity, G**	**Grading Rules Agency**
Coast Sitka Spruce	0.43	NLGA
Yellow Cedar	0.46	NLGA

1111 Nineteenth Street, NW, Suite 800 - Washington, DC 20036 - 202 463-4713 - Fax: 202 463-2791 - www.awc.org
America's Forest & Paper People® - *Improving Tomorrow's Environment Today* ®
AMERICAN WOOD COUNCIL